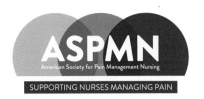

ASPMN
American Society for Pain Management Nursing

SUPPORTING NURSES MANAGING PAIN

T0290838

FOURTH EDITION

CORE CURRICULUM

FOR PAIN MANAGEMENT NURSING

EDITORS

Helen N. Turner

DNP, PMGT-BC, PCNS-BC, AP-PMN, FAAN
Assistant Dean for APRN DNP Programs
Oregon Health & Science University, School of Nursing
Portland, Oregon

Michelle L. Czarnecki

MSN, PMGT-BC, CPNP-PC, AP-PMN
Pediatric Pain Management Advanced Practice Nurse
Jane B. Pettit Pain and Headache Center
Children's Wisconsin
Milwaukee, Wisconsin

ELSEVIER

ELSEVIER
3251 Riverport Lane
St. Louis, Missouri 63043

**CORE CURRICULUM FOR PAIN MANAGEMENT NURSING,
FOURTH EDITION**

ISBN: 978-0-323-79437-4

Previous edition copyrighted 2018

Senior Content Strategist: Yvonne Alexopoulos
Content Development Manager: Danielle Frazier
Senior Content Development Specialist: Maria Broeker
Publishing Services Manager: Deepthi Unni
Senior Project Manager: Kamatchi Madhavan
Design Direction: Ryan Cook

Printed in India
Last digit is the print number: 9 8 7 6 5 4 3 2 1

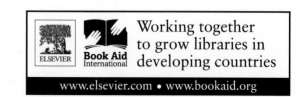

Dedicated to:
Nurses!
We thank you for your commitment as
the unsung heroes of pain care everywhere!

Also dedicated to:
Our families, who are our unsung heroes!

Helen N. Turner and Michelle L. Czarnecki

PRESIDENTIAL FOREWORD

I am honored to write this foreword for the American Society for Pain Management Nursing (ASPMN®) *Core Curriculum for Pain Management* Nursing, 4th Edition. I have known the editors, Dr. Helen Turner and Michelle Czarnecki, MSN, for over 15 years and admire their contributions to the advancement of pain management in general and pain management nursing specifically. Dr. Turner has traveled abroad to China to share her expertise while Ms. Czarnecki is well published, with varied experience in nursing research. Both serve on the editorial board for the *Pain Management Nursing* journal. They have also acted as mentors to me, contributing to my growth in pain management nursing.

The expertise of all the contributors, from section editors to chapter authors, is impressive. Each has contributed to the body of knowledge of pain management through research, publication, clinical work, teaching, and advocacy. This team of ASPMN members has created the go-to reference for nurses who wish to advance their knowledge in caring for patients with pain. The work provides both foundational information and new, expanded bench and clinical science to support nursing practice.

My mantra is: "pain management is a team sport." We know that an integrative approach is the most effective way to address the biopsychosocial complexity of the pain experience. Nurses do not practice pain management in a silo but rather with many other disciplines, including physicians, physician's assistants, physical and occupational therapists, social workers, psychologists, acupuncturists, chiropractors, integrative medicine specialists, and others.

This edition of the *Core Curriculum* should be a required text, not only for nurses but also for all clinicians working with patients experiencing pain. From this text one can gain a breadth and depth of knowledge not found in any other pain management reference. One of my physician colleagues continually tells his peers that if they really want to learn about caring for these patients, they should look to the ASPMN for knowledge and expertise.

I want to extend my thanks to all the contributors to this book, especially to Dr. Turner and Ms. Czarnecki, who persevered through the COVID-19 pandemic, supported the section editors and chapter authors, and produced an impressive reference that will stand out in the field of pain management.

Teri Reyburn-Orne, MSN, PPCNP-BC,
CPNP-AC, PMGT-BC, AP-PMN
President, ASPMN®

PREFACE

Pain management nursing is a relatively young nursing specialty, yet a primary tenet of nursing practice is to maximize patients' comfort and minimize their pain and distress. Our knowledge and understanding of pain and its treatment are constantly evolving and will continue to inform our practice. Through research, a better understanding of mechanisms and types of pain have led to significant changes in treatment. The evidence amassed has allowed us to expand our efforts with pain assessment, treatment, and prevention using a biopsychosocial and spiritual framework, resulting in care that is balanced and focused on harm reduction. Concern for opioid overuse, misuse, and abuse has driven a shift in treatment focus away from opioids toward a multimodal and more integrative approach.

The next three sentences from the third edition's preface bear repeating. "Pain management nurses are truly the unsung heroes in healthcare. Not only are we members of the most trusted profession, but we embrace the hard work of caring for and advocating for vulnerable populations.

This hard work involves clinical care, education, and research as we lead the way in providing evidence based, compassionate, and responsible care." We had planned to have this edition published sooner, but as with many things, there were delays and disruptions related to the COVID-19 pandemic. This fourth edition of the *Core Curriculum* is separated into four sections. Section One provides readers with foundational concepts regarding pain management nursing, Section Two describes professional roles in pain management nursing, Section Three focuses on assessments related to pain management, and Section Four covers the broad spectrum of management options. Our authors and section editors *donated countless* hours of research, writing, review, and editing. It is this knowledge, expertise, and dedication that makes the *Core Curriculum* possible. We hope you find this edition informative and useful to your nursing practice, because every nurse is a pain management nurse!

Helen N. Turner and Michelle L. Czarnecki

SECTION EDITORS

Maureen F. Cooney, DNP, FNP-BC, ACHPN, AP-PMN
Nurse Practitioner
Department of Pain Management
Westchester Medical Center;
Instructor of Anesthesiology
Department of Anesthesia
New York Medical College
Valhalla, New York;
Adjunct Associate Professor
Lienhard School of Nursing
Pace University, College of Health Sciences
New York, New York

Ann Schreier, PhD, BSN, MSN, RN
Professor Emeritus
Department of Nursing Science
East Carolina University
Greenville, North Carolina

Sharon Wrona, DNP, PMGT-BC, CPNP-PC, PMHS, AP-PMN, FAAN
Director
Comprehensive Pain Services
Nationwide Children's Hospital
Columbus, Ohio

Jinbing Bai, PhD, RN, FAAN
Assistant Professor
Nell Hodgson Woodruff School of Nursing
Emory University
Atlanta, Georgia

Michael C. Barnes, JD
Chairman
Center for U.S. Policy;
Managing Attorney
Sequel Health Law PLLC
Washington, District of Columbia

Marilyn Ann Bazinski, DNP, AGCNS, RN, PMGT-BC
Clinical Nurse Specialist
Center for Nursing Excellence and Innovation
University of California, San Francisco
San Francisco, California

Esther I. Bernhofer, PhD, RN, PMGT-BC
Associate Professor
Frances Payne Bolton School of Nursing
Case Western Reserve University;
Associate Professor
Department of Bioethics, School of Medicine
Case Western Reserve University
Cleveland, Ohio

Staja Q. Booker, PhD, RN
Assistant Professor
Department of Biobehavioral Nursing Science
University of Florida
Gainesville, Florida

Chasity Brimeyer, PhD, EdS
Pediatric Psychologist and Associate Professor
Department of Anesthesiology
Medical College of Wisconsin
Milwaukee, Wisconsin

Mary Milano Carter, MS, NP-BC, AP-PMN, PMGT-BC
Nurse Practitioner
Department of Anesthesiology/Pain Management
North Shore University Hospital/Northwell Health
Manhasset, New York;
Nurse Practitioner
Department of Anesthesiology/Pain Management
Long Island Brain & Spine
Smithtown, New York

Angela T. Casey, BSc, MPhil
Vice President
Scientific Services
PharmaCom Group
Stamford, Connecticut

Ann Quinlan-Colwell, PhD, MSN
Pain Management Educator and Consultant Pain
    Management Clinical Nurse Specialist
Independent, AQC Pain Educator and Consultant
Wilmington, North Carolina

Wade Delk, BA
Director
Governmental Affairs
American Society for Pain Management Nursing
Leesburg, Virginia

Theresa J. Di Maggio, MSN, CRNP, PPCNP-BC
Pain Management Nurse Practitioner
Department of Anesthesiology/Pain Management;
Pediatric Nurse Practitioner
Department of Gastroenterology
Children's Hospital of Philadelphia
Philadelphia, Pennsylvania

Danielle Dunwoody, BSc, BScN, MS, PhD
Assistant Professor
Department of Nursing
Brock University
St. Catharines, Ontario, Canada

Mechele Fillman, MSN, NP-C, PMGT-BC
Acute Pain Service Lead Nurse Practitioner
Department of Anesthesia
Christus St. Vincent
Santa Fe, New Mexico

Laura Habighorst, BSN, RN, CAPA, CGRN, NPD-BC
Consultant/Educator
GI, Pain, Perianesthesia, Bariatrics, ERAS, Self-Employed
Hermitage, Missouri;
Clinical Nurse Educator
Surgical Services
North Kansas City Hospital
North Kansas City, Missouri

Karen P. Hall, MSN, MSHSA, RN-BC
Pain Management and Palliative Care Resource Nurse
    Retired
Department of Nursing
Community Hospice
Modesto, California

Ann L. Horgas, PhD, RN, FAAN, FGSA
Professor
Department of Biobehavioral Nursing Science
College of Nursing
University of Florida
Gainesville, Florida

Kim Anderson Khan, PsyD
Associate Professor of Anesthesiology
Department of Anesthesiology
Medical College of Wisconsin;
Pediatric Psychologist
Children's Wisconsin
Milwaukee, Wisconsin

Theresa L. Kapke, PhD
Assistant Professor
Department of Anesthesiology
Medical College of Wisconsin
Milwaukee, Wisconsin

Jennifer Kawi, PhD, MSN, APRN, FNP-BC, CNE
Associate Professor
School of Nursing
University of Nevada, Las Vegas
Las Vegas, Nevada

Tracy Klein, PhD, ARNP, FAAN, FAANP
Associate Professor
Department of Nursing
Washington State University
Vancouver, Washington

Connie Luedtke, MA, RN, PMGT-BC
Retired Ambulatory Nurse Manager
Department of Nursing
Mayo Clinic
Rochester, Minnesota

Karen V. Macey-Stewart, DNP, AGNP-C, PMGT-BC
Undergraduate Program Director
School of Nursing
Loyola University New Orleans
New Orleans, Louisiana

Pamela Madrid, BSN, RN, CCE
Founder and CEO
Joytrek 153 Enterprises LLC
San Tan Valley, Arizona

Robert Montgomery, DNP, PMGT-BC, ACNS-BC
Associate Professor
Department of Anesthesiology
University of Colorado Anshcutz Medical Campus
Aurora, Colorado

Tara Michelle Nichols, DNP, ARNP, CCNS, AGCNS, PMGT-BC
CEO and Clinician
Consulting and Private Practice
Matters of Comfort
Mason City, Iowa;
Program Director–RN-BSN
Nursing, Waldorf University
Forest City, Iowa;
Research Nurse Manager
Department of Psychiatry
Oregon Health & Science University
Portland, Oregon

Susan Kathleen O'Conner-Von, PhD, RN-BC, CNE, FNAP
Professor
School of Nursing
University of Minnesota
Minneapolis, Minnesota

Christine H. Peltier, DNP, APRN, FNP-BC, PMGT-BC
APRN
Department of Acute Pain
M Health Fairview University of Minnesota
    Medical Center
Minneapolis, Minnesota

Janet A. Pennella-Vaughan, MS, FNP, BC-Pain
Senior Nurse Practitioner
Anesthesia Pain Services;
Director of Clinical Research
Department of Anesthesiology;
Clinical Associate
School of Nursing, University of Rochester
    Medical Center
Rochester, New York

Mallory A. Perry-Eaddy, PhD, RN, CCRN
Assistant Professor
School of Nursing
University of Connecticut
Storrs, Connecticut;
Assistant Professor
Department of Pediatrics
School of Medicine
University of Connecticut
Farmington, Connecticut;
Registered Nurse
Pediatric Intensive Care Unit
Connecticut Children's Medical Center
Hartford, Connecticut

Teri Reyburn-Orne, MSN, APRN, PPCNP-BC, CPNP-AC, PMGT-BC, AP-PMN
Senior Instructor–APN
Department of Anesthesiology;
Associate Director, Pain Services and Advanced Practice
Division of Pediatric Anesthesia
University of Colorado, Anschutz Campus,
    School of Medicine
Aurora, Colorado

Patricia Kelly Rosier, MS, RN, ACNS-BC, PMGT-BC
Surgical Clinical Nurse Specialist
Clinical Development
Berkshire Medical Center
Pittsfield, Massachusetts

Jason Sawyer, RN-EC, BScN, MN, NP
Nurse Practitioner
Acute Pain Service
Sunnybrook Health Sciences Centre
Toronto, Ontario, Canada

Melanie H. Simpson, PhD, MSN, PMGT-BC, OCN
Call Center Nurse Consultant
Central Nurse Triage Team
The University of Kansas Health System
Kansas City, Kansas

Donna Sipos Cox, MSN, FNP-C, ONC, PMGT-BC,
AP-PMN
Pain Management Family Nurse Practitioner
Department of Anesthesiology
NYU Health–Long Island
Mineola, New York

Timothy Joseph Sowicz, PhD, RN
Assistant Professor
Division of Advanced Nursing Practice and Science
University of Arizona
Tucson, Arizona

Marsha Stanton, PhD, RN
Independent Consultant
Education, Self-Employed
Los Alamitos, California

Robert Twillman, PhD
Pain Management Psychologist
Behavioral Health
Saint Luke's Health System
Kansas City, Missouri;
Clinical Associate Professor (Volunteer Faculty)
Department of Psychiatry and Behavioral Sciences
University of Kansas School of Medicine
Kansas City, Kansas

Linda Mary Vanni, MSN, NP, ACNS-BC, PMGT-BC,
AP-PMN
Nurse Practitioner, Pain Management
Sole Proprietor
Professional Pain Education & Consulting, LLC
Troy, Michigan

Marian Wilson, PhD, MPH, RN, PMGT-RN
Associate Professor
College of Nursing
Washington State University
Spokane, Washington

Kimberly Wittmayer, MS, APRN-FPA, PCNS-BC,
PMGT-BC, AP-PMN
Advanced Practice Nurse
Pediatric Pain Management/Palliative Care
Advocate Children's Hospital
Oak Lawn, Illinois

REVIEWERS

Jeffrey Boon, PhD, APRN, AGACNP-BC
Nurse Practitioner
Vanderbilt University Medical Center
Nashville, Tennessee

Sarah E. Giron, PhD, CRNA, FAANA
Clinical and Didactic Instructor
Kaiser Permanente Anesthesia Technology
   Program Director
Kaiser Permanente School of Anesthesia
California State University, Fullerton School of Nursing
Pasadena City College
Pasadena, California

Céline Gélinas, RN, PhD, FCAN
Full Professor
Ingram School of Nursing, McGill University
Montreal, Québec, Canada

Robert Hutchison, PharmD
Licensed Pharmacist
Board Certified Ambulatory Care Pharmacist
Clinical Associate Professor
Texas A&M University School of Pharmacy
Round Rock, Texas

Elizabeth M. Hutzel-Dunham, BSN, RN, CPN
Registered Nurse
University of Cincinnati
Cincinnati Children's Hospital Medical Center
Cincinnati, Ohio

Kimberly Dupree Jones, Phd, FNP-BC, RN, FAAN
Professor with Indefinite Tenure
Associate Dean for Academic Advancement
Nell Hodgson Woodruff School of Nursing,
   Emory University
Atlanta, Georgia

Zeynep Karaman Özlü, PhD
Associate Professor
Ataturk University
Erzurum, Turkey

Jennifer E. Lee, PhD
Director and Associate Professor (ret.)
The University of Iowa
Iowa City, Iowa

Kathleen L. Lemanek, PhD
Professor of Pediatrics
Pediatric Psychologist
College of Medicine, The Ohio State University
Nationwide Children's Hospital
Columbus, Ohio

Elizabeth A. Loomis, DNP, RN, FNP-BC
Surgical Nursing, Emergency Nursing, Assistant
   Professor
Eastern Michigan University
Ypsilanti, Michigan

Susan Lynch, RN, MSN, PhD, NEA-BC, CNOR,
CSSM, CNAMB
Director of Nursing
Penn Medicine Chester County Hospital
West Chester, Pennsylvania

Richard Pembridge, ACNP-C
Acute Care Nurse Practitioner through ANCC
Board Certification–Advanced Diabetes Management–
   ANCC
Doctorate of Education in Health Care Administration
AGACNP Program Director
Grand Canyon University
Phoenix, Arizona

Peter D. Smith, BA, MSN, RN, CNE
Instructor
Lindenwood University
Saint Charles, Missouri

Joy Susan Pendergrass, MSN, MEd, APRN, FNP-BC
Nurse Practitioner
Florida Department of Health, Nassau County
Yulee, Florida

Linda Wilson, PhD, RN, CPAN, CAPA, NPD-BC, CNE,
CNEcl, CHSE-A, FASPAN, ANEF, FAAN, FSSH
Assistant Dean for Continuing Education
Simulation and Events & Clinical Professor, Division of
   Nursing
Drexel University, College of Nursing and Health
   Professions
Philadelphia, Pennsylvania

Richard Wilson, DNAP, CRNA
Assistant Program Director
University of South Carolina, School of Medicine
Graduate Program in Nurse Anesthesia
Greenville, South Carolina

Sharon Wrona, DNP, PMGT-BC, CPNP-PC, PMHS,
AP-PMN, FAAN
APRN and Director
Comprehensive Pain and Palliative Care Services
Nationwide Children's Hospital
Columbus, Ohio

CONTENTS

CHAPTER 1

Physiology of Pain

Robert Montgomery, DNP, PMGT-BC, ACNS-BC
Christine H. Peltier, DNP, PMGT-BC, FNP-BC
Mechele Fillman, MSN, NP
Sharon Wrona, DNP, PMGT-BC, CPNP-PC, PMHS, AP-PMN, FAAN*

Introduction

Pain is a dynamic phenomenon. Mounting evidence supports a biological, genetic, and environmental basis to explain individual variations in inflammation and neuropathic pain responses. As we learn about neuromechanisms that cause painful conditions and increasingly understand variations previously referred to as "pain of unknown etiology," we elevate our clinical practice. We look forward to increasing our options for analgesia as neuroscience research continues to explore the territories of pain mechanisms and pain perception.

I. Physiological Pain

A. Nociceptive pain (see Table 1.1)
 1. Pain resulting from ongoing activation of primary afferent nociceptors (i.e., pain nerve fibers) in response to noxious stimuli (i.e., tissue damage)
 2. Pain often consistent with degree of tissue injury and may be long-lasting, even after painful stimuli subsides
 3. Types of nociceptive pain
  a. First pain
   1) Transmitted by A delta (Aδ) fibers
   2) Fast pain: rapidly transmitting input to the somatosensory cortex
   3) Sharp and pricking quality
  b. Second pain
   1) Transmitted by C fibers
   2) Slow pain
   3) Dull, aching, or burning quality
 4. Subtypes of nociceptive pain
  a. Somatic: originating from nociceptor activation in skin, subcutaneous tissue, bones, muscles, and blood vessels; typically well localized and described as sharp, aching, or throbbing
  b. Visceral: originating from nociceptor activation in organs, linings of the organs, and body cavities; described as more diffuse gnawing or cramping
B. Neuropathic pain (see Table 1.1)
 1. Non-nociceptive, pathological pain believed to be sustained by aberrant somatosensory processing in peripheral (PNS) or central nervous system (CNS)
 2. Pain can result from injury to or dysfunction of PNS or CNS.
  a. Typically involves more than one mechanism and may result from abnormal peripheral nerve function and processing of impulses from abnormal neuronal receptor and mediator activity
  b. Subtypes of neuropathic pain
   1) Central: deafferentation pain (e.g., central pain or phantom pain) or sympathetically maintained pain (complex regional pain syndrome [CRPS])
   2) Peripheral: originating in nerve root, plexus, or nerve (e.g., polyneuropathies or mononeuropathies)
C. Mixed pain (see Table 1.1)
 1. Combined pain state including both nociceptive and neuropathic inputs
 2. Complex overlap of different pain types acting simultaneously and/or concurrently to cause pain in the same body area

II. Neurophysiology of Pain

A. Introduction
 1. Pain is essential to human survival.
 2. Pain sensation involves the periphery, ascends through spinal cord and brainstem, and is ultimately perceived in cortex of brain.
 3. Once perceived, pain is modulated by descending pathways.
B. Nociception
 1. Nociception is encoding and processing of noxious stimuli resulting in pain.
 2. Nociceptors (Table 1.2)

---

*Section Editor for the chapter.

Table 1.1

Physiological Sources of Pain

Nociceptive Pain

Somatic Pain
- Sensations: Constant, achy
- Location: Well localized in skin, subcutaneous tissues; less well localized in bone, muscle, blood vessels, connective tissues
- Examples: Incision pain, bone fractures, bony metastases, degenerative joint or spinal disease, osteoarthritis, rheumatoid arthritis, peripheral vascular disease, chronic stasis ulcers

Visceral Pain
- Sensations: Cramping, splitting
- Location: Originates in internal organs or body cavity linings; poorly localized, diffuse, deep
- Examples: Chest or abdominal tubes, drains; bladder distention or spasms; intestinal distention; pericarditis; constipation; organ metastases; spastic bowel; inflammatory bowel disease; hiatal hernia; chronic hepatitis

Neuropathic Pain (non-nociceptive pain)
- Sensations: Shooting, burning, electric shock–like, sharp, numb
- Location: Originates in injury to peripheral nerve, spinal cord, brain; poorly localized
- Examples: Radiculopathy, diabetic neuropathy, postherpetic neuralgia, tumor-related nerve compression, phantom limb pain, trigeminal neuralgia, central poststroke pain

Mixed Pain
- Sensations: Combination of nociceptive and neuropathic pain
- Location: Can be anywhere neuropathic and nociceptive pain occur
- Examples: Complex regional pain syndrome, fibromyalgia, osteoarthritis, low back pain, cancer pain

Table 1.2

Nerve Fibers

Fiber	Description (size)	Location	Sensations Produced
Aδ	• Small, thinly myelinated • Diameter: 2 to 5 micrometers (μm) • Conduction velocity: 10 to 40 m/sec • Respond to mechanical (pressure) stimuli	• Skin and subcutaneous tissue • Corneas • Teeth • Joint capsules • Mucous membranes • Respiratory and digestive system • Muscles, tendons, and fascia • Bone periosteum • Urogenital system (kidneys and organs of reproduction) • Solid abdominal organs (liver, spleen, and pancreas) • Brain meninges and scalp • Cardiac muscle • Blood vessel walls	• Well-localized pain sensations • Sharp • Fast pain
Aβ	• Large and myelinated • Conduction velocity: 40 to 50 m/sec	• Motor and sensory pathways	• Fine touch and proprioception fibers
C	• Small, unmyelinated • Diameter: 0.3 to 3 μm • Conduction velocity: <2 m/sec • Activated by high-intensity mechanical, chemical, and thermal stimulation	• Widely distributed in the somatic sensory system	• Poorly localized painful sensations • "Slow" pain

a. Sensory receptors for pain stimuli
b. Located in PNS (e.g., muscle, fascia, blood vessels, joints, viscera)
c. Respond differentially to intense, potentially harmful stimuli of thermal, chemical, or mechanical nature
d. Unspecialized free nerve endings of primary afferent nerves categorized according to their axon properties

1) A fiber nociceptors Aδ and A beta (Aβ) evoke pricking pain, sharpness, and aching pain.
2) C fiber nociceptors evoke burning pain sensation.

3. Nociceptor subtypes
   a. Aδ fibers (first pain): thinly myelinated and produce rapid transmission of impulse to spinal cord

1) Mechanosensitive: receptive to mechanical stress or damage (e.g., distention, irritation, or infection)
2) Mechanothermal: receptive to thermal (heat and cold) stressors
3) Cold receptors:
   a) Reduction of skin temperature to approximately 59°F (15°C) or less evokes sensation of pain.
   b) Sensations include cold, burning, pricking, and aching.
   c) Sensations are dependent on intensity, duration, rate of stimulation, and location of cold stimulus.
4) Mechano-insensitive receptors:
   a) Some may be insensitive to any mechanical stimulus.
   b) Some may respond when pressure is greater than 600 kPa (60 g/mm^2).
  b. Aδ fibers: Low-threshold mechanical stimulation occurs through fine touch or tactile stimuli.
  c. C fibers (second pain): unmyelinated; produce 10-fold slower transmission of impulse to spinal cord than Aδ fibers
   1) Polymodal nociceptors activated by cold, heat, pressure, and chemicals
    a) Heat activation occurs in range of 102.2°F to 123.8°F (39°C to 51°C).
    b) Cold activation occurs in range of −0.4°F to 57.2°F (−18°C to 14°C).
    c) May develop ongoing discharge after sensitization
    d) Mechanical activation may not be changed by heat and chemical activity.
   2) Mechano-insensitive may be:
    a) Insensitive or may respond to pressure
    b) More responsive after inflammation
    c) Chemospecific (responding to specific chemical stimuli)
    d) May respond to intense heat or cold
  d. Silent or sleeping nociceptors
   1) Include both Aδ and C fibers
   2) Contained in skin, deep tissues, and viscera
   3) Normally unresponsive to noxious mechanical and thermal stimuli but can be activated (i.e., responsive) by onset of inflammation in surrounding tissue, mechanical stimulation during inflammation, and after tissue injury in presence of inflammation and chemical sensitization
   4) When activated, silent nociceptors may discharge vigorously in response to nominal stimuli of pressure or temperature.

  e. Other nociceptors
   1) Articular nociceptors
    a) Located in joints and contain nearly twice as many unmyelinated as myelinated afferent axons
    b) Respond to excess, noxious joint rotation
    c) Can be sensitized by inflammation, causing response to even slight joint movements not in noxious range
   2) Muscle nociceptors are polymodal receptors activated by strong mechanical stimuli, such as trauma or overloading, and by endogenous inflammatory mediators.

III. Nociceptive Pain Messaging

A. Nociceptive pain messaging (Fig. 1.1) involves transduction, transmission, perception, and modulation. Each of these components will be summarized in the *In Brief* boxes and detailed in the following sections.
B. Transduction (Step 1):
  1. Transduction begins when noxious stimuli (mechanical, thermal, or chemical) in PNS is sufficient to damage tissues and cause release of neurochemical mediators along with substances synthesized at site of injury.
  2. These neurochemical mediators include bradykinin, cytokines, histamine, serotonin (5-HT), substance P (SP), hydrogen and potassium ions, arachidonic acid, nerve growth factor, and calcitonin gene–related peptide.
  3. The noxious stimulus energy is converted into electrical impulse by action potential in neuronal membranes.
  4. Sodium (Na$^+$) and calcium (Ca2$^+$) channels open, causing depolarization of nerve endings and release of an electrical signal that is propagated along the nerve fiber.

In Brief: Transduction (Step 1)

Mechanical, thermal, or chemical stimuli activate nociceptors, which stimulate primary afferent fibers. The intensity of stimuli may be strong enough to damage tissues and cause release of neurochemical mediators (e.g., K$^+$, substance P, bradykinin, prostaglandin, histamine, and serotonin [5-HT]), which sensitize or activate nociceptors. Once activated, nociceptors transform energy of stimulus (transduction), causing neuron to respond. This energy transformation generates influx of Na$^+$ and efflux of K$^+$ across neuronal membrane. This ion exchange results in an action potential along neuronal membrane of afferent fibers.

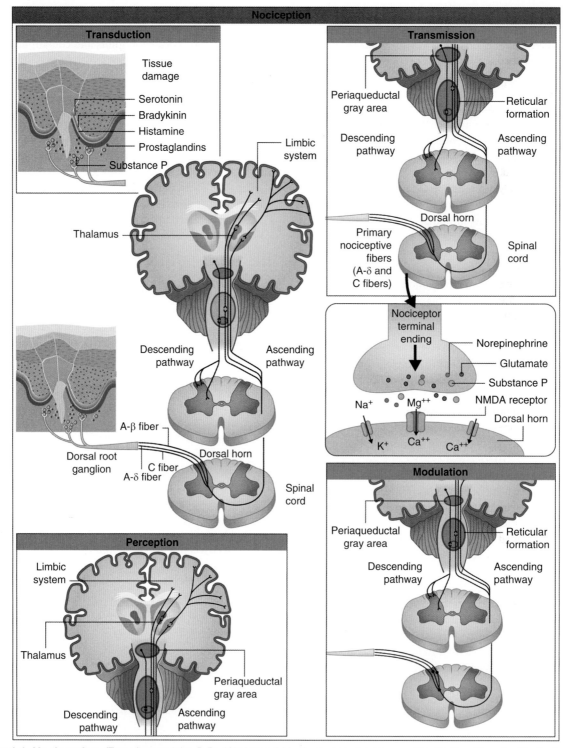

Figure 1.1 Nociception. (From Ignatavicius D.D., Workman M.L. Assessment and care of patients with pain. Medical-surgical nursing: patient-centered collaborative care. 8th edition. St Louis, [MO]: Elsevier; 2016. pp. 24–49.)

C. Transmission (Step 2): nociceptive messaging along neuron
  1. Transmission begins with generation of impulse (action potential) initiated by transduction in PNS.
  2. Nociceptive impulses are transmitted along primary afferent "first order" fibers through dorsal

root ganglia (DRG) to dorsal horn of spinal cord.
  3. In dorsal horn, afferent fibers release a variety of neurotransmitters that bind with receptors on postsynaptic secondary neurons to continue transmission through CNS.

4. These central neurotransmitters include SP, glutamate, aspartate, vasoactive intestinal peptide (VIP), cholecystokinin, somatostatin, and calcitonin gene–related peptide.

In Brief: Transmission (Step 2)

Primary afferent nociceptive fibers terminate in dorsal horn at presynaptic junction. When signal is generated and transmitted, these afferent fibers release neuropeptides, such as substance P (SP), somatostatin, vasoactive intestinal polypeptide, and a large quantity of other neurotransmitters. Some of these chemicals, including SP, bind with receptors on postsynaptic secondary neurons, creating action potential. Opioid receptors (mu [μ], kappa [κ], delta [δ]) are also located in dorsal horn on the end of afferent nociceptor fibers. Endogenous opioids bind to these receptors, resulting in inhibition of release of neurotransmitters, which can stop nociceptive impulse from being communicated to next-order neuron.

5. CNS: spinal cord transmission activity
   a. Transmission continues in CNS starting in spinal cord dorsal horn.
   b. Primary afferent fibers from DRG project into dorsal horn. The dorsal horn is inner, butterfly-shaped gray matter of spinal cord. Gray matter is organized by laminae, or thin cellular layers. There are ten laminae, identified as I though X.
   c. These layers were named "Rexed laminae" due to discovery of Bror Rexed in the 1950s, who identified layers of gray matter in spinal cord arranged by structure and function instead of simple location.
   d. Primary afferent fiber "first-order" neurons terminate in specific laminae, connecting both with longer central "second-order" neurons projecting to brain and with shorter, local-only laminar interneurons. These interneurons connect various laminae and spinal cord segments and can be either excitatory or inhibitory.
   e. Laminae I, II, V, and X have significant nociceptive input from various pain fibers.
   f. Neurotransmitter receptors at synapse of these fibers in spinal cord modulate presynaptic and postsynaptic activity.
      1) Presynaptic receptor types include:
         a) Opioid receptors mu, kappa, and delta: 75% of opioid receptors are presynaptic
         b) Gamma (γ)-aminobutyric acid (GABA) B
         c) 5-HT
         d) Alpha-2 adrenergic
         e) Neurokinin-1 (NK-1)
      2) Postsynaptic receptor types include:
         a) Opioid receptors mu, kappa, and delta—25% of opioid receptors are presynaptic
         b) GABA A
         c) 5-HT
         d) Alpha-2 adrenergic
         e) NK-1
         f) Adenosine
         g) Glutamate: N-methyl-D-aspartate (NMDA), kainate, α-amino-3-hydroxy-5-methyl-4-isoxazolepropionic acid (AMPA)
   g. Neurotransmitters and modulators in spinal cord can be excitatory or inhibitory.
      1) Excitatory substances
         a) Substance P
         b) Glutamate and aspartate, amino acids
         c) Cholecystokinin
         d) Calcitonin gene–related peptide
         e) Vasoactive intestinal polypeptide
         f) Nitric oxide
      2) Inhibitory substances
         a) Endogenous opiates: dynorphin, enkephalin, β-endorphin
         b) Norepinephrine
         c) 5-HT
         d) Somatostatin
         e) GABA
         f) Glycine
6. Ascending nociceptive transmission pathways (Fig. 1.2)
   a. Spinothalamic tract (STT):
      1) Relays sensory information from spinal cord to thalamus, the main site for sensory information integration
      2) Axons cross dorsal and ventral commissures of spinal cord, reaching to contralateral side.
      3) Axons are concentrated in two areas: middle of lateral STT and middle of anterior STT. These tracts ascend in white matter of ventrolateral and lateral STT.
         a) Lateral STT projects to ventroposterolateral nucleus of thalamus and then to somatosensory cortex for location, intensity, and duration of pain.
         b) Medial STT, which also includes input from spinoreticular tract and spinomesencephalic tract, projects to medial thalamus, with projections to reticular formation, pons, midbrain, periaqueductal gray, hypothalamus, various other thalamic nuclei, and other areas of brain.

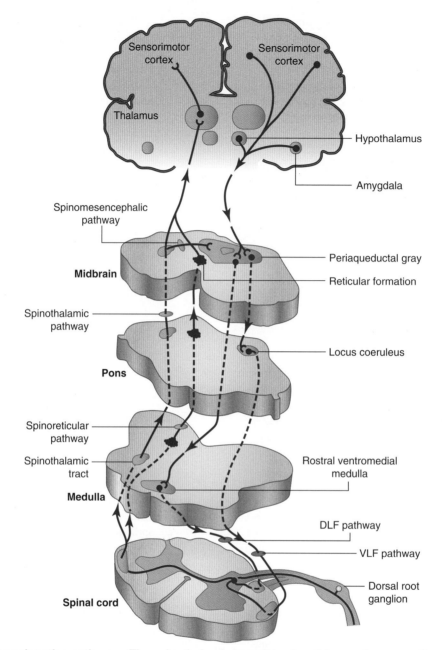

Figure 1.2 Major nociceptive pathways. The spinothalamic tract (blue tract) is a major ascending spinal projection that transmits nociceptive, thermal, and nondiscriminative touch information to several thalamic nuclei, including the ventral posterolateral nucleus, the intralaminar nuclei, and the posterior thalamic nucleus. Descending pain pathways transmit information from several brain regions, including the cortex, hypothalamus, and amygdala, to the periaqueductal gray (PAG) in the midbrain (red tract). Activation of the PAG neurons activates neurons within the rostroventral medulla (RVM). From the RVM (green tract), serotonin- and enkephalin-containing neurons project to the dorsal horn of the spinal cord via the dorsolateral funiculus and exert their inhibitory influences on nociceptive transmission. PAG neurons also activate noradrenergic-containing neurons within the locus coeruleus. This noradrenergic pathway (orange tract) descends in the ventrolateral funiculus to also have an inhibitory effect on the nociceptive transmission within the dorsal horn. (© 2017 American Academy of Pain Medicine. From Irvine, K. A., & Clark, J. D. [2018]. Chronic pain after traumatic brain injury: pathophysiology and pain mechanisms. Pain medicine, 19(7), 1315–1333. https://academic.oup.com/journals/pages/about_us/legal/notices)
This work is written by U.S. Government employees and is in the public domain in the U.S.

b. Spinoreticular tract:
   1) Projection axons from spinal cord provide innervation to regions of brainstem.
   2) Projects to neurons with larger receptor fields that may cover wider areas of body, making it responsible for arousal and autonomic responses to pain
c. Spinomesencephalic tract: primarily nociceptive-specific
d. Ventral STT: plays indirect role in nociception

D. Perception (Step 3): centers in brain receiving nociceptive input
1. Hypothalamus: integrates autonomic arousal and neuroendocrine responses, relates to emotional responses, a strong activator of motivational inputs
2. Thalamus
   a. Controls relay messaging to higher centers of brain
   b. Provides cutaneous awareness for localization and discrimination
   c. Plays role in motor control and increased cortical activity
3. Cerebral cortex
   a. Cortical modulation of pain
   b. Somatotopically arranged cells help with fine sensory discrimination.
4. Limbic system
   a. Generates purposeful, goal-directed behavior
   b. Affects mood states
   c. Generates incentive and motivational reactions
5. Reticular formation
   a. Mediates motor, autonomic, and sensory functions
   b. Triggers arousal and alertness
   c. Adds to emotive responses, including aversive drive (i.e., pain behaviors)
   d. Tectum: enhanced reflexes and learned behavior patterns
6. Basal ganglion
   a. Sensory-discriminative dimension of pain
   b. Affective and cognitive dimension of pain
   c. Sensory gating of nociceptive information to higher motor areas

In Brief: Perception (Step 3)

STT neurons are combined in portion of spinal cord called anterolateral quadrant. These ascending neurons continue to transmit nociceptive messages through to thalamus and midbrain. From thalamus, fibers transmit nociceptive messages to somatosensory cortex, parietal lobe, frontal lobe, and limbic system. At this level of processing, individual perceives the painful sensation. Stimulation of limbic system in area of anterior cingulate gyrus may produce emotional reaction to pain.

E. Modulation (Step 4) (descending) of pain (Fig. 1.2)
1. Periaqueductal gray brain region
   a. Receives input from multiple brain centers; consists of multiple neuron types and receptors: enkephalin, β-endorphin, SP
   b. Releases neurotransmitters that exert inhibitory antinociceptive effects: enkephalin, dynorphin, 5-HT, neurotensin
2. Nucleus raphe dorsalis and mesencephalic reticular formation
   a. Contribute to serotoninergic input by way of dorsolateral STT to all dorsal horn laminae
   b. Consist of multiple neuron types and neurotransmitters: enkephalin, dynorphin, 5-HT, neurotensin
3. Medulla (primarily the rostroventral medulla)
   a. Receives multiple inputs from periaqueductal gray
   b. Releases 5-HT, norepinephrine, enkephalin, SP, and other peptides
   c. May produce dynorphin
   d. Believed to have bidirectional control over nociceptive inputs via on-cells and off-cells that may facilitate or inhibit transmission of pain-related information to brain
4. Pons: Neurons primarily release norepinephrine and 5-HT.
5. Descending modulation control
   a. Noradrenergic tract (norepinephrine tract) seems to have crucial role in opioid-induced analgesia.
   b. Hypothalamospinal tract:
      1) Primary neuronal action mediated by neuropeptides vasopressin and oxytocin with effect on the posterior pituitary
      2) Minor neuronal chemistry input includes enkephalin.
   c. Periaqueductal gray to spinal projections: primarily 5-HT and noradrenergic neurotransmitters
   d. Dorsal horn neurons may contain endogenous opioids and other substances.
      1) Enkephalin-releasing cells (endogenous opiate or endorphin)
      2) Dynorphin-releasing cells exhibit effects primarily through the κ-opioid receptor
   e. Endogenous 5-HT release may be affected by many factors.
      1) Factors that may increase 5-HT release:
         a) Pain
         b) Acupuncture
         c) Exercise
         d) Sexual response
         e) Short-term stress
      2) Factors that may decrease endorphin release:
         a) Prolonged stress

b) Anxiety in acute and persistent pain
c) Depression in persistent pain
d) Suffering or severe distress caused by loss
e) Alcohol use in excess
f) Prolonged pain

f. Other factors affecting pain perception and processing
1) Age-related changes are poorly understood. Sensitivity in sensory systems (e.g., hearing, taste, vision) decrease with advancing age, which is somewhat due to reduction in number of specialized peripheral receptors and deterioration of supporting tissues. There is also reduction in myelinated and unmyelinated fibers as well as damage to these fibers.
2) In early adulthood, number and size of sensory neurons in DRG increase and peak at midlife and then decrease. In addition, in spinal cords of old animals and postmortem humans, a decreased expression of neurotransmitters has been observed.
3) Sex
   a) Sex differences in mechanisms of pain perception are not well elucidated because of limited number of female-driven studies in preclinical literature (i.e., animal models).
   b) Females consistently report increased pain following multiple forms of postoperative pain, musculoskeletal pain, and pain in response to disease states.
   c) Testosterone is thought to serve protective role in persistent pain conditions.
   d) Estradiol-level fluctuations may aid in development of pain states in females, whereas stability of estradiol levels may serve protective role against nociceptive signaling.
   e) Prolactin has been linked to female-specific role in multiple pain conditions and is known to be increased in response to different stressors.
4) Genetics
   a) Growing evidence suggests genes play critical role in determining pain sensitivity, pain reporting, development of persistent pain syndromes, and response to postsurgical pain.
   b) Studies of monozygotic twins' response to experimental and musculoskeletal pain models showed strong correlation, compared to dizygotic twins, demonstrating strong genetic component to pain heritability.
   c) Voltage-gated sodium channels (Na_v) in sensory neurons are subject to wide variety of mutations, both inherited and via single nucleotide polymorphisms, that can lead to hypo-/hyper-excitability in pain-related conditions. Sodium-channel changes in neuropathic pain involve complex patterns of both up- and down-regulation.
   d) Alterations in genes that encode for voltage-gated sodium channels (Na_vs) are implicated in small-fiber neuropathy (Na_v 1.7), peripheral neuropathy (Na_v 1.8), and in alterations in pain perception (Na_v1.9).
   e) Genetic variations in mu-opioid receptor gene are associated with variations in opioid requirements and response in postoperative, cancer, and noncancer pain.
   f) Rare gene variants in angiotensin pathway were associated with differences in pain sensitivity in experimental heat pain-threshold testing.
5) Race/ethnicity
   a) Experimental pain sensitivity studies show significant differences in pain tolerance between non-Hispanic White, African-American, Asian, and Hispanic subjects, with results influenced by pain catastrophizing, coping, and depression/anxiety/stress.
   b) African-Americans report greater pain sensitivity and reduced pain tolerance to variety of quantitative sensory testing methods compared to non-Hispanic Whites, including thermal pain, cold pressor pain, and ischemic pain.
   c) Hispanic-Americans endorse more severe clinical pain and demonstrate greater pain sensitivity and less tolerance for experimental pain compared to non-Hispanic Whites.
   d) Asian–Americans demonstrate lower pain tolerance and threshold and greater pain sensitivity compared to White individuals.
   e) There is some evidence Native Americans are less pain sensitive than White individuals.

In Brief: Modulation (Step 4)

Midbrain activation by nociceptive input causes fibers with descending projections to dorsal horn of spinal cord to modulate pain through descending pathway activation.

This system often works to decrease amount of pain and can explain why some individuals in the face of devastating and painful injuries may not feel pain. It also explains basis for why nonpharmacological approaches, such as visual imagery, distraction, hypnosis, and relaxation, reduce pain. Serotonin (5-HT) is released in the brain by specific neurons, particularly within nucleus raphe magnus, and binds and activates neurons of descending analgesic tract. 5-HT is then released by descending neuron back into synaptic cleft, where reuptake occurs. Neurons that play a role in descending analgesic system in medulla and pons release norepinephrine in the same manner. When reuptake of norepinephrine and 5-HT is inhibited by medications, descending analgesic system is enhanced, resulting in improved inhibition of transmission of nociceptive messages within dorsal horn.

IV. Pathophysiology of Pain

A. Overview
  1. In contrast to physiological pain, pathophysiological pain results from change in baseline somatosensory sensitivity.
  2. Pathophysiological pain can be caused by specific disease (e.g., diabetes or cancer) or painful condition (e.g., low back pain, headache syndromes, postherpetic neuralgia, phantom limb pain, or fibromyalgia).
      a. When there is tissue or nerve damage in an area, there may be increased sensitivity around and extending beyond site of injury.
      b. This increased sensitivity, or hyperalgesia, may serve as an adaptive process to remind the individual to protect injured area.
      c. If pain persists after healing has taken place, it can become persistent pain, associated with changes in how pain is processed and perceived.
  3. For various types of pathophysiological pain states, see Box 1.1.
B. Peripheral sensitization (Fig. 1.3)
  1. Definition: increased sensitivity and spontaneous activity of nociceptors resulting in hyperalgesia and pain
  2. Process:
      a. Injured tissues release several activating substances from mast cells, white blood cells, and damaged tissues.
      b. Inflammatory mediators such as bradykinin, 5-HT, and prostaglandin E_2 potentiate peripheral sensitization by directly affecting nociceptors or sensitizing them to touch (allodynia) or movement. This may even occur in areas distant from inflammatory field.

Box 1.1

Pathophysiological Pain States

Helpful Distinctions

Referred pain seems to have components of central sensitization, such as expansion of receptive fields after inflammatory injuries in areas such as colon, joints, bladder, and esophagus. This is possible because large percentage of spinal neurons (possibly 90%) receive convergent input from visceral and somatic afferents.

Sympathetic mediated pain occurs when sympathetic afferents play role in peripheral inputs that maintain pain.

Sympathetic independent pain describes pain syndrome in which sympathetic afferents *do not play* significant role in maintenance of pain but pain apparently is supported by other peripheral inputs, such as collateral sprouting in dorsal horn and ephaptic connections.

Phantom limb pain is mediated by nerves severed by removal of a body part but continue to generate sensory input to central nervous system. There are some central features to phantom limb pain, which would explain pain memories felt in phantom body part that existed before amputation or avulsion of body part. This syndrome can develop and be expressed when nonlimb areas of body in which pain was felt are removed by surgery or avulsion, including teeth, breasts, stomach areas removed because of ulcers, special sense organs, uterus (may feel labor pains or cramps), rectum, bladder, and cornea. Amputees can be pain free for years and then suddenly have their previous pain return after peripheral stimulus to amputated limb site, which implies presence of quiescent central sensitized neuronal pathways for pain.

---

  1) Cyclooxygenase (COX) also plays important role in both peripheral and central sensitizations.
  2) COX-2 is among enzymes produced with inflammation and converts arachidonic acid into prostaglandins, which in turn increases sensitivity of peripheral nociceptor terminals.
      c. Tissue injury promotes likelihood of peripheral stimulus activating nociceptor and increasing nociceptors' receptive fields.
          1) After tissue injury and inflammatory response, nociceptor thresholds are lowered; pain hypersensitivity often occurs.
          2) Reduction in pain thresholds and increase in responsiveness of nociceptor neurons can lead to nociceptors firing with increased

Part 1

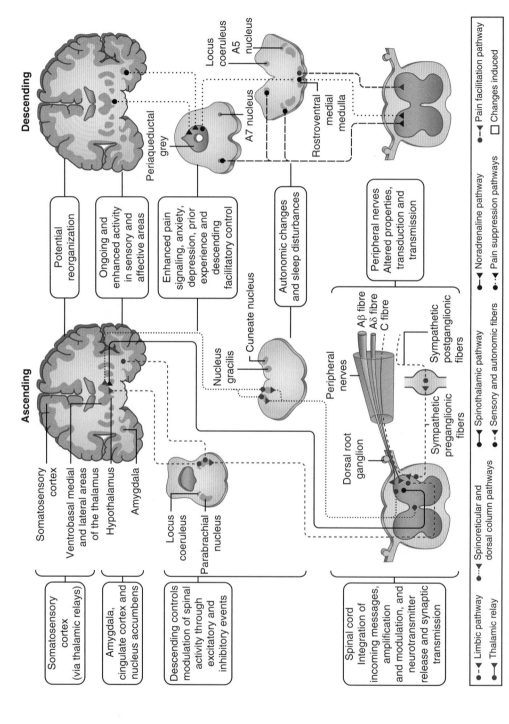

Figure 1.3 Peripheral and central sensitization. (From Anand, P., Dickenson, A., Finco, G., Marinangeli, F., Polati, E., Romualdi, P., et al. [2019]. Novel insights on the management of pain: highlights from the 'Science of Relief' meeting. *Pain Management, 9*(6), 521–533. https://doi.org/10.2217/pmt-2019-0031. Reproduced with permission from *Pain Management* as agreed by Future Medicine Ltd.)

frequency to both noxious and non-noxious stimuli.

3) Enhanced transmission of nociceptive inputs to brain associated with loss of discriminatory processing of noxious and non-noxious stimuli also occurs.

4) Cumulatively, this results in nociceptors being more sensitive, firing more often, and having enhanced transmission of noxious and non-noxious stimuli, resulting in increased pain.

d. Sensitization of primary afferent nociceptors may occur directly through thermal, mechanical, or chemical stimulation or through chemical toxins (e.g., interleukin-1 released from bacteria). It may also occur indirectly through other inflammatory mediators.

1) Nociceptors fire in response to weaker stimuli than usual.

2) Nociceptors may generate more frequent impulses than usual to supra-threshold stimuli.

3) "After-discharge" (e.g., neuron continues to fire after stimulus removed) can occur following repeated or intense stimuli.

4) Nociceptor sensitization occurs within approximately 5 to 10 mm of injury site.

5) Silent nociceptors can become responsive; they may discharge with normal movement and show changes in their receptive field size. *Of note*, silent nociceptors do not respond to nociceptive stimuli until sensitization has occurred.

e. Sites of action for neurochemicals involved in mediating pain vary; some have specific actions in periphery, and others act on receptors in dorsal horn. Some neurochemicals derived from inflammatory response may directly activate nociceptors even in absence of any other stimuli. For example:

1) 5-HT acts differently in PNS and CNS.
   a) Peripherally, it has a hyperalgesic effect, participating with other neurochemicals to exert pro-nociceptive effect.
   b) Centrally, its action is anti-nociceptive by facilitating descending pathway pain modulation.

2) Second messenger system mediated by cyclic adenosine monophosphate has major role in development of primary afferent hyperalgesia.

3. Peripheral sensitization, if maladaptive, may represent failure of inflammatory response feedback loop.

4. Ectopic nerve impulses
   a. Damaged peripheral nerve axons can produce ectopic nerve impulses or paroxysmal firing.
   b. Damaged afferent neurons can transmit normal signals but can also produce impulses initiated from abnormal sites or processes (e.g., originating from somewhere other than transduction of nociceptive stimulus acting on nociceptor).

1) Ectopic firing of injured nerves observed with neuropathic pain syndromes can produce electric shock–like pain or stabbing pain.

2) Ectopic firing can cause nerve fibers that typically do not transmit pain (e.g., A-β touch fibers) to become responsive to pain. This sensitization occurs when DRG cells also become hypersensitive to nerve pain impulses and is further complicated by windup in spinal cord dorsal horn cell bodies (described more in C.5).

c. Activation of glutamate-specific postsynaptic NMDA receptors, which are located in dorsal horn, increases painful inputs.

d. Mechanisms contributing to ectopic discharge in nerves along length of peripheral afferent neuron distal to cell body are as follows:

1) Damaged nerves sprout, and these sprouts can cause neuromas, often a site of ectopic impulse generation and mechanosensitivity (e.g., seen in diabetic neuropathy and amputation).

2) Neuromas:
   a) May be trapped in scar tissue and cause ongoing activations (often referred to as "neuromas in continuity")
   b) Typically form after limb amputations where nerve sheaths are breached
   c) Can form on both myelinated and unmyelinated nerve fibers
   d) Rate of spontaneous discharge from neuromas on *myelinated* neurons increases with warming and decreases with cooling.
   e) Rate of spontaneous discharge from neuromas on *unmyelinated* neurons increases with cooling and is suppressed by heat. This may be basis for cold intolerance often observed in amputees.

3) When myelinated nerves are damaged, myelin sheath retreats, exposing longer length of neuronal membrane than originally present.
   a) This results in demyelinated areas along myelinated nerves.
   b) Can be caused by diabetes, chemotherapeutic or neurotoxic drugs, trauma,

progressive neurological disease, and heavy metal toxicity

   c) Characteristics of demyelinated areas along myelinated nerves:

     (1) Exhibit spontaneous impulse discharge

     (2) Hyperexcitable to mechanical stimuli

4) Constricted nerves develop mechanosensitive hot spots.

5) Up-regulation of alpha-adrenergic receptors (increased numbers) may occur in damaged neuron's membrane. This may partially explain mechanisms for CRPS.

   a) Adrenergic receptors may fire when exposed to norepinephrine from sympathetic nerve fiber activity or from circulating epinephrine.

   b) They may bring threshold of nociceptive afferent nerve closer to firing, enhancing hyperalgesia to thermal and mechanical stimuli.

6) Imbalance in Na^+ channels may be evident in damaged neuron's membrane.

   a) Number of channels per unit length along neuronal membrane may increase as neuron sends more than usual replacement components in an effort to repair damaged neuron.

   b) Passive influx of Na^+ through increased number of channels may initiate impulses without stimulus.

7) Up-regulation and increased numbers of stretch-activated receptors in damaged neuron's membrane result in impulse generation with light pressure (e.g., allodynia in amputation residual limb [stump] area).

8) Ephaptic communication or cross-talk of C fibers in injured zones can occur.

   a) Electrical transmission event whereby transected neuron can short-circuit insulation of neighboring undamaged neuron

   b) Results in inducing electrical impulse on the other neuron, increasing number of pain messages to CNS

9) Collateral neuronal sprouting may occur. Neurons sharing a common border with a damaged nerve may send sprouts into damaged nerve's territory, perhaps secondary to nerve growth factor, and become exposed to chemicals of sensitization.

10) Antidromic impulses (impulses in axon conduction opposite to normal) occur when ectopic impulses are initiated midaxon or from DRG (e.g., impulse may run toward periphery and toward CNS).

   a) These impulses may stimulate release of neurochemicals in periphery, such as substance P, causing local vasodilation leading to warmth, redness, and edema, and are often called neurogenic inflammation.

   b) May play role in trophic changes seen in CRPS II

11) A crushed nerve may cause less disruption than a cut nerve because sprouts from crushed nerves are more likely to come into contact with Schwann cells (myelin-producing cells) than are sprouts on cut nerve. Schwann cells provide source of nerve growth factor that helps damaged nerve recover.

5. Ectopic mechanisms in DRG cell bodies can occur.

  a. These cells have inherent normal rhythmical discharges, but magnitude of discharge can be enhanced in nerve-damage states, causing sensitization.

  b. Mechanical pressure on DRG (e.g., as from herniated disk) may increase neuronal discharge.

  c. Sympathetic nerve activity can cause innervation of DRG, activating primary afferent nociceptive neurons. This mechanism is due to noradrenergic sprouting in DRG after peripheral nerve damage.

  d. DRG cells may develop ephaptic coupling after herpes zoster infection, which is possibly involved in mechanisms causing postherpetic neuralgia.

C. Central sensitization (Fig. 1.3)

1. Definition and description:

  a. A complex condition defined by increase in excitability of neurons within CNS so that normal sensory inputs cause abnormal sensing and responses to painful and nonpainful stimuli; plays crucial role in pathogenesis of persistent pain

  b. Refers to formation of spontaneous impulses and/or increased sensitivity of somatosensory neurons in dorsal horn of spinal cord to pain and occurs after intense peripheral noxious input from tissue injury or nerve damage

  c. Central processing circuits of nervous system are disrupted, including development of spontaneous impulses.

  d. Some aspects of central sensitization can persist after peripheral inputs cease; however, peripheral and central neural mechanisms are involved in causing central sensitization and can be a long-lasting problem.

2. Distinctions between initial sensitization and ongoing central sensitization:

  a. Initial central sensitization is result of afferent barrage that can be short-lived.

b. Ongoing central sensitization is sustained by peripheral inputs caused by severe tissue injury.

3. Process by which acute, unrelieved pain leads to central sensitization and subsequently persistent pain syndromes:

    a. Acute tissue injury produces a cascade of events that involves release of neurotransmitters; electrophysiological, intracellular stress; and structural and neuropsychological responses.

    b. Even brief intervals of acute pain are capable of inducing long-term neuronal remodeling and sensitization ("plasticity"), persistent pain, and lasting psychological distress.

4. Dorsal horn mechanisms play a role in central sensitization (these mechanisms are strongly linked to ongoing peripheral input).

    a. Sprouting of nerve endings into adjacent laminae after peripheral nerve damage results in activation of central pain pathways by neurons communicating non-nociceptive information as light touch (e.g., sprouting of Aβ fibers from lamina III into laminae I and II has been observed).

    b. Unmasked latent synapses within dorsal horn, active only in state of sensitization, result in activation of central pain pathways through neurons communicating non-nociceptive information as light touch or in recruitment of additional second-order nociceptive neurons, increasing number of pain signals going to the brain.

    c. Chemical sensitization occurs when nitric oxide and COX-2, released from second-order neurons after intense stimulation, diffuse into primary afferents and cause increased release of glutamate.

        1) Glutamate excites NMDA receptors and further activates second-order neurons. This positive feedback loop contributes to pain sensitization.

        2) Glutamate also plays major role in central sensitization, which produces hyperexcitability (reduction in threshold for action potential firing).

    d. Dorsal horn neurons whose receptive fields are adjacent to injury sites may expand their receptive fields following tissue damage so they react to stimuli elicited within damaged area itself.

    e. When sensitized, wide dynamic-range neurons that usually discriminate between nociceptive and non-nociceptive stimuli may signal pain with light tactile stimuli (allodynia).

    f. Prolonged activation of non-NMDA receptors (i.e., AMPA and neurokinin receptors) on second-order neurons prime NMDA receptors into state of activation.

    g. Sustained activation of NMDA receptors leads to changes in CNS, playing an important role in persistent pain states.

        1) Central sensitization occurs where nociceptive neurons in dorsal horn of spinal cord become sensitized by peripheral tissue damage or inflammation, leading to increased sensitivity of dorsal horn to stimuli.

        2) Long-term potentiation suggests cellular memory for pain may lead to future increased responses to nociceptive stimuli.

        3) Facilitation is development of state in which, because of repeated stimulation of a neuron, impulse threshold is reduced and intensity of response is increased.

        4) Receptive field alterations in periphery are orchestrated from dorsal horn.

    h. Hyperalgesia (an exaggerated response to painful stimuli that are typically painful) may be evident in different ways, probably depending on source of peripheral input. People with neuropathic pain generally experience cutaneous hypersensitivity and increased pain from thermal or mechanical stimuli.

    i. Other cutaneous manifestations associated with neuropathic pain may include painful numbness, redness, swelling, or warmth in injured area.

        1) Some may have sensitivity to heat and find relief with cold, while others may seek comfort with warmth and experience pain from exposure to cold.

        2) Some improve with standard nerve blocks (Aβ and C fiber) and others with sympathetic nerve blocks.

    j. Changes may occur in spinal cord, resulting in central pain (some of these changes may be independent of peripheral inputs).

        1) If contralateral ascending spinal pathways for pain (i.e., spinothalamic, spinoreticular, and spinomesencephalic) are surgically or chemically severed in an effort to treat pain. This may result in pain messages being carried by latent ipsilateral (same side) pathway that eventually takes over.

            a) This explains why immediate pain relief occurring after such a procedure may continue for some time before pain returns.

            b) This includes results of neuroablative procedures, such as neurectomy, cordotomy, and rhizotomy.

        2) Trauma on or near to spinal cord at any level for any cause (ischemic, transection, neoplastic, hemorrhagic, compression, radiation, or surgery) can cause damage to

any part of spinothalamic, spinoreticulotha-
lamic, or spinomesencephalic pathways.

3) Disease processes such as myelitis or multiple sclerosis may injure cord directly.

k. Changes may occur in supraspinal CNS neurons independent of peripheral inputs.

1) Possible direct causes of changes to supraspinal CNS neurons that may lead to central
pain are stroke or other ischemic injury to
thalamus or other areas of brain, surgical or
traumatic lesions, malignancy invasion, and
radiation damage.

2) Role of supraspinal structures may change
with central sensitization or CNS injury.

a) Thalamus

(1) Positron emission tomography (PET)
shows increased thalamic activity with
acute pain but decreased thalamic
activity in patients with persistent or
cancer pain.

(2) Regional blood flow changes with
neuropathic pain.

(3) Development of spontaneous neuronal hyperactivity

(4) Somatotopic organization is altered.

b) Cortex

(1) Neuronal sprouting occurs.

(2) Intracortical connections are
unmasked.

(3) Gene expression changes after
peripheral nerve injury.

(4) Regional blood flow increases.

c) Cingulate cortex shows activation and
increased regional blood flow.

d) Right gyrus cinguli is activated in some
neuropathic pain states.

5. Windup

a. Definition/description:

1) Windup can be described as progressive
increase in magnitude of C-fiber–evoked
responses of dorsal horn neurons
produced by repetitive activation of
C-fibers.

2) Windup, however, is different from central
sensitization; it can be short-lasting,
whereas central sensitization and
hyperalgesia persist over time.

b. Process

1) Windup, like central sensitization and
hyperalgesia, is induced by C-fiber inputs
and is attenuated by NMDA and NK-1
receptor antagonists.

2) These inputs create many problems, including sprouting of wide dynamic range neurons and induction of glutamate-dependent
NMDA receptors.

3) Synaptic processes that produce windup are
capable of causing central sensitization, but
reverse is not true. Central sensitization
does not produce windup.

6. Neuroplasticity

a. Refers to intricate group of processes that allow
neurons in brain to compensate for injury and
adjust their responses to new situations or
changes in their environment.

b. Process

1) Brain-derived neurotrophic factor (BDNF)
is well-known regulator of synaptic plasticity and is involved in descending
pain-control pathway to inhibit pain.

2) Following peripheral nerve injury, dynamic
changes occur in capabilities of descending
pain pathways to modulate pain.

a) After tissue injury, BDNF and neurotrophic tyrosine kinase receptor signaling in brainstem are rapidly activated.

b) Animal models demonstrate that with
persistent pain, transmission is facilitated. Functional, chemical, and structural plasticity of neurons can contribute
to adaptive mechanisms in reducing
pain and to maladaptive mechanisms
enhancing pain.

3) Genetic makeup and variability among individuals may play important roles in synthesis
and function of proteins affecting plasticity
of CNS. This may explain interpatient differences in pain responses and development of
many persistent pain conditions.

7. Hyperalgesia

a. Primary hyperalgesia occurs at site of tissue
injury. Sensitized primary afferent nociceptors
are partially responsible for increased response
to stimuli such as heat.

b. Secondary hyperalgesia occurs in surrounding
uninjured tissue areas and is thought to be
related to central sensitization rather than to
peripheral sensitization.

1) Presence of inflammatory mediators in tissues may cause recruitment of large and
small fibers outside injured area to be
sensitized.

2) Can extend 10 to 20 cm beyond injured
area

3) Characterized by hyperalgesia to mechanical stimuli but not heat stimuli

a) Mechanical hyperalgesia is similar to
hyperalgesia commonly noted in people
with neuropathic pain.

b) Mechanical hyperalgesia can be in
response to stimuli from light stroking
(allodynia).

8. Opioid-induced hyperalgesia (OIH)
   a. A state of nociceptive sensitization due to chronic opioid exposure
   b. Characterized by paradoxical response in which people exposed to opioids become more sensitive to certain painful stimuli and have increased pain.
   c. OIH can occur with treatment of both acute and persistent pain.
      1) Exact mechanism for this phenomenon is not clearly understood but is believed to be related to neuroplastic changes in PNS and CNS, leading to sensitization of pro-nociceptive pathways.
      2) OIH may explain why opioids tend to lose their effectiveness in certain people over time.

V. Immune/Nervous System Interaction

A. Persistent pain may be a result of aberrant neuronal activity and sensitization of neurons in the CNS. However, pain research over past several decades has revealed critical role of immune system in development, maintenance, and recovery of persistent pain.

B. Mounting evidence exists indicating bidirectional modulatory signaling between nervous system neuronal and immunocompetent cells plays critical role in persistent and neuropathic pain.
   1. Research revealed that nerve injury/damage activates pain transmission through primary afferent neurons in PNS and subsequently triggers biochemical changes in DRG of spinal cord. These changes are initiated and maintained by neuropeptide signaling between neurons and immunocompetent cell.
      a. Nociceptors are sensitized to produce pain by immune cell inflammatory mediators and, in turn, nociceptors release neuropeptides from their terminals to affect shape and function of immune cells.
      b. Nerve injury–induced immune cells and glial cells are activated in PNS and CNS. In response to injury, non-neuronal cells release neuromodulatory substances near peripheral nerve terminals, which will either improve or create maladaptive pain, depending on specific type of mediator.
   2. Neuronal–immune system cellular interaction is initiated and maintained by immune cells and glial cells.
      a. Immune cells located in blood and peripheral tissue at site of injury include mast cells, macrophages, neutrophils, lymphocytes, and endothelial cells.
      b. Glial cells of nervous system include Schwann cells in PNS, satellite glial cells in periphery and DRG, microglia, astrocytes, and oligodendrocytes in spinal cord and brain.
         1) Under normal/healthy conditions, these cells do not play role in pain modulation (Table 1.3).
         2) In resting state, they surround and provide silent support to neurons during nociceptive processes.
         3) Glial activation occurs following nerve injury and plays vital role in pain modulation.
         4) Microgliosis and astrogliosis are nonspecific reactive changes of microglia and astrocyte cells in response to nerve injury and tissue insult involving rapid, distinct, observable morphologic changes characteristic of reactive microglia and astrocytes, including hypertrophy and extension of process, cell proliferation, and increased glial fibrillary acidic protein expression.
      c. When activated, glial cells contribute significantly to abnormal neuronal excitability, resulting in extensive immune response around intact as well as damaged cell bodies of sensory nerves.
      d. Proximity of glial cells to neurons facilitates neuroimmune interaction (cross-talk) and maintenance of persistent inflammatory and neuropathic pain.
      e. Additionally, pain-activated microglia immune-related activities include their activation of toll-like receptors (TLRs), interferon-mediated stimulation, and release of cytokines and other immune-modulating chemicals to allow communication with T cells.
   3. Mediators (Table 1.4) and receptors generated during inflammation
      a. Non-neuronal cells produce pro-nociceptive and anti-nociceptive mediators that directly or indirectly contribute to development and regulation of pain.
         1) Adenosine triphosphate (ATP)
            a) Released by damaged neurons upon injury
            b) Triggers secretion of proinflammatory cytokines from satellite glial cells
            c) Activates microglia to state of reactive gliosis
            d) Key energy-carrying molecule that activates certain purinergic receptors, allowing cell-to-cell, bidirectional, microglial-neuron communication
            e) Evidence supports ATP-stimulated microglia as pro-nociceptive

Table 1.3	
Immune Cells in Normal Physiologic State	
Innate Immune System	
Cell Type	
Mast cells	• Important as initiator of innate immunity • Located close to primary nociceptive neurons • First responders to peripheral inflammation • Contribute to nociceptor sensitization through release of histamine, tumor necrosis factor, and other chemicals that cause pain when primary afferent nerves are damaged
Macrophages	• Derived from peripheral monocytes • Active in tissues • Become phagocytic almost immediately after injury • Engulf and destroy microbes, leukocytes, and damaged cells
Neutrophils	• Most abundant white blood cell type in blood • Engulf and destroy microbes, leukocytes, and damaged cells by phagocytosis • Are not found in healthy nerves; are recruited to site of inflammation following nerve injury
Schwann cells	• Glial cell in peripheral nervous system • Produce myelin sheath around axons • Enhance release of inflammatory cytokines • Show similarities to astrocytes
Satellite cells	• Function almost equivalent to that of astrocytes of central nervous system • Glial cell found in both periphery and dorsal root ganglia • Encapsulate cell bodies of neurons in sensory, sympathetic, and parasympathetic ganglia
Astrocytes	• Most abundant cell type in central nervous system • Provide structural support to neurons • Enable formation of blood-brain barrier • Play active role in pre- and postsynaptic processes contributing to synaptic transmission • Provide neuronal energy supply through trophic support
Oligodendrocytes	• Form myelin sheath covering central nervous system axon, making electrical impulses to brain possible
Microglia	• Survey central nervous system environment, and when a signal or event is detected, they transition to activated state of reactive gliosis • Highly reactive to changes in local environment • Specialized macrophage-like cells of central nervous system • Provide structural integrity support for neurons • Tissue-specific phagocyte: clear cellular debris, remodel synapse upon damage
Adaptive Immune System	
T-lymphocytes (T-cell)	• Regulate neuronal function in central nervous system and peripheral nervous system • Function is directly influenced by nociceptor neurotransmitters and neuropeptides regulating their immunologic activity. • Play important role in bidirectional communication between nervous and immune systems
B-lymphocytes (B-cell)	• Mature in bone marrow into plasma cells and secrete antibodies • Located in extracellular body fluid • Memory B-cells remain after first exposure, so antibody response is quicker and prolonged with repeat exposure.

neurotransmitter with potential to change output from ascending nociceptive pathways, thus contributing to symptoms of neuropathic pain.

2) Cytokines
   a) Small low-molecular-weight protein mediators (peptides) released from non-neuronal immunocompetent cells
   b) Increased production and release induced by conditions such as tissue injury and inflammation, which cause activation of these cells in PNS and CNS
   c) Function as immunomodulating agents that engage immune-signaling between immune and neuronal cells
   d) Display properties both proinflammatory and anti-inflammatory
      (1) In neuropathic pain modulation, cytokines are either predominately algesic or analgesic mediators.

Table 1.4
Mediators

Predominant Cytokine Neural Mediators Involved in Persistent Pain

Proinflammatory	Anti-inflammatory
ATP	IL-4
IL-1	IL-10 (Th2)
IL-1β (beta)	IL-2
IL-6	IL-4
IL-15	IL-10
IL-17	IL-13
IL-18	
IFN-γ (gamma)	TGF-1
TNF	TNF-6
CXCL1	IFN-1α (alpha)
CCL2 (also known as MCP-1)	
CCL5, CCL7	
CX3CL1 (fractalkine)	
NGF-β (beta)	
BDNF	

ATP, adenosine triphosphate; *BDNF*, brain-derived neurotrophic factor; *CCL2,5,7, CX3CL1*, chemokine ligands; *IFN*, interferon; *IL*, interleukin; *NGF*, nerve growth factor; *TGF-1*, transforming growth factor-1; *TNF*, tumor necrosis factor

    (2) In persistent pain, there is often imbalance between algesic and analgesic mediators released by non-neuronal immune cells.
- e) Certain inflammatory cytokines and chemokines can directly and indirectly impact inflammatory response. They are involved in nerve-injury and inflammation-induced central sensitization and play a crucial role in neuropathic pain.
- f) Strongly linked to development of inflammatory and neuropathic pain, development of persistent pathologic pain states, and pain behaviors
    - (1) Glial cells are major source of cytokines and chemokines in spinal cord.
    - (2) Astrocytes and microglia activated by cytokine and chemokines result in their adopting proinflammatory phenotype, directly contributing to induction and maintenance of central sensitization.
    - (3) Macrophages produce and release inflammatory cytokines during immune challenge in periphery and DRG.

3) Cytokine subtypes
- a) Tumor necrosis factor (TNF)
    - (1) Proinflammatory cytokine produced in response to injury
    - (2) Important mediator in acute and chronic inflammation
    - (3) TNF secretion leads to production of other cytokines.
- b) Interleukin (IL)
    - (1) IL-2, IL-4, IL-10, IL-13 preclinical evidence of anti-inflammatory effect
    - (2) IL-1β (beta), IL-6, IL-15, IL-17, IL-18 evidence for proinflammatory effect
- c) Interferon: IFN-γ (gamma): implicated in persistent pain states
- d) Colony-stimulating factor-1: released by injured afferent nerves and will trigger microglial proliferation in spinal cord and ATP
- e) Transforming growth factor (TGF): potent anti-inflammatory cytokine
- f) Chemoattractant cytokines (chemokines) and their receptors
    - (1) Large group of small cytokine-type proteins; released locally from peripheral blood cells at site of inflammation; serve as small messenger molecules between cells of immune system during homeostatic and pathologic conditions
    - (2) Believed to be significant mediators in neuron-to-glial cross-talk implicated in neuropathic pain states and pain sensitivity
    - (3) Bind to surface G-protein–coupled receptors (GPCRs) to trigger intracellular signaling pathways
    - (4) May contribute to neuronal-immune modulation of affective mood
- g) Neurotrophic growth factors (NGF) and BDNF
    - (1) Can induce sprouting of peripheral neurons and nociceptive transduction signaling when released by immune cells during inflammation
    - (2) Neurotrophic growth factors
        - (a) Regulator of immune system, excreted as part of inflammatory response to tissue and nerve injury
        - (b) Causes peripheral sensitization through nociceptor sensory afferent tropomyosin receptor kinase A binding

(c) Can induce allodynia and hyperalgesia when released by mast cells and macrophages during inflammation

(3) Brain-derived neurotrophic factor

  (a) Dramatically increased in microglia following nerve injury

  (b) Can be pronociceptive in normally inhibitory spinal neurons when released by activated microglia

  (c) Contributes to persistent pain hypersensitivity

4) TLRs

  a) Pathogen recognition receptors that sense danger signals from tissue injury, then translate signal into immune signal interpreted and responded to by neurons and immunocompetent non-neuronal cells within CNS

  b) When activated, mediate proinflammatory cytokine production, which leads to enhanced immune signaling implicated in exaggerated pain transmission

  c) TLR-4

    (1) Found in spinal microglia and astrocytes

    (2) Activation of TLR-4 contributes to opioid-induced hyperalgesia, in addition to development and maintenance of inflammatory pain.

    (3) Clinical evidence supports role of TLR-4 in human pain states and development of morphine tolerance.

5) Neurokinin-1 receptor (NK-1R)

  a) GPCR expressed by leukocytes within CNS

  b) Receptor selective to SP, a neurotransmitter of pain

  c) SP and NK1R interactions have been associated with severe neuroinflammation and neuronal damage in number of studies.

6) Purinergic receptors

  a) Microglia express numerous subtypes of P2 puringenic receptors.

  b) ATP-mediated purinergic signaling via P2X4, P2X7, and P2Y12 contributes to development of neuropathic pain.

    (1) Disruption of P2X7 receptor completely suppressed inflammatory and neuropathic pain. Additionally, hyperalgesia was prevented by blockade of this receptor by oxidized ATP.

    (2) Peripheral nerve injury (PNI) in mice and rats causes microglial

activation in spinal cord and long-lasting pain hypersensitivity in ipsilateral hind paw. It is worth noting pharmacological blockage or genetic manipulation of these molecules substantially decreases excitability of dorsal horn pain pathway, leading to suppression of pain hypersensitivity. Therefore, phenotypic switch of microglia to reactive state in spinal dorsal horn is crucial event underlying pathogenesis of neuropathic pain after PNI.

C. Dysregulation of immune system in pathologic pain (Fig. 1.4)

  1. In periphery, when damage occurs to peripheral nerve by trauma or inflammation, local response involves release of peripheral chemical mediators that trigger sensory neurons.

    a. Peripheral immune cell response activates innate and adaptive immune systems.

    b. Inflammatory cells, including Schwann cells, mast cells, neutrophils, resident macrophages, and T cells, contribute to peripheral sensitization and hyperexcitability of injured afferent nerve fibers and proliferate to uninjured primary afferent nerve fibers sharing same innervation territory.

    c. Input from resident immune cells recruits systemic immune cells, leading to peripheral sensitization.

    d. Immune response is further perpetuated by direct and indirect action of inflammatory mediators.

  2. Peripheral immune cells involved in nociception during inflammation:

    a. Schwann cells

      1) First-responder glial cells to nerve injury

      2) Play crucial role in development and maintenance of neuropathic pain

      3) Release glial cell mediators, including growth factors, cytokines, chemokines, and ATP

      4) Begin process of breaking down myelin sheath at injury site

    b. Mast cells

      1) Have role in initial stages of inflammation and pain hypersensitivity

      2) Surrounding peripheral neurons release histamine and 5-HT. Damaged nerves release TNF, NGF, and other cytokines, all of which sensitize nociceptors of damaged primary afferent nerves.

    c. Neutrophils

      1) Recruited by nociceptors to release inflammatory mediators

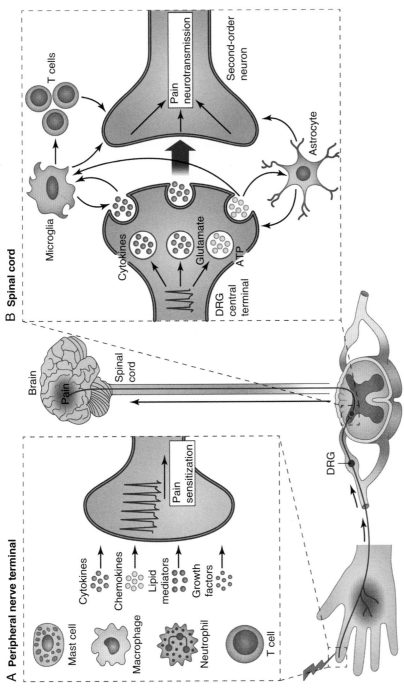

Figure 1.4 Neuroimmune interactions at peripheral nerve terminals and spinal cord in pain. (A) During inflammation, immune cells (mast cells, macrophages/monocytes, neutrophils, and T cells) release mediators (cytokines, chemokines, lipid mediators, and growth factors) that act on peripheral nerve terminals of nociceptor neurons. Action potentials are transduced via the dorsal root ganglia (DRG) to the spinal cord and relayed to the brain to be processed as pain. (B) In the spinal cord dorsal horn, neuroimmune interactions contribute to central mechanisms of pain. Primary DRG nociceptive afferents (presynaptic) release glutamate, adenosine triphosphate, and chemokines from their central terminals, mediating neurotransmission to second-order postsynaptic neurons that relay signals to the brain. T-cells, microglia, and astrocytes also produce proinflammatory cytokines and growth factors that act on both presynaptic and postsynaptic nerve terminals to increase neurotransmission and mediating central pain sensitization. (From Baral, P., Udit, S., & Chiu, IM. [2019] Pain and immunity: implications for host defence. Nature Reviews Immunology, 19(7), 433–447.)

2) Acutely infiltrate site of injury to release chemicals that sensitize nociceptors, leading to recruitment of macrophage and T-cell infiltration
d. Macrophages
1) Play active role in pathologic pain, including inflammatory and/or neuropathic components in periphery
a) Release multiple proinflammatory mediators that regulate activity and "talk to" nociceptors
b) Macrophages also "listen to" nociceptors through neuropeptides, ATP, and macrophage-stimulating factor that regulate their activity.
c) Along with Schwann cells, macrophages continue to degenerate axons and myelin sheaths of nerves through cytokines and chemokines.
2) Infiltrate injured nerve and DRG
3) Can produce analgesic effect through:
a) Phagocytic clearance of debris
b) Expression of inflammatory mediators (IL-10)
c) By production of specialized pro-resolving mediators
e. T-lymphocytes (T-cells)
1) T-cell infiltration plays important role in communication between nervous and immune systems and development of pain.
2) Implicated in neuropathic pain
3) Infiltrate DRG
a) CD4+ T-helper cells infiltrate injured nerve, spinal cord, and DRG, where they promote pain responses.
b) CD8+ regulatory T-cells are important contributors to pain recovery.
4) After nerve injury, T-cells infiltrate and release proalgesic mediator (leukocyte elastase [LE]) in DRG resulting in mechanical allodynia.
f. B-lymphocytes (B-cells) are involved in signaling of TLRs and infiltrating B-cells are implicated in initiation of pain.
D. Sensory ganglia and inflammation
1. Following nerve injury, macrophages and T-cells release chemokines to trigger more macrophage and T-cell recruitment to DRG, which in turn contribute to initiation and maintenance of neuropathic allodynia.
2. Cell bodies of injured and uninjured sensory neurons lie in DRG, where they are exposed to proinflammatory mediators released by macrophages and glial cells. These mediators increase DRG neuronal excitability.

3. When neural barriers, such as blood-nerve barrier and blood–spinal cord barrier, are disrupted after nerve injury, entry of blood-borne molecules and cells occurs.
4. Endothelial cells also release proinflammatory mediators that enhance inflammatory response leading to neuropathic pain.
5. Activated immunocompetent cells (e.g., mast cells, microglia, satellite glial cells, and astrocytes) produce multiple bioactive substances and inflammatory mediators allowing glial cells to:
a. Establish communication among other glial cells
b. Increase expression of surface receptors
c. Proliferate, undergo morphological changes
d. Communicate with adjacent peripheral nerves in DRG and spinal cord to provide autoregulatory feedback
6. Studies continue to support postulation that CNS glial cells, nervous system non-neuronal components, and chemical mediators are associated with neuronal hyperexcitability associated with persistent pain conditions.
7. Glial cells of spinal cord and CNS
a. Microglia
1) Macrophage-like cells distributed throughout CNS, but only microglia on spinal cord are activated following peripheral nerve injury
a) In the presence of abnormal signals from neurons and other glial cells, they undergo microgliosis.
b) Subsequently, they migrate to areas of damage, which leads to release of multiple proinflammatory mediators, neuromodulators, and growth factors, inducing hyperexcitability in pain-signaling pathways.
2) Microglia within rostral ventromedial medulla (RVM) at spinal cord dorsal horn become activated and contribute to descending facilitation and enhanced pain related to nerve injury.
3) Spinal microglia, activated after nerve injury, contribute to pathologic pain processing.
4) Microglia are also found in thalamus, somatosensory cortex, and limbic regions of brain and are likely associated with affective mood component of pain response.
b. Astrocytes
1) Respond to damaged areas
2) Involved in regulation of persistent pain
3) Following noxious stimuli and nerve injury, undergo changes in morphology, and function in process known as astrogliosis

a) Astrocyte becomes reactive.
b) Astrocyte transformation from steady state to reactive state is activated through signaling molecules, including cytokines, chemokines, ATP, and growth factor.
c) Reactive astrocytes are classified according to function as A1 and A2.
   (1) A1 reactive neuroinflammatory astrocytes induce rapid death of neurons and oligodendrocytes through secretion of neurotoxins.
   (2) A2 reactive neuroprotective astrocytes promote neuronal protection and tissue-reparative function.

7. Bidirectional intracellular microglia-astrocyte communication occurs through cytokines, chemokines, ATP, and growth factors.

8. Microglia and astrocytes produce numerous neuromodulators to drive persistent pain by inducing synaptic and neuronal plasticity.
   a. Soluble mediator molecules released by immunocompetent cells bind to pre- and postsynaptic terminals to modulate inhibitory and excitatory neural synaptic transmission, resulting in neuronal nociceptive hypersensitivity.
   b. It is hypothesized the release of substances resulting from microglial activation excite spinal nociceptive neurons through direct or indirect means and promote release of other transmitters that act on nociceptive neurons.

E. CNS response to neuroimmune interaction
1. Repeated stressors activate bidirectional communication between CNS and peripheral immune system.
2. Heightened neuroinflammatory environment occurs in CNS and PNS.
   a. Growing evidence suggests neuroinflammation is involved in central sensitization.
   b. Neuroinflammation involves activation and infiltration of leukocytes and glial cells, leading to increased production of proinflammatory cytokines and chemokines, leading to transition from acute to persistent pain and maintenance of pain.
   c. Exact mechanism of immune cell contribution to persistent pain at spinal cord level is still debated and uncertain. Mechanisms put forth in literature include release of cytokines, reactive oxygen species, or inflammasomes.
   d. Research reveals microglia are highly plastic and activation activity goes beyond resting versus activated state.

3. Further evidence of role in immune dysregulation activation
   a. Glial cell activation in CNS is related to inflammatory injury and pain.
   b. Increased proinflammatory cytokines have distinct mechanisms in dorsal horn neurons either by increasing excitatory synaptic transmission or decreasing inhibitory synaptic transmission, resulting in ongoing neuronal activity.
   c. Proinflammatory cytokines, chemokines, and growth-factor prime adjacent central nociceptive neurons and glia.

4. Neuroinflammatory environment and stress response stimulate activity in sympathetic nervous system and hypothalamic-pituitary-adrenal (HPA) axis.
   a. HPA axis is primary stress response regulator.
   b. HPA activation leads to release of circulating glucocorticoids, mainly cortisol.
   c. Cortisol exerts major effect on suppression of immune response by reducing number and activity of inflammatory cells.
   d. Abnormal increased or decreased output from HPA axis that induces important proinflammatory effects in periphery and CNS may play critical roles in maladaptive responses to persistent pain.

F. Stress and immune function
1. Affective dimension in pain
   a. Growing evidence suggests association between neuroinflammation, negative affect, and persistent pain experience, as well as contributory comorbidity to both conditions.
      1) Elevated inflammatory markers were found in persons with persistent pain and depression.
      2) Human imaging studies (e.g., PET) reveal evidence of CNS glial cell activation in presence of comorbid persistent pain and depression.
   b. Anterior cingulate cortex (ACC) appears to participate in diverse autonomic functions, such as blood pressure and heart rate regulation, and rational cognitive functions, including reward anticipation, decision-making, empathy, impulse control, and emotion. ACC is also involved in neuropathic pain conditions.
      1) Animal studies demonstrated that prolonged astrocyte activation following nerve injury and release of proinflammatory cytokines may be associated with pain sensitivity and affective mood in persistent pain.
      2) From pharmacologic perspective, there are limited therapeutic agents targeting astrocyte activation; therefore, to maintain balanced immune response, most effective method may be to modulate cytokine signaling by providing balance between

pro- and anti-inflammatory cytokines through blockade of certain proinflammatory cytokines and/or enhancing anti-inflammatory cytokines.

2. Evidence suggests CNS immune response to stress has two phases, and type of response is dependent on nature of stress and whether acute or persistent.

   a. First immune response to stress is inflammatory, rapid, and transient (e.g., blood counts for inflammatory mediators are elevated following 2 hours of stress and persist for time-limited course of several hours). It is mediated primarily by glia.

   b. Second immune response to stress is sluggish with slow onset, buildup, and decay. It has been suggested second event is sensitization event, where glia are primed to subsequent stimulation.

G. Pain and stress

1. Effect of pain on immune function

   a. Research over past decade has begun to unravel signaling pathways and processes that engage microglial response to injury.

      1) Microglia are primed by early life injury and subsequently by consequences of pain responses during adulthood.

      2) Stress during early life may have effect on microglia to shift toward proinflammatory profile later in life.

   b. Acute injury-related pain

      1) Surgical injury produces inflammation, skin damage, and peripheral nerve injury.

      2) Tissue trauma initiates non-neuronal processes with physiologic impact. Acute pain activates HPA axis. A wide range of undesirable immunologic effects occurs as result of release of different hormones and glucocorticoids.

      3) Pain is likely component of immunologic effects of surgical stress, such as reduced neurokinin cell activity, depressed cell-mediated immunity and lymphocyte proliferation, and production of proinflammatory cytokines.

   c. Severe insults from both infectious and noninfectious origins are known to induce immune failure and increase risk of hospital-acquired infection. In this framework, initial pathophysiologic responses to insult suggest endogenous danger signals may contribute to development of immune dysfunctions.

   d. Persistent pain is associated with organized organism-wide changes in DNA methylation, including in CNS and immune system.

H. Implications of neuroimmune interface and select pain conditions

1. Pain is physiologic mechanism serving a highly adaptive function. Under normal circumstances, it protects individual from harm and encourages recuperative behaviors. However, when pain becomes persistent, it serves no adaptive or physiologic relevance. Neuropathic pain is form of pathologic pain arising from trauma, infection, or inflammation of peripheral nerves.

2. Clinical pain is not simply consequence of pain system being turned on in periphery by particular injury or pathology but instead is dynamic interaction. Compelling evidence from research over the past 20 years with animal models strongly suggests pathogenesis of neuropathic pain involves immune cells in and around peripheral nerves. Also, immune-like glial cells in spinal cord are key in bidirectional signaling between immune and nervous systems.

   a. Studies continue to support CNS glial cells, chemical mediators, and other non-neuronal components of nervous system are associated with neuronal hyperexcitability associated with persistent pain conditions.

   b. The few human studies available suggest elevated levels of proinflammatory cytokines and/or decreased levels of anti-inflammatory cytokines may be associated with enhanced pain states.

3. Sickle cell disease (SCD) and persistent pain

   a. Involves neuroimmune and neurovascular interactions

   b. Mechanisms by which different non-neuronal immunocompetent cells contribute to pain show overlap in common inflammatory mediators, leading to activation of pain pathway and inflammation.

   c. Mast cells are major contributor to biologic pathology in SCD and pain.

   d. Inhibition of mast cells has been beneficial in reducing pain associated with SCD.

   e. Further research needs to elucidate molecular and pro-nociceptive interactions.

4. CRPS is multi-mechanistic disease with pathology including neuroinflammation (inflammation occurring in CNS or PNS) and immune dysregulation that presents new therapeutic targets for symptomatic people.

5. Neuropathic pain

   a. Caused after lesion or disease of somatosensory nervous system occurs. When pain stimulus occurs, pain cycle begins.

      1) Cause of stimulus can be direct injury or damage due to neurotoxin.

      2) Pain signal is transmitted by afferent neurons to CNS.

3) During pain transmission, glial cells surrounding neurons are activated and generate oxygen radicals and proinflammatory cytokines.

4) Injured primary afferent nerves release ATP, chemokines, and other molecules that activate microglia via surface receptors.

5) Radicals and cytokines support modulation and amplification of pain signals transmitted by neurons.

b. New findings relevant to painful neuropathy include:

1) Significant impact T-cells have on development of neuropathic pain

2) Insights into role of natural killer cells. Degeneration of injured neurons by natural killer cells are mediated by ligand activating natural killer cell receptor, which is upregulated in DRG neurons.

3) Macrophages from one class promote sensitization, and a different class inhibit sensitization, promote healing, and are attributed to pathophysiology of neuropathic pain.

I. Sex differences, immune responses, and pain

1. Sex is one variable that influences innate and adaptive immune responses, and yet sex differences in mechanisms of pain perception are not well studied.

2. Evidence in preclinical animal studies suggests role of microglia in neuropathic pain is sex dependent.

a. Absence of microglial role in mediating neuropathic pain in female mice

b. Astrocyte cell morphology is different between male and female mice.

c. Animal model showed that spinal toll-like receptor 4 proteins (a transmembrane protein), expressed specifically on microglia in CNS, contribute to PNI-induced pain hypersensitivity in male mice but are not actually required for pain hypersensitivity in female mice.

3. Sex differences reported in circulating T-cell populations indicate females have higher cluster of differentiation 4 (CD4$^+$) counts, helper T-cell counts, and CD4:CD8 ratios than males, and males have higher natural killer cell frequencies than females.

J. Sickness response

1. Classic example of the importance of inflammatory mediators producing behavior is sickness response.

2. Inflammatory mediators (including cytokines and chemokines) contribute to brain function and behavior, have ability to affect neurotransmitter systems, and in turn alter behavior.

a. Afferent peripheral nerve immune-activated signaling to CNS provokes sickness response.

b. Release of proinflammatory cytokines by immune cells occurs in response to inflammation and trauma. These proinflammatory cytokines play a role in signaling brain to produce neurochemical, neuroendocrine, neuroimmune, and behavioral changes related to inflammation, triggering cascade of unpleasant activity-limiting symptoms. This "sickness behavior" is characterized by fever, malaise, fatigue, poor concentration, excessive sleep, decrease in appetite and libido, pain, and depression.

c. Release of inflammatory products within CNS during acute, time-limited immune challenge is beneficial, whereas in chronic immune activation, inflammatory mediators alter neuronal plasticity, transmission, and integrity and are not beneficial.

d. Hyperalgesia may be related to contributions from spinal microglia and astrocytes.

e. Most research implicates spinal glial activation and proinflammatory cytokines in enhanced pain. Conclusions are based on animal models of pain enhancement following intrathecal injection of proinflammatories, while knocking out IL-1 signaling and glial and cytokine inhibitors preventing and/or reversing those pain enhancements.

f. "Sickness response" and peripheral inflammation is well-described, with an abundance of evidence showing people with major depressive disorder exhibit immune system involvement and elevated levels of circulating proinflammatory cytokines. Proinflammatory cytokines participate in innate immune response and inflammation, metabolic and endocrine effects, and neural plasticity.

K. Drug misuse and substance use disorder (SUD)

1. Conjecture exists suggesting microglia and astrocytes have role in development and maintenance of SUD.

2. Neuroimmune mechanisms may contribute to opioid use disorder (OUD). Substances of abuse can activate microglia and astrocyte immune receptor signaling, which influences neuronal function and potentially directly affects remodeling of synapses.

3. It is postulated that glia can be directly influenced by certain compounds through interactions at surface receptors sensitive to compound or to neighboring neurons through microglia or astrocyte communication. In turn, glial responses potentially result in synaptic plasticity. Moreover, neurons serve as cells responsible for behavior, and glia serve supportive role; therefore, it is possible these neural-glial interactions also have a role in development and maintenance of SUD.

L. Epigenetic mechanisms involved in neuroimmune interaction
   1. Activated glial cells remaining in "primed" state undergo epigenetic changes that enhance their transcriptional processes.
   2. Increased likelihood of immune priming involves factors such as stress, aging, illness, injury, and opioid consumption, which in turn leads to transition from acute to persistent pain.
M. Impact of opioids on immune system
   1. Mounting evidence from opioid analgesic studies indicates exogenous opioid administration is associated with suppression of immune response and development of inflammatory mechanisms that enhance persistent pain.
   2. Immune cells (i.e., neutrophils, macrophages, and T-cells) secrete endogenous opioid peptides. In animal studies on neuropathy, injection of exogenous mu, kappa, and delta opioids can activate opioid receptors on leukocytes, which then release multiple endogenous opioid peptides at site of injection, inducing analgesia, by binding to peripheral opioid receptor sites.
   3. Evidence from different models, including preclinical, healthy volunteer, and surgical models suggests different opioids have variable impact on tumor progression through their inhibitory influence on immune surveillance mechanisms. However, data derived from cancer populations are inconclusive and cannot be used to make definitive recommendations.
   4. Immunosuppressive effect depends on type of opioid, with effect independent of potency or duration of action. Little relevant evidence in humans and growing yet incomplete evidence from animal studies indicate use of exogenous morphine, fentanyl, methadone, and codeine has strong immunosuppressive effect, while oxycodone, hydromorphone, and tramadol have weak effect, and smallest effect noted with buprenorphine.
   5. Studies suggest morphine induces immune suppression by directly regulating adaptive and innate immune cells, and indirectly regulating in CNS and HPA axis.
   6. Opioid-induced adrenal insufficiency (OIAI) is due to suppression of HPA communication from wide range of opioids, including fentanyl, oxycodone, tramadol, methadone, and heroin.
      a. Estimated prevalence of OIAI in people receiving long-term opioid therapy for analgesia ranges from 9% to 29%.
      b. Risk factors for developing OIAI are currently unknown, and time of onset varies.
      c. Time to recovery or lowest dose at which HPA axis recovers is currently unknown.
      d. Current approaches to OIAI include careful consideration of possibility in people who exhibit signs and symptoms of adrenal insufficiency.
      e. FDA safety statement in "Warnings and Precautions" section about adrenal insufficiency on all opioid labels suggests:
         1) Providers should perform diagnostic testing when adrenal insufficiency is suspected.
         2) Treat with corticosteroids when adrenal insufficiency is confirmed.
         3) Consider opioid taper or cessation if appropriate.
         4) If opioid can be discontinued, follow-up assessment of adrenal function should be performed to determine if corticosteroids can be discontinued.
   7. Use of high-dose and long-term opioid therapy for nonmalignant persistent pain correlates to higher susceptibility to infection, and opioids have influence on development of carcinogenesis. However, further studies are needed to determine importance and clinical relevance in humans. Despite uncertainty regarding effects of exogenous opioids on immune function, adequate cancer-related pain control remains an important consideration; therefore, use of opioids continues to be recommended
   8. Growing evidence for the role of opioids in development of hyperalgesia, tolerance, and dependence
      a. Evidence exists implicating opioids as activators of CNS resident glial cells (i.e., microglia and astrocytes), which leads to production and release of proinflammatory cytokines that promote neuroimmune activation and can sensitize central terminals of primary afferent and second-order neurons. This in turn results in overall increase in neuroexcitability.
      b. Repeated morphine administration has been shown to result in increased glial release of cytokines, making these excitatory substances key players in development of opioid tolerance and opioid-induced pain sensitivity.
   9. Immune mechanism involvement in opioid hyperalgesia and tolerance
      a. Well-established research exists in terms of midbrain ventrolateral pariaquedcutal gray being primary substrate for analgesic effects of morphine and development of morphine tolerance. Limited research exists as to glial activation role in facilitation of pain transmission and opposition to morphine analgesia.
      b. Growing evidence indicates that glia regulate morphine analgesia, tolerance, and dependence/withdrawal. Glia may also contribute to morphine reward system.

c. Growing evidence in animal models indicates opioids activate astrocytes, microglia, and glial cell activity at spinal cord level, which induces proinflammatory cytokines, enhancing neuro-excitability; however, little is known about ventrolateral pariaquedcutal gray glia.

d. Additionally, TLR4 (class of innate immune receptors) may be integral component of tolerance, with its underlying role in opioid-induced CNS glial activation.

10. Bidirectional communication between opioids and central neuroimmune signaling has been identified during in vitro studies, and evidence exists that naloxone and naltrexone inhibit TLR-4 signaling.

N. Neuroimmunopharmacology: therapeutic opportunities in pain management

1. Research in bidirectional communication between immune and nervous systems suggests pain might be relieved by targeting immune system.

2. Research in animal models has established role of neuroimmune signaling in development of neuropathic pain. It is postulated blockade of proinflammatory signaling could be an effective way to suppress central sensitization and alleviate persistent pain.

3. Human imaging studies are consistent with research findings and evidence of glial activation in brains of people who are experiencing persistent pain.

4. Animal studies with glial modulating compounds, such as fluorocitrate, minocycline, propentofylline, and ibudilast (an anti-inflammatory medication used in Japan; development code, AV-411), formed strong foundation of preclinical data supporting role of glia in several pathologic pain models and for potential therapeutic strategies in treatment of persistent pain in humans.

a. While preclinical trials were promising for minocycline effectiveness in reducing allodynia and hyperalgesia, it has shown little efficacy in pain amelioration in humans. This may be related to its pharmacokinetics and limited sensitivity to the drug, yet it is more likely that potential benefit is limited by the drug's effect on nonmicroglial targets that may counteract its analgesic properties.

b. Propentofylline also with promising preclinical data has shown little benefit for pain in people with postherpetic neuralgia, with proposed explanation of rat-to-human species difference in microglial activation.

c. Pharmacologic agents, such as ibudilast and cannabinoids, show promise as analgesics for people with neuropathic pain, although studies are still in preliminary stages.

5. Traditional Chinese мedicine: Sinomenine is an analgesic agent purified from roots of the plant *Sinomenium acutum.*

a. Widely used for treatment of rheumatoid arthritis in China but not approved in the United States

b. Active substance has anti-inflammatory and anti-hyperalgesic properties.

6. Use of local anesthetics or spinal NMDA receptor blockers following peripheral nerve injury attenuates some microglia and astrocyte response in animal models.

a. Beneficial effects on pain and cytokine production were seen with preemptive epidural analgesia containing local anesthetics.

b. Lidocaine has anti-inflammatory properties demonstrated through decreased upregulation of proinflammatories and increased secretion of anti-inflammatory cytokine IL-1 receptor antagonist.

7. Other pharmacological therapies being explored due to effect on neuroimmune interaction include such currently available medications as amitriptyline, ceftriaxone, methotrexate, and rifampin.

8. Enhanced production of endogenous IL-10 using gene therapy has been shown to produce long-term pain relief in neuropathic pain in clinically relevant animal models.

9. Potential use of soluble anti–TNF-blocking formulation as adjuvant tool accompanying opioid therapy to act as countermeasure to opioid-induced neuroinflammation and changes to glutamatergic signaling in spinal cord shown to accompany development of morphine tolerance.

10. PNI in mice and rats causes microglial activation in spinal cord and long-lasting pain hypersensitivity in ipsilateral hind paw. Pharmacological blockage or genetic manipulation of these molecules substantially decreases excitability of dorsal horn pain pathway, leading to suppression of pain hypersensitivity.

11. Clinical trials

a. Anti-TNF drugs such as infliximab and etanercept have been associated with successful treatment of pain in Crohn's disease, depressive bipolar disorder, rheumatoid arthritis, and CRPS. However, TNF antagonist as monotherapy did *not* show benefit in treatment of low back pain related to intervertebral disc degeneration.

b. Strategies targeting specific chemokines or chemokine receptors involved in neuron-to-glial interactions may offer new therapeutic potential for management of neuropathic and persistent pain.

c. Pharmacological, interventional, and nonpharmacological therapies aimed at targeting proinflammatory mediators contributing to both acute and persistent pain by providing acute pain relief and promoting pain resolution

1) In small study, interventional approaches using targeted, selective pulsed radiofrequency treatment to DRG for people with lumbosacral radicular pain were associated with reduced pain intensity and improved function in 9 of 10 patients.

2) It was also associated with altered lymphocyte populations and inflammatory cytokine levels in treatment responders' cerebrospinal fluid at 3 months posttreatment.

O. Implications for pain management nursing

1. Addressing and targeting mechanisms of pain transmission, including the immune system, allows clinicians opportunity to use multimodal analgesia to provide efficacious pain management and diminish side effects.

2. Knowledge that pain is immunosuppressive with potentially significant consequences if undertreated, especially in immunocompromised individuals and people with metastatic disease, makes it imperative pain management nurses and other healthcare professionals incorporate appropriate preemptive and multimodal pain management strategies.

3. Understanding neuroimmune communication and role of immune system in contributing to neuropathic pain may expose potential targets and analgesic treatment approaches.

Bibliography

Aich, A., Jones, M. K., & Gupta, K. (2019). Pain and sickle cell disease. *Current Opinion in Hematology, 26*(3), 131–138. https://doi.org/10.1097/MOH.0000000000000491.

Albrecht, D. S., Ahmed, S. U., Kettner, N. W., Borra, R. J. H., Cohen-Adad, J., Deng, H., et al. (2018). Neuroinflammation of the spinal cord and nerve roots in chronic radicular pain patients. *Pain, 159*(5), 968–977. https://doi.org/10.1097/j.pain.0000000000001171.

Allen, N. J., & Eroglu, C. (2017). Cell biology of astrocyte-synapse interactions. *Neuron, 96*(3), 697–708. https://doi.org/10.1016/j.neuron.2017.09.056.

Anand, P., Dickenson, A., Finco, G., Marinangeli, F., Polati, E., Romualdi, P., et al. (2019). Novel insights on the management of pain: highlights from the 'Science of Relief' meeting. *Pain management, 9*(6), 521–533. https://doi.org/10.2217/pmt-2019-0031.

Apkarian, A. V., Mutso, A. A., Centeno, M. V., Kan, L., Wu, M., Levinstein, M., et al. (2016). Role of adult hippocampal neurogenesis in persistent pain. *Pain, 157*(2), 418–428. https://doi.org/10.1097/j.pain.0000000000000332.

Baral, P., Udit, S., & Chiu, I. M. (2019). Pain and immunity: Implications for host defence. *Nature Reviews Immunology, 19*(7), 443–447. https://doi.org/10.1038/s41577-019-0147-2.

Bharwani, K. D., Dik, W. A., Dirck, M., & Huygen, F. J. P. M. (2019). Highlighting the Role of Biomarkers of Inflammation in the Diagnosis and Management of Complex Regional Pain Syndrome. *Molecular Diagnosis & Therapy, 23*(5), 615–626. https://doi.org/10.1007/s40291-019-00417-x.

Bannister, K., & Dickenson, A. H. (2017). The plasticity of descending controls in pain: translational probing. *The Journal of physiology, 595*(13), 4159–4166. https://doi.org/10.1113/JP274165.

Blanchet, P. J., & Brefel-Courbon, C. (2018). Chronic pain and pain processing in Parkinson's disease. *Progress in Neuro-Psychopharmacology and Biological Psychiatry, 87*, 200–206. https://doi.org/10.1016/j.pnpbp.2017.10.010.

Boogaard, S., Heymans, M. W., de Vet, H. C., Peters, M. L., Loer, S. A., Zuurmond, W. W., et al. (2015). Predictors of Persistent Neuropathic Pain–A Systematic Review. *Pain Physician, 18*(5), 433–457. https://doi.org/10.36076/ppj.2015/18/433.

Bosma, R. L., Ameli Mojarad, E., Leung, L., Pukall, C., Staud, R., & Stroman, P. W. (2015). Neural correlates of temporal summation of second pain in the human brainstem and spinal cord. *Human Brain Mapping, 36*(12), 5038–5050. https://doi.org/10.1002/hbm.22993.

Burmeister, A. R., Johnson, M. B., Chauhan, V. S., Moerdyk-Schauwecker, M. J., Young, A. D., Cooley, I. D., et al. (2017). Human microglia and astrocytes constitutively express the neurokinin-1 receptor and functionally respond to substance P. *Journal of Neuroinflammation, 14*(1), 245. https://doi.org/10.1186/s12974-017-1012-5.

Burston, J. J., Valdes, A. M., Woodhams, S. G., Mapp, P. I., Stocks, J., Watson, D. J. G., et al. (2019). The impact of anxiety on chronic musculoskeletal pain and the role of astrocyte activation. *Pain, 160*(3), 658–669. https://doi.org/10.1097/j.pain.0000000000001445.

Chen, G., Zhang, Y-Q., Qadri, Y. J., Serhan, C. N., & Ji, R-R. (2018). Microglia in pain: Detrimental and protective roles in pathogensis and resolution of pain. *Neuron, 100*(6), 1292–1311. https://doi.org/10.1016/j.neuron.2018.11.009.

Chen, O., Donnelly, C. R., & Ji, R. R. (2019). Regulation of pain by neuro-immune interactions between macrophages and nociceptor sensory neurons. *Current Opinion Neurobiology, 62*, 17–25. https://doi.org/10.1016/j.conb.2019.11.006.

Chiechio, S. (2016). Modulation of chronic pain by metabotropic glutamate receptors. *Advanced Pharmacology, 75*, 63–89. https://doi.org/10.1016/bs.apha.2015.11.001.

Chou, R., Gordon, D. B., de Leon-Casasola, O. A., Rosenberg, J. M., Bickler, S., Brennan, T., et al. (2016). Management of Postoperative Pain: A Clinical Practice Guideline From the American Pain Society, the American Society of Regional Anesthesia and Pain Medicine, and the American Society of Anesthesiologists' Committee on Regional Anesthesia, Executive Committee, and Administrative Council. *The journal of pain, 17*(2), 131–157. https://doi.org/10.1016/j.jpain.2015.12.008.

Cooper, A. H., Brightwell, J. J., Hedden, N. S., & Taylor, B. K. (2018). The left central nucleus of the amygdala contributes to mechanical allodynia and hyperalgesia following right-sided peripheral nerve injury. *Neuroscience letters, 684*, 187–192. https://doi.org/10.1016/j.neulet.2018.08.013.

Coraggio, V., Guida, F., Boccella, S., Scafuro, M., Paino, S., Romano, D., Maione, S., & Luongo, L. (2018). Neuroimmune-driven neuropathic pain establishment: A focus on gender differences. *International Journal of Molecular Sciences, 19*(1), 281. https://doi.org/10.3390/ijms19010281.

Das, B., Conroy, M., Moore, D., Lysaght, J., & McCrory, C. (2018). Human dorsal root ganglion pulsed radiofrequency treatment modulates cerebrospinal fluid lymphocytes and neuroinflammatory markers in chronic radicular pain. *Brain Behavior and Immunity, 70,* 157–165. https://doi.org/10.1016/j.bbi.2018.02.010.

Defaye, M., Gervason, S., Altier, C, Berthon, J. Y., Ardidi, D., Filaire, E., & Carvalho, F. A. (2020). Microbiota: a novel regulator of pain. *Journal of Neural Transmission, 127*(4), 445–465. https://doi.org/10.1007/s00702-019-02083-z.

DeMarco, G. J., & Nunamaker, E. A. (2019). A review of the effects of pain and analgesia on immune system function and inflammation: Relevance for preclinical studies. *Comparative Medicine, 69*(6), 520–534. https://doi.org/10.30802/AALAS-CM-19-000041.

Devor, M. (2018). Rethinking the causes of pain in herpes zoster and postherpetic neuralgia: the ectopic pacemaker hypothesis. *Pain reports, 3*(6), 1–9. https://doi.org/10.1097/PR9.0000000000000702.

Djouhri, L. (2016). Aδ-fiber low threshold mechanoreceptors innervating mammalian hairy skin: A review of their receptive, electrophysiological and cytochemical properties in relation to Aδ-fiber high threshold mechanoreceptors. *Neurosci Biobehav Rev, 61,* 225–238. https://doi.org/10.1016/j.neubiorev.2015.12.009.

Dodds, K. N., Beckett, E. A. H., Evans, S. F., Grace, P. M., Watkins, L. R., & Hutchinson, M. R. (2016). Glial contributions to visceral pain: implications for disease etiology and the female predominance of persistent pain. *Translational Psychiatry, 6*(9), e888. https://doi.org/10.1038/tp.2016.168.

Donegan, D., & Bancos, I. (2018). Opioid-induced adrenal insufficiency. *Mayo Proceedings, 93*(7), 937–944. https://doi.org/10.1016/j.mayocp.2018.04.010.

Domoto, R., Sekiguchi, F., Tsubota, M., & Kawabata, A. (2021). Macrophage as a Peripheral Pain Regulator. *Cells, 10*(8), 1881. https://doi.org/10.3390/cells10081881.

Donnelly, C. R., Andriessen, A. S., Chen, G., Wang, K., Jiang, C., Maixner, W., & Ji, R-R. (2020). Central nervous system targets: Glial cell mechanisms in chronic pain. *Neurotherapeutics, 17,* 846–860. https://doi.org/10.1007/s13311-020-00905-7.

dos Santos, G. G., Delay, L., Yaksh, T. L., & Corr, M. (2020). Neuraxial cytokines in pain states. *Frontiers, 10*(3061), 1–17. https://doi.org/10.3389/fimmu.2019.03061.

Duque, L., & Fricchione, G. (2019). Fibromyalgia and its new lessons for neuropsychiatry. *Medical Science: Monitor Basic Research, 25,* 169–178. https://doi.org/10.12659/MSMBR.915962.

Eidson, L. N., & Murphy, A. Z. (2019). Inflammatory mediators of opioid tolerance: Implications for dependency and addiction. *Peptides, 115,* 51–58. https://doi.org/10.1016/j.peptides.2019.01.003.

Feldman, E. L., Nave, K. A., Jensen, T. S., & Bennett, D. L. H. (2017). New horizons in diabetic neuropathy: Mechanisms, bioenergetics, and pain. *Neuron, 93*(6), 1296–1313. https://doi.org/10.1016/j.neuron.2017.02.005.

Finnerup, N. B., Kuner, R., & Jensen, T. S. (2021). Neuropathic pain: From mechanisms to treatment. *Physiological Review, 101*(1), 259–301. https://doi.org/10.1152/physrev.00045.2019.

Freynhagen, R., Rey, R., & Argoff, C. (2020). When to consider "mixed pain"? The right questions can make a difference! *Current Medical Research and Opinion, 36*(12), 2037–2046. https://doi.org/10.1080/03007995.2020.1832058.

Ghelardini, C., Di Cesare Mannelli, L., & Bianchi, E. (2015). The pharmacological basis of opioids. *Clin Cases Miner Bone Metab, 12*(3), 9–21. https://doi.org/10.11138/ccmbm/2015.12.3.219.

Grace, P. M., Hutchinson, M. R., Maier, S. F., & Watkins, L. R. (2014). Pathological pain and neuroimmune interface. *Nature Review Immunology, 14*(4), 217–231. https://doi.org/10.1038/nri3621.

Grace, P. M., Tawfik, V. L., Svensson, C. I., Burton, M. D., Loggia, M. L., & Hutchinson, M. R. (2021). The neuroimmunology of chronic pain: from rodents to humans. *Journal of Neuroscience, 41*(5), 855–865. https://doi.org/10.1523/JNEUROSCI.1650-20.2020.

González-Roldán, A. M., Terrasa, J. L., Sitges, C., van der Meulen, M., Anton, F., & Montoya, P. (2020). Age-related changes in pain perception are associated with altered functional connectivity during resting state. *Frontiers in aging neuroscience, 12,* 116. https://doi.org/10.3389/fnagi.2020.00116.

Grossberg, S., Palma, J., & Versace, M. (2016). Resonant Cholinergic Dynamics in Cognitive and Motor Decision-Making: Attention, Category Learning, and Choice in Neocortex, Superior Colliculus, and Optic Tectum. *Frontiers in neuroscience, 9,* 501. https://doi.org/10.3389/fnins.2015.00501.

Goubert, D., Danneels, L., Graven-Nielsen, T., Descheemaeker, F., Coppieters, I., & Meeus, M. (2017). Differences in pain processing between patients with chronic low back pain, recurrent low back pain and fibromyalgia. *Pain physician, 20*(4), 307–318. https://doi.org/10.36076/ppj.2017.318.

Gu, N., Peng, J., Murugan, M., Wang, X., Evo, U. P., Sun, D., et al. (2016). Spinal microgliosis due to resident microglial proliferation is required for pain sensitivity after peripheral nerve injury. *Cell Reports, 32*(5), 605–614. http://dx.doi.org/10.1016/j.celrep.2016.06.018.

Guan, Z., Kuhn, J. A., Wang, X., Colquitt, B., Solorzano, C., Vaman, S., et al. (2016). Injured sensory neuron-derived CSF1 induces microglial proliferation and DAP12-dependent pain. *Nature Neuroscience, 19,* 94–101. https://doi.org/10.1038/nn.4189.

Gulur, P., & Nelli, A. (2019). Persistent postoperative pain: Mechanisms and modulators. *Current Opinion in Anaesthesiolology, 32*(5), 668–673. https://doi.org/10.1097/ACO.0000000000000770.

Hanani, M., & Spray, D. C. (2020). Emerging importance of satellite glia in nervous system function and dysfunction. *Nature Reviews Neuroscience, 21*(9), 485–498. https://doi.org/10.1038/s41583-020-0333-z.

Harte, S. E., Harris, R. E., & Clauw, D. J. (2018). The neurobiology of central sensitization. *Journal of Applied Biobehavioral Research, 23*(2), e12137. https://doi.org/10.1111/jabr.12137.

Hore, Z., & Denk, F. (2019). Neuroimmune interactions in chronic pain–an interdisciplinary perspective. *Brain, behavior, and immunity, 79,* 56–62. https://doi.org/10.1016/j.bbi.2019.04.033.

Hu, Z., Deng, N., Liu, K., Zhou, N., Sun, Y., & Zeng, W. (2020). CNTF-STAT3-IL-6 Axis mediates neuroinflammatory cascade across Schwann cell-neuron-microglia. *Cell reports, 31*(7), 107657. https://doi.org/10.1016/j.celrep.2020.107657.

Hua, S. (2016). Neuroimmune interaction in the regulation of peripheral opioid-mediated analgesia in inflammation. *Frontiers in Immunology, 7*, 293. https://doi.org/10.3389/fimmu.2016.00293.

Ignatavicius, D. D., & Workman, M. L. (2016). *Assessment and care of patients with pain*. In *Medical-surgical nursing: patient-centered collaborative care* (8th edition pp. 24–49). St Louis, MO: Elsevier.

Inoue, K. A. (2018). State-of-the-art perspective on microgliopathic pain. *Open Biology, 8*(11), 180154. https://doi.org/10.1098/rsob.180154.

Irvine, K. A., & Clark, J. D. (2018). Chronic pain after traumatic brain injury: pathophysiology and pain mechanisms. *Pain medicine, 19*(7), 1315–1333. https://doi.org/10.1093/pm/pnx153.

Jain, A., Hakim, S., & Woolf, C. J. (2020). Unraveling the plastic peripheral neuroimmune interactome. *The Journal of Immunology, 204*(2), 257–263. https://doi.org/10.4049/jimmunol.1900818.

Jha, M. K., Jo, M., Kim, J. H., & Suk, K. (2019). Microglia-astrocyte crosstalk: An intimate molecular conversation. *Neuroscientist, 25*(3), 227–240. https://doi.org/10.1177/1073858418783959.

Ji, R. R., Chamessian, A., & Zhang, Y. Q. (2016). Pain regulation by non-neuronal cells and inflammation. *Science, 354*(6312), 572–577. https://doi.org/10.1126/science.aaf8924.

Ji, R. R., Nackley, A., Huh, Y., Terrando, N., & Maixner, W. (2018). Neuroinflammation and central sensitization in chronic and widespread pain. *Anesthesiology, 129*(2), 343–366. https://doi.org/10.1097/ALN.0000000000002130.

Ji, R. R., Donnelly, C. R., & Nedergaard, M. (2019). Astrocytes in chronic pain and itch. *Nature Review Neuroscience, 20*(11), 667–685. https://doi.org/10.1038/s41583-019-0218.

Jiang, B. C., Liu, T., & Gao, Y. J. (2020). Chemokines in chronic pain: Cellular and molecular mechanisms and therapeutic potential. *Pharmacology & Therapeutics, 212*, 107581. https://doi.org/10.1016/j.pharmthera.2020.107581.

Kim, H. J., Greenspan, J. D., Ohrbach, R., Fillingim, R. B., Maixner, W., Renn, C. L., et al. (2019). Racial/ethnic differences in experimental pain sensitivity and associated factors—Cardiovascular responsiveness and psychologicalstatus. *PloS one, 14*(4), e0215534. https://doi.org/10.1371/journal.pone.0215534.

Klein, S., & Flanagan, K. L. (2016). Sex differences in immune response. *Nature Review Immunology, 16*(10), 626–638. https://doi.org/10.1038/nri.2016.90.

Lacagnina, M. J., Riveria, P. D., & Bilbo, S. (2017). Glial and neuroimmune mechanisms as critical modulators of drug use and abuse. *Neuropsychopharmacology, 42*(1), 156–177. https://doi.org/10.1038/npp.2016.121.

Lacagnina, M. J., Watkins, L. R., & Grace, P. M. (2018). Toll-like receptors and their role in persistent pain. *Pharmacology & Therapeutics, 184*, 145–158. https://doi.org/10.1016/j.pharmthera.2017.10.006.

Laedermann, C. J., Abriel, H., & Decosterd, I. (2015). Post-translational modifications of voltage-gated sodium channels in chronic pain syndromes. *Frontiers in pharmacology, 6*, 263. https://doi.org/10.3389/fphar.2015.00263.

Laumet, G., Ma, J., Robison, A. J., Kumari, S., Heijnen, C. J., & Kavelaars, A. (2019). T cells as an emerging target for chronic pain therapy. *Frontiers in Molecular Neuroscience, 12*, 216. https://doi.org/10.3389/fnmol.2019.00216.

Lee, G. I., & Neumeister, M. W. (2020). Pain: pathways and physiology. *Clinics in plastic surgery, 47*(2), 173–180. https://doi.org/10.1016/j.cps.2019.11.001.

Lee, S., Shi, X. Q., Fan, A., West, B., & Zhang, J. (2018). Targeting macrophage and microglia activation with colony stimulating factor 1 receptor inhibitor is an effective strategy to treat injury-triggered neuropathic pain. *Molecular Pain, 14*, 1744806918764979. https://https://doi.org/10.1177/1744806918764979.

Lenert, M. E., Avona, A., Garner, K. M., Barron, L. R., & Burton, M. D. (2021). Sensoryneurons, neuroimmunity, and pain modulation by sex hormones. *Endocrinology, 162*(8), 1–17. https://doi.org/10.1210/endocr/bqab109.

Liddelow, S. A., & Barres, B. A. (2017). Reactive astrocytes: Production, function, and therapeutic potential. *Immunity, 46*(6), 957–967. https://doi.org/10.1016/j.immuni.2017.06.006.

Lim, J. S. Y., & Kam, P. C. A. (2020). Neuroimmune mechanisms of pain: Basic science and potential therapeutic modulators. *Anaesthesia and Intensive Care, 48*(3), 167–178. https://doi.org/10.1177/0310057X20902774.

Lolignier, S., Eijkelkamp, N., & Wood, J. N. (2015). Mechanical allodynia. *Pflugers Archiv: European journal of physiology, 467*(1), 133–139. https://doi.org/10.1007/s00424-014-1532-0.

Malcangio, M. (2019). Role of the immune system in neuropathic pain. *Scandinavian Journal of Pain, 20*(1), 33–37. https://doi.org/10.1515/sjpain-2019-0138. PMID: 31730538.

Mahan, M. A., Yeoh, S., Monson, K., & Light, A. (2019). Rapid stretch injury to peripheral nerves: biomechanical results. *Neurosurgery, 85*(1), E137–E144. https://doi.org/10.1093/neuros/nyy423.

Mappleback, J. C. S., Beggs, S., & Salter, M. W. (2017). Molecules in pain and sex: A developing story. *Molecular Brain, 10*(9), 1–8. https://doi.org/10.1186/s13041-017-0289-8.

Masuda, T., Tsuda, M., & Inoue, K. (2016). Transcriptional regulation in microglia and neuropathic pain. *Pain Management, 6*(2). Editorial. https://doi.org/10.2217/pmt.15.34.

McGill University. (2016, January 28). *Chronic pain changes our immune systems: Epigenetics may bring us a step closer to better treatments for chronic pain*. ScienceDaily. www.sciencedaily.com/releases/2016/01/160128074319.htm.

McMahon, S. B., La Russa, F., & Bennett, D. L. (2015). Crosstalk between the nociceptive and immune systems in host defence and disease. *Nature reviews Neuroscience, 16*(7), 389–402. https://doi.org/10.1038/nrn3946.

Meints, S. M., Cortes, A., Morais, C. A., & Edwards, R. R. (2019). Racial and ethnic differences in the experience and treatment of noncancer pain. *Pain Management, 9*(3), 317–334. https://doi.org/10.2217/pmt-2018-0030.

Miladinovic, T., Nashed, M. G., & Singh, G. (2015). Overview of Glutamatergic Dysregulation in Central Pathologies. *Biomolecules, 5*(4), 3112–3141. https://doi.org/10.3390/biom5043112.

Morales-Soto, W., & Gulbransen, B. D. (2019). Enteric glia: A new player in abdominal pain. *Cellular and Molecular Gastroenterology and Hepatology, 7*(2), 433–445. https://doi.org/10.1016/j.jcmgh.2018.11.005.

Nazıroğlu, M., & Braidy, N. (2017). Thermo-Sensitive TRP Channels: Novel Targets for Treating Chemotherapy-Induced Peripheral Pain. *Frontiers in physiology, 8*, 1040. https://doi.org/10.3389/fphys.2017.01040.

Nijs, J., George, S. Z., Clauw, D. J., Fernández-de-las-Peñas, C., Kosek, E., Ickmans, K., et al. (2021). Central sensitisation in chronic pain conditions: Latest discoveries and their potential for precision medicine. *The Lancet Rheumatology, 3*(5). https://doi.org/10.1016/s2665-9913(21)00032-1.

Petralla, S., De Chirico, F., Miti, A., Tartagni, O., Massenzio, F., Poeta, E., Virgili, M., Zuccheri, G., & Monti, B. (2021). Epigenetics and communication mechanisms in microglia activation with a view on technological approaches. *Biomolecules, 11*(2), 306. https://doi.org/10.3390/biom11020306.

Pinho-Ribeiro, F. A., Verri, W. A., Jr., & Chiu, I. M. (2017). Nociceptor sensory neuron-immune interactions in pain and inflammation. *Trends in Immunology, 38*(1), 5–19. https://doi.org/10.1016/j.it.2016.10.001.

Plein, L. M., & Rittner, H. L. (2018). Opioids and the immune system – friend or foe. *British Journal of Pharmacology, 175*(14), 2717–2725. https://doi.org/10.1111/bph.13750.

Rabin, A., Shmushkevich, Y., & Kalichman, L. (2019). Initial pain and disability characteristics can assist the prediction of the centralization phenomenon on initial assessment of patients with low back pain. *The Journal of manual & manipulative therapy, 27*(2), 66–72. https://doi.org/10.1080/10669817.2018.1542560.

Rajkumar, R., Kumar, J. R., & Dawe, G. S. (2017). Priming locus coeruleus noradrenergic modulation of medial perforant path-dentate gyrus synaptic plasticity. *Neurobiology of learning and memory, 138*, 215–225. https://doi.org/10.1016/j.nlm.2016.07.003.

Rea, P. (2015). *Spinal Tracts–Ascending/Sensory Pathways*. In *Essential Clinical Anatomy of the Nervous System* (pp. 133–160). Philladelphia: Elsevier.

Roeckel, L. A., Le Coz, G. M., Gavériaux-Ruff, C., & Simonin, F. (2016). Opioid-induced hyperalgesia: cellular and molecular mechanisms. *Neuroscience, 338*, 160–182. https://doi.org/10.1016/j.neuroscience.2016.06.029.

Royds, J., & McCrory, C. (2018). Neuroimmunity and chronic pain. *British Journal of Anesthesia, 18*(12), 377–383. https://doi.org/10.1016/bjae.2018.09.003.

Sagi, V., Mittal, A., Gupta, M., & Gupta, K. (2019). Immune cell neural interactions and their contributions to sickle cell disease. *Neuroscience Letters, 699*(23), 167–171. https://doi.org/10.1016/j.neulet.2019.02.008.

Sawicki, C. M., Humeidan, M. L., & Sheridan, J. F. (2021). Neuroimmune interactions in pain and stress: an interdisciplinary approach. *The Neuroscientist, 27*(2), 113–128. https://doi.org/10.1177/1073858420914747.

Sawicki, C. M., Kim, J. K., Weber, M. D., Jarrett, B. L., Godbout, J. P., Sheridan, J. F., et al. (2018). Ropivacaine and Bupivacaine prevent increased pain sensitivity without altering neuroimmune activation following repeated social defeat stress. *Brain, Behavior, and Immunity, 27*(2), 113–123. https://doi.org/10.1177/1073858420914747.

Si, H. B., Yang, T. M., Zeng, Y., Zhou, Z. K., Pei, F. X., Lu, Y. R., et al. (2017). Correlations between inflammatory cytokines, muscle damage markers and acute postoperative pain following primary total knee arthroplasty. *BMC musculoskeletal disorders, 18*(1), 1–9. https://doi.org/10.1186/s12891-017-1597-y.

Silva, C. E. A., Guimaraes, R. M., & Cunha, T. M. (2021). Sensory neuron-associated macrophages as novel modulators of neuropathic pain. *Pain Report, 6*(1), e873. https://doi.org/10.1097/PR9.0000000000000873.

Sofroniew, M. V. (2015). Astrocyte barriers to neurotoxic inflammation. *Nature Review Neuroscience, 16*(5), 249–263. https://doi.org/10.1038/nrn3898.

Sorge, R. E., Mapplebeck, J. C. S., Rosen, S., Beggs, S., Taves, S., Alexander, J. K., et al. (2015). Different immune cells mediate mechanical pain hypersensitivity in male and female mice. *Natural Neuroscience, 18*(8), 1081–1083. https://doi.org/10.1038/nn.4053.

Totsch, S. K., & Sorge, R. E. (2017). Immune system involvement in specific pain conditions. *Molecular Pain, 13*, 1–17. https://doi.org/10.1177/1744806917724559.

Tsuda, M. (2018). Modulation of pain and itch by spinal glia. *Neuroscience Bulletin, 34*(1), 178–185. https://doi.org/10.1007/s12264-017-0129-y.

Treede, R. D. (2016). Gain control mechanisms in the nociceptive system. *Pain, 157*(6), 1199–1204. https://doi.org/10.1097/j.pain.0000000000000499.

United States Food and Drug Administration (FDA). (2016). FDA Drug Safety Communication: FDA warns about several safety issues with opioid pain medicines; requires label changes. https://www.fda.gov/drugs/drug-safety-and-availability/fda-drug-safety-communication-fda-warns-about-several-safety-issues-opioid-pain-medicines-requires.

van den Broeke, E. N., Lenoir, C., & Mouraux, A. (2016). Secondary hyperalgesia is mediated by heat-insensitive A-fibre nociceptors. *The Journal of physiology, 594*(22), 6767–6776. https://doi.org/10.1113/JP272599.

Wang, C., Yu, X., Yan, Y., Yang, W., Zhang, S., Xiang, Y., Zhang, J., & Wang, W. (2017). Tumor necrosis factor-α: a key contributor to intervertebral disc degeneration. *Acta Biochimica et Biophysica Sinica, 49*(1), 1–13. https://doi.org/10.1093/abbs/gmw112.

Willis, W. D. (2019). *Anatomy, Physiology, and Descending Control of Lumbosacral Sensory Neurons Involved in Tactile and Pain Sensations*. In *Handbook of Behavioral State Control* (pp. 463–485). CRC Press.

Xu, M., Bennett, D. L. H., Querol, L. A., Wu, L. J., Irani, S. R., Watson, J. C., Pittock, S. J., & Klein, C. J. (2018). Pain and the immune system: emerging concepts of IgG-mediated autoimmune pain and immunotherapies. *Journal of Neurology Neurosurgery and Psychiatry, 91*(2), 177–188. https://doi.org/10.1136/jnnp-2018-318556.

Zhang, Z.-J., Jiang, G.-C., & Gao, Y-J. (2017). Chemokine in neuron glial cell interaction and pathogenesis of neuropathic pain. *Cellular and Molecular Life Sciences, 74*(18), 3275–3291. https://doi.org/10.1007/s00018-017-2513-1.

CHAPTER 2

Current Pain Theories: How We Arrived Here

Melanie H. Simpson, PhD, MSN, PMGT-BC, OCN
Sharon Wrona, DNP, PMGT-BC, CPNP-PC, PMHS, AP-PMN, FAAN*

Introduction

Pain is truly a complex, dynamic, and unique individual experience. Early pain theories focused on locating the cause of pain. Later, when surgical interventions failed to control pain, other explanations were explored. Identifying the distinction between contributors to and causes of pain led to a more comprehensive approach to treatment. The interaction between pain practice and research has advanced our understanding of and ability to manage pain. Current pain theories explain pain as a physical, psychological, social, cognitive, affective, and behavioral experience. Nursing interventions must be individualized and multidimensional to capture these aspects of pain for each individual.

I. Overview

A. Theories of pain, like all science, evolve because of new facts, which then require a new theory to incorporate them.
  1. Theoretical frameworks have been proposed to explain the physiological concept of pain, but due to the complexity of pain, the brain, and pain generators, none has completely accounted for all aspects of pain perception.
  2. Main debate among earlier theories was whether pain was mediated by a specific, hardwired pathway or by a nonspecific pathway in the nervous system.
B. Although many pain theories are credited to specific individuals at specific times, the majority continued to change and evolve over numerous years, with major contributions from a variety of scientists.
C. Important to understand evolution of pain theories over the years in order to understand the therapies we currently use to treat pain or those that are being researched for future use.

---

*Section Editor for the chapter.

II. History of Select Pain Theories

A. Cartesian Dualistic Theory by Reneé Descartes in 1644
  1. Hypothesized pain was mutually exclusive phenomenon whereby pain could result from physical or psychological injury (separation of mind and body); however, they did not influence each other.
  2. At that time, religious beliefs influenced people's thoughts and actions.
    a. People believed pain was punishment for committing immoral acts or wrongdoing.
    b. People also believed enduring pain/suffering was a way to repent for their sins.
    c. Descartes incorporated the notion that pain has a connection to the soul to appease the Church.
  3. Cartesian Dualistic Theory:
    a. One of the first pain theories to describe somatosensory pathway in humans and stated the soul of pain was in the pineal gland, thus identifying the brain as moderator of painful sensations
    b. Credited with famous hypothetical drawing that illustrated transmission of pain (e.g., "foot in the fire") via peripheral nerves and spinal cord to ventricles of brain and pineal gland, where conscious perception of painful stimulus was perceived
    c. Provided a new and strong foundation on which future researchers could build
  4. Evidence gap of Cartesian Dualistic Theory: does not explain why two individuals with similar injuries do not have the same pain experience
B. Specificity Theory by Charles Bell in 1811
  1. Identified as one of the first modern theories of pain and considered one of the most influential
  2. Similar to Cartesian Dualistic Theory because it delineated different types of sensations to dedicated pain pathways

3. Suggests brain was much more complex and integral part of pain perception than previously believed
4. Over the next century and a half, many scientists and philosophers continued to study the intricate anatomy and physiology of pain and contributed to the foundation of Specificity Theory.
   a. Johannes Muller in 1840
      1) Developed concept of sensory nerve specificity, known as "law of specific nerve energies"
      2) This explained individual sensations were felt because specific energy was experienced at certain receptors and the brain could distinguish one from another.
   b. Magnus Blix and Adolf Goldscheider in 1884
      1) Identified sensory spots (subcutaneous receptors) on skin, which were small areas that elicited a specific sensation when touched
      2) These spots were specific to cold, heat, pressure, or pain.
   c. Maximillian von Frey in 1894
      1) Continued research on sensory spots (by Blix and Goldscheider) to identify four somatosensory modalities of cold, heat, pain, and touch and went on to say all other skin senses were the result of these four modalities
      2) Developed a still well-known test, "von Frey hairs" (esthesiometer), used to measure force applied to a specific spot to elicit a sensation
   d. Sir Charles Scott Sherrington in 1906
      1) Introduced concept of nociception, which identified tissue injury as a common source of pain
      2) Identified primary function of receptor is to lower excitability threshold of reflex arc for one kind of stimulus and heighten it for all others
      3) Proposed concept of synapse and discovered pre-and postsynaptic components, leading to synaptic transmission and modulation in central nervous system (CNS)
5. Bell's Specificity Theory provided significant advancement in study of pain.
   a. Proposed tissue injury activates specific receptors and fibers that send pain impulses along a spinal pathway to pain center in brain
   b. Understanding pain pathway helped to determine clinical implications of appropriate treatments designed to block activation and transmission of pain messages.
   c. Clinical treatments of pain included cutting pain pathways and blocking generation and transmission of pain messaging through targeted medication therapy.

d. Continued research on Specificity Theory has waxed and waned for many years, but its concepts have continued to survive and provide useful clinical information.
6. Evidence gaps of Specificity Theory
   a. Does not address factors besides physical injury that cause sensation of pain
   b. Lacks clarification for variation in pain tolerance and intensity among individuals with same tissue injury
   c. Does not explain why pain can persist long after initial injury heals
C. Pattern Theory by John Paul Nafe in 1929
   1. Described as "quantitative theory of feeling" and major opponent to Specificity Theory
   2. Identified different patterns of neural activity received from primary afferent nerve fibers in response to different stimulus modalities, such as mechanical, thermal, and chemical, using electrophysiological recordings
   3. Explained all subcutaneous receptors were alike and unique patterns of stimulation at nerve endings caused variability in interpretations of sensory signal received by CNS, resulting in pain experience
   4. Described experiencing pain after termination or summation of stimuli input in CNS as causing neuropathic pain, such as phantom limb pain or allodynia
   5. Widely covered in scientific literature, greatly expanded pain research, and was considered as a group of new theories, which included:
      a. Goldscheider: proposed central summation in dorsal horn is a critical cause of pain
      b. Livingston: postulated a reverberatory circuit in dorsal horn to explain summation, referred pain, and pain that persists long after healing process
      c. Noordenbos: claimed small-diameter fibers were inhibited by large-diameter fibers and substantia gelatinosa in dorsal horn is responsible for summation of incoming nerve impulses, among other dynamic processes
   6. Specifically credited with an explanation for neuropathic pain, although it is not consistent with all types of pain experiences
   7. Evidence gap of Pattern Theory: Further research has proven subcutaneous receptors are unique and specialized for each type of sensation.
D. Gate-Control Theory (GCT) by Patrick Wall and Ronald Melzack in 1965
   1. Identified pain as a complex perceptual individual experience influenced by both physiological and psychological factors
   2. First theory to study pain as a mind-body experience by incorporating central control processes of brain

3. Supported concepts of Specificity (specialized pain and touch fibers) and Pattern (substantia gelatinosa in dorsal horn) Theories yet provided model that explained the opposing views
4. Components of original GCT theory:
   a. Experience of pain is result of signal being sent to brain in complex interaction among three components of spinal cord:
      1) Substantia gelatinosa
      2) Dorsal horn
      3) Transmission cells
   b. Gating mechanism, located in substantia gelatinosa in dorsal horn, modulates transmission of sensory information from primary afferent neurons to transmission cells in spinal cord.
   c. In addition to gating mechanism in substantia gelatinosa, Melzack and Wall determined there was another gating mechanism in cortical regions of brain.
      1) Proposed cortical control centers are responsible for effects of cognitive and emotional factors of pain experience.
      2) Negative thoughts, such as helplessness, hopelessness, and anger, tend to amplify intensity of signals sent to brain. Someone depressed has a gate open more often than someone not depressed. This results in more signals getting through and increases likelihood the person will experience pain from an otherwise normal stimulus.
      3) Unhealthy lifestyle choices, such as poor eating habits, smoking, and lack of exercise, may result in an open gate, which can lead to pain disproportionate to the stimulus.
      4) Promoting healthy behaviors, such as strategies focusing on reducing stress and improved coping, helps to close gate and lessens pain perception.
   d. Gating mechanism is controlled by activity in large and small fibers. The stronger the noxious stimulation, the more active pain fibers become.
      1) Small-fiber (Aδ and C) activity facilitates or opens gate.
      2) Large-fiber (Aβ) activity inhibits or closes gate.
      3) Balance of input between large and small fibers is responsible for determining intensity of pain caused by stimulus.
   e. Activity from descending fibers originating in supraspinal regions and projecting to dorsal horn can also modulate gate mechanism.
   f. When nociceptive information reaches a threshold that exceeds the inhibition elicited, it "opens the gate," and transmission cells activate pathways that lead to subjective experience of pain and related behaviors.

5. Profound discoveries attributed to GCT were endogenous descending pain modulation system and opioid peptide receptors in the CNS.
6. These discoveries created not only a scientific but also a clinical impact on practice of pain management.
   a. Previously, psychological factors had been seen as "reactions to pain" but were now identified as an important part of pain processing, which led to more psychological therapies for pain care.
   b. Analgesic effect of transcutaneous electrical nerve stimulation (i.e., TENS) and dorsal column stimulation through inhibition of large-fiber inputs was well demonstrated.
7. Evidence gaps of Gate-Control Theory
   a. Lacks explanation for other pain mechanisms, such as peripheral inflammation, spinal modulation, midbrain descending control, and the complete etiology of pain
   b. Does not describe role of autonomic nervous system (sympathetic, parasympathetic) on inhibition or facilitation of pain perception

III. Select Current Pain Theories

A. Concepts of the previous pain theories, which continue to be referenced and researched, have contributed greatly to pain care today. However, current pain theories take a much more comprehensive approach, including aspects of psychological and behavioral theories of pain.
B. Neuromatrix Theory of Pain by Ronald Melzack in 1999
   1. Expansion of GCT, stating pain is affected by cognitive and emotional factors in addition to physical factors and suggests the CNS is responsible for producing painful sensations instead of direct sensory input induced by injury, inflammation, or other pathology
   2. Suggests pain is a multidimensional individual experience produced by a "neurosignature," which is patterns of nerve impulses generated by a widely distributed neural network known as the "body-self neuromatrix" in the brain. Neuromatrix is determined by genetic and sensory influences.
      a. Body-self neuromatrix integrates multiple inputs to produce output pattern triggered by pain. Inputs include:
         1) Sensory inputs, such as cutaneous, visceral, and other somatic receptors
         2) Visual and other sensory inputs, which influence cognitive interpretation of situation

3) Phasic, tonic, cognitive, and emotional inputs from other areas of brain
4) Intrinsic neural inhibitory modulation, which is inherent in all brain function
5) Activity of body's stress-regulation systems, including cytokines, in addition to endocrine, autonomic, immune, and opioid systems

   b. The neurosignature, or output of neuromatrix, is composed of patterns of nerve impulses that vary in temporal and spatial dimensions and produce neural programs genetically built into the neuromatrix and determine properties of both pain experience and behavior.

   c. These neurosignature patterns may be generated by sensory inputs or triggered independently of them.

1) Brief noxious inputs that evoke acute pain through sensory transmission mechanisms are generally well understood.
2) Persistent pain syndromes may be characterized by severe pain, yet there may be little or no apparent physical injury or pathology.

3. Introduced the stress component into pain perception and proposes:

   a. Hyperactivity of stress response has direct effect on pain.

   b. When individual has increased levels of stress, they experience higher levels of pain.

   c. Chronic physical or psychological stress routinely accompanies persistent pain, but the relationship is unclear.

4. A new conceptual framework, whereby genetically determined template for body-self neuromatrix is influenced by cognitive, emotional, and physical factors

5. Evidence gap of Neuromatrix Theory: failed to account for social constructs of experience of pain

C. Biopsychosocial Theory by George Engel in 1977

1. Hypothesizes individual experience of pain is consequence of complex interactions between biological, psychological, sociological, and contextual factors.

2. Identifies pain as dynamic process with experiences unique to each individual and acknowledges difference between contributing factors and causes of pain

   a. Negates earlier thoughts of pain as direct linear relationship between sensory input, tissue damage, and expected experience of pain

   b. Supports vast numbers of people who continue to report persistent pain despite laboratory and imaging evaluations yielding negative results

3. Premise: One must use multidimensional holistic approach to treatment and manage whole person instead of focusing on single disease/impairment.

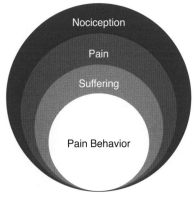

Figure 2.1 Loeser's model of pain. (From Olson K. History of pain: the nature of pain. *Pract Pain Manag*. 2013;*13*[9]).

4. Term *biopsychosocial* is credited to Roy Grinker, a neurologist and psychologist, in 1954.

5. Most prominent physicians to use this approach in association with pain were John Joseph Bonica, an anesthesiologist at an Army hospital and known as founding father of pain medicine, and John D. Loeser, an anesthesiologist at University of Washington.

6. Loeser advocated for use of four dimensions to be evaluated in a person reporting pain: nociception, pain, suffering, and pain behaviors (Fig. 2.1).

   a. Nociception: signal sent to brain from periphery to alert body of tissue injury or damage

   b. Pain: subjective experience as result of brain processing nociceptive input

   c. Suffering: individual's emotional response to nociception

   d. Pain behaviors: response or actions people have, either conscious or unconscious, to pain experience

7. Engel promoted his theory as way to reverse dehumanization of medicine and disempowerment of patients and bring empathy and compassion back to pain care.

8. Use of this theory by wide variety of specialties, including primary care, psychiatry, psychology, pain management, physical therapy, occupational therapy, and disability case management, provides superior outcomes, as evidenced by:

   a. Improved patient satisfaction

   b. A higher degree of restoration of patient function

   c. A more cost-effective process for treating patients with persistent pain

9. Critics of Biopsychosocial Theory point out several weaknesses or evidence gaps:

   a. Considered too broad in nature, lacking ability to operationalize and test because it does not specify which interventions on which to focus.

	Relief	Ease	Transcendence
Physical	Abdominal pain, diarrhea, N/V, lack of mobility	Comfortable resting position (sleep and relaxation), PCA	Pt resumes his ADLS with side effects controlled
Psychospiritual	Anxiety, depression, social stigma	Deep breathing, coaching/role models, reassurance	Pt feels spiritually and emotionally at ease
Environmental	Double-patient rooms, female nurses, temperature, bright lights	Male nurses, single room, low lighting, quiet, privacy provided	Pt feels comfortable changing colostomy bag
Sociocultural	Family not present, financial concerns	Visitors, phone calls, learns more about financial implications	Pt has a supportive network in place, financial issues have been addressed

Figure 2.2 **Dimensions of Kolcaba's Comfort Theory.**

b. Can lead to an overreliance on subjective or psychosocial outcome measures, thus minimizing contributions of traditional biomedical objective outcome measures

c. Can lead to loss of attention to and pathophysiology or under-diagnosis, thereby allowing medically unexplained pain to move too quickly to realm of psychiatry

d. Biopsychosocial Theory is compromised when any component(s) (i.e., biological, psychological, social, contextual) are excluded.

D. Comfort Theory is nursing theory by Katherine Kolcaba in 1994

1. Comfort is a multifaceted concept, a basic individual need, and central to the patient experience. Kolcaba was first to conceptualize and operationalize (measure) comfort.

   a. People have very different responses to painful/uncomfortable stimuli.

   b. Providing comfort is a holistic outcome for nursing care because it improves physical and/or psychological function.

2. Has two dimensions of comfort:

   a. Dimension one: comfort consists of three states:

      1) Relief: experience of having a specific need met, thus allowing one to return to previous function

      2) Ease: state of calm or contentment allowing efficient performance

      3) Transcendence: state in which one can rise above problems or pain

   b. Dimension two: four contexts in which comfort occurs:

      1) Physical: concerning bodily sensations, homeostatic mechanisms, immune function, etc.

      2) Psychospiritual: concerning internal awareness of self, such as esteem, identity, sexuality, meaning in one's life, and relationship to higher order or being

      3) Environmental: concerning external background, temperature, sound, light, smell, color, noise, etc.

      4) Sociocultural: concerning interpersonal, family, and cultural relationships, finances, traditions, rituals, and religious practices

3. Using these two dimensions, a taxonomic structure was developed to guide assessment, measurement, and evaluation of patient comfort (Fig. 2.2).

4. Comfort outcomes are nurse sensitive because they are directly related to nursing interventions.

5. Evidence gaps and limitations of Comfort Theory

   a. Comfort is a complex individual concept and has been difficult to define, operationalize, and evaluate.

   b. No standard definition exists because comfort is used in so many ways, as a noun, verb, adjective, state, process, and outcome.

   c. In absence of a consensual definition of comfort, assessing, measuring, and testing of effectiveness of interventions has limitations.

Bibliography

Adams, L. M., & Turk, D. C. (2018). Central sensitization and the biopsychosocial approach to understanding pain. *Journal of Applied Biobehavioral Research.* http://doi.org/10.1111/jabr.12125.

Cuomo, A., Bimonte, S., Forte, C. A., Botti, G., & Cascella, M. (2019). Multimodal approaches and tailored therapies for pain management: the trolley analgesic model. *Journal of Pain Research, 12,* 711–714. https://doi.org/10.2147/JPR.S178910.

Derbyshire, S. W. (2000). Exploring the pain "neuromatrix." *Current Review of Pain, 4*(6), 467–477. https://doi-org.proxy.kumc.edu/10.1007/s11916-000-0071-x.

Engel, G. (1977). The need for a new medical model: a challenge for biomedicine. *Science, 196*, 129–136. https://dx.doi.org/10.3109/13561828909043606.

Gatchel, R. J., & Maddrey, A. M. (2004). The biopsychosocial perspective of pain. In J. M. Raczynski & L. C. Leviton (Eds.), *Handbook of Clinical Health Psychology: Vol. 2. Disorders of Behavior and Health.* (pp. 357–378). Washington, D.C.: American Psychological Association. https://doi.org/10.1037/11589-011.

Gatchel, R. J., & Howard, K. J. (2008). The biopsychosocial approach. *Practical Pain Management, 8*(4). https://www.practicalpainmanagement.com/treatments/psychological/biopsychosocial-approach.

Katz, J., & Rosenbloom, B. N. (2015). The golden anniversary of Melzack and Wall's gate control theory of pain: celebrating 50 years of pain research and management. *Pain Research and Management, 20*(6), 285–286. https://doi-org.proxy.kumc.edu/10.1155/2015/865487.

Iannetti, G. D., & Mouraux, A. (2010). From the neuromatrix to the pain matrix (and back). *Experimental Brain Research, 205*(1), 1–12. https://doi-org.proxy.kumc.edu/10.1007/s00221-010-2340-1.

Melzack, R. (1999). From the gate to the neuromatrix. *Pain,* (Suppl. 6), S121–S126. https://doi-org.proxy.kumc.edu/10.1016/S0304-3959(99)00145-1.

Melzack, R. (2001). Pain and the neuromatrix in the brain. *Journal of Dental Education, 65*(12), 1378–1382.

Melzack, R. (2005). Evolution of the neuromatrix theory of pain. The Prithvi Raj Lecture: Presented at the Third World Congress of World Institute of Pain, Barcelona 2004. *Pain Practice, 5*(2), 85–94. https://doi.org/10.1111/j.1533-2500.2005.05203.x.

Melzack, R., & Katz, J. (2013). Pain. *Wiley Interdisciplinary Reviews, Cognitive Science, 4*(1), 1–15. https://doi.org/10.1002/wcs.1201.

Melzack, R., & Wall, P. D. (1965). Pain mechanisms: a new theory. *Science, 150*, 971–979.

Mendell, L. M. (2014). Constructing and deconstructing the gate theory of pain. *Pain, 155*(2), 210–216. https://doi-org.proxy.kumc.edu/10.1016/j.pain.2013.12.010.

Miaskowski, C., Blyth, F., Nicosia, F., Haan, M., Keefe, F., Smith, A., et al. (2020). A biopsychosocial model of chronic pain for older adults. *Pain Medicine, 21*(9), 1793–1805. https://doi.org/10.1093/pm/pnz329.

Moayedi, M., & Davis, K. D. (2013). Theories of pain: from specificity to gate control. *Journal of Neurophysiology, 109*, 5–12. https://doi:10.1152/jn.00457.2012.

Moseley, G. L., & Butler, D. S. (2015). Fifteen years of explaining pain: the past, present, and future. *The Journal of Pain, 16*(9), 807–813. https://doi-org.proxy.kumc.edu/10.1016/j.jpain.2015.05.005.

Olson, K. A. (2013). History of pain: a brief overview of the 17th and 18th centuries. *Practical Pain Management, 13*(6). https://www.practicalpainmanagement.com/pain/history-pain-brief-overview-17th-18th-centuries.

Olson, K. A. (2013). History of pain: a brief overview of the 19th and 20th centuries. *Practical Pain Management, 13*(7), 17–22. https://www.practicalpainmanagement.com/treatments/history-pain-brief-overview-19th-20th-centuries.

Olson, K. A. (2013). History of pain: The nature of pain. Practical Pain Management, *13*(9). https://www.medcentral.com/pain/chronic/history-pain-nature-pain.

Papadimitriou, G. (2017). The "Biopsychosocial Model": 40 years of application in psychiatry. *Psychiatriki, 28*(2), 107–110. https://pubmed.ncbi.nlm.nih.gov/28686557/.

Penlington, C., Urbanek, M., & Barker, S. (2019). Psychological theories of pain. *Primary Dental Journal, 7*(4), 24–29.

Trachsel, L. A., Munakomi, S., & Cascella, M. (2020). Pain theory. *StatPearls,* Retrieved from: https://www.ncbi.nlm.nih.gov/books/NBK545194/.

CHAPTER 3

Mental Health Disorders and Pain

Theresa L. Kapke, PhD
Kim Anderson Khan, PsyD
Sharon Wrona, DNP, PMGT-BC, CPNP-PC, PMHS, AP-PMN, FAAN*

Introduction

This chapter focuses on underlying mechanisms and theoretical models to explain co-occurrence of mental health disorders and pain. Descriptions of various mental health conditions commonly observed among individuals with pain are reviewed, allowing readers to understand the prevalence, development, and course of comorbid mental health disorders and pain.

I. Mental Health Disorders and Pain

A. Bidirectional relation
1. Most research has focused on relation between mental health factors and persistent pain, although research on the overlap of mental health factors and acute pain is growing.
2. Persistent pain and severe pain often negatively impact mood, but underlying mental health conditions may also contribute to development of pain conditions, as well as plan of care, patient compliance with treatment recommendations, and treatment outcomes.
3. Pain is influenced by one's thoughts, feelings, and behavioral responses.
4. Early treatment is important.
   a. Identification of pain and mental health disorders reduces risk of persistent pain conditions.
   b. Adequate treatment of acute pain decreases risk of developing depression and anxiety in the long term.
5. Despite high co-occurrence of pain and internalizing mental health disorders, there remains limited understanding of underlying mechanisms, especially for pediatric pain populations. Some proposed theoretical models include cognitive (e.g., attention biases), affective (e.g., anxiety, sensitivity and depression), and behavioral (e.g., avoidance and sleep disturbance) domains.

B. Overall prevalence
1. Adults
   a. Persistent (chronic) pain occurs in 19% to 43% of adults.
      1) Research suggests 5% of adults with persistent pain fall into high-impact chronic pain (HICP) category, in which pain significantly impairs functioning across different domains (i.e., work, social, and/or self-care activities).
      2) For those within HICP population, prevalence rates for most common pain conditions include:
         a) Joint pain (84%)
         b) Back pain (75%)
         c) Leg pain (64%)
         d) Neck pain (51%)
         e) Headache/migraine (41%)
         f) Jaw muscle/joint (19%)
   b. Comorbid persistent pain and a mental health disorder occur in 17% to 20% of adults.
   c. Adults with persistent pain are at increased risk for other poor health outcomes, including suicide, substance use, and sexual violence/relational concerns.
2. Children and adolescents
   a. Persistent pain, which often persists into adulthood, occurs in 11% to 38% of youth. The most common conditions include headache, migraine, back pain, musculoskeletal pain, and abdominal pain.
   b. High levels of psychiatric comorbidity among youth with persistent pain and comorbidities often arise in adolescence.
   c. Of the youth with persistent pain, 3% to 5% have moderate to severe functional disability. Domains include social/extracurricular functioning, sleep, school attendance and performance, and psychological well-being.
C. Biological mechanisms to explain co-occurrence of pain and mental health conditions
1. Overlapping structural brain regions
   a. Neural models include Melzack's neuromatrix and Garcia-Larrea and Peyron's hierarchical pain matrix.

---

*Section Editor for the chapter.

1) Moving away from rigid, single "pain center" in the brain, as the process is more extensive and complex
2) Pain matrix refers to various interrelated brain regions activated by nociceptive stimuli, as well as emotional and behavioral factors.
3) Hierarchical pain matrix
   a) 3-tiered model involves "first-order" processing of nociceptive stimuli in spinothalamic tract; "second-order" processing in anterior cingulate cortex (ACC), insula, prefrontal cortex (PFC), and posterior parietal cortex; and "third-order" processing in orbitofrontal, perigenual ACC, and anterolateral PFC regions.
   b) "Second-order" processing involves developing pain perceptions and memory formation, which are impacted by emotional and psychological factors.
   b. Functional MRI studies
   1) Brain regions involved in processing pain signals also process emotions, learning, memory, and behavioral and emotional responses to pain.
   2) Shared regions include primary and secondary somatosensory cortices, ACC, anterior insula cortex, thalamus, cerebellum, nucleus accumbens, amygdala, and PFC.
   c. Acute pain
   1) Pharmacological analgesia shows effects on cortical and subcortical regions (e.g.,

primary and secondary somatosensory cortices, insula, ACC, PFC, and thalamus).
   2) Other brain areas have been implicated in acute pain perception (e.g., basal ganglia, cerebellum, amygdala, hippocampus, and areas within parietal and temporal cortices).
   d. Brain areas involved in persistent pain include medial prefrontal cortical areas and subcortical limbic regions (e.g., dorsal and ventral basal ganglia, amygdala, and hippocampus).
   e. Changes in one's emotional state, motivation, and reward-related behaviors, as well as the brain circuits involved, can impact the severity and duration of pain. Dysregulation of default mode network (e.g., dorsomedial PFC, ventromedial PFC, posterior cingulate cortex, temporoparietal junction, and superior temporal sulcus) may be present for individuals with comorbid persistent pain and depression.
   f. Shared brain regions are affected by use of pharmacological and nonpharmacological interventions (Table 3.1).
2. Shared neurotransmitters
   a. Chemical substances that impact transmission of neuronal signals across synapses.
   b. Classified according to function (i.e., excitatory or inhibitory), size, or type.
   c. Serotonin, norepinephrine, glutamate, and γ-aminobutyric acid are neurotransmitters involved in depression and pain.

Table 3.1

Corticolimbic Structures Associated With Persistent Pain

Brain Structures	Location	Function
Medial prefrontal cortex	Located in the frontal lobe	Decision making, self-control, regulation of emotion, processing of risk and fear, and regulation of amygdala activity
Amygdala	Located in the frontal portion of the temporal lobe, close to the hippocampus	Memory modulation, decision-making, reward, and emotional responses
Periaqueductal gray	Located around the cerebral aqueduct within the tegmentum of the midbrain	Autonomic function, motivated behavior, behavioral responses to threatening stimuli, and primary control center for descending pain modulation
Anterior cingulate cortex	Located in the frontal part of the cingulate cortex	Autonomic functions, attention allocation, reward anticipation, decision-making, ethics and morality, impulse control, emotion, and registration of physical pain
Hippocampus	Located in the medial temporal lobe	Consolidation of memories, emotion, navigation, spatial orientation, and learning
Nucleus accumbens	Located in the basal forebrain	Cognitive processing of motivation, aversion, reward, reinforcement learning, and significant role in addiction

(From Yang S, Chang. Chronic pain: structural and functional changes in brain structures and associated negative affective states. *Int J Mol Sci, 20*[13]:1–17, 2019.)

d. Pharmacological agents (e.g., gabapentinoids, *N*-methyl-D-aspartate receptor antagonists, and antidepressants) used in pain management target these neurotransmitters.
 1) Antidepressants can inhibit pain via descending pathways in midbrain and brainstem by targeting serotonin or norepinephrine to block pain signals to somatosensory cortex, which may be especially helpful for treating comorbid pain and depression.
 2) Some common antidepressant classes include:
  a) Serotonin-norepinephrine reuptake inhibitors (SNRIs) (e.g., venlafaxine, duloxetine, milnacipran)
  b) Selective serotonin reuptake inhibitors (SSRIs) (e.g., paroxetine, sertraline)
  c) Opioid partial agonist-antagonists (e.g., buprenorphine), antipsychotics (e.g., quetiapine XR)
  d) Tricyclic antidepressants (TCAs) (e.g., amitriptyline)
 3) Antidepressants seem to be especially effective in treating neuropathic pain, headache, and myofascial pain/fibromyalgia but are not as effective in treating musculoskeletal pain.
 e. Use of psychological interventions (e.g., cognitive and behavioral therapy, motivational interviewing, relaxation training, and use of virtual reality) and integrative strategies (e.g., exercise, yoga, and nutrition) are thought to have analgesic effects and impact neurotransmitters involved in pain, anxiety, and mood regulation.
3. Hypothalamic-pituitary-adrenal axis and stress hormones
 a. An increased level of stress hormones (e.g., cortisol and epinephrine) is considered to be a physiological response to pain and depression.
 b. Trauma and toxic and chronic stress (e.g., adverse childhood events [ACEs]) are thought to lead to various physiological changes (i.e., epigenetic, hormonal, and autoimmune) and dysregulation of one's hypothalamic-pituitary-adrenal axis circuit, placing individuals at increased risk for developing mood and anxiety disorders, as well as persistent pain conditions.
4. Immune dysfunction
 a. Depression has been characterized as an inflammatory response/disorder in the brain due to release of proinflammatory cytokines, which have been shown to trigger and exacerbate pain.
 b. Positive emotions, trait positive affect, and positive cognitions are inversely related to pro-inflammatory cytokine levels, highlighting

way in which these protect against inflammation/pain.
 c. However, inflammation is known to negatively impact neural circuitry involved in regulating positive affect, highlighting need for interventions focused on promoting positive coping and behavioral activation.
D. Theoretical models to explain co-occurrence
1. Asmundson and colleagues' shared vulnerability model (SVM)
 a. Similar diathesis-stress model underlies persistent pain and posttraumatic stress disorder (PTSD).
 b. Adults at increased risk for persistent pain and/or PTSD have similar predisposing characteristics and vulnerabilities, including anxiety and injury sensitivity, selective attention to threat, and reduced threshold for alarm.
 c. During times of stress, these factors may lead to negative emotional responses and other processes (e.g., autonomic nervous system/muscular response, avoidance, and cognitive processes) that contribute to disability over time.
2. Jastrowski Mano and colleagues' developmentally informed SVM
 a. Builds upon the SVM and extends to youth
 b. Poses youth at risk for persistent pain and/or anxiety have similar predisposing characteristics and vulnerabilities
 c. Caregiver factors (e.g., pain and mental health history) also impact children's predisposing characteristics.
 1) Fifty percent of parents of youth with persistent pain have persistent pain themselves.
  a) Stone and Wilson's integrative conceptual model of transmission of risk from parents with persistent pain to their children:
   (1) Suggests genetics, early neurobiological development, pain-specific social learning, general parenting and family health, and environmental stressors serve as potential mechanisms for relation between parental and pediatric pain outcomes
   (2) Potential moderating factors for relation between parent and child persistent pain include presence of persistent pain in other parent, parent pain characteristics, and child characteristics (i.e., sex, development, race/ethnicity, and temperament).
 2) Parents of youth with persistent pain report higher lifetime rates of psychiatric disorders (e.g., anxiety and mood disorders) than do parents of youth without pain.

3) Parents of youth with persistent pain and greater functional disability report especially high levels of psychological distress.
d. During times of stress, interaction of these factors leads to negative emotional responses between children and caregivers, which may contribute to disability over time.

E. Assessment and treatment of pain conditions
1. Support for biopsychosocial approach
   a. Historically, traditional Western medicine assessment of pain has focused solely on biomedical and/or physiological causes, which may not fully address and explain the complexity of pain.
   b. Given various factors that impact pain (i.e., biological, psychological, sociocultural, and contextual), modern theory calls for biopsychosocial assessment and treatment of pain.
      1) Biological factors: genetics, physiology, neurochemistry, tissue health
      2) Psychological factors: perceived control, self-efficacy, catastrophic thinking, hypervigilance, depression, anxiety, and anger
      3) Sociocultural factors: socioeconomic status, social factors, skepticism, operant learning, social learning, and social support
      4) It is important to assess these factors in biopsychosocial clinical interview, including role functioning, sleep, other symptoms and adverse events, and patient's global satisfaction with treatment.
   c. Important to consider factors that predispose, initiate, maintain, and exacerbate one's pain and pain-related behaviors
   d. Biopsychosocial approach to pain allows for flexibility over time.
2. Criticism of biopsychosocial approach
   a. Critics emphasize this approach can be too broad/vague, lacks objective and scientific ways to test various factors impacting pain, does not clearly indicate which interventions to prioritize in treatment, and potentially overemphasizes impact of psychological factors.
      1) Focusing solely on psychological component of pain can lead to stigma and blame.
      2) Psychiatric comorbidity does not mean mental health factors cause one's pain condition; living with pain often leads to increased psychological distress over time.
   b. It is important to balance biological, psychological, sociocultural, and contextual aspects of pain in assessment and treatment.
3. Importance of utilizing multiple informants in assessment of pain for youth
   a. Given that multiple factors contribute to development and maintenance of pain during childhood, a multi-informant, biopsychosocial assessment is recommended, including assessment of impaired physical functioning, sleep disturbance, fatigue, cognitive problems (e.g., impaired concentration and attention) that may impair school performance, school absenteeism, and psychiatry comorbidity.
   b. Multi-informant assessment
      1) Caregivers of youth with persistent pain may underreport their children's internalizing symptoms (e.g., anxiety and depression) and other behavioral concerns.
      2) Greater discrepancy between child and caregiver reports is common among youth with worse functional impairment and may point to family functioning concerns.

II. Bipolar Disorder (BD)

A. Overview
1. Bipolar I and II disorders are classified as Bipolar and Related Disorders in *Diagnostic and Statistical Manual of Mental Disorders, Fifth Edition* (*DSM-5*).
2. These disorders include symptoms of depression and mania or hypomania. Mania and hypomania refer to periods of disrupted mood and/or level of activity or energy, such as decreased need for sleep and increased goal-directed activity or risky behavior. For more detail on diagnostic criteria for Bipolar I and Bipolar II Disorders, please see *DSM-5*.

B. Prevalence and co-occurrence of BD and persistent pain conditions
1. Literature often does not distinguish between different kinds of BD.
2. Presence of BD among adults reporting persistent pain ranges from 1% to 21%. A recent review found nearly 30% of individuals with BD reported clinical pain concerns, including persistent pain (approximately 24%) and migraines (approximately 14%).
3. Little research is available regarding children and adolescents and BD.

C. Underlying mechanisms to explain increased pain in individuals with BD
1. Shared polymorphism, novel protein KIAA0564/ Von Willebrand Domain-containing Protein 8 (VWA8) gene, which has been linked to developmental delays, BD with comorbid migraine, and other medical conditions
2. Individuals with BD have increased prevalence of depression, which has been associated with increased physical problems, greater pain sensitivity, and heightened amygdala activity.
3. Serotonergic and noradrenergic pathway involvement

4. Heightened neuroinflammatory mechanisms
5. Limited cognitive flexibility and deficits in memory and executive functioning among individuals with BD may lead to increased risk for persistent pain.

D. Development and prognosis for those with comorbid BD and pain conditions
   1. Treatment implications for adults with comorbid BD and persistent pain
      a. Individuals with BD are more likely to experience persistent pain, impaired recovery, greater functional impairment, poorer quality of life, and increased risk of suicide and are less likely to seek treatment compared with those without pain.
      b. Research suggests individuals with BD reported approximately four pain complaints at any given time.
      c. Individuals with BD who are treatment adherent report significantly lower levels of pain than do those with BD who are treatment nonadherent.
   2. Pharmacological considerations
      a. Be aware of potential for drug-drug interactions between analgesics and medications used to treat mental health disorders, sleep, and appetite, as well as other substances a patient may be using (e.g., cannabidiol [CBD], cannabis, and herbal supplements).
         1) Use of tricyclic antidepressants and stronger analgesic medications (e.g., opioids) with individuals with BD may trigger manic episodes, particularly without use of a mood stabilizer.
         2) Use of nonsteroidal anti-inflammatory medications may contribute to lithium toxicity.
      b. Ketamine
         1) Controlled use of ketamine has shown promising results in treating comorbid persistent pain, treatment-resistant depression, and BD.
         2) Although ketamine has its own adverse effects, use of ketamine may be helpful in managing opioid and benzodiazepine withdrawal and in replacing opioid treatment for persistent pain.

III. Depressive Disorders

A. Overview
   1. Major depressive disorder (MDD) and persistent depressive disorder (PDD) are classified as depressive disorders in *DSM-5*. PDD is a new diagnosis that includes diagnostic criteria from MDD and dysthymia from *DSM-4*.

2. MDD and PDD symptoms include feelings of sadness, emptiness, or increased irritability; disrupted sleep and eating; and other cognitive and behavioral changes, such as loss of interest in activities, concentration difficulties, fatigue, and suicidality. For more detail on diagnostic criteria for MDD and PDD, please see *DSM-5*.

B. Prevalence and co-occurrence of depressive disorders and persistent pain
   1. Depressive disorders and persistent pain often occur together, exacerbate each other, and have overlapping symptoms.
      a. Literature on depressive disorders and persistent pain has largely been focused on MDD.
      b. Across adults with persistent pain, prevalence of MDD is 2% to 61% and dysthymia is 1% to 9%.
      c. Fifty percent or more of adults with fibromyalgia, tem-poromandibular joint disorder, persistent spinal pain, and persistent abdominal pain have depression.
      d. Twenty percent or more of adults with arthritis, migraine headache, and pelvic pain have depression.
      e. Adults with neuropathic pain demonstrate lowest depression comorbidity.
      f. Adults with neck or back pain are 2 to 2.5 times more likely to suffer an episode of depression at 6- or 12-month follow-up than are individuals without pain, and adults with depression are three times more likely to develop persistent pain than are those without depression.
   2. Children and adolescents
      a. Persistent pain and depressive symptoms co-occur at higher rates than in youth without persistent pain.
      b. More frequent pain increases risk for depression in youth.
      c. Depressive symptoms in youth increase risk for pain frequency, persistence, severity, and development of new pain problems over time, including during adulthood.
      d. Youth with persistent pain are at increased risk of developing depression as adults.

C. Impact of depressive disorders on acute pain experience
   1. Individuals with depression experience acute pain more frequently and with increased severity, similar to that of individuals with persistent pain.
   2. Individuals who experience increased severity or greater duration of acute pain are more likely to develop depression, as seen in the postpartum population.
   3. Summary of conflicting data on pain threshold/tolerance and depression and the need for standardized assessments and tools:

a. Some studies show individuals with depression have lower pain thresholds and pain tolerance than do individuals without depression.

b. Other studies show individuals with depression have higher pain thresholds than do individuals without depression.

c. "Paradox of pain" refers to experience of individuals with depression demonstrating a higher threshold for induced pain but a lower threshold for endogenous pain.

D. Underlying mechanisms to explain co-occurrence of depression and pain
   1. Cognitive, affective, and behavioral mechanisms
      a. Cognitive-affective factors: negative affect, emotionality, acceptance, catastrophizing, emotion regulation strategies (e.g., suppression of emotional expression), attentional biases, and other cognitive biases (e.g., interpretation of events and memory formation)
      b. Behavioral: sleep disturbance, avoidance, and behavioral inactivation
   2. Shared neurobiology (see section I.D.1-6 above)
   3. Developmental factors (sex and age)
      a. Females are more likely to experience persistent pain than males and are at increased risk of depression during adolescence and adulthood.
      b. Among youth, pediatric pain concerns increase with age, and onset of pain peaks in adolescence, when youth are at increased risk for depression.
   4. Impact of family and caregiver factors: parental mental health status, pain status, parenting style, parent-child relationship, and genetic factors have been linked to co-occurrence of pain and depression in youth.

E. Development of and prognosis for those with comorbid depressive disorders and pain conditions
   1. Comorbidity of depressive disorders and pain conditions exacerbates physical and psychological symptoms and leads to worse physical functioning, longer duration of symptoms, poorer quality of life, and poorer prognosis than does either condition alone.
      a. This comorbidity includes more functional disability across different domains.
      b. Youth typically demonstrate more school problems.
   2. Depression appears to maintain persistent pain conditions and contributes to transition from acute to persistent pain.

F. Suicidality and persistent pain conditions
   1. Prevalence of suicidality in the United States (2019)
      a. Adults
         1) Total rate of suicide: 13.9 per 100,000 standard population
         2) Males: total rate of suicide: 22.4 per 100,000 standard population
         3) Females: total rate of suicide: 6.0 per 100,000 standard population
      b. Suicide was 10th leading cause of death for all ages, second leading cause of death for ages 10 to 34, and fourth leading cause of death for ages 35 to 54.
   2. Prevalence of persistent pain and suicidality
      a. Adults
         1) Suicidal ideation is reported by 28% to 48% of adults with persistent pain.
         2) Some pain-related risk factors (including comorbid mental health problems, severe pain, and analgesic medication use) increase risk of suicide.
         3) Adults with persistent back pain, migraine headache, and fibromyalgia may be at increased risk for suicide.
         4) Safety assessments should be completed within context of persistent pain management, and providers should be prepared to make use of crisis resources and safety planning as needed.
      b. Youth: There are mixed findings on rates of suicidal ideation among youth with persistent pain, and youth with comorbid persistent pain and depression are at increased risk for suicidal ideation and suicide attempts.

IV. Anxiety Disorders

A. Overview
   1. Separation anxiety disorder, specific phobia, social anxiety disorder (i.e., social phobia), panic disorder (PD), and agoraphobia are classified as anxiety disorders in *DSM-5*.
   2. These anxiety disorders are characterized by developmentally inappropriate levels of fear and anxiety resulting in behavioral and somatic changes, such as avoiding certain objects, tasks, or activities; disrupted sleep; and/or physical complaints. For more detail on diagnostic criteria for anxiety disorders, please see *DSM-5*.

B. Prevalence and co-occurrence of anxiety disorders and pain conditions
   1. Adults
      a. High rates of co-occurrence
         1) Across adults with persistent pain, prevalence of generalized anxiety disorder (GAD) is 1% to 10%, PD is 1% to 28%, and agoraphobia is 1% to 8%.
         2) Approximately 50% of adults with temporomandibular joint disorder, fibromyalgia, or persistent abdominal pain have high levels of anxiety or an anxiety disorder.

3) High levels of anxiety or an anxiety disorder are reported by 35% to 40% of adults with migraine headache, pelvic pain, or arthritis.

4) Migraines

a) Population-based studies have shown adults with migraine are two to three times more likely to be diagnosed with GAD, PD, agoraphobia, or PTSD than are those without migraine headache.

b) Adults with anxiety disorders are two times more likely to develop migraines than are individuals without anxiety disorders.

5) Lowest prevalence of anxiety is among adults with spinal pain or neuropathic pain.

6) Comorbidity with mood disorders is high, which highlights importance of differential diagnosis (e.g., MDD vs. dysthymia) to inform effective treatment.

b. Prevalence of pain among various anxiety disorders and disorder-specific considerations

1) Generalized anxiety disorder

a) Prevalence rates of 9.1% (migraine), 6.2% (back pain), and 5.6% (arthritis)

b) Catastrophizing thoughts and negativistic attitudes are common among people with GAD, which often impacts attitude toward pain.

2) Panic disorder

a) Adults with persistent pain are 4.27 more likely to have PD than are adults without persistent pain.

b) Adults with arthritis or bone/joint disease are two times more likely to have PD than are adults without these diseases.

c) Many individuals with PD go undiagnosed in primary care settings when presenting for chest pain concerns, which may lead to unnecessary medical treatment, increased healthcare costs, and missed opportunities for psychological intervention.

3) Social anxiety disorder (social phobia)

a) One of the lesser studied anxiety disorders in medical populations and requires careful assessment.

b) Eleven percent of disabled workers with persistent pain had social anxiety.

c) Symptoms of social anxiety negatively impact one's social interactions and support network, which may serve as barrier to proper treatment.

2. Youth

a. High rates of co-occurrence of pain and anxiety

1) Younger children with persistent pain report higher levels of separation anxiety and social phobia.

2) Females with persistent pain reported a higher level of panic/somatic symptoms, GAD, and separation anxiety than did males.

3) Research suggests 80% of youth with persistent pain meet criteria for an anxiety disorder based on structured diagnostic interviews.

4) Tran and colleagues found 31% of youth presenting to a tertiary pain clinic with persistent pain reported elevated symptoms of anxiety across a range of anxiety disorders and nearly half reported clinical elevations on at least one anxiety subscale of Screen for Child Anxiety Related Emotional Disorders (SCARED), indicating possible anxiety disorder. Youth report:

a) School phobia (56%)

b) GAD (25%)

c) Separation anxiety (24%)

d) Panic/somatic symptoms (22%)

e) Social anxiety (22%)

b. Prevalence of anxiety among different pain conditions among youth with:

a) Noncardiac chest pain, 56% to 81% reported anxiety.

b) Abdominal pain, 45% reported anxiety.

c) Fibromyalgia, 58% reported anxiety.

d) Complex regional pain syndrome, 20% reported anxiety.

e) Unexplained pain, 18% reported anxiety.

f) Headache, 6% reported anxiety.

g) Youth with abdominal pain reported higher panic/somatic symptoms compared with youth with headaches or extremity and/or joint pain.

c. School avoidance and absenteeism in youth with persistent pain

1) Anxiety is stronger predictor of academic impairment in school setting than pain frequency/severity.

2) School is often source of anxiety for youth with persistent pain, including fears related to academic performance, evaluations by teachers, and relationships with peers.

3) School anxiety often leads to school avoidance for youth with persistent pain; one-third of youth with persistent pain demonstrate anxiety-related school avoidance. School avoidance leads to decreased academic performance and other maladaptive school-related behaviors, which can have long-lasting effects.

4) Youth with persistent pain may demonstrate higher rates of school absenteeism than do youth with other chronic health conditions.

5) It is important to assess school anxiety and avoidance within context of pediatric persistent pain management, as well as parental responses and factors. Parental protectiveness in response to their children's pain may negatively impact school functioning and attendance rates.

C. Impact of anxiety on acute pain experience

1. In general, anxiety is positively associated with acute pain, such that individuals with higher anxiety scores report more severe acute pain.

2. Individuals with more anxiety demonstrate lower pain tolerance and higher pain sensitivity, likely due to increased attention to threatening stimuli and perceived pain.

3. Higher levels of catastrophizing and state anxiety have been linked to greater levels of pain intensity among those presenting in emergency department for acute pain.

4. Anxiety and overemphasis on threat-related stimuli for individuals with acute pain may contribute to decreased functional self-efficacy and increased fear of movement, reinjury, and behavioral deactivation, which may lead to persistent pain and increased disability.

D. Development and prognosis for those with comorbid anxiety and pain conditions

1. Development

a. Research suggests dispositional characteristics (e.g., anxiety sensitivity and tendency to experience negative emotions) may serve as vulnerability factors that place individuals at greater risk for developing persistent pain, anxiety, or both.

b. Individuals with persistent pain and anxiety seem to maintain similar attentional and cognitive biases, such as more sensitivity and attention to and fear of pain, as well as somatosensory amplification and behavioral avoidance.

c. Jastrowski Mano and colleagues' developmentally informed SVM

1) Anxiety sensitivity (i.e., "fear of fear"), intolerance of uncertainty, difficulty with tolerating distress and physical discomfort, experiential avoidance, and low threshold for alarm (i.e., high physiological arousal and low pain threshold) may contribute to co-occurrence of anxiety and pain in youth.

2) Heightened autonomic nervous system arousal, avoidance behavior, and hypervigilance/cognitive biases appear to maintain co-occurrence of anxiety and pain in youth.

2. Overlapping symptoms and treatment

a. Anxiety and pain both involve physiological arousal (e.g., accelerated heart rate, rapid breathing, and muscle tensions), which often leads to overlap of somatic symptoms (e.g., dizziness, nausea, and breathing difficulty).

b. It is important to identify and treat underlying anxiety, as opposed to just attributing one's somatic symptoms to pain. Failing to treat underlying anxiety may result in poor treatment outcome.

V. Trauma and Stressor-Related Disorders

A. Overview

1. Acute stress disorder, PTSD, and adjustment disorder are classified as trauma- and stressor-related disorders in *DSM-5*.

2. These disorders are characterized by development of symptoms and associated changes in mood, cognitions, and behavior in relation to exposure to traumatic or stressful life event(s). Individuals with these disorders may experience intrusive thoughts and memories and changes in cognitions, mood, sleep, arousal, and behavior. For more detail on diagnostic criteria for these disorders, please see *DSM-5*.

3. When evaluating symptoms of trauma and stressor-related disorders following loss or death of a loved one, it is important to distinguish between these symptoms and symptoms of normative bereavement.

B. Trauma

1. Adverse childhood experiences

a. Based on retrospective reports of abuse, a high percentage of patients with persistent pain have a history of childhood physical or sexual abuse.

b. Studies show individuals with pain conditions are more likely than individuals without pain conditions to have been neglected or abused.

c. Three or more ACEs were associated with increased prevalence of medical disorders, including pain-related disorders, throughout one's lifetime.

d. Relation between ACEs, internalizing disorders, and pain

1) Strong dose-response relation between ACEs and internalizing disorders, as well as pain

2) Internalizing disorders as mediator: ACEs contribute to development of internalizing disorders, which may lead to pain.

3) Internalizing disorders as moderator:

a) Individuals with more internalizing disorders and higher number of ACEs report more pain.

b) Presence of internalizing disorders affects reported pain among people with low and high numbers of ACEs.

e. ACEs may serve as an additional barrier to treatment and engagement in multidisciplinary pain management treatment.

2. Sensitization hypothesis

a. Persistent stress associated with ACEs impacts one's physiological and behavioral response to stress, potentially through dysregulating one's hypothalamic-pituitary-axis circuit and autoimmune system. This places individuals at greater risk for developing internalizing problems and pain-related conditions.

b. Trauma exposure sensitizes individuals to subsequent stressors and trauma over course of their lifetimes.

3. Co-occurrence with internalizing disorders and pain conditions

a. Adults

1) There is growing evidence ACEs are related to persistent pain and disability in adults.

2) Adults with higher number of ACEs are at increased risk of developing neck/back pain in adulthood.

3) Adults' self-reported childhood sexual and/or physical abuse is related to development of pain conditions in adulthood.

b. Children and adolescents

1) Youth with persistent pain presenting to a multidisciplinary outpatient pain clinic reported high rates of ACEs (i.e., greater than 80% of youth report one or more ACE in their lifetimes).

2) Youth with persistent pain and history of three or more ACEs reported significantly higher psychosocial impairment than did youth with persistent pain and no reported ACEs.

C. Posttraumatic stress disorder and persistent pain conditions

1. Prevalence and co-occurrence

a. High comorbidity of PTSD and persistent pain exists, likely due to shared underlying factors placing individuals at greater risk for development of these conditions and maintaining them over time.

b. Adults

1) Across adults with persistent pain, prevalence of PTSD is 1% to 23%.

2) Among adults with accident- and/or injury-related pain condition, rates of PTSD are closer to 25%.

c. Children and adolescents

1) Research suggests 20% to 30% of youth with persistent pain demonstrate posttraumatic stress symptoms (PTSS).

a) PTSS (e.g., avoidance, hyperarousal, and re-experiencing) may follow stressful or traumatic life event.

b) Unlike criteria for PTSD and/or acute stress disorder, these triggering events do not necessarily include "actual or threatened death, serious injury, and/or sexual violence."

2) While estimates suggest 20% of youth with persistent pain have experienced some kind of trauma, studies suggest 10% of these youth have comorbid PTSD, which is a higher prevalence than in community samples.

3) Holley and colleagues proposed a developmental model of PTSS and persistent pain:

a) Helps explain severity, co-occurrence, and maintenance of PTSS and persistent pain in youth

b) Outlines various interpersonal factors (i.e., role of parents, family, and peers), neurobiological processes, and shared symptomatology of interest and potential maintaining factors (e.g., trauma, cognitive biases, avoidance and activity limitations, anxiety sensitivity, hyperarousal, depression, and perceived injustice)

2. Given high co-occurrence of PTSS/PTSD and persistent pain in adults and youth, there is need for dually targeted interventions to promote better treatment outcomes.

VI. Obsessive-Compulsive Disorder (OCD)

A. Overview

1. OCD is classified as an obsessive-compulsive and related disorders in *DSM-5*.

2. These disorders are characterized by presence of obsessions and/or compulsions. Obsessions include intrusive and unwanted patterns of thinking; compulsions are recurring behaviors or mental acts that are time-consuming or that negatively impact functioning. For more detail on diagnostic criteria for these disorders, please see *DSM-5*.

B. Prevalence and co-occurrence of OCD and pain conditions

1. Although previous versions of *DSM* included OCD as an anxiety disorder, *DSM-5* includes OCD as its own family of mental health disorders, including obsessive-compulsive and related disorders (i.e., trichotillomania, excoriation disorder, hoarding disorder, body dysmorphic disorder, etc.).

2. Research on co-occurrence of OCD and persistent pain is limited at this time, especially within the child and adolescent populations.

3. One percent to eight percent of adults with persistent pain have OCD. Some individuals experience obsessions related to pain concerns.
4. Co-occurrence of OCD and pain conditions
   a. Individuals with comorbid OCD and persistent pain may obsess over their pain experiences.
   b. Screening and addressing these types of obsessive thoughts and related symptoms within context of pain management treatment may lead to better treatment outcomes.
   c. Considering differential diagnoses
      1) Depression: While individuals with OCD and depression both are known to obsess and/or ruminate about specific thoughts, beliefs, memories, and/or images, individuals with depression are more likely to ruminate over negative content and do not necessarily attempt to suppress these ruminations.
      2) Generalized anxiety disorder: Individuals with GAD experience uncontrollable worry across different domains, as opposed to obsessions, and type of worry may vary.

VII. Somatic Symptom and Related Disorders

A. Overview
   1. Somatic symptom disorder (SSD), illness anxiety disorder, and conversion disorder are classified as somatic symptom and related disorders in *DSM-5*.
   2. These disorders are characterized by presence of somatic symptoms; being overly concerned about having a serious medical illness or condition and related worry; presence of excessive health-related behaviors; and/or associated changes in thoughts, behavior, and motor/sensory functioning. These symptoms cannot be better explained by another underlying medical or mental health disorder.
   3. Factitious disorder imposed on self and factitious disorder imposed on another are classified as somatic symptom and related disorders in *DSM-5*. These disorders are primarily characterized by presenting oneself or another as sick or injured with use of fabricated symptoms and deception.
   4. For more detail on diagnostic criteria for these disorders, please see the *DSM-5*.
      a. SSD replaces three of *DSM-IV* somatoform disorders, including somatization disorder, pain disorder, and undifferentiated somatoform disorder/hypochondriasis.
      b. SSD has received criticism for misdiagnosing pain conditions as mental illness, lacking validity, and being overly inclusive.

   c. Some practitioners argue it is more appropriate to use adjustment disorder and/or other diagnoses when characterizing these disorders and symptoms.
   d. Pain disorder (*DSM-IV*) received criticism for emphasizing idea of "medically unexplained pain" and failing to define associated psychological factors.

B. Development and prognosis for those with comorbid SSD and related conditions and persistent pain conditions
   1. Limited clinical interventions exist for individuals with these diagnoses, likely due to varying definitions over time and lack of representation in psychiatric and mental health settings, as these individuals are more likely to be seen in primary care and medical settings.
   2. Various treatment recommendations have been made for individuals with these comorbid conditions and persistent pain.
      a. For those with persistent physical symptoms, consider these diagnoses as part of diagnostic picture and treatment plan.
      b. Try to avoid unnecessary investigations and interventions to any extent possible.
      c. Assess for psychological factors and symptoms and refer as needed; consider potential use of medication management.
      d. Discuss contextual factors as "amplifiers" of pain instead of "causes" of pain; avoid blame.
      e. Promote functioning and positivity; set realistic goals focused on "coping" as opposed to "cure."
      f. Treat symptoms and remain open to complementary approaches; emphasize importance of multidisciplinary team and integrated approaches, including psychiatry, physical therapy, and engagement in cognitive and behavioral therapy and related therapies.
      g. Maintain regular communication and follow-up with patients and families.
      h. Consult and collaborate with other providers as appropriate.

VIII. Summary of Mental Health Disorders and Pain and Implications for Nursing

A. Comorbidity of mental health diagnoses and persistent pain in adults and youth is high, especially among those with functional disability.
B. Individuals with pain and mental health concerns are at increased risk for other poor health and psychosocial outcomes, including substance use disorders.

C. Persistent pain is a common experience in childhood and adulthood; early intervention is key in reducing risk and fostering a positive trajectory.

D. Appropriate management of acute pain and mental health concerns may help to mitigate transition from acute to persistent pain.

E. A bidirectional relation exists between pain and mental health concerns; various factors likely contribute to this, including shared underlying neural mechanisms (i.e., structural brain regions and shared neurotransmitters), hypothalamic-pituitary-axis system and stress response, immune dysfunction, cognitive and affective processes, modeling of pain and coping behaviors, and behavioral factors (e.g., sleep, nutrition, hydration, and physical activity), all of which can be impacted by psychosocial stressors and adverse life experiences.

F. Regarding assessment and intervention for individuals with pain conditions, it is important to use a biopsychosocial framework and consider potential impact of sociocultural stressors and factors, as well as to involve multidisciplinary team when appropriate (e.g., medical team, mental health, physical therapy, and school liaison/staff).

G. Taking a functional, rehabilitative approach is critical to effective intervention for pain and mental health concerns.

H. When working with youth, gathering information from multiple informants and working with caregivers and other significant attachment figures is critical to case conceptualization and treatment, as well as working to address school plan, avoidance/absenteeism, and factors that may contribute to development of other risky behaviors and/or substance use disorders.

Bibliography

Adams, L. M., & Turk, D. C. (2018). Central sensitization and the biopsychosocial approach to understanding pain. *Journal of Applied Biobehavioral Research, 23*(2), 1–18. https://doi.org/10.1111/jabr.12135.

American Psychiatric Association (APA). (2013). *Diagnostic and statistical manual of mental health disorders* (5th ed.). Arlington, VA: American Psychiatric Association.

Asmundson, G. J. G., & Katz, J. K. (2009). Understanding the co-occurrence of anxiety disorders and chronic pain: state-of-the-art. *Depression and Anxiety, 26*, 888–901. https://doi.org/10.1002/da.20600.

Bussieres, A., Hartvigsen, J., Ferreira, M. L., Ferreira, P. H., Hancock, M. J., Stone, L. S., et al. (2020). Adverse childhood experience and adult persistent pain and disability: protocol for a systematic review and meta-analysis. *Systematic Reviews, 9*(1), 1–9. https://doi.org/10.1186/s13643-020-01474-8.

Cimpean, A., & David, D. (2019). The mechanisms of pain tolerance and pain-related anxiety in acute pain. *Health Psychology Open, 6*(2), 1–13. https://doi.org/10.1177/2055102919865161.

Dimsdale, J. E., Creed, F., Escobar, J., Sharpe, M., Wulsin, L., & Barsky, A. (2013). Somatic symptom disorder: an important change in DSM. *Journal of Psychosomatic Research, 75*(3), 223–228. https://doi.org/10.1016/j.jpsychores.2013.06.033.

Garcia-Larrea, L., & Peyron, R. (2013). Pain matrices and neuropathic pain matrices: a review. *Pain, 154*, (S29–S43). https://doi.org/10.1016/j.pain.2013.09.001.

Groenewald, C. B., Murray, C. B., & Palermo, T. M. (2020). Adverse childhood experiences and chronic pain among children and adolescents in the United States. *Pain Reports, 5*(5), e839. https://doi.org/10.1097/PR9.0000000000000839.

Hassett, A. L., & Finan, P. H. (2016). The role of resilience in clinical management of chronic pain. *Current Pain and Headache Reports, 20*, 1–9. https://doi.org/10.1007/s11916-016-0567-7.

Hedegaard, H., Curtin, S. C., & Warner, M. (2021). *Suicide mortality in the United States, 1999–2019*. Hyattsville, MD: National Center for Health Statistics. NCHS Data Brief, no 398. https://stacks.cdc.gov/view/cdc/101761.

Henningsen, P. (2018). Management of somatic symptom disorder. *Dialogues in Clinical Neuroscience, 20*(1), 23–31. https://doi.org/10.31887/DCNS.2018.20.1/phenningsen.

Holley, A. L., Wilson, A. C., Noel, M., & Palermo, T. M. (2016). Post-traumatic stress symptoms in children and adolescents with chronic pain: a topic review of the literature and a proposed framework for future research. *European Journal of Pain, 20*(9), 1372–1383. https://doi.org/10.1002/ejp.879.

Hooten, W. M. (2016). Chronic pain and mental health disorders: shared neural mechanisms, epidemiology, and treatment. *Mayo Clinic Proceedings, 91*(7), 955–970. https://doi.org/10.1016/j.mayocp.2016.04.029.

IsHak, W. W., Wen, R. Y., Naghdechi, L., Vanle, B., Dang, J., Knosp, M., et al. (2018). Pain and depression: a systematic review. *Harvard Review of Psychiatry, 26*(6), 352–363. https://doi.org/10.1097/HRP.0000000000000198.

Jastrowski Mano, K. E. (2017). School anxiety in children and adolescents with chronic pain. *Pain Research and Management*, 1–9. https://doi.org/10.1155/2017/8328174.

Jastrowski Mano, K. E., O'Bryan, E. M., Gibler, R. C., & Beckmann, E. (2019). The co-occurrence of pediatric chronic pain and anxiety: a theoretical review of a developmentally informed shared vulnerability model. *Clinical Journal of Pain, 35*(12), 989–1002. https://doi.org/10.1097/AJP.0000000000000763.

Jordan, K. D., & Okifuji, A. (2011). Anxiety disorders: differential diagnosis and their relationship to chronic pain. *Journal of Pain & Palliative Care Pharmacotherapy, 25*(3), 231–245. https://doi.org/10.3109/15360288.2011.596922.

Katz, J., Rosenbloom, B. N., & Fashler, S. (2015). Chronic pain, psychopathoolgy, and the *DSM-5* somatic symptom disorder. *Canadian Journal of Psychiatry, 60*(4), 160–167. https://journals.sagepub.com/doi/pdf/10.1177/070674371506000402.

Liossi, C., & Howard, R. F. (2016). Pediatric chronic pain: biopsychosocial assessment and formulation. *Pediatrics, 138*(5). https://doi.org/10.1542/peds.2016-0331.

Melzack, R. (1999). From the gate to the neuromatrix. *Pain, S6*, S121–S126.

Martel, M. O., Shir, Y., & Ware, M. A. (2018). Substance-related disorders: a review of prevalence and correlates among patients with chronic pain. *Progress in Neuropsychopharmacology & Biologial Psychiatry, 87*, 245–254.

Martin, S. R., Zeltzer, L. K., Seidman, L. C., Allyn, K. E., & Payne, L. A. (2020). Caregiver-child discrepancies in reports of child emotional symptoms in pediatric chronic pain. *Journal of*

Pediatric Psychology, 45(4), 359–369. https://doi.org/10.1093/jpepsy/jsz098.

Michaelides, A., & Zis, P. (2019). Depression, anxiety and acute pain: links and management challenges. *Postgraduate Medicine, 131*(7), 438–444. https://doi.org/10.1080/00325481.2019.1663705.

Miller, M. M., Meints, S. M., & Hirsh, A. T. (2018). Catastrophizing, pain, and functional outcomes for children with chronic pain: a meta-analytic review. *Pain, 159*(12), 2442–2460. https://doi.org/10.1097/j.pain.0000000000001342.

Nelson, S., Simons, L. E., & Logan, D. (2018). The incidence of adverse childhood experiences (ACEs) and their association with pain-related and psychosocial impairment in youth with chronic pain. *Clinical Journal of Pain, 34*(5), 402–408. https://doi.org/10.1097/AJP.0000000000000549.

Nelson, S., Smith, K., Sethna, N., & Logan, D. (2019). Youth with chronic pain and a history of adverse childhood experiences in the context of multidisciplinary pain rehabilitation. *Clinical Journal of Pain, 35*(5), 420–427. https://doi.org/10.1097/AJP.0000000000000686.

Nelson, S. M., Cunningham, N. R., & Kashikar-Zuck, S. (2017). A conceptual framework for understanding the role of adverse childhood experiences in pediatric chronic pain. *Clinical Journal of Pain, 33*(3), 264–270. https://doi.org/10.1097/AJP.0000000000000397.

O'Neal, M. A., & Baslet, G. (2018). Treatment for patients with a functional neurological disorder (conversion disorder): an integrated approach. *Treatment in Psychiatry, 175*(4), 307–314. https://doi.org/10.1176/appi.ajp.2017.17040450.

Pitcher, M. H., Von Korff, M., Bushnell, M. C., & Porter, L. (2019). Prevalence and profile of high-impact chronic pain in the United States. *The Journal of Pain, 20*(2), 146–160. https://doi.org/10.1016/j.jpain.2018.07.006.

Raja, S. N., Carr, D. B., Cohen, M., Finnerup, N. B., Flor, H., Gibson, S., et al. (2020). The revised International Association for the Study of Pain definition of pain: concepts, challenges, and compromises. *Pain, 161*(9), 1976–1982. https://doi.org/10.1097/j.pain.0000000000001939.

Sachs-Ericsson, N. J., Sheffler, J. L., Stanley, I. H., Piazza, J. R., & Preacher, K. J. (2017). When emotional pain becomes physical: adverse childhood experiences, pain, and the role of mood and anxiety disorders. *Journal of Clinical Psychology, 73*(10), 1403–1428. https://doi.org/10.1002/jclp.22444.

Soltani, S., Kopala-Sibley, D. C., & Noel, M. (2019). The co-occurrence of pediatric chronic pain and depression: a narrative review and conceptualization of mutual maintenance. *Clinical Journal of Pain, 35*(7), 633–643. https://doi.org/10.1097/AJP.0000000000000723.

Stahlschmidt, L., Rosenkranz, F., Dobe, M., & Wager, J. (2020). Posttraumatic stress disorder in children and adolescents wtih chronic pain. *Health Psychology, 39*(5), 463–470. https://doi.org/10.1016/S1056-4993(18)30375-4.

Stone, A. L., & Wilson, A. C. (2016). Transmission of risk from parents with chronic pain to offspring: an integrative conceptual model. *Pain, 157*(12), 2628–2639. https://doi.org/10.1097/j.pain.0000000000000637.

Stubbs, B., Eggermont, L., Mitchell, A. J., De Hert, M., Correll, C. U., Soundy, A., et al. (2015). The prevalence of pain in bipolar disorder: a systematic review and large-scale meta-analysis. *Acta Psychiatrica Scandinavica, 131*, 75–88. https://doi.org/10.1111/acps.12325.

Tran, S. T., Jastrowski Mano, K. E., Anderson Khan, K., Davies, W. H., & Hainsworth, K. R. (2016). Patterns of anxiety symptoms in pediatric chronic pain as reported by youth, mothers, and fathers. *Clinical Practice in Pediatric Psychology, 4*(1), 51–62. https://doi.org/10.1037/cpp0000126.

Yang, S., & Chang, M. C. (2019). Chronic pain: structural and functional changes in brain structures and associated negative affective states. *International Journal of Molecular Sciences, 20*(13), 1–17. https://doi.org/10.3390/ijms20133130.

Williams, L. J., Pasco, J. A., Jacka, F. N., Dodd, S., & Berk, M. (2012). Pain and the relationship with mood and anxiety disorders and psychological symptoms. *Journal of Psychosomatic Research, 72*(6), 452–456. https://doi.org/10.1016/j.jpsychores.2012.03.001.

CHAPTER 4

Essential Ethics for Pain Management Nursing

Esther I. Bernhofer, PhD, MA, RN, PMGT-BC
Sharon Wrona, DNP, PMGT-BC, CPNP-PC, PMHS, AP-PMN, FAAN*

Introduction

Since ancient times, philosophers and theologians have written about pain, agony, misery, existential meaning, and the moral duty to do all one can to relieve the suffering of others. Nurses embody the human response of caring for those who suffer and must be vigilant in providing optimal care for patients with pain. The management of pain is a moral endeavor with ethical implications and thus requires the use of ethical frameworks. As members of one of the most trusted professions, nurses must continue to be worthy of patient trust for providing ethical, optimal pain care. In this chapter, moral obligations, ethical frameworks, social issues, and the application of ethics on behalf of patients with pain will be discussed.

I. Current State of Pain in the United States

A. Pain is experienced by everyone, yet each person's pain is unique to them. It is this combination of ubiquity and subjectivity that makes pain an epistemological puzzle, leaving sufferers to rely on the good moral agency of others for understanding and resolution.

B. According to Centers for Disease Control and Prevention (CDC), in 2019, 20.4% of adults in the United States reported persistent pain, with 7.4% having high-impact persistent pain, which negatively affects daily life.

C. *Acute Pain-Market Insights, Epidemiology and Market Forecast to 2028* reported the prevalence of acute pain in the United States was the highest of seven Western countries and accounted for 74.3% (88,900,931) of 119,619,121 international acute pain cases studied.

D. Inadequately treated persistent and acute pain may result in serious consequences, including poor health outcomes, increased healthcare costs, psychosocial and behavioral issues, depression, disability, and lower quality of life.

E. Examples of factors contributing to undertreatment of pain:
1. Declining numbers of interprofessional pain care programs in the United States, largely due to lack of insurance coverage, other reimbursement, or funding
2. Concerns of patients, families, healthcare providers (HCPs), and policy makers that overuse of opioids to treat acute pain could lead to opioid use disorder (OUD), despite unrelieved pain contributing to poor physical and mental health outcomes
3. Lack of pain management education for nurses and other HCPs. Neglecting to provide pain management education is ethically inappropriate because it impedes clinicians' ability to uphold their duty to provide relief from suffering
4. Social determinants of health hindering access to optimal pain care

F. There are promising advances in pharmacology, technology, psychiatry, procedures, and integrative and complementary therapies for pain management. Availability and usefulness of these advances will depend, in large part, on ethical decision-making along the way, including research funding, politics, government and institution policies, cost, and availability of treatment.

II. Ethics Frameworks Relevant to Pain Care

A. *Ethics* and *morality* are often used interchangeably, but there are important distinctions.
1. Ethics is the application of a society's or community's moral code.
2. Ethical frameworks should assist in guiding pain care in both practice and policy-making.
3. Morality is defined as deeply held personal beliefs that are normative and often instilled by religious faith or other deep convictions.

---

*Section Editor for the chapter.

4. Given that pain management is considered a moral endeavor with ethical applications, optimal pain care must include consideration of moral or ethical frameworks for assessment and treatment.
B. Ethical dilemmas occur when a choice must be made between two or more opposing moral options.
   1. Pain care often encounters ethical dilemmas due to moral goal of alleviating pain through use of treatments with potentially harmful side effects. For example, should a patient continue in pain or potentially be exposed to the risk of developing a substance use disorder (SUD)?
   2. Nurses often take on the role of moral agent, facilitating these decisions.
C. Principlism is the most commonly used ethical framework in pain management. While described by Beauchamp and Childress in the 1980s to initially address the need for ethical research and protection of human subjects, principlism quickly became an ethical framework for clinical practice. Principlism includes four major ethical principles:
   1. Autonomy or respect for persons
      a. Autonomy is defined as the right to self-determination.
      b. Nurses' ethical obligation in respecting patient autonomy is to listen, educate, and advocate as necessary. Examples of autonomy:
         1) Allowing a person with pain to request and/or refuse treatment after being fully informed of benefits and risks
         2) Autonomy is exemplified when patients are fully educated on risks and benefits of pain medications before agreeing to them (e.g., providing patients who are prescribed opioids with information on risks of misuse and other side effects, balanced with potential benefit of pain relief in their individual situation).
      c. Autonomy is frequently challenged in patients with pain when they ask for specific medication or seek other HCPs' opinions because they do not believe their needs are being met.
   2. Beneficence
      a. Beneficence is doing good for the welfare of others.
      b. Examples of beneficence:
         1) Nurse making pain management a priority
         2) Advocating for patients' optimal pain management
      c. Beneficence is often used as the principle promoting an acceptable quality of life. However, care must be taken so quality of life is determined by the patient and not by others (e.g., HCPs, family members).

3. Nonmaleficence
   a. Nonmaleficence is to refrain from doing harm.
   b. Examples of nonmaleficence:
      1) Preventing harm of unmanaged pain
      2) Ensuring patients prescribed opioids are also given naloxone (and educated on its use) to limit/prevent potential harm of overdose
   c. Nonmaleficence may be seen as the opposite of beneficence and used to justify poorly managed pain under the guise of "do no harm" by not administering analgesics because of their risks and side effects.
4. Justice
   a. Justice means fair and equitable treatment of all people in similar situations with similar needs. The principle of justice in pain management includes treating all patients equitably, regardless of their personal characteristics, race, gender, gender identity, socioeconomic status, or any other demographic.
   b. Examples of justice:
      1) Providing access to full and complete assessment and treatment of pain regardless of personal characteristics and socioeconomic status
      2) Engaging in policy-making at organizational and governmental levels to ensure policies are equitable for all
D. Ethical principles applied to patient/healthcare professional (HCP) relationship
   1. Fidelity
      a. Fidelity requires one remain faithful to their commitments and keep their promises, including protection of confidentiality.
      b. Example of fidelity: keeping a promise to bring a patient their pain medication on time
   2. Veracity
      a. The principle of veracity obliges one to tell the truth, albeit with kindness and insight.
      b. Example of veracity: Informing a patient of expected benefits and risks of pain treatment and answers patient's questions truthfully and completely.
      c. Use of placebos in place of analgesics without informing a patient and obtaining informed consent is a violation of veracity and autonomy. Doing so deceives the patient and undermines trust, the foundation of the nurse/patient relationship. There is no place for use of placebos for pain management beyond situations in which patients have given informed consent.
E. Deontology is an ethical theory associated with Immanuel Kant, an 18th century philosopher, and states all rational beings are ethically bound to act out of duty and adherence to moral rules and to take ethically right action, despite the outcome.

1. Deontology in pain management is useful to describe acting to mitigate pain in even the smallest way, knowing optimal pain control may not realistically be achieved.
2. Deontology is also used to justify high doses of opioids at end of life to quell severe pain even if death may occur, an action known as doctrine of double effect.
   a. Double effect is a term used to describe action of doing good (duty) even if a bad outcome results (consequentialism), whether the outcome was anticipated or not, as long as the bad outcome was not the intention of the act.
   b. Double effect describes ethical permissibility of aggressive pain management with opioids at end of life even if death may be an outcome because the good action to provide adequate analgesia for the patient was the intention.

F. Consequentialism is an ethical theory stating ethics of action is determined by consequences (outcomes); if consequences are good and desirable, then no matter what the actions, they are ethical. This is often colloquially described as "the ends justify the means."
1. Utilitarianism is a subcategory of consequentialism describing the philosophy that the ethical choice is the one that does the most good for the most people.
2. An example of utilitarianism is limiting everyone's access to opioids, regardless of benefit, in hope of reducing OUD and opioid-related deaths.

G. Ethics of care is an ethical theory acknowledging interdependent relationships, such as those between nurse and patient.
1. Focuses on characteristics of compassion, love, concern, and sympathy, all of which are useful for determining ethically permissible actions toward patients with pain
2. Example: nurses getting to know their patients more fully as individuals, to learn more about each patient's life and goals, how pain impacts them, and how relief of pain would benefit them.

H. Virtue ethics is a theory emphasizing the character and virtue of a moral agent who cares for a patient.
1. Premise: Moral virtues of a caregiver will lead to ethically right actions being made for a patient. If one is virtuous, then their actions will be ethical.
2. Foundation of good pain management nursing relies on patient/nurse relationship built on integrity and nursing virtues, such as patience, respect, intellectual honesty, benevolence, fortitude, and compassion.

I. Narrative ethics is a relationship-based theory considering the person's individual story.
1. Respecting the unique history and story of an individual and their context can be helpful in deciding the ethically acceptable way to manage their pain.

2. Example: Nurses take extra time to listen to patient's story of how persistent pain first came to be, listening for contextual cues surrounding that time in order to potentially identify treatable biopsychosocial and spiritual reasons for persistent pain.

III. Official Statements on Ethics and Pain Care

A. Professional pain management organizations
1. American Society for Pain Management Nursing (ASPMN) has several position statements addressing ethics in pain management, including:
   a. *Pain Management at the End of Life*
   b. *Pain Assessment of the Patient Unable to Self-Report*
   c. *Deceptive use of Placebo in the Assessment and Management of Pain*
2. American Nurses Association (ANA) provides two documents useful for ethics and pain management.
   a. *Code of Ethics for Nurses* (2016) holds nurses to nine provisions for ethical practice.
      1) Provision 1 most directly addresses management of pain and suffering.
         a) Provision 1: "The nurse practices with compassion and respect for the inherent dignity, worth, and unique attributes of every person" (p. 1).
         b) Provision 1.3, part 1: "Optimal nursing care enables the patient to live with as much physical, emotional, social, and religious or spiritual well-being as possible and reflects the patient's own values" (p. 2).
         c) Provision 1.3, part 2: "Supportive care is particularly important at the end of life to prevent and alleviate the cascade of symptoms and suffering that are commonly associated with dying" (p. 2).
         d) Provision 1.3, part 3: "Nurses are leaders who actively participate in assuring the responsible and appropriate use of interventions to optimize the health and well-being of those in their care. This includes acting to minimize unwarranted, unwanted, or unnecessary medical treatment and patient suffering" (p. 2).
         e) Provision 1.4: "The nurse should provide interventions to relieve pain and other symptoms in the dying patient consistent with palliative care practice standards and may not act with the sole intent to end life" (p. 3).
   b. Position statement *Ethical Responsibility to Manage Pain and the Suffering It Causes* (2018) was written "...to provide ethical guidance and

support to nurses as they fulfill their responsibility to provide optimal care to persons experiencing pain" (American Nurses Association Center for Ethics and Human Rights, 2018, p. 1) and reviews several important topics of ethical pain care (e.g., moral disengagement, knowledge deficits, biases, environments not conducive to optimal practice, economic limitations) with recommendations.

3. *Pain Management Nursing: Scope and Standards of Practice*, (2016) 2nd Edition, provides examples of all nine provisions of the *ANA Code of Ethics for Nurses* (2016) for pain management nursing.

4. American Academy of Pain Medicine is an inter-professional pain management organization. Their document, "Ethical Practice of Medicine," states that physicians have an ethical duty to provide pain relief, and this requires comprehensive assessment, facilitation of access to care through organization support, professional education, research, policy, and advocacy development.

5. International Association for the Study of Pain (IASP) is a global interprofessional pain management organization. IASP's "Declaration of Montreal," stated pain management was insufficient worldwide and declared pain management to be a human right.

B. Government organizations
   1. Institute of Medicine
      a. "Relieving Pain in America" is a 382-page report about acute and persistent pain in the United States and begins with the major premise for better pain management that management of pain is a moral endeavor, thus setting the stage for moral obligation for healthcare clinicians to commit to optimal pain management for all patients.
   2. The Joint Commission
      a. The Joint Commission (TJC) is the main standard-setting, regulating body of hospital accreditation in the United States.
      b. TJC publishes program-specific requirements, rationale, and reference reports on pain assessment and management standards.
   3. CDC has published statements and guidelines on assessment and treatment of acute and persistent pain but does not include any ethical or moral obligation to follow those guidelines, although that sentiment may be implied.

IV. Select Social Issues and Ethical Implications for Pain Management

A. Opioid crisis
   1. Prevalence of OUD and opioid-related deaths in the United States had been decreasing in the two years prior to the COVID-19 pandemic.

However, as the pandemic began to take hold across the world, the highest number of opioid deaths over a 12-month period in the United States was recorded in May 2020: over 81,000 deaths primarily due to illicitly manufactured drugs.
   a. The tragedy of opioid abuse and related deaths has been linked to prescription opioids used for pain management; however, the reality is most opioid-associated deaths result from a combination of substances, and they have increased with a different trajectory from that of the persistent pain epidemic.
   b. Ethical questions related to use of opioids for pain in context of a high level of OUD in the community are ones of acceptable risks versus potential benefits.

2. History of pain and opioid use and misuse goes back to ancient times.
   a. Ethical questions of prescribing opioids for pain began when overuse and misuse became apparent in those treated with various opiate preparations. Throughout time, people have used varying degrees of legal methods in order to "protect the public" from those who misused substances.
   b. In early 20th century, the American Medical Association blamed physicians who prescribed too many opioids as "mis-prescribers" and suggested they were one of 4Ds: dated, duped, disabled, or dishonest. A new 3C (careless, corrupt, or compromised) model appeared with similar moral intonations. There is also the insinuation that patient behaviors are unethical, implying patients had ulterior motives and "duped" their physicians.
   c. Nurses' ethical struggle to care for patients with pain while working to prevent substance use disorder has also been long-standing.

3. A middle-range nursing theory developed by Marion Good in 1998 describes a balance between providing adequate pain relief and preventing serious adverse events (e.g., OUD) and is important for ethical and humanitarian reasons.

B. Social stigma
   1. Stigmatization or "othering" is a destructive social construct.
      a. Stigmatization occurs when one group ("in group") assigns another group ("out group") a shared characteristic and judges them as "less than" or socially deviant. Moral judgment and blame occur.
      b. When the "out group" is people with pain, their pain is "… denied, invalidated, and delegitimized" (Goldberg, 2020 p. 1).
   2. Pain-related stigma comes from HCPs, family, friends, insurers, employers, and policymakers. For people with pain, stigmatization results in added

suffering, decreased quality of care, and lack of trust in caregivers and those who create pain management policies and guidelines.

3. People who experience long-term stigmatization die sooner than others and are often sicker throughout their lives because stigma is a barrier to receiving proper care. Goldberg (2020) writes, "In addition to being bad for physical health, stigma is also morally bad. It is among the most antisocial and alienating experiences humans can inflict on each other. It isolates people, causes suffering, and violates basic obligations to treat people fairly and with dignity. Accordingly, we should intervene to alleviate it" (p. 4).

C. Social determinants of health and pain care disparities

1. According to the ANA *Code of Ethics for Nurses,* (2016) nurses are "ethically obligated to take action against the disparities associated with access to pain management" (p. 28).

   a. Nurses must seek to understand disparities in pain care experienced by marginalized people.
      1) Marginalization results from stigmatization and othering and is a significant contributor to social determinants of health, including access to care.
      2) People who are marginalized face significant barriers to receiving adequate pain management.
      3) Every patient is an individual with a unique experience of pain requiring compassionate assessment and equitable, culturally acceptable treatment options without regard to race, ethnicity, gender, sexual preference, immigration status, employment status, socioeconomic status, literacy level, geographic location, cognitive function, or any other characteristic that might result in disparities in pain care.

   b. Factors contributing to disparities
      1) Implicit (an unconscious belief) and explicit (an acknowledged attitude/belief) bias against others influences pain assessment and prevents or erodes mutual trust.
      2) Long-held myths regarding biological differences and experiences (e.g., Blacks do not experience pain as much as Whites do)
      3) Negative stereotypes and labeling behaviors without investigating their source
      4) Lack of pain research involving minorities or other marginalized people
      5) HCPs not believing patients' pain reports because of different communication styles and expression
      6) Persistent stress and lack of access to health care because of marginalization may result in exacerbation of persistent pain conditions not being reported.

7) Clinicians may be condescending in tone, have patients wait longer to receive care, and make assumptions about drug use and adherence to other treatments, thereby causing patients with pain to avoid healthcare and thus receive poor or nonexistent pain care.
8) Language barriers, cultural differences, differences in styles of communication, and health literacy issues contribute to lack of understanding, care, and treatment.

V. Moral Distress in Pain Management

A. Moral distress occurs when a person experiences distress (physical, psychological, or spiritual discomfort or anxiety) related to a decision or dilemma that challenges deeply held moral beliefs of right or wrong. There are several types of moral distress, but two are most often experienced by nurses caring for patients with pain.

1. Moral distress occurs when one knows the morally correct action to take but is prevented from doing so. Example: Nurses, who know their patients and understand what they require for optimal pain care but are prevented from providing it due to institutional or hierarchal constraints, may thus experience moral distress.
2. Moral uncertainty is a type of moral distress that may be more prevalent than classic moral distress and occurs when nurses face a moral dilemma in pain care and do not know the "right thing to do." Example: distress over such things as how much analgesia a patient should receive near end of life, or whether or not to reveal patient's past opioid use to provider who may then refuse to provide analgesics to a patient with severe acute pain

B. Nurses must be aware that all types of moral distress can be damaging and, if experienced too often, can lead to burnout or compassion fatigue.
C. Nurses must stay vigilant and talk with trusted colleagues, mentors, and friends to help resolve stress related to moral and ethical decision-making.

VI. Practical Applications of Ethics in Pain Management Nursing

A. Practical application of ethics is the moral responsibility of every nurse.

1. Providing the most ethical pain management begins with being as educated as possible regarding pain, its treatment and policies, and how it affects populations.

2. Lack of pain management education for nurses and other HPCs is ethically unacceptable because every clinician is duty-bound to be fully knowledgeable about their patients' conditions and all available treatments; there is a moral obligation to be up to date with the science of pain management and population needs.

B. Every nurse must review their values surrounding pain, treatment, and patient population served and be aware of personal biases. It is important to know what one finds ethically acceptable or unacceptable based on one's personal moral principles so that pain management dilemmas can be dealt with honestly.

C. Nurses must take the time to ascertain a patient's values surrounding pain because pain is interpreted and ascribed moral meaning differently by different people. Understanding what is important to a patient will help to reduce stigma, increase the relationship-based ethics of care, lead to advocacy, and improve pain management outcomes.

D. Applying a combination of ethical frameworks for difficult situations when medical and biopsychosocial models do not seem to work may lead to solutions and resolve quagmires in pain care. Ethical reasoning should be used to solve ethical dilemmas regarding poorly managed pain. Nurses must also advocate for pain management policies based on ethical frameworks.

1. Principlism can be used when questioning if respect for patient's autonomy will provide the most beneficence for their pain situation. Are patient's preferences given highest priority? What must be done to reduce risks of harm and still provide the best analgesia?

2. When caring for someone in a marginalized population, the principle of justice and framework of the ethics of care may provide support for effective problem-solving. Use of narrative ethics allows for listening to patient stories to lessen stigma, discrimination, and judgment.

Bibliography

Abd-Elsayed, A. (October 30, 2019). *Disparities in Care for LGBTQ patients.* American Society of Regional Anesthesia and Pain Medicine. https://www.asra.com/guidelines-articles/original-articles/article-item/asra-news/2019/10/30/disparities-in-care-for-lgbtq-patients.

American Nurses Association. (2016). *Code of Ethics for Nurses with Interpretive Statements.* Silver Spring, MD: American Nurses Association.

American Nurses Association Center for Ethics and Human Rights. (2018). *American Nurses Association position statement: The Ethical Responsibility to Manage Pain and the Suffering It Causes.* https://www.nursingworld.org/~495e9b/globalassets/docs/ana/ethics/theethicalresponsibilitytomanagepainandthesufferingitcauses2018.pdf.

American Nurses Association and Association for Pain Management Nursing. (2016). *Pain Management Nursing: Scope and Standards of Practice.* (2nd ed.). Silver Spring, MD: American Nurses Association.

Azadfard, M., Huecker, M. R., & Leaming, J. M. (2020). *Opioid Addiction. Stat Pearls [Internet].* https://www.ncbi.nlm.nih.gov/books/NBK448203/.

Beauchamp, T. L., & Childress, J. F. (2013). *Principles of Biomedical Ethics.* (7th ed.). New York, NY: Oxford University Press.

Bernhofer, E. (2011). Ethics: ethics and pain management in hospitalized patients. *OJIN: The Online Journal of Issues in Nursing,* *17*(1), 11. https://doi:10.3912/OJIN.Vol17No01EthCol01.

Bernhofer, E. I., & Sorrell, J. M. (2015). Nurses managing patients' pain may experience moral distress. *Clinical Nursing Research,* *24*(4), 401–414. https://doi.org/10.1177/1054773814533124.

Boerner, K. E., Chambers, C. T., Gahagan, J., Keogh, E., Fillingim, R. B., & Mogil, J. S. (2018). Conceptual complexity of gender and its relevance to pain. *Pain, 11*(159), 2137–2141. https://doi.org/10.1097/j.pain.0000000000001275.

Brannan, C. (2021). What's the difference between morality and ethics? *Britannica.* https://www.britannica.com/story/whats-the-difference-between-morality-and-ethics.

Buchman, D. Z., Leece, P., & Orkin, A. (2017). The epidemic as stigma: the bioethics of opioids. *The Journal of Law, Medicine & Ethics,* *45*(4), 607–620. https://journals.sagepub.com/doi/abs/10.1177/1073110517750600?journalCode=lmec.

Centers for Disease Control and Prevention. (2020). *Overdose Deaths Accelerating During COVID-19.* https://www.cdc.gov/media/releases/2020/p1218-overdose-deaths-covid-19.html.

Carvalho, A. S., Pereira, S. M., Jácomo, A., Magalhães, S., & Araújo, J., et al.(2018). Ethical decision making in pain management: a conceptual framework. *Journal of Pain Research, 11,* 967–976. https://doi.org/10.2147/JPR.S162926.

Craig, K. D., Holmes, C., Hudspith, M., Moor, G., Moosa-Mitha, M., Varcoe, C., et al. (2020). Pain in persons who are marginalized by social conditions. *Pain, 161*(2), 261–265. https://doi.org/10.1097/j.pain.0000000000001719.

Dahlhamer, J., Lucas, J., Zelaya, C., Nahin, R., Mackey, S., DeBar, L., et al. (2018). Prevalence of chronic pain and high-impact chronic pain among adults—United States, 2016. *Morbidity and Mortality Weekly Report, 67*(36), 1001. https://www.ncbi.nlm.nih.gov/pmc/articles/PMC6146950/.

Dineen, K. K., & Ruggles, A. J. (2018). Legal regulation of prescription opioids and prescribers. In J. F. Peppin, J. J. Coleman, K. K. Dineen, & A. J. Ruggles. (Eds.), *Prescription Drug Diversion and Pain: History, Policy, and Treatment* (pp. 17–38). New York, NY: Oxford University Press.

Dowell, D., Haegerich, T. M., & Chou, R. (March 18, 2016). CDC guideline for prescribing opioids for chronic pain—United States, 2016: Recommendations and reports. *Morbidity and Mortality Weekly, 65*(1), 1–49. http://dx.doi.org/10.15585/mmwr.rr6501e1external icon.

Ghoshal, M. (2020). Special report: race, pain management, and the system. *Practical Pain Management, 20*(5). https://www.practicalpainmanagement.com/resources/practice-management/special-report-race-pain-management-system.

Goldberg, D. S. (2014). *The Bioethics of Pain Management: Beyond Opioids.* Oxfordshire, UK: Routledge.

Goldberg, D. (January 23, 2020). *Pain doesn't stigmatize people. We do that to each other.* STAT. https://www.statnews.com/2020/01/23/pain-doesnt-cause-stigma-we-do-that-to-each-other.

Good, M. (1998). A middle-range theory of acute pain management: use in research. *Nursing Outlook, 46*(3), 120–124. https://doi.org/10.1016/s0029-6554(98)90038-0.

Gross, J., & Gordon, D. B. (2019). The strengths and weaknesses of current US policy to address pain. *American Journal of Public Health, 109*(1), 66–72. https://doi.org/10.2105/AJPH.2018.304746.

Hoffman, K. M., Trawalter, S., Axt, J. R., & Oliver, M. N. (2016). Racial bias in pain assessment and treatment recommendations, and false beliefs about biological differences between blacks and whites. *Proceedings of the National Academy of Sciences, 113*(16), 4296–4301. https://doi.org/10.1073/pnas.151604711.

Institute of Medicine. (2011). *Relieving Pain in America: A Blueprint for Transforming Prevention, Care, Education, and Research*. Washington, DC: The National Academies Press. https://doi.org/10.17226/13172.

The Joint Commission. (2021). *Pain Assessment and Management Standards*. https://www.jointcommission.org/resources/patient-safety-topics/pain-management-standards-for-accredited-organizations/#a98ee961a3184ec899b62579053a24a7.

Jungquist, C. R., Vallerand, A. H., Sicoutris, C., Kwon, K. N., & Polomano, R. C. (2017). Assessing and managing acute pain: a call to action. *AJN The American Journal of Nursing, 117*(3), S4–S11. https://doi.org/10.1097/01.naj.0000513526.33816.0e.

Lazaridou, A., Paschali, M., & Edwards, R. R. (2020). Future directions in psychological therapies for pain management. *Pain Medicine, 21*(11), 2624–2626. https://doi.org/10.1093/pm/pnaa335.

Link, B., & Hatzenbuehler, M. L. (2016). Stigma as an unrecognized determinant of population health: research and policy implications. *Journal of Health Politics, Policy and Law, 41*(4), 653–673. https://doi.org/10.1215/03616878-3620869.

Loeser, J. D., & Schatman, M. E. (2017). Chronic pain management in medical education: a disastrous omission. *Postgraduate Medicine, 129*(3), 332–335. https://doi.org/10.1080/00325481.2017.1297668.

Meints, S. M., Cortes, A., Morais, C. A., & Edwards, R. R. (2019). Racial and ethnic differences in the experience and treatment of non-cancer pain. *Pain Management, 9*(3), 317–334. https://doi.org/10.2217/pmt-2018-0030.

Morley, G., Bradbury-Jones, C., & Ives, J. (2020). What is 'moral distress' in nursing? A feminist empirical bioethics study. *Nursing Ethics, 27*(5), 1297–1314. https://doi.org/10.1177/0969733019874492.

Peppin, J., Dineen, K., Ruggles, A., & Coleman, J. (Eds.). (2018). *Prescription Drug Diversion and Pain: History, Policy, and Treatment*. New York, NY: Oxford University Press.

PR Newswire. (September 30, 2019). *Global Acute Pain Market Insights, Epidemiology and Market Forecast to 2028*. https://www.prnewswire.com/news-releases/global-acute-pain-market-insights-epidemiology-and-market-forecast-to-2028-300927702.html.

Reinisch, C. (2019). Ethical patient care overview for doctoral nursing students. *Montclair State University Digital Commons*. https://digitalcommons.montclair.edu/cgi/viewcontent.cgi?article=1002&context=nursing-facpubs.

Schatman, M. E. (Ed.). (2016). *Ethical Issues in Chronic Pain Management*. Boca Raton, FL: CRC Press.

Singh, S., Kumar, A., & Mittal, G. (2021). Ketamine-polymer based drug delivery system for prolonged analgesia: recent advances, challenges and future prospects. *Expert Opinion on Drug Delivery, 18*(8), 1117–1130. https://doi.org/10.1080/17425247.2021.1887134.

Summers, K. M., Deska, J. C., Almaraz, S. M., Hugenberg, K., & Lloyd, E. P. (2021). Poverty and pain: low-SES people are believed to be insensitive to pain. *Journal of Experimental Social Psychology, 95*, 104116. https://doi.org/10.1016/j.jesp.2021.104116.

Turk, D. C., Fillingim, R. B., Ohrbach, R., & Patel, K. V. (2016). Assessment of psychosocial and functional impact of chronic pain. *The Journal of Pain, 17*(9), T21–T49. https://doi.org/10.1016/j.jpain.2016.02.006.

WHO revision of pain management guidelines. (August 27, 2019). https://www.who.int/news/item/27-08-2019-who-revision-of-pain-management-guidelines.

Vallerand, A. H. (2018). Pain-related disparities: are they something nurses should care about? *Pain Management Nursing, 19*(1), 1–2. https://doi.org/10.1016/j.pmn.2017.11.009.

Van Dijk, J. F., Schuurmans, M. J., Alblas, E. E., Kalkman, C. J., & van Wijck, A. J. (2017). Postoperative pain: knowledge and beliefs of patients and nurses. *Journal of Clinical Nursing, 26*(21–22), 3500–3510. https://doi.org/10.1111/jocn.13714.

Volkow, N. (November 12, 2020). *Rising Stimulant Deaths Show that We Face More than Just an Opioid Crisis*. https://www.drugabuse.gov/about-nida/noras-blog/2020/11/rising-stimulant-deaths-show-we-face-more-than-just-opioid-crisis.

Zappaterra, M., & Nanda, U. (2020). Future research in pain. In S. Pangarkar, Q. G. Pham, & B. B. Eapen. (Eds.), *Pain Care Essentials and Innovations* (pp. 255–267). New York, NY: Elsevier.

Zelaya, C. E., Dahlhamer, J. M., Lucas, J. W., & Connor, E. M. (2020). *Chronic Pain and High-Impact Chronic Pain among US Adults, 2019*, NCHS Data Brief, no. 390. Hyattsville, MD: National Center for Health Statistics.

CHAPTER 5

Impact of Pain and Benefits of Pain Management

Tara Michelle Nichols, DNP, ARNP, CCNS, AGCNS, PMGT-BC
Sharon Wrona, DNP, PMGT-BC, CPNP-PC, PMHS, AP-PMN, FAAN*

Introduction

What is the impact of pain on the individual, their social structures (e.g., family, community, work), society, and other unknown entities? "Impact" can be described as one object coming forcibly into contact with another. Thus, impact of pain causes a forceful action when encountered by those undergoing the experience. Impact of pain has been predominately discussed from an economic perspective; however, the benefit of pain as a warning signal is important and should be acknowledged. Because pain is a warning sign, more emphasis should be placed on elevating patient comfort, increasing functioning, and maximizing safety. Emphasizing these three aligns with the call for a biopsychosocial (BPS) approach to pain and consideration of nonpharmacological treatment as first-line. The literature identifies both barriers and enablers to application of a BPS approach and corresponding impact and benefits when employed. Developing predictive analytical models (structural, mathematical, and over-aggregated) is a tool that could establish more precise costs of pain and treatments, including psychosocial factors, impact of social determinants of health, and adverse childhood events (ACEs). With more holistic and precise measures of impact of pain, treatment of pain can be improved for the person in pain in partnership with healthcare professionals (HCPs).

I. Impact and Prevalence of Pain

A. Benefit of pain
   1. Benefit of pain is often negated by negative impact of severe and persistent pain, but in reality, pain is considered a warning signal, an alarm something is wrong. When pain functions in this manner, impact and benefit can save our lives.
   2. When pain signal is firing continually, as with persistent pain syndromes, pain no longer functions as a warning but delivers stimulus that overcomes benefit of pain.
   3. Benefit of experiencing pain is rarely discussed in the literature.
      a. People, mostly children with congenital insensitivity to pain, are unable to experience pain, and others with asymbolia for pain can lose their ability to recognize a painful or threatening stimulus. Congenital insensitivity to pain can result in a life with wounds, bruises, broken bones, and other deficits and usually premature death.
      b. Thus, inability to experience pain results in another illness. From this premise, one can derive there is benefit to pain when it functions as a warning system.
   4. This premise supports approach of rather than focusing on "no pain," focus should be on increasing comfort and preventing progression of acute pain to persistent pain.
B. The complexity of describing impact of pain is reflected in the following statements from the International Association for the Study of Pain (IASP) supporting pain as a BPS phenomenon:
   1. Pain is personal, influenced to varying degrees by BPS factors.
   2. Pain and nociception are different phenomena; thus, pain cannot solely be defined by activity in sensory neurons.
   3. Verbal description is only one way to express pain; thus, inability to communicate (human or nonhuman animal) does not negate ability to experience pain.
   4. Pain experience is learned through life experiences.
   5. A person's self-reported pain experience should be respected.
C. Pain impacts various dimensions of a person's quality of life (Fig. 5.1).
   1. Physical well-being and symptoms
   2. Psychological well-being

---

*Section Editor for the chapter.

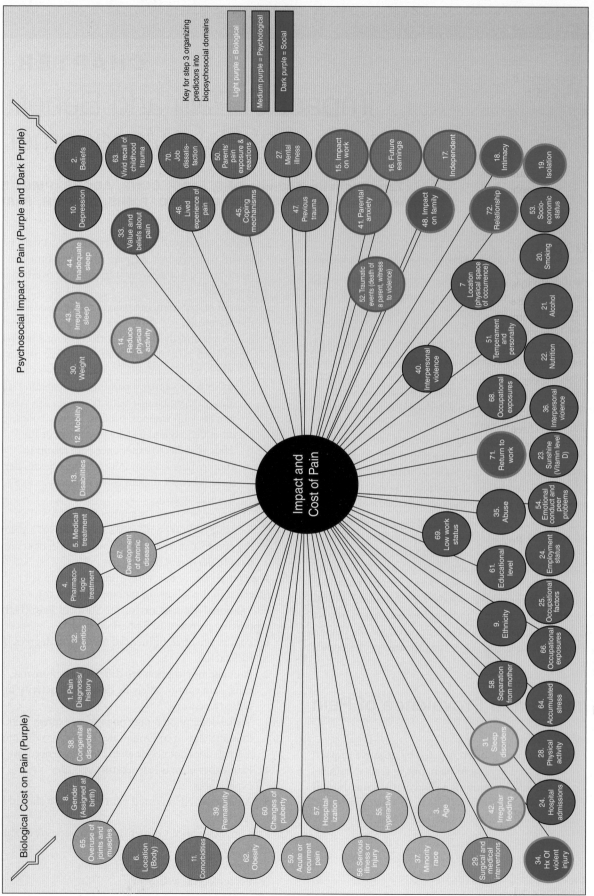

Psychosocial Impact on Pain (Purple and Dark Purple)

Biological Cost on Pain (Purple)

Key for step 3 organizing
predictors into
biopsychosocial domains

Light purple = Biological
Medium purple = Psychological
Dark purple = Social

Figure 5.1 Impact and cost of pain structural model. (From Dr. Tara Nichols, Mason City, Iowa.)

3. Social well-being
4. Spiritual well-being

D. Financial impact:

1. Annual estimated cost of pain in the United States has ranged between $560 billion and $635 billion since 2010.

2. Cost related to treatment:

   a. Agreement exists that nonpharmacological treatments should be used as first-line and are grounded in a BPS approach. Many studies point out cost as one barrier to implementation of nonpharmacological treatments. Yet a study analyzing insurance claims found when first contact for low back pain (LBP) was a chiropractor, physical therapist, or acupuncturist, opioid use was markedly reduced. This study estimated cost savings of $200 million a year with 30% to 50% increase of these therapies being used as first-line treatments.

   b. A systematic review evaluated current evidence for cost-effectiveness of pain management services for persistent back pain.

      1) Cross-study comparison was difficult due to wide variation in interventions, intensity, and duration of program use from study to study.

      2) Three studies found pain management was cost-effective, and two found pain management was not cost-effective.

      3) Review also highlighted:

         a) Gap between learning about BPS approach and adoption of guidelines and protocols into practice

         b) Provider bias against following guidelines and protocols, some due to system issues and others due to personal beliefs

         c) Lack of adequate or accessible assessment tools to assess psychosocial issues and determine corresponding risk and treatment

         d) Many treatments appropriate for psychosocial issues may not be accessible and are costly.

         e) Big data are allowing review and analysis of insurance information to identify trends and patterns supporting broader approach to interprofessional treatment.

E. Prevalence of pain

1. Prevalence of pain varies depending on study methodology.

   a. Most people will experience acute pain at some point in their lives.

   b. Estimates of persistent pain occurrences nationally and globally are summarized in Table 5.1.

Table 5.1

Global Estimates of Persistent Pain

Region	Estimates
United States	• In secondary analysis of *National Longitudinal Study of Adolescent to Adult Health*,[a] results found 4.3% of subjects reported physical disabilities and had significantly higher reports of pain (27.2%) compared to able-bodied peers (15.6%). However, reports of persistent pain and its co-occurrence with depressive symptoms, anxiety, or insomnia were independent of disability status.
United Kingdom	• Persistent pain affects 13% to 50% of adults. • Of those living with persistent pain, 10.4% to 14.3% have moderate to disabling pain. • New cases of persistent pain in one region were estimated at 8% per year.
France	• Over 2-week period, reports collected from 1,805 cancer patients during clinic appointments revealed overall prevalence of persistent pain was at 28.2% (95% CI: 26.3 to 30.5), with neuropathic characteristics present in 20.9% of patients.
Globally	• Study from 42 countries found common persistent pain reports in at least two sites (e.g., headache, stomach, and backache) was 20.6% of 11 to 15-year-olds (varied from 13.2% in Armenia to 33.8 % in Israel). There was higher incidence of multi-site complaints with female adolescents than male adolescents. • Results of systematic analysis of the *Global Burden of Disease* study in 2017, involving 195 countries and territories, found leading causes of YLD in 2017 independent of sex are low back pain, headache disorders, and depressive disorders.

[a]https://www.icpsr.umich.edu/web/DSDR/studies/21600
CI, confidence interval; *YLD*, years lived with disability

---

2. The literature supports the complex interrelationship of advancing age and comorbidities, with some comorbidities being independently associated with persistent pain.

3. A higher prevalence of persistent pain is found in aging populations compared to younger populations.

   a. Number of adults in the United States experiencing various types of pain ranges between 50 to 100 million or more, and 19.6 million people also experience high-impact persistent pain, interfering with life and work. However, controversy exists whether these U.S. values are over- or under-estimations.

   b. In 2017, a 195-country study (*Global Burden of Disease*) reviewed prevalence, incidence, and years lived with disability (YLD) surrounding 354 diseases and injuries.

1) LBP, headache, and depressive disorders were leading causes of YLD for both males and females and have prevailed as leading causes of YLD for over three decades.
2) Recently diabetes emerged as fourth leading cause of YLD, which involves pain from diabetic neuropathy, pain associated with vascular insufficiency, and onset of phantom pain associated with amputations.
3) Other types of pain (e.g., neck pain, arthritis) impacted YLD, but globally, musculoskeletal pain (MSP), when experienced during working years, has major impact on individual's finances.
   a) Global mean prevalence of LBP was found to be 11.9%.
   b) In United Kingdom, MSP is leading cause of persistent pain, with LBP and osteoarthritis comprising half of all cases.
   c) Financial impact of MSP focuses on direct and indirect costs, including both healthcare treatment cost and workplace productivity cost.
   d) Economic burden from this directly impacts many countries' gross domestic product per capita.
   e) Prevalence and burden of MSP disease (and corresponding pain) are anticipated to increase worldwide.
4. Genetics, sex, and comorbidity
   a. Study summarizes reports identifying pain-related role of estrogens and sex-specific differences in pain-related genes. Differences in pain perception based on sex assigned at birth are incomplete and lean toward females having increased sensitivity and reporting of persistent pain.
   b. People with comorbidity, especially those related to mobility issues and chronic mental illness, have greater probability of suffering from persistent pain than do those without comorbidity.
      1) It is common for people with persistent pain to also have other chronic conditions (e.g., increase in people having persistent pain, depression, and cardiovascular disease together).
      2) One study found in people with other medical comorbidities, persistent pain is independent risk factor for all-cause mortality (i.e., death from any cause). This review also stressed impact of co-occurrence of persistent pain and depression, which studies have found can cluster in families and manifest with anxiety and negative beliefs about pain.

3) Comorbidity with persistent pain can limit optimization of traditional pain management treatment options.
c. Percentage of disability is increased when depression and anxiety are added, as they coexist in 30% to 50% of people in pain.

II. Determining Biopsychosocial Impact of Pain

A. BPS approach to pain
1. Although impact of pain is often discussed in terms of economic values, understanding the full impact of pain is much more complex than simply economic impact.
2. BPS approach to pain is described as a clinical approach systematically considering biological, psychological, and socioenvironmental factors and complex interactions in understanding pain.
3. When using BPS model, clinicians focus on both disease and illness, where illness includes interplay of BPS factors.
4. Most clinicians are aware of the biology (neurobiology of nociception process) and psychology (both emotions [immediate response to pain, which is more midbrain focused] and cognitions [where meaning is attached to response]) of pain; however, the social impact of pain has been less defined.
   a. To illustrate BPS impact of pain, consider potential effects of persistent pain: mobility issues, loss of independence, chronic opioid use, difficulty weaning from opioids, anxiety, depression, poor health, financial difficulty, poor relationships, isolation, difficulty with intimacy, difficulty with returning to work, and poor quality of life in general.
   b. Systematic review of BPS approach to MSP found a substantial gap between HCPs learning about BPS approach and adoption of this approach into practice.
B. Often biological aspects of pain drive discussions of the impact of pain.
1. Many types of pain, including MSP, are caused by a combination of BPS risk factors summarized in Table 5.2.
2. Increase in acute or persistent pain, persistent pain with comorbidities, and persistent pain with mental illness (with and without substance use disorder) has made determining impact of pain even more complex.
3. Persistent pain is one of the most common reasons adults seek medical care. However, there is mismatch in evidence-based practice calling for BPS approaches to pain management and implementation of (and adherence to) BPS clinical practice guidelines.

Table 5.2
Risk Factors for Development of Persistent Pain Aligned With Social Determinants of Health

Risk Factors	SDOH	IOM Report (2011)	SDOH
Demographics		**From Birth**	
• Age • Gender • Ethnicity • Cultural background • Employment status • Occupational factors	• Economic stability • Education access and quality • Healthcare access and quality • Neighborhood and environment • Social and community context	• Genetics • Female sex • Minority race or ethnicity • Congenital disorders • Prematurity • Parental anxiety • Irregular feeding and sleeping • Parents' pain exposure and reactions • Temperament and personality	• Education access and quality • Healthcare access and quality • Social and community context
Lifestyle and Behaviors		**Childhood**	
• Smoking • Alcohol • Physical activity • Nutrition • Sunshine and vitamin D	• Economic stability • Education access and quality • Healthcare access and quality • Social and community context	• Physical/sexual abuse • Traumatic events (death of a parent, witness to violence) • Low socioeconomic status • Emotional, conduct, and peer problems • Hyperactivity • Serious illness or injury, hospitalization • Separation from mother • Acute or recurrent pain experience	• Education access and quality • Healthcare access and quality • Social and community context
Clinical		**Adolescence**	
• Pain • Multi-morbidity and mortality • Mental health • Surgical and medical interventions • Weight • Sleep disorders • Genetics	• Education access and quality • Healthcare access and quality • Neighborhood and environment	• Changes of puberty • Gender roles • Education level • Injuries • Obesity • Low levels of fitness	• Economic stability • Education access and quality • Healthcare access and quality • Neighborhood and environment • Social and community context
Psychosocial (other)		**Adulthood**	
• Attitudes and beliefs about pain • History of violent injury • Abuse • Interpersonal violence	• Economic stability • Education access and quality • Healthcare access and quality • Social and community context	• Vivid recall of childhood trauma • Lack of social support accumulated stress ("allostatic load") • Surgery • Overuse of joints and muscles • Occupational exposures • Job dissatisfaction • Low work status • Development of chronic disease • Aging	• Economic stability • Healthcare access and quality • Neighborhood and environment • Social and community context

IOM, Institute of Medicine; *SDOH,* social determinants of health
Mills, S., Nicolson, K. P., & Smith, B. H. (2019).

4. Biological impact of pain
   a. Biological impact of pain includes relationship of pain to morbidity and mortality, which are complex and difficult to determine. In most instances, morbidity and mortality rates of people in pain are associated with co-occurring diagnoses.
   b. Risk factors are associated with development of persistent pain (Table 5.2).
      1) One report outlined similar risk factors that can predispose individuals to development of persistent pain from birth throughout the lifespan.
      2) These risk factors have also been aligned with several social determinants of health (SDOH) categories (i.e., environmental conditions where people are born, live, learn, work, play, worship, and age that affect health, functioning, and quality-of-life outcomes and risks).
      3) Identification of risk factors provides new insight into treatment and potential prevention strategies that may alter course and impact of pain.

C. Within past 5 years, psychological factors have gained prominence in study, assessment, and treatment of pain, the associated "opioid crisis," and the increase in substance use disorder (SUD) and opioid use disorder (OUD).
  1. Diagnosis of depression may be an independent predictor of persistent pain. Depression impacts treatment and management of pain and associated outcomes.
  2. Many types of pain can lead to suffering and cause overwhelming life burden. For example, MSP has reoccurring nature, many times an undetermined trigger, spontaneous resolution with or without treatment, and functional disabilities that impact an individual's quality of life.

D. Psychosocial and relational impact of pain
  1. Systematic review identified five themes representing BPS impact of pain (Table 5.3).
    a. Each theme reveals psychosocial impact of pain, which for many is unquantifiable in economic terms and, as importantly, offers a window into experience of those who suffer silently and alone in pain.
    b. Complexity of quantifying psychological and social costs should not deter effort to identify their impact.
  2. Clinician-patient relationship
    a. BPS approach highlights importance of relationships. A clinician partnering with person in pain is one of the most important parts of treatment.

Table 5.3

Biopsychosocial Themes Related to Pain

Theme	Summary	Domain (Biological, Psychological, Social)	Focus
Activities	**Decline in functioning**: • ADLs, domestic chores, recreational activities, ability to plan ahead **Subthemes:** • Domestic issues, difficulty with leisure activities, rest, sleep, unpredictability of future activities, coping with pain needs	Declining functioning can be associated with biological aspect of pain, but resulting impacts are psychological and social domains.	Focus not only on functioning or mobility but also on psychological and social impact of not being able to complete ADLs' daily chores, or simple activities, as well as unpredictable future
Relationships	**Damaged relationships (with close contacts) subthemes:** • Feelings of isolation, family and cohabitation difficulties, issues with sexual relationships • Issues with social interactions, paradoxical need/desire for support and distance for close relationships while in pain, avoidance of family activities to not ruin it for others, feeling unsupported, concerned about engagement in activities known to exacerbate symptoms and impact on loss of credibility and being believed, dependency, activity limitations negatively impacting relationships marriages where cohabitation became unviable, absence of sexual activity associated with perception of damaged relationship, social withdrawal precipitated by cognitive dissonance of being social and fear of toll of being social (being in uncomfortable social activities, perception of others, fear of sitting for long periods in pain, and spoiling event for others)	Psychological and social domains	Range from feelings of isolation to loss of intimacy to worries of not being believed
Work	**Work needs and fears:** • Need to modify work task • Fear of losing a job • Interpersonal challenges associated with disbelief of coworkers **Subthemes:** • Anxiety • Modifications to work-related activities • Interpersonal relationships • Time off sick • Financial worries (including losing a home and descent into poverty)	Psychological and social domains	Encompassing mental exhaustion of how to modify work, fear of losing job, resulting financial implications, to navigating interpersonal challenges associated with disbelief from coworkers about legitimacy of pain

Table 5.3

Biopsychosocial Themes Related to Pain—cont'd

Theme	Summary	Domain (Biological, Psychological, Social)	Focus
Stigma	**Concerns of legitimacy, credibility, and validation:** • "Being believed" • Establishing themselves as credible **Subthemes:** • Delegitimization (consider in relationship to absence of identifiable pathology or diagnosis) • Frustration from lack of diagnosis • Struggles with ability to meet expectation • Worries of no pathological reason for pain and no diagnosis increased struggles to be believed. • Strong stigmatization led to self-doubt about pain, amplification of symptoms, or self-isolation.	Psychological and social domains	Focus on "being believed" was repeated in almost every theme. "Being believed" was associated with delegitimization (no identifiable pathology or diagnosis associated with no reason for pain).
Changing Outlook	**Changing and accepting outlook:** Adapting and changing outlook led to increased ability to cope. **Subthemes:** Searching for diagnosis: • A different secondary diagnosis gave rise to anger and confusion, especially if diagnosis implied psychosomatic origin. • Obtaining diagnosis facilitated empowerment and adaption when in form of radiographic evidence. Psychological and emotional experiences: • Anger, depression, determination, embarrassment, fear of pathology, feeling imprisoned, feelings of inadequacy, frustration, hopelessness, despair, identity threats, insomnia, irritability, isolation, kinesophobia, mood swings, self-loathing, shame, uselessness Adaptation: • "Listening" to their back • Avoiding certain situations or tasks • Adopting certain postures • Doing certain activities • Relying on faith and positive thoughts • Prioritizing their back • Portraying themselves differently • Acceptance	Psychological and social domains	These sub-themes play a central role in cognition and perception of pain. The focus is on adaption based on individuals change outcome creating improvements in coping.

ADLs, activities of daily living

b. Pain management has been predominately assessed, treated, and researched from perspective of the person in pain, leaving out clinician and importance of clinician-patient relationship.

c. Reports have indicated pain treatment and plans of care depend on strength of clinician-patient relationship, and shared decision-making happens only in a partnering relationship.

1) Pain and its management can be influenced by clinician-patient relationship.

2) Not focusing on importance of clinician-patient relationship extends to not focusing on therapeutic use of self by clinician. This may then extend to not focusing on importance of essential relational skills beyond compassion and empathy.

3. Researchers have attempted to understand obstacles to returning to work as perceived by people with persistent nonmalignant pain and employers.

a. For most individuals, their identity is connected to their work and social status; in children, this concept may apply to their role in the school setting. HCPs managing individuals' pain or ability to return to work/school with pain can help them prepare and navigate return-to-work challenges.

b. People attempting to return to work/school with pain must navigate three main issues: managing pain, managing relationships, and making work/school place adjustments.

1) These aspects of returning to work/school are influenced by societal expectations, self-legitimacy, autonomy, health/illness/

pain representations, prereturn to work/school support and rehabilitation, and system factors (i.e., healthcare, work/school place, and social security).

    2) A mismatch has been found in expectations, and work/school was most stressful with person feeling judged and having difficulty asking for help. Availability of a supportive "other" (person) may be helpful in preparing to handle and accommodate needs of person in pain.

  c. These obstacles make it difficult for person in pain to share times of decreased pain for fear of not being believed when a flare-up occurs. From employer/teacher and coworker/classmate perspective, this interpersonal conflict may cause mistrust and become a barrier to returning to work/school. This may lead to feeling need to justify absenteeism, pain, and limitations.

  d. Return to work/school was most successful (depending on type of work and ability to make accommodations) and when belief accommodations were not burdensome for employer/school. People in pain consistently report feelings of not being believed or having their pain illegitimatized, whereas managers/teachers report feeling person with pain was taking advantage of system.

III. Using Predictive Analytics in Pain Management

A. Why use predictive analytics to study impact of pain?

1. Predicting impact of pain is more complex than just economics.
2. Predictive analytics is a category of data analytics aimed at making predictions about future outcomes based on historical data and analytics techniques (e.g., statistical modeling, machine learning).
3. Developing a predictive model of impact may help quantify pain and impact of BPS approach to pain management.
4. Several organizations have attempted to quantify impact of pain and present compelling analyses, but most fell short of a holistic analysis.
5. Building on economic definition from Institute of Medicine (IOM) and including cost of psychosocial impact of pain, a holistic definition of the

impact of pain would be economic cost + psychosocial cost.

B. Predictive analytics applied to pain

1. Proposing a predictive model focused on impact of pain aligns with National Pain Strategy (2015) calling for more precise estimates.
2. Existing literature reinforces importance of using a predictive analytic framework to help understand BPS interdependence of pain.

  a. One study looked at patient-reported outcome measures at 12 months after elective lumbar fusion and found prediction tools could provide insight for shared decision-making. Main predictive variables (i.e., risk factors) were age, sex, race, insurance status, and smoking status.

  b. Aim of another study was to systematically summarize current evidence on the topic and facilitate interdisciplinary collaboration.

  c. Yet another study focused on creating a pain information model from 51,000 records of adults admitted to clinical and surgical units between 2015 and 2019 using predictive analytics.

    1) Goal was to review pain assessments, interventions, goals, and outcomes to determine patients most likely to be discharged with self-reported pain.

    2) Predictive modeling can guide nurses' and other health professionals' decision-making in effective pain treatments.

3. Long-term application of predictive models may facilitate personalized treatments, reduce cost, and improve health outcomes.

C. A proposal for developing a predictive model of the impact of pain from a BPS perspective uses Nelson's Methodology for Healthcare Analytics (NMHA).

1. Simply, Nelson's methodology involves:

  a. Phase I: Building specified model
  b. Phase II: Data discovery and mathematics
  c. Phase III: Examine data
  d. Phase IV: Respecify model and repeat
  e. Phase V: Machine learn, automate, and forecast

2. See Box 5.1 for specifics of each phase

D. Application of Nelson's Methodology for Healthcare Analytics

1. Proposing BPS structural and measurement model: cost of pain

  a. NMHA methodology was developed in quest to improve healthcare outcomes, cost, care, and staff engagement in context of theory, mission, and vision of organization.

Box 5.1

Nelson's Methodology (16 steps) for Healthcare Analytics

Phase I: Building a Specified Model

Step 1: Identify variable of interest (the outcome variable).

Step 2: Identify things that relate things to variable of interest (the predictor variables).

Step 3: Organize predictor variables by similarity in a structural model.

Step 4: Rank variables based on how directly they appear to relate to variable of interest (outcome variable).

Step 5: Structure predictor variables in model that visually communicates their relationship to variable of interest (outcome variable).

Phase II: Data Discovery and Mathematics

Step 6: Evaluate if and/or where data on predictor variables are already being collected (this is also referred to as data discovery).

Step 7: Find ways to measure predictor variables not currently being measured.

Step 8: Select an analytic method (it may or may not be predictive analytics).

Step 9: Collect retrospective data right away and take action if possible.

Phase III: Examine the Data

Step 10: Examine data before analysis (i.e., clean data and look for outliers).

Step 11: Analyze the data.

Step 12: Present data to staff; get their interpretation of results.

Phase IV: Respecify Model and Repeat

Step 13: Respecify measurement model as needed (add or subtract variable discovered to be important to variable of interest).

Step 14: Repeat steps 2–13 if explained variance declines (indicating resolution of risk predictors).

Phase V: Machine Learn, Automate and Forecast

Step 15: Interface and automate.

Step 16: Write predictive mathematical formulas electronically to manage outcomes in real time and even proactively by using forecasting of risk.

due to pain + value of lost productivity [days of worked missed + hours of work lost + lower wages]) to include the psychosocial impact.

1) Impact of pain has only recently considered psychological perspectives; thus, only biological and psychological perspectives are predominately reported in the literature.

2) Social aspect of pain is rarely reported, and absence of social consideration creates an incomplete picture of the impact of pain. Leaving these perspective measures out will result in inaccurate conclusions.

3) Fig. 5.2 represents over-aggregated models, which take form as similar variables are grouped together in remaining steps and can be used to communicate predictive model to others.

2. Nelson's methodology has ability to bring simplicity to complex ideas and transform them into elegant scientific predictive models.

   a. Models are best designed by interprofessional teams, from a place of empathy, with end user in mind. Consider benefits, not just to people in pain but to people who spend hours caring for them, to have a way to consider a true BPS approach to pain.

      1) Perhaps one of the most powerful illustrations of predictive analytics is ACEs study, which translated many psychosocial predictors into a numeric score.

      2) ACEs survey outlines ten types of childhood trauma with potential lifelong impacts.

         a) Five ACE items are personal and include verbal abuse, physical abuse, sexual abuse, physical neglect, and emotional neglect.

         b) Five more ACE items relate to other family members and include alcoholics, mothers who were victims of domestic violence, incarcerated family members, mental illness, and parental loss through divorce, death, or abandonment.

   b. Using NMHA to guide model development of impact of pain, the potential impact of ACEs is revealed and now can be integrated into a scientific formula to predict the impact.

   c. Interprofessional team should consider relationship of ACE scores on impact of pain because it has been proposed that the higher the ACE score, the greater the impact of pain not only to the individual but to family, healthcare, and society at large.

3. An expanded theory of impact of pain might be that pain is a BPS phenomenon.

   a. Impact should be evaluated based on this theoretical premise (including clinician-patient

   b. Four foundational principles support 16 steps contained within Nelson's methodology (Table 5.4): data, theory, operations, and leadership.

   c. Proposed model would attempt to expand definition of the impact of pain beyond the economic cost (i.e., incremental cost of medical care

Table 5.4

Measurement Model: Impact of Pain Illustrating Data Discovery

Measurement model illustrating biopsychosocial predictors and data discovery
Note: Numbers in front of predictors represent ranking of impact of predictor variable on outcome variable of interest. Ranking is step four in the NMHA process.

Biological Predictor Variables	Specific Measurement (Data Point)	Data Discovery
1. Pain diagnosis/history	ICD 11 code	Demographics from medical record
3. Age	Selection 1 to 100	
6. Location (body part of pain)	List of selection of body parts up to three	
8. Gender (assigned at birth)	Female = 1 Male =2	
9. Ethnicity	Team discuss if 9 and 37 needed	
11. Comorbidities (DM, CVD, COPD)	ICD 11 code	
37. Minority race	White = 1 Nonwhite = 2 with follow-up questions with specific race	
30. Weight	Kilograms	
13. Disabilities	ICD 11 code	
56. Serious illness and injury	ICD 11 code	
4. Pharmacologic treatments	List of top 15 to 20 pharmacologic treatments	Pharmacy medical records/billing or insurance (inpatient) Prescription monitoring–(outpatient)
5. Medical treatments	List of top medical treatments and diagnostic test (10 each)	Medical records/billing or insurance
27. Pain	—	—
12. Mobility	Independent = 1 Partial independent = 2 Dependent = 3	Medical records–nurse assessment (inpatient) Patient self-report clinic assessment (outpatient)
Psychosocial Predictor Variables	**Specific Measurement (Data Point)**	**Data Discovery**
2. Beliefs (specifically what kind of beliefs)	Team to discuss if domain predictor If 2 and 33 are needed How represented by person in pain and clinician	Patient/clinician self-report survey
10. Depression	ICD 11 code	Medical records
27. Mental health (other than depression)	ICD 11 code	Medical records
33. Attitudes and beliefs about pain	Team to discuss if domain predictor If 2 and 33 are needed; how represented by person in pain and clinician	Patient/clinician self-report survey
45. Coping mechanisms	Team to discuss how to measure	Patient/clinician self-report survey
7. Location (physical space of occurrence of pain)	Home = 1 Hospital = 2 with follow-up question of unit Work = 3 with follow-up question of type of work	Medical record, patient portal, or self-report survey question
35. Abuse	ACEs score	ACEs survey
34. History of violent injury		
61. Educational level		
24. Employment status		
52. Traumatic events (death of a parent, witness to violence)		
53. Socioeconomic status		
58. Separation from mother or parent		
19. Isolation		
54. Emotional conduct and peer problems		
40. Interpersonal violence		
63. Vivid recall of childhood trauma		

(From Dr. Tara Nichols, Mason City, Iowa.)
ACEs, adverse childhood events; *COPD,* chronic obstructive pulmonary disorder; *CVD,* cardiovascular disease; *DM,* diabetes mellitus; *ICD 11, International Classification of Diseases,* 11th edition; *NMHA,* Nelson's Methodology for Healthcare Analytics

Variable of interest–Impact and cost of pain

Theory:
1. Pain is a biopsychosocial phenomenon, and the impact and cost should be evaluated based on this theoretical premise to improve treatment, cost, and shared decision-making. However, the cost of pain has predominantly only been evaluated from a biological perspective. Since one definition of the economic cost of pain is: incremental cost of medical care duo to pain + value of lost productivity (days of worked missed + hours of work lost + hours of work lost) + lower wages. The proposed model would attempt to expand this definition to the economic cost (as defined above) + the psychosocial impact.
2. Even less reported on in the literature is the impact of the clinician-patient relationship and the impact of the beliefs and values of the patient and clinician; how these aspects may influence the impact and cost of pain.
3. In this model, it is believed that the clinician-patient relationship and the beliefs and values of the patient and clinician are dominate predictors influencing the biopsychosocial impact and cost of pain and each other.

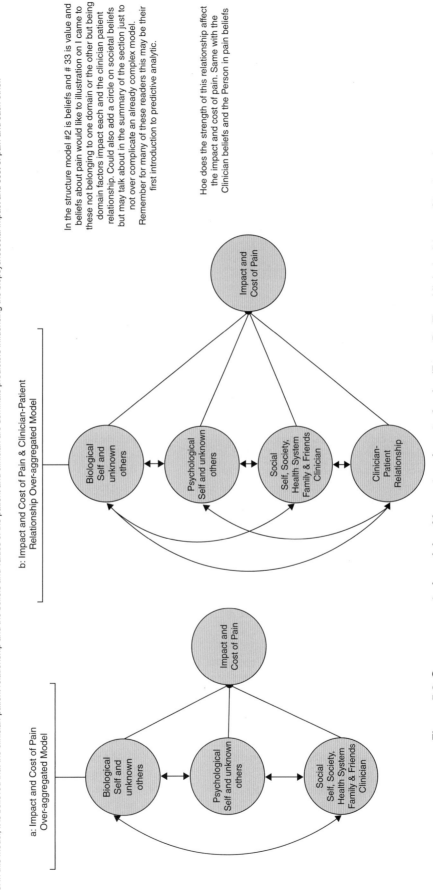

Figure 5.2 Over-aggregated models of impact and cost of pain. (From Dr. Tara Nichols, Mason City, Iowa.)

relationship, beliefs and values of patient and clinician) to improve treatment, cost, and shared decision-making.
  b. Using NMHA, a structural, mathematical, and over-aggregated predicative model of cost and impact of pain has been proposed.
    1) Within the analysis of predictive variables in mathematical model, connection between psychosocial factors and ACEs is exposed.
    2) Next steps would be to bring together an interprofessional team of HCPs, computer scientists, statisticians, and people in pain to continue to build and refine model for a pilot before implementation. See Table 5.4 for an example.

IV. Benefits of Pain/Comfort Management

A. Biopsychosocial approach to pain assessment and treatment
  1. The BPS approach:
    a. Highlights importance of clinician-patient relationship and promotion of comfort as outcome
    b. Enhances importance of independent and interdependent role of nurse within interprofessional team
    c. Causes shift from just pain management to pain and comfort management, whereby care of person in pain is focused on increasing comfort to dampen pain for a productive life. In this approach, comfort is more than just the absence of pain.
  2. One theory of comfort provides HCPs a powerful resource when working to relieve pain to create an experience that strengthens another by having needs for relief, ease, or transcendence met in physical, psychospiritual, environmental, and social contexts.
  3. Nurses must know their dependent, independent, and interdependent roles within healthcare team in pain and comfort management. Table 5.5 outlines modifiable factors that impact pain, which nurse can work with interprofessional team and person in pain to address.
B. Development of pain and comfort management plan
  1. Identify types of pain:
    a. Nociceptive pain (somatic or visceral)
    b. Acute
    c. Persistent
    d. Neuropathic (central or peripheral)
    e. Inflammatory
    f. Psychogenic
    g. Sensory hypersensitivity pain

Table 5.5	
Modifiable Life Factors Impacting Pain	
Physical Factors	**Psychological Factors**
• Posture • Function and occupation • Neuroplasticity • Strength/endurance/pacing • Mobility/movement • Sleep/rest/fatigue • Diet/nutrition	• Mindfulness • Anxiety/depression • Cognition/attention • Happiness/enjoyment • Self-efficacy/meaning/purpose • Sense of safety/sense of place • Self-image/shame
Social Factors	**Spiritual Factors**
• Caregiver burden • Roles and responsibilities • Social support/isolation • Transportation	• Suffering • Meaning of pain • Faith/religiosity • Hope/despair

(Reprinted with permission from Oregon Health Authority.)

  2. Screen emotional descriptors and identify types of traumatic experiences/toxic stressors that can contribute to pain experience, as these can lead to altered processing of sensory stimuli and emotional processing of pain opposed to nociceptive processing of pain.
    a. War
    b. Abuse
    c. Assault
    d. Neglect
    e. Environment
  3. Identify and treat sources of other discomforts. Multiple studies report people with pain are willing to endure slightly higher pain scores to decrease associated discomforts.
    a. Nausea
    b. Itching
    c. Constipation
    d. Emesis
    e. Temperature sensitivity
    f. Isolation
    g. Depression
    h. Fear
    i. Anger
    j. Restless
    k. Anxiety
    l. Insomnia
  4. In consideration of BPS approach to pain, consider how to elevate assessment and treatment of psychosocial factors.
    a. The following tools were identified for people newly diagnosed with persistent pain to assess (predict) risk of developing persistent pain disability:

1) Örebro Musculoskeletal Pain Screening Questionnaire (ÖMPSQ)
   a) Developed for adults with acute and persistent MSP and predicts long-term disability and work absenteeism
   b) ÖMPSQ subgroupings resulted in one of two intervention approaches: 1) cognitive behavioral therapy (CBT) pain and disability treatment, or 2) early workplace program where psychosocial variables identified in screening were addressed.
      (1) Results of CBT group (high risk) compared to treatment as usual showed both improved cost-effectiveness and benefit.
      (2) CBT group had nine-fold reduction in long-term absenteeism and fewer healthcare visits, even after 5 years (with 97% participation rate). This group also had less pain, was more active, and had higher quality of life compared to treatment-as-usual group.
2) STarT Back Screening Tool is used for screening physical and psychosocial prognostic indicators (risk factors) for persistent, disabling back pain.
   b. The higher the score on both tools indicates increased risk, and results are stratified as low, medium, and high risk.
      1) Study found both tools are acceptable for discriminating disabilities, and ÖMPSQ had an 83% average for predicting absenteeism outcomes.
      2) Once person in pain has been screened with one of these tools and stratified into risk group, interventions are selected for pain and psychosocial risk factors.
      3) For example, low risk on StarT Back Screening Tool would result in conservative treatment (education on self-management, reassurance, education on activity, and, when appropriate, medication), whereas those with medium risk receive physical therapy treatment aimed at reducing pain and disability while increasing physical capacity. Those stratified to high risk saw a physical therapist who used simple cognitive behavioral techniques, and these three groups were compared to treatment as usual.
      4) Study found medium- and high-risk groups had clinically important results.
   c. With an aggressive model to consider full impact and benefits of BPS approach to pain

and comfort management within context of strong clinician-patient relationship, all will benefit.
   d. Using the BPS approach to assess, manage, and treat pain within context of therapeutic clinician-patient relationship has many benefits and can minimize impact of pain.
C. Benefits of effective pain treatment plan:
   1. Improved quality of life
   2. Improved sleep
   3. Physical impact
   4. Improved social relationships
   5. Increased ability to return to work and or school
   6. Improved clinician-patient relationship
D. Morbidity and mortality of improper or inadequately treated pain
   1. Undertreatment of persistent pain: the silent epidemic
      a. Large percentage of U.S. citizens suffer from persistent pain, resulting in one of top reasons people are seen in outpatient clinics.
      b. Combination of inadequately treated persistent pain and OUD can result in significant morbidity and mortality.
      c. Prevalence of people with comorbidity combinations of trauma, depression, and/or anxiety with persistent pain:
         1) Over 67% of patients with persistent pain suffer from comorbid psychiatric disorders.
         2) Over 100 million people in the U.S. suffer from debilitating persistent pain.
         3) Research showed between 5% and 14% lifetime prevalence for suicide attempts of people with persistent pain, and 20% experience suicidal ideation. Of people with persistent pain who committed suicide, 53.6% died of firearm-related injuries, while 16.2% died by opioid poisoning.
      d. Inadequate treatment also impacts range of motion, morning stiffness, weakness, and change in muscle strength; patients should be asked about discomforts like spasms, aches, bloating, gas, and temperature changes that may not be associated with pain.
      e. Inadequate treatment and pain can impact functioning and activities of daily living, relationships, and recreational activities, which can lead to isolation and depression. As result of these and other symptoms that can occur with inadequate treatment of pain, people experience lost work productivity, reduced quality of life, and stigma.
      f. Inadequate treatment of cancer-related pain during or following cancer treatment due to

stigma of using opioid medications and resistance to trying nonpharmacologic treatments

1) Recent studies found one-third of women develop persistent pain after breast cancer surgery or radiation (e.g., persistent nerve pain in chest wall, armpit, and arm after surgery).

2) Survivors of leukemias may experience chronic graft-versus-host disease, causing host of changes to integumentary system, including joint pain and dry eyes, mouth, and vagina. These types of pains and discomforts are often overlooked or inadequately treated.

3) In January 2019, it was estimated 16.9 million individuals with history of cancer were alive, living up to 30 years beyond their diagnosis. Most common side effects of cancer and treatment are pain, fatigue, and emotional distress (trauma). Yet even more distressing is these people are no longer being actively treated, so surveillance on their quality of life or pain management is not being monitored. These people are at high risk for substance misuse without proper HCP assistance to sort out different types of pain and devise plan for proper treatment.

g. Self-rated health (SRH) is major predictor of mortality. Relationship of SRH and pain is not well understood. One study looked at relationship of SRH, age, and pain.

1) Study found a 4 to 5 times lower SRH score ($p < 0.001$) for those reporting pain than those without pain.

2) People with fibromuscular dysplasia (FMD) (an enlargement or narrowing of medium-sized arteries) can find themselves experiencing severe discomfort and poor treatment outcomes.

3) People with FMD complain of migraine, neck pain, and flank pain, which are associated with decrease in mental functioning. Migraine and neck pain were also associated with lower physical ability.

4) Reports of abdominal pain by these people are associated with higher levels of depression compared to people without FMD. Additionally, abdominal pain and pulsatile tinnitus were associated with greater anxiety. Migraine was also associated with lower SRH. Participants with history of stroke/transient ischemic attack are at 2.42 times the odds of poor SRH compared to those without stroke/transient ischemic attack.

h. Persistent pain in the elderly is associated with debilitation, isolation, and suffering when treatment is inadequate.

1) Due to cognitive impairment and dementia, the elderly may not be able to self-report their pain.

2) Many pharmaceutical treatments are contraindicated or ineffective and present a host of side effects (i.e., urinary retention, constipation, sedation, mental impairment, and safety risk).

2. Increase in illicit drug use

a. In 2019, the Food and Drug Administration (FDA) published a safety announcement warning of reports of serious harm to patients who are physically dependent on opioids suddenly having the medicines discontinued or the dose reduced. The announcement warned of serious withdrawal symptoms, uncontrolled pain, psychological distress, and suicide.

1) FDA warned that due to the onset of uncontrolled pain or withdrawal symptoms, people may turn to other sources of relief, which may be confused with misuse and abuse.

2) The announcement went on to warn of the use of illicit opioids, such as heroin and other substances, to treat pain or withdrawal symptoms.

b. Studies have found more than half of people taken off long-term high-dose prescribed opioids were not weaned but discontinued suddenly. Nearly 50% of those who had opioids abruptly discontinued had an opioid-related event, and less than 1% received OUD treatment.

3. Inequities in pain and comfort treatment

a. Inequities in pain management exist on many levels and in many situations. However, studies report disproportionately less pain treatment provided to Blacks compared to Whites for same type of pain.

1) Meta-analysis of 20 years of studies on pain management in numerous settings found Blacks were 22% less likely than Whites to receive any pain medication for same type of pain.

2) Blacks receiving less pain treatment than Whites was seen in cancer pain, postpartum pain, and acute pain in emergency department.

3) In Blacks, multidisciplinary care has been shown to decrease depressive symptoms and improve functioning related to pain but not reported pain severity.

4) Due to inadequate pain treatment, Blacks are more likely to resort to repeat emergency department visits to manage their pain.

5) Reason for differences in treatments are influenced by:

a) Implicit bias: automatic unintentional favoring that impacts one's judgment, decisions, and behaviors

b) False beliefs: A study found large number of lay people and medical students held false beliefs that Black skin was thicker than White skin and Blacks' nerve endings were less sensitive than Whites'.

c) Communication

(1) Older Blacks compared to older Whites are more hesitant to discuss pain or may feel discussing pain will only intensify pain, thus preferring to ignore pain.

(2) Blacks may struggle to have quality provider-patient communication compared to Whites.

(d)Long history of distrust of Blacks and healthcare (e.g., story of Henrietta Lacks and Tuskegee syphilis study)

b. Very little research exists on inequities in pain and comfort treatment for the lesbian, gay, bisexual, transgender, or queer (LGBTQ+) population. In 2020, one in six adults in Gen Z identified as LGBTQ+.

1) Studies have found people who identify as LGBTQ+ experience more frequent functional limitations due to pain from multiple sites compared to cisgender heterosexuals.

2) Pain types were headache; migraines; abdominal pain; digestive issues; back, shoulder, and neck pain; and arthritis.

3) High prevalence (51.8% to 69.1%) of persistent pain and depression

4) LGBTQ+ adolescents have higher incidences of depression, anxiety, and increased suicidal behavior than do non-LGBTQ+ adolescents. These comorbidities create unique challenges in treating persistent pain in this population.

Bibliography

Abd-Elsayed, A., Heyer, A. M., & Schatman, M. E. (2021). Disparities in the treatment of the LGBTQ population in chronic pain management. *Journal of Pain Research, 14*, 3623. https://doi.org/10.2147/JPR.S348525.

AlMazrou, S. H., Elliott, R. A., Knaggs, R. D., & Al Aujan, S. S. (2020). Cost-effectiveness of pain management services for chronic low back pain: a systematic review of published studies. *BMC Health Services Research, 20*(1), 1–11. https://doi.org/10.1186/s12913-020-5013-1.

American Cancer Society. (2019). *Cancer Treatment and Survivorship Facts and Figures 2019–2021*. Atlanta, GA: American Cancer Society. https://www.cancer.org/content/dam/cancer-org/research/cancer-facts-and-statistics/cancer-treatment-and-survivorship-facts-and-figures/cancer-treatment-and-survivorship-facts-and-figures-2019-2021.pdf.

Bennett, D. (2022). The pain of trauma the trauma of pain: breaking down the silos to address the opioid crisis. In, *ASPMN National Conference,* September 14–17. http://aspmn.org/education/annualconference/Pages/Program.aspx.

Blyth, F. M., Briggs, A. M., Schneider, C. H., Hoy, D. G., & March, L. M. (2019). The global burden of musculoskeletal pain—where to from here? *American Journal of Public Health, 109*(1), 35–40. doi:10.2105/AJPH.2018.304747.

Bonnie, R. J., Ford, M. A., & Phillips, J. K. (2017). National Academies of Sciences, Engineering, Medicine. Pain management and the opioid epidemic: balancing societal and individual benefits and risks of prescription opioid use. Washington, DC: *National Academies of Science.* https://doi.org/10.17226/24781.

Dahlhamer, J., Lucas, J., Zelaya, C., Nahin, R., Mackey, S., DeBar, L., et al. (2018). Prevalence of chronic pain and high-impact chronic pain among adults — United States, 2016. *MMWR Morbidity and Mortality Weekly Report, 67*, 1001–1006. http://dx.doi.org/10.15585/mmwr.mm6736a2.

de la Vega, R., Groenewald, C., Bromberg, M. H., Beals-Erickson, S. E., & Palermo, T. M. (2018). Chronic pain prevalence and associated factors in adolescents with and without physical disabilities. *Developmental Medicine & Child Neurology, 60*(6), 595–601. https://doi.org/10.1111/dmcn.13705.

Dinoff, B. L. (2019). Ethical treatment of people with chronic pain: an application of Kaldjian's framework for shared decision-making. *British Journal of Anaesthesia, 123*(2), e179–e182. https://doi.org/10.1016/j.bja.2019.04.042.

Domenichiello, A. F., & Ramsden, C. E. (2019). The silent epidemic of chronic pain in older adults. *Progress in Neuro-Psychopharmacology and Biological Psychiatry, 93*, 284–290.

Dydyk, A., Sizemore, D., Trachsel, L., Dulebohn, S., & Porter, B. (2022). Tennessee controlled substance prescribing for acute and chronic pain. *StatPearls [Internet].*

Fayaz, A., Croft, P., Langford, R. M., Donaldson, L. J., & Jones, G. T. (2016). Prevalence of chronic pain in the UK: a systematic review and meta-analysis of population studies. *BMJ Open, 6*(6), e010364. https://doi.org/10.1136/bmjopen-2015-010364.

Froud, R., Patterson, S., Eldridge, S., Seale, C., Pincus, T., Rajendran, D., et al. (2014). A systematic review and meta-synthesis of the impact of low back pain on people's lives. *BMC Musculoskeletal Disorders, 15*, 50. https://doi.org/10.1186/1471-2474-15-50.

Gaedke Nomura, A. T., de Abreu Almeida, M., Johnson, S., & Pruinelli, L. (2021). Pain information model and its potential for predictive analytics: applicability of a big data science framework. *Journal of Nursing Scholarship, 53*(3), 315–322. https://doi.org/10.1111/jnu.12648.

Grant, M., O-Beirne-Elliman, J., Froud, R., Underwood, M., & Seers, K. (2019). The work of return to work. Challenges of returning to work when you have chronic pain: a meta-ethnography. *BMJ Open, 9*(6), e025743. https://doi.org/10.1136/bmjopen-2018-025743.

Gobina, I., Villberg, J., Välimaa, R., Tynjälä, J., Whitehead, R., Cosma, A., et al. (2019). Prevalence of self-reported chronic pain among adolescents: evidence from 42 countries and regions. *European Journal of Pain, 23*(2), 316–326. https://doi.org/10.1002/ejp.1306.

Interagency Pain Research Coordinating Committee (IPRCC). (2015). *National Pain Strategy: A Comprehensive Population Health-Level Strategy for Pain.* Washington, DC: Department of Health and Human Services. Retrieved from https://www.iprcc.nih.gov/sites/default/files/documents/NationalPainStrategy_508C.pdf.

Linton, S. J., & Kienbacher, T. (2020). Psychological subgrouping to assess the risk for the development or maintenance of chronic musculoskeletal pain: Is this the way forward? *The Clinical Journal of Pain, 36*(3), 172–177. https://doi.org/10.1097/AJP.0000000000000787.

Liu, D., Cheng, D., Houle, T. T., Chen, L., Zhang, W., & Deng, H. (2018). Machine learning methods for automatic pain assessment using facial expression information: protocol for a systematic review and meta-analysis. *Medicine, 97*(49), e13421. https://doi.org/10.1097/MD.0000000000013421.

Mark, T. L., & Parish, W. (2019). Opioid medication discontinuation and risk of adverse opioid-related health care events. *Journal of Substance Abuse Treatment, 103*, 58–63.

Meints, S. M., & Edwards, R. R. (2018). Evaluating psychosocial contributions to chronic pain outcomes. *Progress in Neuro-Psychopharmacology & Biological Psychiatry, 87*(Pt B), 168–182. https://doi.org/10.1016/j.pnpbp.2018.01.017.

Mills, S., Nicolson, K. P., & Smith, B. H. (2019). Chronic pain: a review of its epidemiology and associated factors in population-based studies. *British Journal of Anaesthesia, 123*(2), e273–e283. https://doi.org/10.1016/j.bja.2019.03.023.

National Academies of Sciences, Engineering, and Medicine; Health and Medicine Division (2019). Board on Global Health; Board on Health Sciences Policy; Global Forum on Innovation in Health Professional Education; Forum on Neuroscience and Nervous System Disorders. In Stroud, C., Posey Norris, S. M., & Bain, L. (Eds.), *The Role of Nonpharmacological Approaches to Pain Management: Proceedings of a Workshop.* Washington, DC: National Academies Press (US). https://doi.org/10.17226/25406.

National Quality Forum. (2015). *National Quality Partners Playbook: Opioid Stewardship.* Retrieved from https://www.qualityforum.org/Home.aspx.

Nelson, J. W., Felgen, J., & Hozak, M. A. (Eds.). (2021). *Using Predictive Analytics to Improve Healthcare Outcomes.* Hoboken, NJ: Wiley.

Nichols, T., & Nelson, J. W. (2021). Theory and Model Development to Address Pain Relief by Improving Comfort. In Nelson, J. W., Felgen, J., & Hozak, M. A. (Eds.), *Using Predictive Analytics to Improve Healthcare Outcomes* (pp. 171–182). Hoboken, NJ: Wiley. https://doi.org/10.1002/9781119747826.ch13.

Nichols, T. (2018). Comfort as a multidimensional construct for pain management. *Creative Nursing, 24*(2), 88–98. https://doi.org/10.1891/1078-4535.24.2.88.

Ng, W., Slater, H., Starcevich, C., Wright, A., Mitchell, T., & Beales, D. (2021). Barriers and enablers influencing healthcare professionals' adoption of a biopsychosocial approach to musculoskeletal pain: a systematic review and qualitative evidence synthesis. *Pain, 162*(8), 2154–2185. https://doi.org/10.1097/j.pain.0000000000002217.

Olavsrud, J., & Edwards, J. (2023) What is predictive analytics? Transforming data into future insights. Retrieved from https://www.cio.com/article/3273114/what-is-predictive-analytics-transforming-data-into-future-insights.html.

Pizzo, P., Clark, N., Carter-Pokras, O., Christopher, M., Farrar, J. T., Follett, K. A., et al. *Relieving Pain in America: A Blueprint for Transforming Prevention, Care, Education, and Research.* Washington, DC: The National Academies Press. https://doi.org/10.17226/13172.

Quddusi, A., Eversdijk, H., Klukowska, A. M., de Wispelaere, M. P., Kernbach, J. M., Schröder, M. L., et al. (2020). External validation of a prediction model for pain and functional outcome after elective lumbar spinal fusion. *European Spine Journal, 29*(2), 374–383. https://doi.org/10.1007/s00586-019-06189-6.

Raja, S. N., Carr, D. B., Cohen, M., Finnerup, N. B., Flor, H., Gibson, S., et al. (2020). The revised International Association for the Study of Pain definition of pain: concepts, challenges, and compromises. *Pain, 161*(9), 1976–1982. https://doi.org/10.1097/j.pain.0000000000001939.

Sabin, J.A. (2020). How we fail black patients. Retrieved from https://www.aamc.org/news-insights/how-we-fail-black-patients-pain.

Siegmund, L. A., Gornik, H. L., Mahlay, N. F., Hornacek, D., Bena, J., & Morrison, S. (2022). The relationship among pain location, complications, and quality of life in individuals with fibromuscular dysplasia. *Pain Management Nursing, 23*(3), 273–280.

Stevens, J. E. (2015). "Got your ACE score?." Retrieved from http://acestoohigh.com/got-you-ace-score/.

Telusca, N., Gaisey, J. N., Woods, C., Khan, J. S., & Mackey, S. (2022). Strategies to promote racial healthcare equity in pain medicine: a call to action. *Pain Medicine, 23*(7), 1225–1230.

US Department of Health and Human Services. (2019). *Pain Management Best Practices Inter-Agency Task Force Report: Updates, Gaps, Inconsistencies, and Recommendations.* Retrieved from US Department of Health and Human Services website: https://www.hhs.gov/sites/default/files/pmtf-final-report-2019-05-23.pdf.

US Food and Drug Administration. (2019). FDA identifies harm reported from sudden discontinuation of opioid pain medicines and requires label changes to guide prescribers on gradual, individualized tapering. https://www.fda.gov/drugs/drug-safety-and-availability/fda-identifies-harm-reported-sudden-discontinuation-opioid-pain-medicines-and-requires-label-changes.

CHAPTER 6

Nursing Process for Pain Management

Donna Sipos Cox, MSN, FNP-C, ONC, PMGT-BC, AP-PMN
Ann Schreier, PhD, BSN, MSN, RN*

Introduction

The nursing process is the cornerstone of all nursing practice. This chapter will explore each step of the process, including principles of assessment, North American Nursing Diagnosis Association International (NANDA-I) diagnoses surrounding pain, and the importance of synthesizing assessment data to formulate an evidenced-based, holistic, individualized plan for pain management. Nursing interventions for specific patient populations as well as nursing responsibilities in the evaluation of pain management interventions will be discussed.

I. Nursing Process Overview

A. The nursing process is a problem-solving approach used by nurses to meet patient needs and is the guiding framework for nursing practice.
B. As an evidence-based method, the nursing process uses critical thinking, scientific reasoning, clinical judgment, and problem-solving.
C. Critical knowledge competencies must be understood within nursing practice prior to the assessment and accurate performance of the nursing process. Critical competencies needed to apply to persons' pain experience include:
  1. Theories of pain
  2. Related concepts in pathophysiology (e.g., depression, fatigue)
  3. Manifestation of pain
  4. At-risk populations
D. Interrelated steps of the nursing process include:
  1. Assessment
  2. Diagnosis
  3. Planning
  4. Implementation
  5. Evaluation
E. Most professions have a common language shared within the profession. In nursing, a shared language exists between NANDA-I and University of Iowa classifications.

1. NANDA-I develops and revises nursing diagnoses.
2. University of Iowa develops and revises the Nursing Interventions Classification (NIC) and Nursing Outcomes Classification (NOC).
3. NANDA-I diagnoses were incorporated into recent editions of NIC and NOC.

II. Assessment

A. Assessment involves collection of pertinent information related to a patient's pain, health, and situation.
B. Pain management theories provide a framework for the collection of information.
  1. Intrinsic and extrinsic factors influence behavioral responses.
  2. Previously, the Biopsychosocial (BPS) model was widely accepted given that pain is a dynamic and complex interaction within biology, psychology, and social factors.
  3. Biopsychosocial-spiritual model provides more holistic approach to pain.
    a. Expands on previous BPS model by including spiritual factors, which have been associated with improved coping.
    b. This model may strengthen therapeutic relationship through increased connectedness.
C. Individual assessment considerations
  1. Use developmentally, culturally, and literacy sensitive pain-assessment tools as appropriate for each person.
  2. Identify barriers and adapt communication considering age, cultural, financial, literacy, physical and psychosocial factors.
  3. Discuss preferences; allow patient to express needs.
  4. Discuss current treatments to reduce pain.
    a. Assess use of prescribed and nonprescribed medication, supplements, herbals, and illicit substances.
    b. Assess use of complementary/alternative therapies.

---

*Section Editor for the chapter.

D. Family assessment–immediate environment
1. Involve family/significant others in culturally sensitive, holistic data collection.
2. Assess family dynamics affecting patient's health, pain, and wellness.
E. Environment
1. Assess global and environmental factors: assessment parameters are identified in other organizations that influence pain management.
   a. Healthy People 2030
      1) Reduction in proportion of adults with chronic (persistent) pain
      2) Reduction of persistent pain and misuse of prescription medications
   b. Centers for Disease Control "Opioid Prescribing Guideline Recommendations and Guiding Principles"
2. Use ethical, legal, and privacy guidelines and policies.
F. Nurse self-assessment
1. Personal experience, attitudes, values, and beliefs can impact care.
2. Honor patient's preferences in care.

III. Diagnosis

A. Assessment data are analyzed to determine actual or potential diagnoses, issues, and problems.
B. NANDA-I: nursing diagnoses
1. Definition: clinical judgment regarding health condition or response to health condition by person, family, community, or group
2. Each diagnosis concerns individual, caregiver, family, group, or community.
3. Problem-focused diagnosis: undesirable response to current health condition or life process
4. Risk diagnosis: how susceptible person, family, community, or group is to developing an undesirable response to health condition
5. Health promotion diagnosis: desire and motivation to enhance well-being and health promotion
6. Syndrome diagnosis: grouping of nursing diagnoses treated with similar interventions
   Example: Persistent pain syndrome may include the following nursing diagnoses:
   a. Persistent pain
   b. Fatigue
   c. Social isolation
   d. Disturbed sleep pattern
C. Nursing responsibilities
1. Use data, clinical decision tools, standardized classification systems, and technology to formulate actual or potential diagnoses, issues, and problems related to pain.
2. Prioritize pain-related and other diagnoses, issues, and problems based on patient-discussed goals across health-illness continuum.

3. Identify actual or potential risks to health and safety or barriers, which include cultural, environmental, interpersonal, or systematic circumstances.
4. Document diagnoses, issues, and problems that facilitate outcomes and the plan.

IV. Plan

A. Nurses' responsibility in creating a plan outlining pain management strategies and measurable outcomes
1. Develop an evidenced-based, holistic, individualized pain management plan, including patient, family, and healthcare team.
2. Advocate for appropriate and responsible use of interventions to minimize unwanted or unwarranted treatment and/or patient suffering.
3. Prioritize elements of plan based on patient assessment.
4. Use evidence-based strategies in plan to address pain diagnoses, issues, or problems. Strategies may include:
   a. Health promotion and restoration
   b. Improvement of function
   c. Prevention of pain-producing disease, illness, or injury
   d. Supportive care
   e. Cultural considerations
5. Provide continuation of plan across the care system.
6. Ensure that plan complies with current standards, rules, and regulations.
7. Identify economic implication(s) of plan.
8. Modify plan according to assessment and evaluation of patient responses and outcome indicators.
9. Document using agreed-upon language and terminology.
B. Nurses' responsibility in outcome identification
1. Involve patient, family, and team to recognize expected outcomes, including favorable pain management goals.
2. Using assessment data and identified diagnosis, formulate expected pain-related, culturally sensitive outcomes.
   a. Use current evidenced-based practice and clinical expertise to recognize course of pain and related health benefits, risk, and costs.
   b. Develop time frame to attain pain-related outcomes.
   c. Modify outcomes after evaluation of patient's pain.
3. Using measurable goals, document progress toward expected outcomes.

C. Nursing outcome classification
1. A nursing outcome is behavior or perception in response to a nursing intervention of an individual, family, or community.
2. Every outcome has the following:
   a. Definition
   b. Measurement
   c. Associated indicators
   d. Supporting references
3. Standardized outcomes allow for study of nursing interventions' effect on patient outcomes.
4. Nurse establishes baseline prior to and after intervention across settings and time using five-point Likert scale (never demonstrated = 1 to consistently demonstrated = 5).
5. Example outcome: pain control: personal actions to eliminate or reduce pain. Some indicators to choose are:
   a. Recognizes pain onset
   b. Describes pain
   c. Sets pain relief goals with healthcare professional (HCP)
   d. Uses pain-preventive measures
   e. Avoids medication misuse
   f. Reports changes in pain symptoms to HCP
   g. Keeps appointments with HCPs
   h. Has access to recommended pain treatment

V. Implementation

A. Nurses' responsibilities in executing pain management plan:
1. Work with patient to implement plan in effective, efficient, equitable, patient-centered, and timely manner.
2. Ensure treatment plan is appropriately based on assessment.
3. Administer prescribed interventions and non-pharmacological strategies as standard of care.
4. Integrate interprofessional team through communication and collaboration across continuum of care.
5. Develop therapeutic relationship via caring and nonjudgmental behaviors.
6. Provide patient-centered, holistic, culturally compatible care across lifespan for diverse populations.
7. Implement strategies promoting multimodal pain management, medication administration safety, health, and self-management approaches to pain management.
8. Use care transitions and community resources to implement plan safely.
9. Advocate for patients in reaching treatment goals.
10. Integrate critical thinking and technological solutions to implement nursing process.
11. Document implementation and evaluation of plan.

B. Nursing Interventions Classification (NIC)
1. NIC is standardized language recognized by American Nurses Association and used by several healthcare agencies in development of care plans, competencies, and educational curricula.
2. Nursing interventions are treatments based on clinical knowledge and judgment performed to improve patient outcomes.
3. Every intervention has the following:
   a. Name
   b. Definition
   c. Activities related to performing intervention
   d. Supporting references
4. NIC captures nurses' expertise in all specialties and in all settings.
5. Interventions include management of psychosocial and physiological conditions and provision of health promotion, illness prevention, and treatment.
6. Intervention example: analgesic administration: use of medications to decrease or eliminate pain (not a complete list of interventions)
   a. Holistic approach to pain management
   b. Use appropriate pain assessment tool to determine current and desired comfort level.
   c. Verify opioid dose appropriateness (e.g., opioid-naïve patient is prescribed a lower starting dose than is opioid-tolerant patient).
   d. Explore patient and family concerns or misconceptions regarding pain medication, including risk of overdose and addiction.

VI. Evaluation

A. Assess progress toward achievement of pain outcomes and goals at intervals appropriate to each step.
B. Each step in nursing process should be evaluated for effectiveness of interventions and achievement of outcomes.
C. Nurses' responsibilities
1. Conduct evaluation of goals and outcomes in systematic, holistic manner within timeline of plan.
2. Collaborate with patient and others (e.g., family, other healthcare providers) in evaluation process.
3. Determine if strategies are patient-centered, effective, equitable, and safe in response to plan and outcomes related to pain management.
4. Revise diagnoses, plan, outcomes, and implementation strategy with ongoing assessments.
5. Provide evaluation data and conclusions in accordance with state and federal laws and regulations with patient and other stakeholders.
6. Document evaluation.

VII. NANDA-I Diagnoses: Domain 12, Comfort. Class 1, Physical Comfort. Nursing Intervention Classification and Nursing Outcome Classification

A. Impaired comfort: perceived lack of relief or ease within biopsychosocial-spiritual model and cultural dimensions
1. Defining characteristics (no minimum required for diagnosis)
   a. Anxiety
   b. Crying
   c. Difficulty relaxing
   d. Expresses discontentment with situation
   e. Expresses fear
   f. Expresses feeling cold, warm; itching
   g. Expresses psychological distress
   h. Irritable mood
   i. Moaning
   j. Psychomotor agitation
   k. Reports altered sleep-wake cycle
   l. Reports hunger
2. Related factors
   a. Inadequate control over environment
   b. Inadequate health resources
   c. Inadequate situational control
   d. Insufficient privacy
   e. Unpleasant environmental stimuli
3. Associated conditions
   a. Illness-related signs and symptoms
   b. Treatment regimen
4. NIC (examples of potential interventions below)
   a. Environmental management: comfort
   b. Activities include:
      1) Discover patient and family goals for maximum comfort.
      2) Create supportive and relaxing environment.
      3) Adjust lighting for maximum comfort (e.g., lighting should not be directly in eyes).
      4) Assist patient with hygiene activities for comfort, including oral care, etc.
      5) Provide education materials and resources on illness and injury management to patient's family.
5. NOC (not all outcomes listed below)
   a. Comfort status: individual overall ease and safety within biopsychosocial, spiritual, and cultural environment dimensions
   b. Comfort status: environment: comfort, ease, and safety of surroundings
   c. Comfort status: physical: physical sensations and homeostasis at ease and comfortable

   d. Comfort status: psychospiritual: emotional well-being related to self-concept, the meaning and purpose of the patient's life
6. Readiness for enhanced comfort: defining characteristics: all begin with "Expressed desire to enhance …"
   a. Comfort
   b. Feeling of contentment
   c. Relaxation
   d. Resolution
7. NIC and NOC as above in Impaired comfort
B. Acute pain: International Association for the Study of Pain definition: Pain has a duration of less than 3 months of any intensity with a foreseen and predictable completion.
1. Defining characteristics
   a. Altered physiological parameters
   b. Appetite change
   c. Diaphoresis
   d. Distraction behavior
   e. Evidence of pain using standardized pain behavior checklist for those unable to communicate verbally
   f. Expressive behavior and/or facial expression of pain
   g. Guarding behavior
   h. Positioning to ease pain
   i. Proxy report of activity or pain behavior changes
   j. Patient reports intensity and pain characteristics using standardized pain instrument.
2. Related factors
   a. Biological injury
   b. Inappropriate use of chemical agent
   c. Physical injury agent
3. NIC: Pain Management. Sample interventions for acute pain:
   a. Medicate patient before pain is severe and prior to pain-inducing activities.
   b. Medicate patient after trauma, injury, or surgery every 4 hours (for 24 to 48 hours), except if patient is sedated or compromised in respiratory status.
   c. Use multimodal analgesics to treat pain.
   d. Select and use personalized interventions tailored to patient's preference, risks, and benefits to enable pain relief.
   e. Provide family with accurate information about patient's pain experience.
4. NOC: Pain Management. Sample outcomes for acute pain:
   a. Ambulation
   b. Comfort status
   c. Knowledge: medication
   d. Knowledge: pain management
   e. Medication response

f. Post-procedure recovery

g. Surgical recovery: immediate postoperative

C. Chronic (persistent) pain: International Association for the Study of Pain definition: Pain has a duration of more than 3 months of any intensity without a foreseen and predictable completion.

1. Defining characteristics

a. Altered ability to continue activities

b. Anorexia

c. Use of standardized pain behavior checklist demonstrates pain for nonverbal persons

d. Expressed fatigue

e. Proxy report of activity or pain behavior changes

f. Reports intensity and pain characteristics using standardized pain instrument

g. Self-focused

2. Related factors

a. Body mass index above normal range

b. Fatigue

c. Ineffective sexuality pattern

d. Injury agent

e. Malnutrition

f. Prolonged computer use

g. Psychological distress

h. Repeated handling of heavy loads

i. Social isolation

3. At-risk population

a. Age >50 years

b. History of abuse, genital mutilation

c. History of indebtedness

d. History of static work postures

e. History of substance misuse

f. History of vigorous exercise

g. Female

4. Associated conditions

a. Bone fractures

b. Central nervous system sensitization

c. Chronic musculoskeletal diseases

d. Contusion

e. Imbalance of neurotransmitters, neuromodulators, and receptors

f. Impaired metabolism

g. Neoplasms

h. Nerve compression syndromes

i. Nervous system diseases

j. Post-trauma related condition

k. Soft-tissue or spinal cord injuries

5. NIC: Pain Management. Sample interventions for persistent pain:

a. Determine effect of pain experience on quality of life (e.g., sleep, appetite, activity, cognition, mood, relationships, job performance, and role responsibilities).

b. Evaluate effectiveness of past pain control measures with patient.

c. Encourage patient to monitor pain and use self-management.

d. Prevent and manage medication side effects.

e. Watch for signs of depression (e.g., sleeplessness, not eating, flat affect, states of depression, or suicidal ideation).

f. Watch for signs of anxiety or fear (e.g., irritability, tension, worry, fear of movement).

g. Incorporate multidisciplinary approach to pain management when appropriate.

h. Consider referrals for patient and family to support groups and other resources as appropriate.

6. NOC: Pain Management. Sample outcomes for persistent pain:

a. Ambulation

b. Comfort status

c. Discomfort level

d. Knowledge:

1) Medication

2) Musculoskeletal rehabilitation

3) Pain management

e. Musculoskeletal rehabilitation participation

f. Pain: adverse psychological response

g. Disruptive effects of pain

h. Self-management: chronic disease

D. Chronic (persistent) Pain Syndrome: Persistent pain at least 3 months in duration and significantly affects well-being and activities of daily living

1. Defining characteristics

a. Anxiety

b. Constipation

c. Disturbed sleep pattern

d. Fatigue

e. Fear

f. Impaired mood regulation

g. Impaired physical mobility

h. Insomnia

i. Social isolation

j. Stress overload

2. Related factors

a. Body mass index above normal

b. Fear of pain

c. Fear-avoidance beliefs

d. Inadequate knowledge of pain management behaviors

e. Sleep disturbances

3. NIC: Pain Management. Sample interventions for Chronic Pain Syndrome:

a. NIC sample interventions listed in VII C 5 above (Not all outcomes listed below):

b. Use valid and reliable chronic (persistent) pain assessment tool (e.g., Brief Pain Inventory [Short Form], McGill Pain Questionnaire Short-Form, and Fibromyalgia Impact Questionnaire).

    c. Explore patient's knowledge and beliefs about pain, including cultural influences.

    d. Question patient regarding level of pain that allows a state of comfort and appropriate function and attempt to keep pain at or below identified goal.

    e. Encourage appropriate use of nonpharmacologic techniques (e.g., biofeedback, transcutaneous electrical nerve stimulation [TENS], hypnosis, relaxation, guided imagery, music therapy, distraction, play therapy, activity therapy, acupressure, heat and cold application, and massage) and pharmacological options as pain-control measures.

4. NOC: Pain Management Sample outcomes for Chronic Pain Syndrome: NOC sample outcomes listed in VII C 6

    a. Anxiety level

    b. Depression level

    c. Self-care: activities of daily living

    d. Self-care: instrumental activities of daily living

    e. Stress level

E. Labor pain: emotional and sensory experience in accordance with labor and childbirth

  1. Defining characteristics

    a. Altered blood pressure, heart rate, muscle tension, neuroendocrine functioning, respiratory rate, and urinary functioning

    b. Anxiety

    c. Appetite changes

    d. Diaphoresis

    e. Distraction or expressive behavior

    f. Facial expression of pain

    g. Perineal pressure

    h. Positioning to decrease pain

    i. Uterine contraction

    j. Nausea/Vomiting

  2. Related factors

    a. Behavioral: insufficient fluid intake or supine position

    b. Cognitive

      1) Fear of childbirth

      2) Inadequate knowledge

      3) Inadequate preparation

      4) Low self-efficacy

      5) Perception of labor pain as:

        a) Negative

        b) Threatening

        c) Unnatural

        d) Meaningful

    c. Social: interference in decision-making or unsupportive companionship

    d. Unmodified environment

      1) Noisy delivery room

      2) Overcrowded delivery room

      3) Turbulent environment

3. At-risk populations

    a. Persons experiencing emergency situation during labor

    b. Persons from cultures with negative perspective

    c. Persons giving birth in a disease-based healthcare system.

    d. Persons with history of prepregnancy dysmenorrhea

    e. Persons with history of sexual abuse during childhood

    f. Persons without supportive companion

4. Associated conditions

    a. Cervical dilation

    b. Depression

    c. Fetal expulsion

    d. High maternal trait anxiety

    e. Prescribed mobility restriction

    f. Prolonged duration of labor

5. NIC: Pain Management. Sample interventions for labor pain:

    a. Family integrity promotion: childbearing family

      1) Identify family interaction patterns.

      2) Assist family in developing adaptive coping mechanisms to deal with transition to parenthood.

      3) Encourage family to use support systems as appropriate.

      4) Offer to be advocate for family.

    b. Intrapartum care

      1) Monitor pain level during labor per protocol.

      2) Explore positions that improve maternal comfort and maintain placental perfusion.

      3) Provide alternative methods of pain relief consistent with patient's goals (e.g., simple massage, effleurage, aromatherapy, hypnosis, TENS).

      4) Assist labor coach or family in providing comfort and support during labor.

      5) Administer analgesics to promote comfort and relaxation during labor.

    c. Medication administration: intraspinal

      1) Determine patient's knowledge of medication and understanding of method of administration.

      2) Monitor epidural or intrathecal catheter insertion site for signs of infection.

      3) Document medication administration and patient response according to agency protocol.

6. NOC: Women's Health and Obstetrics. Sample outcomes:

    a. Family coping and function

    b. Knowledge: labor and delivery

    c. Pain level

Bibliography

American Nurses Association, Association of Pain Management Nursing. (2016). *Pain Management Nursing: Scope and Standards of Practice* (2nd Ed.). Silver Spring, MD: American Nurses Association, Association of Pain Management Nursing.

Butcher, H. K., Bulechek, G. M., Dochterman, J. M., & Wagner, C. M. (Eds.). (2018). *Nursing Interventions Classification (NIC)* (7th ed.). New York, NY: Elsevier.

Centers for Disease Control and Prevention. (2022). Opioid Prescribing Guideline Recommendations and Guiding Principles. https://www.cdc.gov/opioids/healthcare-professionals/prescribing/guideline/recommendations-principles.html.

Gallagher-Lepak, S., & Lopes, C. T. (2021). Nursing diagnosis basics. In T. H. Herdman, S. Kamitsuru, & C. T. Lopes. (Eds.). *NANDA International, Inc. Nursing Diagnoses: Definitions and Classification 2020–2023* (12th Ed., pp. 78–92). New York, NY: Thieme.

Matteliano, D., St Marie, B. J., Oliver, J., & Coggins, C. (2014). Adherence monitoring with chronic opioid therapy for persistent pain: a biopsychosocial-spiritual approach to mitigate risk. *Pain Management Nursing, 15*(1), 391–405. https://doi.org/10.1016/j.pmn.2012.08.008.

Moorhead, S., Swanson, E., Johnson, M., & Maas, M. L. (Eds.). (2018). *Nursing Outcomes Classification (NOC): Measurement of Health Outcomes* (6th ed.). New York, NY: Elsevier.

NANDA International (NANDA-I) (2021). Domain 12. Comfort. Sense of mental, physical, or social well-being or ease. In T. H. Herdman, S. Kamitsuru, & C. T. Lopes (Eds.), *NANDA International, Inc. Nursing Diagnoses: Definitions and Classification 2020–2023* (12th Ed., pp. 549–561). New York, NY: Thieme.

Shewangizaw, Z., & Mersha, A. (2015). Determinants towards implementation of nursing process. *American Journal of Nursing Science, 4*(3), 45–49. https://doi.org/10.11648/j.ajns.20150403.11.

US Department of Health and Human Services Office of Disease Prevention and Health Promotion. (n.d.) Healthy People 2030 Building a healthier future for all. https://health.gov/healthypeople/.

Part 2

CHAPTER 7

Research and Quality Improvement in Pain Management Nursing

Patricia Kelly Rosier, MS, RN, ACNS-BC, PMGT-BC
Jinbing Bai, PhD, RN, FAAN
Ann Schreier, PhD, BSN, MSN, RN*

Introduction

Pain management research can provide guidance on best approaches to topics such as pain assessment, management, and evaluation. This chapter outlines the importance of having a foundation in nursing research, evidence-based practice (EBP), and quality improvement (QI) to provide quality pain management nursing. Regardless of their role, all nurses play a critical role in advancing the quality and science of pain systems improvement. As pain management nursing advances, it is important to follow guiding principles of knowledge-based, patient-centered, and system-minded care.

I. Impact of Research Utilization and Quality Improvement on Pain Management

A. Nurses engage in activities along a continuum of research practice.
   1. An understanding of nursing research can improve nurses' professional practice and contribute to quality patient care.
   2. At one end of spectrum, nurses are consumers of nursing research. At other end of spectrum, nurses identify areas of need and design and conduct nursing research.
B. Research utilization contributes to practice by:
   1. Building professionalism that defines parameters of practice
   2. Providing accountability to patients, healthcare agencies, and third-party payers
   3. Demonstrating efficacy of nursing in changing healthcare arena
   4. Promoting critical thinking and reflective practice
   5. Expanding knowledge related to pain management nursing
   6. Validating efforts of researchers
   7. Improving patient outcomes

C. Contributions to pain management guideline, policy, and position statement development such as:
   1. *American Society of Pain Management Nursing (ASPMN) Position Statements*
      a. *Pain Assessment in the Patient Unable to Self-Report*
      b. *Prescribing and Administering Opioid Doses Based Solely on Pain Intensity*
      c. *Pain Management and Substance Use Disorders*
   2. *ASPMN Guidelines on Monitoring for Opioid-Induced Advancing Sedation and Respiratory Depression: Revisions.*
   3. *Guidelines on Managing Postoperative Pain: A Clinical Practice Guideline from the American Pain Society, the American Society of Regional Anesthesia and Pain Medicine, and the American Society of Anesthesiologists' Committee on Regional Anesthesia*
   4. *Pain Management Best Practices Inter-Agency Task Force Report*
   5. *Recommendations on Chronic Pain Practice during the COVID-19 Pandemic. A Joint Statement by American Society of Regional Anesthesia and Pain Medicine and European Society of Regional Anesthesia and Pain Therapy*
D. Helpful distinctions
   1. Research is diligent, systematic inquiry or investigation to validate and refine existing knowledge and generate new knowledge.
   2. Nursing research is formal inquiry through quantitative, qualitative, or mixed-methods research that validates and refines existing knowledge and generates new knowledge that directly and indirectly influences delivery of evidence-based nursing practices.
   3. Translational research is an evolving concept defined by the National Institutes of Health as translation of basic scientific discoveries into practical applications.

*Section Editor for the chapter.

E. Research utilization is process of synthesizing, disseminating, and using research-generated knowledge to impact a change in practice.
F. Evidence-based practice
1. In delivery of quality and cost-effective healthcare, EBP is conscientious integration of best research evidence with clinical expertise and patient values and needs.
2. EBP centers are universities and healthcare agencies identified by the Agency for Healthcare Research and Quality (AHRQ) as centers for performance, communication, and synthesis of research knowledge in selected areas to promote evidence-based healthcare.
3. EBP guidelines are rigorous and explicit clinical guidelines based on best research evidence available, supported by consensus from recognized national experts and affirmed by outcomes obtained by clinicians.
G. Quality improvement
1. Healthcare quality is generally described in terms of attributes and outcomes of care provided by practitioners and received by patients.
2. Quality healthcare has been defined as the kind of healthcare expected to maximize an inclusive measure of patient welfare after considering balance of expected gains and losses that accompany process of care in all its parts.
3. The Institute of Medicine (IOM) defined quality healthcare as "the degree to which health services for individuals and populations increase the likelihood of desired health outcomes and are consistent with current professional knowledge" (Medicare, & Lohr, K. N. (Eds.). (1990)).
   a. The IOM is now the National Academy of Medicine.
   b. The IOM revisited these seminal definitions and statements, redefining the phrase "desired health outcomes" to specifically include health outcomes that patients desire.
4. Patient satisfaction is a recommended measure in most evaluations of quality.
   a. There is a paradox in many hospital patient-satisfaction studies that patients often report high pain intensity and high satisfaction with their pain management. It is generally accepted that patient satisfaction does not always equate with quality pain management.
   b. Patient satisfaction with pain may be more representative of the quality of interpersonal relationships between caregivers and patients than of actual quality of care or outcomes, as research shows both patient satisfaction and outcomes improve when patients are directly involved in their care.
   c. Evaluation of quality pain care should include questions about the adequacy of pain-related

information provided, patient education, and ability to participate in care decisions. These questions may be a better measure than general patient satisfaction questions.
5. Definition of quality depends on the purpose of measurement and perspective of measurer.
H. The most prominent nurse-developed models used to guide nursing clinical practice change are:
1. Stetler Model of Research Utilization to facilitate EBP: a five-step process emphasizing critical thinking and decision-making to facilitate safe and effective use of research findings.
2. Iowa Model of Evidence-Based Practice:
   a. Provides direction for development of EBP in a clinical agency that reflects consideration of the patient, provider, and infrastructure of the healthcare organization
   b. Responds to triggers
3. Promoting Action on Research Implementation in Health Services model: emphasizes that successful implementation of evidence recommendations is a product of complex relationships among evidence, context, and facilitation
I. Steps in integrating EBP
1. Identify and frame answerable question
2. Search for relevant research evidence
3. Appraise and synthesize evidence
4. Integrate evidence with other factors, such as patient preferences and values
5. Assess effectiveness and outcomes of practice change
J. Sources of evidence
1. Journals
2. Textbooks
3. Guidelines
4. Expert opinion
5. Electronic searchable databases
   a. The Joanna Briggs Collaboration is a useful source of systemic reviews in nursing and other health fields (http://joannabriggs.org/).
   b. The AHRQ awarded contracts to establish EBP centers that issue evidence reports (www.ahrq.gov).
   c. Cochrane Database of Systematic Reviews (http://www.cochrane.org)
   d. PubMed (http://www.ncbi.nlm.nih.gov/pubmed)
   e. Cumulative Index to Nursing and Allied Health Literature (CINAHL) database via academic health libraries
K. The hierarchy of evidence table lists items based on strength of evidence
1. Grading the strength of a body of evidence incorporates three domains
   a. Quality: extent to which a study's design, conduct, and analysis have minimized selection, measurement, and confounding biases

b. Quantity: number of studies that have evaluated the question, sample size across studies, and magnitude of treatment effects

c. Consistency: whether investigators with both similar and dissimilar study designs report similar findings

II. Types of Research Design

A. Definition and purpose
1. Research design is the overall strategy used to integrate different components of a study in a coherent and logical way.
2. The purpose of research design is to address a research problem effectively via collection, measurement, and analysis of data.

B. Types of research design:
1. Quantitative research involves systematic collection of numeric information under conditions of considerable control and analysis of that data. It involves manipulation of such data through statistical procedures for the purpose of describing phenomena or assessing the magnitude and reliability of relationships among them. Types of quantitative research designs:
   a. Case-study design involves intensive exploration of a single unit of study, which will be a person, family, group, community, population, or institution.
   b. Descriptive study design focuses on accurate portrayal of characteristics of people, situations, or groups and the frequency with which certain phenomena occur.
      1) A summary includes mean and standard deviation.
      2) No manipulation of variables occurs.
   c. Correlational study design explores interrelationships among variables of interest without any active interventions by researcher.
   d. Observational study design involves researcher observing effect of a risk factor, treatment, or other intervention without trying to manipulate it. Cohort and case-control studies are two types of observational studies.
   e. Cross-sectional design examines relationship between variables of interest as they exist in a defined population at a single point in time or over a short period of time.
   f. Longitudinal design involves conducting several observations of the same subjects over specified time period. Benefit is researchers can detect developments or changes in characteristics of target population.
   g. Quasi-experimental study design examines causality. Although researcher does manipulate independent variable and exercises certain controls to enhance internal validity of results, subjects cannot be assigned randomly to treatment conditions, and threats to internal validity may exist.
   h. Experimental study design examines causality by controlling independent variable and randomly assigning subjects to different conditions.
      1) Involves essential elements of random sampling, researcher-controlled manipulation of independent variable, and control of experimental situation, including a control group. Key components are manipulation, control, and randomization.
      2) Threats to validity may also exist. Tightly controlled inclusion and exclusion criteria may result in threats to external validity and affect ability to generalize study findings to other populations.

2. Qualitative research is a systematic, interactive, subjective approach used to describe and give meaning to life experiences.
   a. Characteristics of qualitative research:
      1) Its purpose is to describe or generate theories so they may be used to develop hypotheses or study phenomena about which little is known.
      2) It has a purposeful sample; participants are selected because they have characteristics in common.
      3) The researcher is involved closely with participants but maintains an objective perspective.
      4) Involves inductive data analysis
      5) Uses narrative approach to report findings
   b. Types of qualitative studies:
      1) Phenomenology considers the lived experience of people (e.g., study of the phenomenon of pain flare in a population of persons with persistent pain).
      2) Ethnography focuses on the culture of a people.
      3) Grounded theory is an approach to data collection with the purpose of developing theories about phenomena under study.
      4) Historical research is focused on looking for patterns and relationships from the past in a systematic way to evaluate past occurrences.
      5) Content analysis provides systematic means of measuring frequency, order, or intensity of occurrence of words, phrases, or sentences because of their theoretical importance.
      6) Narrative inquiry is a lens through which study takes form. It is often used in marginalized and vulnerable populations. Results of this method can be used to affect social policy.

3. Additional research and study designs
   a. Evaluation research: This form of applied research identifies how well a program, policy, procedure, or practice is working.
   b. Methodological research: Controlled investigations explore ways of obtaining, organizing, and analyzing data. These studies address development, validation, and evaluation of measurement tools or methods.
   c. Quality improvement project: Not considered a research design but involves systematic investigations of working hypotheses on how a process in a healthcare system might be improved, and frequently uses analytic tools to evaluate process and outcome improvement
   d. Translational research/implementation science: investigates how research evidence can effectively be integrated into agency and individual practice, leading to meaningful health outcomes
   e. Big data science: use of large volumes of high-velocity, complex, and variable data that require advanced techniques and technologies to enable the capture, storage, distribution, management, and analysis of information to explore health trends and populations
   f. Comparative effectiveness research: direct comparison of existing healthcare interventions to determine which work best for which patients and which pose the most benefit and harm for patients

III. Generating Evidence: Research Process

A. Research involves a systematic process that leads to the generation of new knowledge, refinement of knowledge, or extension of knowledge that contributes to the discipline of nursing, including pain management nursing.
B. Purpose of research:
   1. Describe: depict characteristics of individuals, groups, situations, and health states
   2. Explore: investigate dimensions of a phenomenon
   3. Explain: attempt to understand underpinnings of phenomena and their interrelationships
   4. Predict and control: forecast how combinations of variables will operate in different circumstances involving different groups of individuals
C. Limitations of research process
   1. Every study has limitations based on design and sampling techniques.
   2. Moral and ethical constraints, protection of human subjects, and institutional review board (IRB) are imposed limitations.

3. Measurement and data collection can face difficulties.
4. Obstacles such as extraneous variable(s) prevent complete control of research environment.
5. Complexity of humans adds another level of intricacy.
D. Steps in research process
   1. Identify gaps based on:
      a. Experience in clinical setting
      b. Literature
      c. Theories and conceptual frameworks
      d. External resources such as government agencies, task forces, and research guidelines
   2. Narrow a topic by generating a list of researchable questions.
   3. Evaluate research problems.
      a. Identify the significance and relevance of a problem.
      b. Assess ability to research the identified problem.
         1) Does the problem have an empirical reality or objective focus (i.e., evidence rooted in understandable, predictable, or controllable fashion and gathered through data collection by using senses to generate knowledge)?
         2) Does it explain defined concepts?
         3) Is it able to capture the phenomena being studied?
      c. Determine feasibility of research by considering the following factors:
         1) What are the time (e.g., project will be completed in allotted time frame) and timing (e.g., subjects will be available during period study takes place)?
         2) Does it have an empirical reality or objective focus?
         3) Does it employ defined concepts?
         4) Is it able to capture the phenomena being studied?
         5) What is availability of financial resources, including funding?
         6) What is experience of researcher or research team?
         7) What are ethical considerations?
   4. State research problem
      a. Delineate problem: Statement of the research problem guides the development of the study and must be presented clearly.
         1) Research problems become refined further by reviewing the literature to discover what research has been conducted on a topic, focusing on research designs and sampling techniques.
         2) The research purpose is generated from the problem. As the problem identifies a knowledge gap in a selected area, its purpose

clarifies knowledge that will be produced from a specific investigation.

3) In a quantitative study, purpose statements should indicate independent and dependent variables of study population.

4) In a qualitative study, the purpose is to identify a phenomenon of interest and study population.

b. Ask a research question: From the research problem, the purpose of the study and research questions are generated.

1) Many research studies contain a general statement of purpose and several more specific research questions.

2) The research question(s) directs methodology.

5. Build research hypothesis

a. Hypotheses are a means of generating knowledge through testing of theoretical statements or relationships that have been identified in previous research, proposed by theorists, or observed in practice.

1) Must be empirically testable and inferred from measured and observable phenomena

2) Translates problem statements into predictions of expected outcomes

3) Not used in descriptive research because descriptive research describes instead of explains phenomena

4) Hypotheses are never proven; they are only supported.

b. Characteristics of workable hypotheses

1) Testable

a) Hypotheses have measurable variables.

b) Predict relationship between at least two variables

c) Are statistically testable

2) Justifiable

a) Specific instances are observed, collated, and combined into a general statement.

b) Deductive reasoning moves from general to specific or from general premise to particular conclusion.

6. Review the literature

a. Purpose

1) Can be a source of research ideas.

2) Researchers can understand current state of science for a particular phenomenon using literature.

3) Documents the prevalence and significance of a research problem.

4) Provides a conceptual framework or theory to guide study design and data interpretation.

5) Supports a choice of study variables.

6) Can identify studies to determine previous methods, research instruments, and samples.

b. Sources for literature review

1) A primary source is a description written by person(s) conducting the study.

2) A secondary source is a description of a study written by someone other than an original researcher. It is less desirable than a primary source.

c. Locating relevant literature for research review

1) Review of available literature from sources such as CINAHL, PubMed, Medline, Embase, PsychINFO, Cochrane Database of Systematic Reviews

2) Examples of journals relevant to pain management nursing:

a) *Pain Management Nursing*

b) *Pain*

c) *Pain Medicine*

d) *Journal of Pain and Symptom Management*

e) *Nursing Research*

f) *Oncology Nursing Forum*

g) *Cancer Nursing*

h) *Clinical Journal of Pain*

i) *Research in Nursing and Health*

j) *Journal of Hospice and Palliative Nursing*

k) *Journal of Palliative Medicine*

3) Federal agencies, foundations, or other website resources

a) National Institute of Health (www.nih.gov)

b) American Cancer Society (www.cancer.org)

c) Centers for Disease Control and Prevention (CDC) (www.cdc.gov)

d) International Association for the Study of Pain (www.iasp-pain.org)

e) Joanna Briggs Institute (https://jbi.global)

IV. Evaluating Existing Research for Clinical Decision-Making

A. Key principles for critical appraisal of research

1. Examine research, clinical, and educational backgrounds of the authors.

2. Examine organization and presentation of research report.

3. Read and critique entire study.

4. Examine the significance of the study problem for nursing practice and knowledge.

5. As strengths and weaknesses of study are identified, provide specific examples of and rationale(s) for identified strengths and weaknesses of the study.

6. If study resulted in valid and trustworthy findings, examine the usefulness or transferability to practice.
7. Suggest ideas and modifications for future studies.

B. Evidence should be appraised before taking clinical action.
1. What is the quality of evidence?
   a. Were study methods sufficiently rigorous?
2. What was the magnitude of effect?
   a. Are results clinically important?
   b. What is effect size?
3. How precise is estimate of effects (i.e., relevant with quantitative research)?
4. What evidence is there of side effects or side benefits?
5. What is financial cost of applying (or not applying) the evidence?
6. Is there evidence relevant to a particular clinical situation?
7. Possible actions based on evidence appraisals
   a. Continue with usual care.
   b. Apply new evidence.
   c. Design another study (e.g., larger population, broader application).
   d. Ask a new question.

C. Elements of a critique of a quantitative study
1. Does the title suggest a key phenomenon and group being studied?
2. Does the abstract clearly and concisely summarize key features of study?
3. Introduction and problem statement
   a. Is problem clearly stated and easy to identify?
   b. Does problem statement build a clear indication for new study?
   c. Is problem significant for nursing?
   d. Was quantitative approach appropriate for this study?
4. Hypothesis or research question
   a. Is there a good fit between research question and method used to study it?
   b. Were research questions and/or hypotheses explicitly stated?
   c. Were key variables clearly stated?
5. Literature review
   a. Was the literature review current and mainly based on primary sources?
   b. Did the literature review synthesize the evidence of the problem?
6. Conceptual framework
   a. Was there a clearly articulated conceptual framework?
   b. Did the conceptual framework fit the research question?
7. Methods
   a. Were human subjects appropriately protected?
   b. Were an IRB review and approval obtained?

c. Did study design minimize risks and maximize benefits to the subjects?
d. Was the most rigorous possible design used?
e. Was the population identified, and was a sample described in sufficient detail?
f. Was the best possible sampling method used?
g. Were steps taken to minimize biases and threats to validity?
h. Was blinding used?
i. Was sample size adequate and based on power analysis?
j. Were key variables measured using an appropriate method?
k. Were research instruments adequately described?
l. Was there evidence that the data collection methods yielded data that were reliable, valid, and responsive?
m. If there was intervention, was it clearly described and rigorously developed?
n. Were data collected in a manner that minimized bias?
o. Were the staff who collected data appropriately trained?

8. Results
   a. Were appropriate statistical methods used for analysis?
   b. Were Type I and Type II errors avoided or minimized?
   c. Was an intent-to-treat analysis performed?
   d. Were missing values or data evaluated and explained?
   e. Was statistical significance presented?
   f. Were tables and figures used to summarize key findings?
   g. Were the findings presented in a manner that facilitates their use as EBP?

9. Discussion
   a. Were the findings discussed in the context of a literature review and conceptual framework?
   b. Was the clinical significance of results discussed?
   c. Was generalizability of results discussed?
   d. Were implications for nursing practice or future research presented?
   e. Were limitations of the study addressed?

10. Dissemination
    a. Peer-reviewed journals
    b. Impact factor
    c. Citation analysis

D. Elements of a review of a qualitative study
1. Does title suggest key phenomenon and group being studied?
2. Does abstract clearly and concisely summarize key features of the study?
3. Is problem clearly stated and easy to identify?

4. Does problem statement build a clear indication for a new study? Is the problem statement significant for nursing?
5. Was the qualitative approach appropriate for this study?
6. Was the research question clearly stated and consistent with the philosophical basis of study?
7. Did the literature review adequately summarize existing knowledge on the topic and provide a strong basis for a new study?
8. Were key concepts adequately defined conceptually?
9. Ethical considerations
   a. Was IRB approval obtained?
   b. Were the rights of subjects adequately protected?
   c. Was the study designed to minimize risks and maximize benefits to the subjects?
10. Design considerations
   a. Was the identified research tradition congruent with data collection methods?
   b. Was an adequate amount of time spent with the study subjects?
   c. Was there an adequate number of contacts with the study subjects?
   d. Did the design unfold during data collection, allowing researchers opportunities to take advantage of early understandings?
   e. Was study population adequately described?
   f. Were setting and sample described in sufficient detail?
   g. Was participant recruitment approach appropriate and productive?
   h. Was the sampling method designed to enhance the richness of information and address the needs of the study?
   i. Was sample size adequate?
   j. Was saturation achieved?
   k. Was the data collection method appropriate?
   l. Were the data gathered with two or more methods to achieve triangulation?
   m. Did the researcher ask correct questions or make correct observations?
11. Data collection considerations
   a. Were data recorded in an appropriate manner?
   b. Was there a sufficient amount of data collected?
   c. Were data sufficient in depth and richness?
   d. Were data collection methods and recording procedures adequately described?
   e. Were data collected in a manner to minimize bias?
   f. Was the data collection staff adequately trained?
   g. Were strategies used to enhance the trustworthiness and integrity of the study effective?
   h. Did the researcher document research procedures and decision processes sufficiently, such that results are auditable and confirmable?

12. Results
   a. Were data management and analysis methods adequately described?
   b. Was the data analysis strategy compatible with the nature and type of data collected?
   c. Did data analysis yield an appropriate "product"?
   d. Did data analysis suggest any possibility of bias?
   e. Were the data effectively summarized?
   f. Were excerpts of the data used effectively to support the data?
   g. Did the themes adequately capture the meaning of the data?
   h. Did the researcher satisfactorily conceptualize themes or patterns in the data?
   i. Did analysis yield an insightful, authentic, and meaningful picture of the phenomenon being studied?
   j. Were the themes or patterns logically connected to each other to form integrated whole?
   k. Were figures, maps, or models effectively used to summarize concepts?
   l. If a conceptual framework was used to guide the study, were the themes or patterns cogently linked to it?
13. Discussion
   a. Were findings interpreted within the appropriate social or cultural context?
   b. Were major findings discussed within the context of prior studies?
   c. Were implications for clinical practice or future research discussed?
14. Dissemination
   a. Peer-reviewed journals
   b. Impact factor
   c. Citation analysis

V. Applying Evidence to Clinical Practice by Implementing an Evidence-Based Practice Project

A. EBP projects use a systematic process involving use and dissemination of research-generated information to influence or change nursing practice.
   1. Clinical relevance: Is the evidence relevant for your clinical situation? Does it apply to your patients?
   2. Scientific merit
      a. Each study must be critiqued to determine if findings and conclusions are accurate and generalizable. Can the study influence clinical practice?

   b. Have replication studies been conducted and resulted in the same or different findings?
   c. Were the studies conducted in a clinical setting?
3. Implementation potential
   a. Transferability: Does it make sense to implement innovation in a practice setting?
   b. Feasibility addresses practical concerns such as availability of staff and resources, organizational climate, need for and accessibility of external assistance, and potential for clinical evaluation.
   c. The cost-benefit ratio must be carefully assessed in regard to implementing proposed changes to clients, nurses, and the organization.
B. Process for initiating an evidence-based project
   1. Select a relevant clinical problem.
      a. A problem-focused trigger arises from a clinical practice problem in need of solution. This could occur in the normal course of clinical practice.
      b. A knowledge-focused trigger comes from research evidence, such as a new clinical guideline.
   2. Address the practical issues in organizational EBP efforts.
      a. Organizational support
      b. Structure and composition of the team
      c. Solicit support of stakeholders.
   3. Find and appraise evidence.
      a. Use existing clinical practice guidelines, care bundles, or other decision-support tools if available.
      b. Use a guideline appraisal tool to evaluate evidence.
      c. Guidelines often change more slowly than evidence; examine the literature for more recent evidence if the guidelines are greater than 3 years old.
   4. Make decisions based on evidence appraisals.
      a. Is the evidence sufficient to recommend practice change?
      b. Can it be adapted locally?
   5. Assess implementation potential and environmental readiness.
   6. Develop a protocol. Consider the need for IRB approval.
   7. Implement.
      a. Staff education is essential.
      b. Identify potential barriers.
   8. Evaluate.
      a. Identify desired outcomes.
      b. Develop a measurement plan.
      c. Measure and revise as needed.

9. Disseminate an evaluation of the protocol to other nursing and healthcare professionals.

VI. Creating a Culture of Research Utilization and Evidence-Based Practice in Pain Management

A. Barriers to using research and quality-improvement projects in nursing practice.
   1. Research barriers
      a. Lack of research evidence evaluating the effectiveness of many nursing interventions
      b. Lack of extensive knowledge based on valid, reliable, and generalizable study results
      c. Dearth of reported replication studies
      d. Limited systemic reviews and meta-analysis in nursing compared to other disciplines
   2. Organizational barriers
      a. Lack of resources (e.g., time, financial, journals, and databases)
      b. Resistance to change
      c. Fear of "cookbook" approach
      d. Lack of institutional commitment to research
   3. Nursing profession barriers
      a. Lack of time for clinical nurses to perform the steps in the research utilization process
      b. Lack of skills in a critical appraisal
      c. Shortage of appropriate role models
      d. Lack of authority or support to change patient care based on research
      e. Minimal incentives for providing evidence-based care
B. Strategies for improving the use of research and QI in practice requires all involved take an active role.
   1. Reflective inquiring approach
   2. Read research reports (look for translational research reports).
   3. Attend professional conferences.
   4. Expect evidence that procedures and practices are effective.
   5. Offer and participate in journal clubs.
   6. Participate in research, EBP initiatives, and translational research.
   7. Use credible research findings to change practice.
   8. Compare and contrast mythical or outdated concepts to concepts that are well-grounded in research.
   9. Collaboration between academic nurse educators, researchers, and clinical nurses.
      a. Researchers should collaborate with clinicians with clinical knowledge and questions. Convert questions to actual research projects.
         1) Collaboration enhances research process and usage.
         2) Collaborate with "seasoned" researchers to enhance likelihood of receiving research grant funding.

3) Collaboration can facilitate research for bedside nurses because time and workload constraints inhibit full participation in the research process.

4) Invite faculty/researchers to participate in hospital research committees and journal clubs.

   b. Encourage nursing students to critically read and review nursing research. Foster interest in nursing research and build a foundation on which to grow.

   c. Incorporate advanced practice nursing students' academic research and QI projects into the work arena.

10. Facilitate organizational EBP.

   a. Organizational goals should include use of evidence to promote excellence.

   b. Job descriptions and performance appraisals should incorporate use of EBP.

   c. Charters for nursing committees, task forces, and councils should include use of EBP.

   d. Allot time, funds, and resources to support nursing research at all levels of nursing practice.

   e. Consider offering incentives for EBP (e.g., prizes, books, journal subscriptions, or conference registration).

VII. Dissemination

A. The last step in research and QI processes is dissemination.

1. Ensure that nurses conducting research within the institution share their results with nursing staff.

2. Findings can be presented at local, regional, national, and international conferences.

B. Select communication outlets.

1. Podium/oral presentations

2. Poster presentation

3. Written report or manuscript

4. Grand rounds or clinical rounds

5. Podcasts or webinars

6. Hospital, organizational, or professional meetings

7. Health policy issue briefs

8. News media

9. Community events

10. Blogs

C. Know your audience.

1. Nursing

2. Healthcare providers

3. Policymakers

4. Consumers

D. Develop a plan and be prepared for and anticipate questions.

E. Disseminate findings as a journal article. Consider the following when choosing a journal:

1. Is the journal peer-reviewed?

2. Impact factor

3. Editorial process

4. Ethical standards

VIII. Attributes of Healthcare Quality

A. To manage quality, quality must be defined, and attributes must be specific and measurable.

1. Approach may vary with circumstances and purpose.

2. Donabedian (1992) defined six important attributes of healthcare quality (Table 7.1).

3. The degree of attention given to any attribute varies depending on the aspect of quality being assessed.

   a. Technical quality consists of "doing the right thing right"—that is, performing the right tests or providing the right services to accomplish desired result.

   b. Attributes of patient-provider interaction include communication, trust, empathy, sensitivity, and honesty.

Table 7.1	
Attributes of quality healthcare	
Attribute	**Description**
Effectiveness	The ability to attain the greatest improvement in health now achievable by the best care
Efficiency	The ability to lower cost of care without diminishing attainable improvements in health
Optimality	The balancing of costs against the effects of care on health (or on the benefits of healthcare, meaning the monetary value of improvements in health) so as to attain the most advantageous balance
Acceptability	Conformity to the wishes, desires, and expectations of patients and responsible members of their families
Legitimacy	Conformity to social preferences as expressed in ethical principles, values, norms, laws, and regulations
Equity	Conformity to a principle that determines what is just or fair in the distribution of healthcare and its benefits among the members of a population

(From Donabedian, A. (1992). The role of outcomes in quality assessment and assurance. *Quality Review Bulletin*, (11), 356–360.)

B. Quality assurance
1. Quality assurance (QA) encompasses processes that systematically monitor different aspects of service or facility.
2. Standards of care are norms on which quality of care is judged.
3. A major limitation of QA is that feedback comes too late in the process and does little to explain differences in practice or outcomes.
4. The primary source of QA review data is medical records that are often incomplete and an insufficient source of information needed to evaluate the quality of pain management.
5. The traditional formula of education and QA was insufficient to improve pain management and treatment outcomes.
C. Quality improvement
1. Evolved from QA as a framework used to systematically improve care delivery within systems
2. Focuses on improving practices and processes within an organization or patient population
3. Not intended to generate new knowledge beyond the specific context of study
4. Data can be collected to help understand systems' processes and uncover root causes of any inconsistencies or variations contributing to problems with quality.
   a. A system is a group of related processes or a sequence of tasks necessary to achieve a particular outcome.
   b. Organizations are complex systems designed to serve customers (e.g., patients, providers, the community, regulators).
   c. There is no predetermined or final yardstick of quality; instead, the goal is continuous improvement.
5. Compilation of methods adapted from many disciplines to avoid errors, eliminate variations in practice, and improve production of goods and services
6. Depends on development and implementation of care standards in healthcare and generation of data for performance measurement
   a. Data must be generated and reviewed against an established norm or baseline to make care consistent and reduce statistical errors.
   b. Use of data to track and monitor trends has been shown to be critical for hospital-based QI activities to succeed.
7. Requires knowledge of the system being improved and involves enlisting entire organization; all disciplines must work together
8. Select approaches to QI: all use similar principles
   a. Juran quality improvement methodology
   b. Six Sigma
   c. Lean Thinking (Toyota)
   d. Verzuh's steps

9. Select the tools available to assist in QI projects:
   a. Institute for Healthcare Improvement offers a toolkit that describes some commonly used tools: the *Quality Improvement Essentials Toolkit*
   b. Failure Modes and Effects Analysis (FMEA)
      1) FMEA is used to conduct a systematic, proactive analysis of a process in which harm may occur.
      2) Emphasis on prevention may reduce risk of harm.
      3) FMEA is particularly useful in evaluating a new process prior to implementation (e.g., prior to implementing use of new pain pump).
   c. Plan-Do-Study-Act (PDSA) cycle
      1) Useful for documenting test of change
      2) In many improvement projects, a team will test several different changes; each change may go through several PDSA cycles.
   d. Pareto Principle (80/20 rule)
      1) In any group of factors that contribute to the overall effect, roughly 80% of the effect comes from 20% of the causes.
      2) The Pareto chart arranges various factors in order from largest to smallest contribution, which helps identify key factors warranting most attention.
10. Quality indicators should demonstrate room for improvement and should be relevant, actionable, valid, unambiguous, reliable, and feasible to collect data for.
11. It is important to understand the complexity of a system or issue being studied and improved. Lack of awareness of all aspects can contribute to failure or challenges in an improvement project.
D. Clinical practice and EBP guidelines
1. Clinical practice guidelines are evidence-based, combining synthesis and appraisal of research evidence with specific recommendations for clinical decisions.
2. Limited evidence exists on the most effective method to disseminate and implement guidelines.
   a. Translating best evidence regarding effectiveness and safety recommendations from guidelines into usable care bundles (e.g., central line bundle) has been a successful approach.
   b. This approach allows all providers to hold each other accountable.
3. Guidelines may be translated into performance measures to assess delivery of care by administrators, regulators, and payers.
E. Public accountability
1. Performance measures are rate-based and reported as fractions or percentages of the total number of eligible events.
2. Performance indicators (PI)s are used to facilitate QI activities, as well as for reporting to external

agencies, both voluntary and required. Many measures are publicly reported.
3. Healthcare purchasers use PIs to compare services and may be used in negotiating payments.
4. PIs should measure variations and improvements in performance and should include concerns of all stakeholders: patients, providers, regulators, insurers, and accreditation agencies.
5. PIs reported back to healthcare purchaser or consumer can have a significant impact on healthcare choices.
6. Several leaders in the development of broad-based national performance data sets include:
   a. Agency for Healthcare Research and Quality
      1) 2002: AHRQ partnered with the Centers for Medicare and Medicaid Services (CMS) to create a standardized survey instrument and data collection methodology for measuring patients' perspectives on hospital care, termed *Hospital Consumer Assessment of Healthcare Providers and Systems (HCAHPS, or Hospital CAHPS).*
      2) Hospital Value-Based Purchasing (Hospital VBP) links a portion of hospital payment from CMS to performance on HCAHPS.
      3) HCAHPS initially included pain composite questions.
         a) 2017: CMS removed pain management dimension from the Hospital VBP program based on stakeholder feedback that linking survey questions on pain management to hospital payment could create incentives to prescribe more opioids.
         b) 2018: CMS removed pain management questions and replaced them with questions on provider communication with patients about pain.
         c) Due to continued concerns, communication about pain questions were removed and responses were no longer publicly reported.
         d) Patient satisfaction questions regarding pain are included in some patient satisfaction platforms, such as Press Ganey or Force.
      4) The National Committee for Quality Assurance is an independent, nonprofit agency working to improve quality of healthcare that highlights top performers.
      5) The Commission on Accreditation of Rehabilitation Facilities is an independent, nonprofit accreditor of health and human services in areas such as behavioral health, rehabilitation services, and opioid treatment programs.
      6) The Joint Commission is largest standard-setting agency that accredits and certifies healthcare organizations and programs in the United States.
      7) The National Quality Forum is a nonprofit organization whose measures and standards serve as the foundation for initiatives to enhance healthcare value, improve patient safety, and achieve better outcomes.
      8) Leapfrog collects, analyzes, and publishes data on safety and quality to promote high-value care and informed healthcare decisions.

IX. American Nurses Association Nursing Sensitive Quality Indicators for Acute Care Settings

A. The American Nurses Association (ANA) launched quality indicators in 1994 as a multiphase initiative to investigate impact of healthcare restructuring on safety and quality of patient care, as well as on nursing.
B. ANA safety and quality initiative
   1. Focuses on educating registered nurses about QI
   2. Informs the public and purchasing and regulating constituencies about safe, quality healthcare
   3. Investigates research methods and data sources to evaluate safety and quality patient care
C. 1998: ANA provided funding to develop a national database to house data collected using nursing sensitive quality indicators; this became the National Database of Nursing Quality Indicators (NDNQI).
D. Research has shown that some patient quality and safety measures are significantly affected by nursing care or "nurse-sensitive" measures. These are collected through a combination of medical record review and administrative data. NDNQI is the leading voluntary system for collection and analysis of data.
E. 2015: NDNQI was acquired by Press Ganey, with plans to carry on and expand the efforts of the ANA to advance the quality of the patient experience and achieve higher quality and more coordinated care.
F. Nurse-sensitive quality indicators include hospital-acquired conditions and adverse events subject to CMS nonpayment rule, such as:
   1. Catheter-associated urinary tract infection (CAUTI)
   2. Central line-associated bloodstream infection (CLABSI)
   3. Patient falls
   4. Pressure injuries
   5. Ventilator-associated pneumonia events (VAP, VAE)
   6. Pediatric Pain Assessment/Intervention/Reassessment (AIR) Cycle
   7. Pain-impairing function
G. Tracking these indicators can provide actionable insights based on structure, process, and outcome data.

X. ANA and American Society for Pain Management Nursing Scope and Standards of Practice (2016)

A. *The aim of the ANA and ASPMN Scope and Standards* is to provide standards and responsibilities for all professional nurses in their delivery of safe care and advocacy for care directed at alleviating pain and suffering across the lifespan, in every practice setting and for all healthcare consumers.

B. Competencies accompany each standard. Whether the standard applies depends on the clinical setting and situation. Competencies are presented for registered nurse (RN)–level practice in all settings. Additional competencies are presented for RNs educated at graduate level and for advanced practice registered nurses (APRNs).

1. Standards of professional performance include:
   a. EBP and research: RN integrates evidence and research findings into pain management practice.
   b. Quality of practice: RN contributes to quality pain management nursing practice (Box 7.1).

Box 7.1

Competencies for Standard 14: Quality of Practice

The Registered Nurse (RN):
- Ensures that nursing practice is safe, effective, efficient, equitable, timely, and patient-centered
- Identifies barriers and opportunities to improve pain management safety, effectiveness, efficiency, equitability, timeliness, and patient-centeredness
- Recommends strategies to enhance nursing care of patients, especially those in pain
- Uses creativity and innovation to improve and enhance nursing care and pain management
- Participates in quality improvement activities
- Collects data to monitor the quality of pain management nursing
- Contributes in efforts to improve the efficacy of care, including pain management
- Provides critical review and/or evaluation of policies, procedures, and guidelines to improve the quality of care and pain management
- Engages in formal and informal peer review process
- Collaborates with the interprofessional team to implement quality improvement plans and interventions
- Documents nursing practice in a manner that supports quality and performance improvement initiatives
- Obtains and maintains professional certification in pain management nursing

There are additional competencies for the graduate-level prepared specialty nurse and the advanced practice registered nurse (APRN).

---

c. Resource utilization: RN uses appropriate resources to plan, provide, and sustain evidence-based pain management nursing services that are safe, effective, and fiscally responsible.

XI. Quality Improvement in Pain Management

A. High-quality pain management includes elements of structure, process, and outcome.
1. Appropriate assessment includes screening for presence of pain, completion of a comprehensive initial assessment, and frequent reassessments of response to treatment.
2. Interprofessional, collaborative care planning includes patient input.
3. Appropriate treatment is efficacious, cost-conscious, culturally and developmentally appropriate, and safe.
4. Access to specialty care is provided as needed.

B. Complicating factors in the discussion of quality pain management
1. Pain is highly subjective and difficult to quantify, resulting in challenges in defining and measuring quality of pain care.
2. Emotional impact of pain and accompanying suffering increase the difficulty of quantifying and comparing pain experience and treatment among individuals.

C. Patient outcome QI survey designed to appraise six aspects of quality was validated in 2010 by Gordon et al. and includes measures of:
1. Pain severity and relief
2. Impact of pain on activity, sleep, and negative emotions
3. Side effects of treatment
4. Helpfulness of information about pain treatment
5. Ability to participate in pain treatment decisions
6. Use of nonpharmacologic strategies

D. Institutions should develop an interprofessional QI team and use a structured approach to assess and improve quality of pain care.

E. Key elements to improve pain care as a starting point for institutional responsibility include:
1. Recognize and treat pain promptly.
   a. Avoid focusing on unidimensional aspects of pain, such as the pain rating; this has been found to be problematic.
   b. Comprehensive assessments appropriate to population and setting are necessary.
   c. Analgesics should be preemptive and multimodal.
2. Involve patients in pain care plan and promote collaborative, shared decision-making.

3. Improve pain care patterns.
   a. Transition from as-needed dosing to preemptive and around-the-clock dosing when appropriate.
   b. In most situations, multimodal analgesia is recommended. Include combinations of analgesics with different mechanisms of action, along with nonpharmacologic interventions.
   c. Ensure that treatments are safe.
   d. Implement evidence-based advancements for regimens sensitive to the type of pain and the treatment setting.
4. Reassess and adjust pain care plan as needed.
   a. Establish realistic goals with a focus on function and quality of life for acute and persistent pain.
   b. The burden of treatment on quality of life and resources should also be considered.
5. Monitor processes and outcomes of pain care using questions to frame QI evaluations.
   a. Why do we do what we do?
   b. How do we know it works?
   c. How can we do it better?
6. Where possible, use standardized measures that have validity and reliability.
7. A meta-analysis of 20 pain QI studies performed at eight large U.S. hospitals identified quality indicators for hospital-based pain management. Select indicators include:
   a. Intensity of pain is documented with a numeric or descriptive rating scale.
   b. Pain intensity is documented at frequent intervals.
   c. Pain is treated with regularly administrated analgesics, and a multimodal approach is used when possible.
   d. Pain is prevented and maintained to the degree that facilitates function and quality of life.
   e. Patients are adequately informed and knowledgeable about pain management.
F. Example of a pain QI project
1. Topham and Drew (2017) describe a project to replace the numeric rating scale with a Clinically Aligned Pain Assessment (CAPA) tool.
   a. Goal was to improve patients' experience with pain management as measured by Press Ganey satisfaction scores.
   b. Verzuh's steps were used to implement use of the tool.
      1) Define scope of project.
      2) Identify and manage risks: Key clinical leaders were contacted early to enlist support to replace long-standing use of numeric pain rating scale in healthcare.
      3) Break down and schedule work: A major component of scheduling work included education sessions for all nurses and healthcare providers.

      4) Multiple communication methods were used.
      5) Progress was measured.
         a) Weekly compliance reports for each unit on use of CAPA tool
         b) Press Ganey patient satisfaction scores
         c) Press Ganey scores were variable and trended upward. Eighty percent of staff felt communication with patients improved with the use of CAPA.

XII. Applying Guidelines to Clinical Practice

A. Techniques used to implement EBP can be used to apply clinical practice guidelines to a practice.
B. To determine credibility, guidelines should demonstrate:
1. Expertise of the panel that developed the guidelines
2. Incorporation of patient perspectives
3. Evidence of systematic review, including all scientifically credible studies that address the question at hand
4. Assessment of the strength of each individual recommendation
5. Consideration of outcomes and implementation
6. Recency of development, or evidence of review and updating
7. Endorsement by respected national bodies, such as the ASPMN
8. Review by experts outside sponsoring organization
9. Disclosure of any conflict(s) of interest (financial or otherwise) for each panel member
10. Any disagreement among guidelines developed on same topic by different organizations
11. Pluralism: The United States has guidelines developed by a variety of organizations, rather than a single version prepared by the federal government.
C. Select an appropriate appraisal tool.
1. Determine the type of evidence being reviewed.
2. Examples of tools:
   a. Joanna Briggs Institute Manual for Evidence Implementation (https://doi.org/10.46658/JBIMEI-20-01)
   b. Johns Hopkins has research and nonresearch evidence appraisal tools: 2022 EBP models and tools (hopkinsmedicine.org).
   c. Rapid critical appraisal checklists can be used with clinical practice guidelines.

XIII. Developing a QI Pain Project

A. QI projects focus on making incremental changes measured at regular intervals to test the impact of change.

1. Determine aim or purpose of the project.
2. Summarize current situation that triggered the project or what needs improvement.
3. Plan to engage team, patients, and other stakeholders.
4. Describe baseline data.
5. Identify improvement strategy.
6. Implement change(s).
7. Measure impact of change(s).
8. Provide feedback.
9. Continue to monitor.

B. Once implemented, continue to monitor and evaluate for any necessary adjustments and to ensure sustainability.

Bibliography

American Nurses Association, American Society for Pain Management Nursing. (2016). *Pain Management Nursing: Scope and Standards of Practice* (2nd Ed.). Silver Spring, MD: American Nurses Association, Association of Pain Management Nursing.

American Nurses Association Center for Ethics and Human Rights. (2018*). American Nurses Association position statement: The Ethical Responsibility to Manage Pain and the Suffering It Causes.* https://www.nursingworld.org/~495e9b/globalassets/docs/ana/ethics/theethicalresponsibilitytomanagepainandthesufferingitcauses2018.pdf.

Black, K., & Revere, L. (2006). Six Sigma arises from the ashes of TQM with a twist. *International Journal of Health Care Quality Assurance Incorporating Leadership in Health Services, 19*(2–3), 259–266. https://doi.org/10.1108/09526860610661473.

Buccheri, R. K., & Sharifi, C. (2017). Critical appraisal tools and reporting guidelines for evidence-based practice. *Worldviews on Evidence-Based Nursing, 14*(6), 463–472. https://doi.org/10.1111/wvn.12258.

Chou, R., Gordon, D. B., de Leon-Casasola, O. A., Rosenberg, J. M., Bickler, S., Brennan, T., et al. (2016). Management of postoperative pain: a Clinical Practice Guideline from the American Pain Society, the American Society of Regional Anesthesia and Pain Medicine, and the American Society of Anesthesiologists' Committee on Regional Anesthesia, Executive Committee, and Administrative Council. *The Journal of Pain, 17*(2), 131–157. https://doi.org/10.1016/j.jpain.2015.12.008.

Chou, R., Wagner, J., Ahmed, A. Y., Blazina, I., Brodt, E., Buckley, D. I., et al. (2020). *Treatments for Acute Pain: A Systemic Review.* Comparative Effectiveness Review, No. 240. Report No. 20 (21)-EHC006. Rockville, MD: Agency for Healthcare Research and Quality. https://doi.org/10.23970/AHRQEPCCER240.

Donabedian, A. (1968). Promoting quality through evaluating the process of patient care. *Medical Care, 6*(3), 181–202. http://www.jstor.org/stable/3762934.

Gordon, D., Polomnao, R., Pellino, T., Turk, D., McCracken, L., Sherwood, G., et al. (2010). Revised American Pain Society patient outcomes questionnaire (APS-POQ-R) for quality improvement of pain management in hospitalized adults: preliminary psychometric evaluation. *The Journal of Pain, 11*, 1172–1186. https://doi.org/10.1016/j.jpain.2010.02.012.

Gray, J., Grove, S., & Sutherland, S. (2017). *Burn's and Grove's The Practice of Nursing Research: Appraisal, Synthesis, and Generation of Evidence* (8th ed.). St. Louis, MO: Elsevier.

Haber, L. A., DeFries, T., & Martin, M. (2019). Things We Do for No Reason™: discontinuing buprenorphine when treating acute pain. *Journal of Hospital Medicine, 14*(10), 633–635. https://doi.org/10.12788/jhm.3265.

Herr, K., Coyne, P. J., Ely, E., Gélinas, C., & Manworren, R. (2019). ASPMN 2019 Position Statement: Pain Assessment in the Patient Unable to Self-Report. *Pain Management Nursing,* (5), 402–403. https://doi.org/10.1016/j.pmn.2019.07.007.

Institute for Healthcare Improvement. (2017). *Quality Improvement Essentials Toolkit.* www.ihi.org/resourcespages/tools/quality-improvement-essentials-toolkit.aspx.

Institute of Medicine (US) Committee to Design a Strategy for Quality Review and Assurance in Medicare, & Lohr, K. N. (Eds.). (1990). Medicare: A Strategy for Quality Assurance. National Academies Press (US).

The Joint Commission. (2021). Joint Commission Resources. Oakbrook Terrace, IL. E-dition. https://e-dition.jcrinc.com.

Jungquist, C. R., Quinlan-Colwell, A., Vallerand, A., Carlisle, H. L., Cooney, M., Dempsey, S. J., et al. (2020). American Society for Pain Management Nursing Guidelines on Monitoring for Opioid-Induced Advancing Sedation and Respiratory Depression: Revisions. *Pain Management Nursing, 21*(1), 7–25. https://doi.org/10.1016/j.pmn.2019.06.007.

Juran, D. (2021). *The Juran Model and Excellence Framework.* https://www.juran.com/approach/the-juran-model/.

Kim, C. S., Spahlinger, D. A., Kin, J. M., & Billi, J. E. (2006). Lean health care: what can hospitals learn from a world-class automaker?. *Journal of Hospital Medicine, 1*(3), 191–199. https://doi.org/10.1002/jhm.68.

Medicare Learning Network. (2017). *Hospital value-based purchasing.* Centers for Medicare and Medicaid Services. https://www.cms.gov/Outreach-and-Education/Medicare-Learning-Network-MLN/MLNProducts/downloads/Hospital_VBPurchasing_Fact_Sheet_ICN907664.pdf.

Melnyk, B. M., & Fineout-Overholt, E. (2015). *Evidence-Based Practice in Nursing and Healthcare* (3rd ed.). Philadelphia, PA: Lippincott Williams & Wilkins.

Mendelson, A., Kondo, K., Damberg, C., Low, A., Motúapuaka, M., Freeman, M., O'Neil, M., Relevo, R., & Kansagara, D. (2017). The effects of pay-for-performance programs on health, health care use, and processes of care: a systematic review. *Annals of Internal Medicine, 166*(5), 341–353. https://doi.org/10.7326/M16-1881.

Montalvo, I. (2007). The National Database of Nursing Quality Indicators™ (NDNQI®). *Online Journal of Issues in Nursing.* 12(3), Manuscript 2. https://doi.org/10.3912/OJIN.Vol12No03Man02.

Pasero, C., Quinlan-Colwell, A., Rae, D., Broglio, K., & Drew, D. (2016). American Society for Pain Management Nursing Position Statement: Prescribing and Administering Opioid Doses Based Solely on Pain Intensity. *Pain Management Nursing, 17*(5), 291–292. https://doi.org/10.1016/j.pmn.2016.08.002.

Polit, D. F., & Beck, C. T. (2017). *Nursing Research: Generating and Assessing Evidence for Nursing Practice.* (10th ed.). Philadelphia, PA: Wolters Kluwer.

Press Ganey. July 14, 2015. https://www.prnewswire.com/news-releases/press-ganey-acquires-national-database-of-nursing-quality-indicators-ndnqi-262538811.html.

Saunders, H. (2015). Translating knowledge into best practice care bundles: a pragmatic strategy for EBP implementation via moving postprocedural pain management nursing guidelines into clinical practice. *Journal of Clinical Nursing, 24*(13–14), 2035–2051. https://doi.org/10.1111/jocn.12812.

Shanthanna, H., Cohen, S.P., Strand, S., Lobo, C., Eldabe, S., Bhatia, et al. (2020). *Recommendations on Chronic Pain Practice during the COVID-19 Pandemic. A Joint Statement by American Society of Regional Anesthesia and Pain Medicine and European Society of Regional Anesthesia and Pain Therapy (ESRA).* https://www.asra.com/page/2903/recommendations-on-chronic-pain-practice-during-the-covid-19-pandemic.

Siriwardena, A. N., & Gillam, S. (2013). Measuring for improvement. *Quality in Primary Care, 21*(5), 293–301.

Stetler, C. B. (1994). Refinement of the Stetler/Marram model for application of research findings to practice. *Nursing Outlook, 42*(1), 15–25. https://doi.org/10.1016/0029-6554(94)90067-1.

Titler, M. G., Kleiber, C., Steelman, V. J., Rakel, B. A., Budreau, G., & Everett, L. Q. (2001). The Iowa Model of evidence-based practice to promote quality care. *Critical Care Nursing Clinics of North America, 13*(4), 497–509.

Topham, D., & Drew, D. (2017). Quality improvement project: replacing the numeric rating scale with a Clinically Aligned Pain Assessment (CAPA) Tool. *Pain Management Nursing, 18*(6), 363–371. https://doi.org/10.1016/j.pmn.2017.07.001.

U.S. Department of Health and Human Services. (2019). *Pain Management Best Practices Inter-Agency Task Force Report: Updates, Gaps, Inconsistencies, and Recommendations.* https://www.hhs.gov/ash/advisory-committees/pain/reports/index.html.

Verzuh, E. (2021). *The Fast Forward in Project Management* (6th ed.). Hoboken, NJ: John Wiley & Sons.

Zoëga, S., Gunnarsdottir, S., Wilson, M. E., & Gordon, D. B. (2016). Quality pain management in adult hospitalized patients: a concept evaluation. *Nursing Forum, 51*(1), 3–12. https://doi.org/10.1111/nuf.12085.

CHAPTER 8

Advocacy in Pain Management Nursing

Marsha Stanton, PhD, RN
Pamela Madrid, BSN, BS
Michael C. Barnes, JD
Robert Twillman, PhD
Wade Delk, BA
Angela T. Casey (professional writer)
Ann Schreier, PhD, BSN, MSN, RN*

Introduction

Social, political, and ethical issues drive policy and impact the ability of nurses and other healthcare professionals (HCPs) to provide effective, patient-centered pain management. This chapter will differentiate between policies that promote or hinder care of people with pain and aid readers in developing and implementing strategies to effectively advocate for people with pain in a clinical, peer community, and wider stakeholder settings. Readers will gain insight into how to actively engage with people affected by pain, colleagues, legislators, and other stakeholders to better understand the impact of current policies and identify areas future policies should address. Lastly, American Society for Pain Management Nursing (ASPMN) position statements and advocacy statements to improve pain care and enhance pain management practices will be shared.

I. Types of Advocacy

A. Advocacy is defined as the act or process of pleading for, supporting, or recommending a cause or course of action.
   1. Advocacy for patient rights, health, and safety is part of nurses' ethical obligation.
   2. As the largest group of HCPs in the United States, and ranked by the public for the nineteenth consecutive year as the most honest and ethical profession, nurses are in a unique position to influence the health of communities they serve.
B. Nurses can engage in different types of advocacy in a variety of arenas.
   1. Individual patient level
      a. Nurses' close patient contact allows a more patient-centered versus disease-centered view, making them the most likely HCPs to act as patient and family advocates.

b. Nurses can ensure patients receive evidence-based care aligned with best practices. Examples may include advocating for changes to an ineffective pain management regimen or advocating for patients who are denied insurance coverage by submitting documentation to the insurance company outlining why the treatment is most appropriate, cost-effective, and provides other benefits, such as avoiding emergency department visits.
   2. Practice settings
      a. Nurses can advocate for patient-focused pain management practice changes to improve patient care for an entire patient population (e.g., within practice setting; with certain diagnosis). This might involve working with committees and leadership to decide on practice change (e.g., implementing an ASPMN position statement [noted in Resources VIII.A.2]) and subsequently championing change among colleagues.
   3. Healthcare profession
      a. Should be priority for all nurses and involves:
         1) Role-modeling and mentoring next generation of nurses
         2) Acting to promote pain management nursing profession
         3) Advocating for patients as mandated by American Nurses Association (ANA) Code of Ethics
      b. Professional advocacy could also include efforts aimed at changing federal or state legislation around scope of practice or professional education barriers.
   4. Community
      a. Nurses can serve on boards (e.g., county health or hospital board), where they can leverage nursing perspectives to advocate for the health of communities they serve.
      b. Nurses could participate and advocate in discussions surrounding the allocation of

---

*Section Editor for the chapter.

resources to support those with mental health or substance use disorders (SUDs).

5. Coalition(s)
   a. Coalitions involve people coming together to achieve a common goal (e.g., improved pain management) and may include members from:
      1) Healthcare
      2) Social services
      3) Educational organizations
      4) Accreditation agencies
      5) Insurers
      6) Employers
      7) Foundations
      8) Patient-advocate organizations
   b. A wide variety of nursing organizations generate greater influence with a larger collective voice.
      1) ASPMN has been involved in nursing coalition actions, such as engaging with members of Congress to request allocation of funds for nursing programs and to support legislation promoting improved pain management.
      2) Other activities may include training or participating in public awareness campaigns to promote core messages.

6. Federal-, state-, or local-level legislation
   a. Influencing policy agenda
   b. Working on introduction or amending legislation
   c. Opposing a bill
   d. Advocating to fund an enacted law (see section III.B.1).
   e. At all levels, nurses can influence agencies responsible for interpreting and implementing laws related to health of communities, patient populations, or nursing profession (see section III.B.2).

7. Media
   a. Raise awareness of a problem.
   b. Encourage other professionals and community members to learn more and get involved.
   c. Influence policy by shaping the debate (i.e., changing the way people talk about a particular public health problem).
   d. Advance policy by informing and influencing policymakers.
   e. Transmit information to general public through:
      1) Broadcast (television, radio, streaming audio, and video)
      2) Print (newspapers, magazines)
      3) Online media
   f. Social media (e.g., blogs, Facebook, Instagram, LinkedIn) involvement with 24/7 availability:
      1) Share information (e.g., ASPMN position statements, legislative updates).
      2) Express support (e.g., comment on other posts); can be as simple as "liking" or "following" posts of individuals or groups.
      3) Integrate social media into organizations' advocacy campaigns in systematic way, using analytics to guide efforts to reach, engage with, and activate target audiences.

C. Nurses who have successfully engaged in advocacy efforts in any of these areas can and should share their experiences to inspire other nurses to engage in advocacy and ultimately lead to positive change in the lives of people with pain.
   1. Publish in *Pain Management Nursing* or other professional journals.
   2. Present at conferences (e.g., ASPMN or other professional organizations).

II. Factors Complicating Pain Management in the United States

A. Opioid-related public health crisis
   1. The United States is in the midst of an opioid-related public health crisis, characterized by misuse, opioid-use disorder (OUD), and deaths due to overdoses involving prescription and nonprescription opioids.
   2. While deaths associated with prescription opioids declined from 2013 to 2019, provisional data from Centers for Disease Control and Prevention (CDC) show this trend was reversed in the first 8 months of 2020, potentially exacerbated by COVID-19 pandemic.
   3. Deaths involving synthetic opioids (largely illicit fentanyl), psychostimulants with abuse potential (e.g., methamphetamine), and cocaine have increased in recent years, particularly since 2013.

B. Inadequately treated pain and patient suffering
   1. Behind the headline-making opioid crisis, there is a second, less publicized continuing public health crisis of inadequately treated pain and patient suffering.
   2. In 2019, 20.4% of U.S. adults (more than 52 million) reported persistent pain, and 7.4% of U.S. adults (18.9 million) had persistent pain limiting life or work activities. A Human Rights Watch report found patients with persistent pain face challenges in obtaining appropriate care.
   3. Many patients have been left with debilitating pain due to the opioid-related public health crisis because prescribers increasingly saw these patients as a potential source of liability and avoided prescribing opioids, even when indicated.

C. Multiple policies at federal, state, and payer level have been implemented to reduce unsafe prescribing of opioids.
   1. Many policies cite 2016 *CDC Guideline for Prescribing Opioids for Chronic Pain* to provide

recommendations for prescribing opioid analgesics for adults in primary care settings. However, these guidelines have been misinterpreted and misapplied, creating unintended patient consequences (as discussed later; see section V.A.3.a/b).

2. A balanced approach to opioid prescribing is necessary to avoid opioid-related harms, support more judicious opioid prescribing, and decrease patient harm. This involves using opioids where appropriate in combination with evidence-supported non-opioid and nonpharmacological therapies, which are often underutilized due to inadequate insurance coverage and reimbursement.

D. Solving these problems requires sustained, coordinated, multipronged approach by relevant stakeholders.
   1. Nurses have an opportunity and obligation to participate in development and evaluation of proposed policies and legislation surrounding pain management to help ensure that unintended consequences and harm do not occur.
   2. Research evaluating the impact of policies (once implemented) is imperative.

III. Policy

A. Public health policies are authoritative decisions regarding health or pursuit of health made in legislative, executive, or judicial branches of government. Legislators decide on laws, federal agencies of executive branch decide on rules to implement and enforce laws, and judges review interpretations and applications of laws to individual cases.
   1. Health policies are established at federal, state, and local levels of government and can take several forms, including:
      a. Laws enacted at any level of government
      b. Rules or regulations established by administrative agencies in executive branch to guide implementation of laws passed in legislative branch. Rulemaking is processes by which agencies write rules to implement and enforce laws.
      c. Implementation decisions address how to implement or enforce rules and regulations.
      d. Judicial decisions address applicability of laws to specific situations or appropriateness of actions by implementing organizations.
   2. Unlike policies that are authoritative decisions, guidelines are official statements and do not have the force of law.
      a. Guidelines may be issued by a professional association, licensing board, or government agency to express its position on particular topics.
      b. State medical boards have issued guidelines defining conduct the board considers to be

within accepted standards of medical practice regarding legitimate use of opioids for pain.
      c. Guidelines may also be referred to as position or policy statements and may be published in reports, journal articles, letters, or newsletters.
   3. Public policymaking is a dynamic process including three interconnected phases in cyclical flow:
      a. Formulation: setting policy agenda and developing legislation that leads to or modifies public laws
      b. Implementation: designing, rulemaking, operating, enforcing and evaluating
      c. Modification: revisiting and potentially changing prior decisions

B. There are many opportunities for nurses to influence policy to support their work of improving health for patients or populations.
   1. Influencing policy formulation
      a. Know your legislators and where they stand on issue(s) in question.
         1) To identify your U.S. representative and senator, use websites noted in the Resources section (VIII.D.1).
            a) Their biographies will provide background information, such as hometown, education, profession, and interests, while press releases, official statements, and voting record will help to identify their positions on policies affecting nursing, healthcare, and pain.
            b) Most legislators' websites also include committee and subcommittee assignments, caucus memberships, and bills they support.
         2) Subscribe to their newsletter and follow them on social media to stay informed.
      b. Communicating with legislators (See ASPMN Legislative Toolkit at ASPMN.org)
         1) Request and prepare for meeting.
            a) Plan how to introduce yourself.
            b) Set goals for meeting and create a half- to one-page summary.
            c) Know issue well, including all sides of argument.
            d) Provide context with personal stories about how issue affects your patients and nursing profession.
            e) Connect issue back to legislator's congressional district or state as much as possible.
            f) For an in-person or video meeting;
               (1) Arrive early; be patient and flexible.
               (2) State your position clearly and concisely.
               (3) Make your "ask."

(4) Be prepared to explain technical terms and answer questions.

g) Advocacy does not end after your visit, so keep in regular contact with relevant staff.

2) Email is quickest way to communicate with legislator.

3) Share your email with colleagues on social media; ask them to send similar message to their legislators.

2. Influencing policy implementation

a. Much of federal- and state-level advocacy is geared toward numerous governmental departments and agencies that interpret, implement, and enforce legislation affecting the nursing profession and patients' health. It is important the voice of nursing be heard during decision-making processes. Examples of relevant federal departments and agencies include:

1) U.S. Department of Health and Human Services (HHS)

a) Administration for Community Living (ACL)

b) Agency for Healthcare Research and Quality (AHRQ)

c) Centers for Disease Control and Prevention (CDC)

(1) National Center for Chronic Disease Prevention and Health Promotion (NCCDPHP)

(2) National Center for Injury Prevention and Control (NCIPC)

d) Centers for Medicare & Medicaid Services (CMS)

e) Health Resources and Services Administration (HRSA)

f) Indian Health Service (IHS)

g) National Institutes of Health (NIH)

(1) National Institute on Aging (NIA)

(2) National Institute on Drug Abuse (NIDA)

(3) National Institute of Nursing Research (NINR)

h) Substance Abuse and Mental Health Services Administration (SAMHSA)

i) U.S. Food and Drug Administration (FDA)

2) U.S. Department of Veterans' Affairs (VA)

a) Veterans' Health Administration

3) U.S. Department of Justice (DOJ)

a) U.S. Drug Enforcement Administration (DEA)

4) Defense Health Agency (DHA)

b. Commenting on proposed rules or proposed amendments to existing rules, which are published in the *Federal Register* (www.federalregister.gov)

for review by those who will be affected by them, is one of the most active points of involvement in policymaking.

1) Regulatory officials from agency review all public comments received within open comment period, which may result in revision of proposed rule before it is published as a final rule, becomes part of *Code of Federal Regulations*, and is enforced.

a) Federal government also provides a website, www.regulations.gov, to facilitate public participation in rulemaking, where stakeholders can electronically submit comments on proposed new or amended rules.

b) Medicare Payment Advisory Commission accepts comments on proposed rules to update Medicare payment systems at www.MedPAC.gov; meetings notices are also posted here.

c) State governments publish public notices and proposed administrative rules in official state publications or electronic regulation system. Notices include instructions for submission of electronic or written comments on proposed new rules or amendments, together with deadlines for submission.

2) When submitting regulatory comments on proposed rules, nurses should:

a) Briefly describe professional background and relevant work or personal experience. Include name, professional credentials, and contact information.

b) Clearly state issue, your position, and offer suggestions for alternative solutions if you disagree with proposed rule.

c) Include real-world examples showing how proposed policy may affect patient care and nursing practice, and, if appropriate, cite supporting studies and data.

d) Do not include anything confidential because comments are public.

c. Participating with policy advisory bodies and commissions

1) Nurses can also influence policy by serving on, or interacting with, health agency advisory bodies and commissions. Agencies also seek public input through workshops and meetings, some of which are available by webcast.

a) Notices of public meetings and requests for nominees to federal panels are published in the *Federal Register*. To make an oral presentation during open public hearing portion of an advisory committee meeting, register with agency before meeting.

b) State agencies also provide information on public hearings in official state government publications or electronic regulation systems.

(1) State practice acts and licensure boards enact laws affecting nursing profession. Nurses should take any opportunity to develop relationships with licensure board members, attend their meetings if public, and seek appointment to serve on board.

(2) Nurses looking to influence state policy may also consider involvement in groups such as state attorney general's task force to prevent prescription overdose deaths to advocate and develop relationships with legislators and others on task force who have interest in opioid issue.

c) At federal level, National Institute of Nursing Research (NINR) has become the leader in pain research initiatives. NINR has developed its 2022–2026 strategic plan that:

(1) Describes future research goals and its vision for field of nursing science

(2) Encourages nurses to check their webpage (www.ninr.nih.gov/about-ninr/ninr-mission-and-strategic-plan) for updates on providing input to the future of nursing science

(3) Welcomes ideas about research directions via email at NINRstrategicplan@mail.nih.gov

2) The Recognize, Assist, Include, Support, and Engage (RAISE) Family Caregivers Act of 2017 became law in 2018 and directs HHS to develop a national Family Caregiving Strategy to support family caregivers.

a) Planning and implementation phase is ongoing, supported by Family Caregiving Advisory Council, which was established to support development and execution of national strategy (https://acl.gov/programs/support-caregivers/raise-family-caregiving-advisory-council).

b) Nurses should advocate for this national strategy to recognize needs of and provide support to family caregivers of people with pain.

C. In response to opioid overdose deaths, many states have enacted legislation and guidelines affecting use of opioid analgesics.

1. From 2015 to April 2021:

a. Thirty-nine states enacted a total of 92 laws related to opioid prescription limits (18 states have a total of 39 bills pending in 2021). Most of this legislation limits first-time opioid prescriptions to a certain number of days; a few states also set dosage limits.

b. Forty-six states enacted a total of 191 bills related to prescription drug monitoring program (PDMPs) (five states have a total of six bills pending).

c. Thirty-three states enacted a total of 85 bills related to provider education (12 states have a total of 28 bills pending).

2. In addition to state laws, opioid prescribing can also be limited by state-level Medicaid program requirements and limits and state licensing board guidelines and rules.

3. Ongoing efforts to study impact of state-level laws suggest there is no easy policy solution to decrease incidence of OUD, opioid overdose, and mortality.

D. Policy made by private organizations, healthcare systems, health insurance companies, and pharmacy benefit managers (PBMs) also affect pain management. For example, decisions made by:

1. Healthcare systems about services provided or medications on their formularies

2. Insurance companies and PBMs about provided coverage

a. Some insurers and PBMs developed further restrictions by expanding on the *CDC Guideline for Prescribing Opioids for Chronic Pain* (despite its limited scope and fact the recommendations were not intended to be mandatory).

b. In 2017, the trade association of health insurers, America's Health Insurance Plans (AHIP), launched its Safe, Transparent Opioid Prescribing (STOP) initiative, which includes a data analysis tool to identify opioid-prescribing patterns inconsistent with the guideline. This is problematic when applied to nonprimary care settings, and it ignores patients' individual needs.

3. Accreditation organizations:

a. The Joint Commission's (TJC) revised pain assessment and management standards became effective in 2018 for hospitals and in 2019 for all other types of healthcare settings. TJC provides opportunities for HCPs to comment on draft standards.

b. National Committee for Quality Assurance (NCQA) Healthcare Effectiveness Data and Information Set (HEDIS) collected data from health plans and healthcare organizations to assess and improve performance. Measures used assess potentially high-risk opioid prescribing practices, such as the proportion of adult members who, during the measurement year:

1) Received high-dose prescription opioids (average daily morphine milligram equivalent dose ≥90) for ≥15 days

2) Received prescription opioids for ≥15 days from multiple providers

3) Had a new episode of opioid use, putting them at risk for continued opioid use:

   a) ≥15 days of prescription opioids in 30-day period

   b) ≥31 days of prescription opioids in 62-day period

c. Commission on Accreditation of Rehabilitation Facilities (CARF) accredits interdisciplinary pain rehabilitation programs, requiring them to conform to quality standards.

IV. Politics

A. Policymaking is a highly political process affected by ideology and priorities of those who participate in the process. Health policy is also influenced by numerous external factors, such as economic conditions, heightened awareness of a problem, media pressure, and the influence of special interest groups and advocacy organizations.

B. When a new Congress convenes or a new president takes office, new policy preferences may arise and motivate efforts to modify, undermine, or eliminate policy. In addition, leaders of most federal departments and agencies implementing and regulating policy within the framework of laws passed by Congress are chosen by White House and are often replaced with a new administration. Therefore, transitions in political power affect funding, development, and implementation of policies, and can impact realization of national initiatives to improve pain management practices, such as the HHS's 2019 *Pain Management Best Practices Inter-Agency Task Force Report: Best Practices: Updates, Gaps, Inconsistencies, and Recommendations.*

V. Recent Legislation and Public Policy

A. Administration activity

1. HHS published *Pain Management Best Practices Inter-Agency Task Force Report: Updates, Gaps, Inconsistencies, and Recommendations* in 2019.

   a. The Task Force recommendations provide policymakers with essential blueprint to improve pain management and reduce opioid risks by achieving a system of effective, safe, high-quality, evidence-based pain care.

   b. Efforts are underway to ensure the government appropriates necessary resources to disseminate and implement recommendations.

2. NIH Helping to End Addiction Long-Term (HEAL) Initiative is in the process of funding projects nationwide to improve pain management and prevention and treatment of OUD.

   Nurses can submit suggestions on research to address opioid crisis through HEAL Idea Exchange at https://nih-heal.ideascalegov.com/a/campaign-home/216.

3. The CDC formed an Opioid Workgroup in 2020 to revise the *CDC Guideline for Prescribing Opioids for Chronic Pain* ("Guideline"). The CDC was forced to act following pushback against the misapplication of the original Guideline:

   a. An American Academy of Pain Medicine (AAPM) consensus report on challenges with implementation of the Guideline noted:

      1) Since its release, several polices were developed that go beyond the Guideline's intent.

      2) Lack of flexibility in application of recommended ceiling doses, prescription durations, and abrupt opioid taper or cessation in physically dependent, opioid-treated patients (despite CDC's support for empathically reviewing benefits and risks of continued therapy and collaboration with developing a tapering plan)

      3) The report urged that the appropriate role of regulatory and policymaking bodies be clarified regarding Guideline implementation.

   b. In 2019, Guideline authors acknowledged many of the challenges described may have caused harm to patients, stating some policies and practices purportedly derived from the Guideline had been inconsistent with and went beyond intended recommendations, including:

      1) Misapplication to populations outside the Guideline's scope

      2) Misimplementation of recommended dosage thresholds to justify hard limits

      3) Abrupt tapering or sudden discontinuation of opioids

   c. In 2022, the CDC issued its updated *Clinical Practice Guidelines for Prescribing Opioids for Pain*. Dosage and duration limits were removed, and it was clarified the recommendations should not be applied as inflexible standards of care across patient populations. Critics warn the Guideline's recommendations may be misinterpreted and are unlikely to have their intended effect of easing restrictions on prescription opioids. Additionally, some critics have expressed concern that the recommendations place too much emphasis on reducing opioid prescriptions, which can lead to undertreatment of persistent pain in some patients.

4. In 2022, the Consolidated Appropriations Act, 2023 removed the federal requirement that advanced practice registered nurses (APRNs) and physician assistants complete 24 hours of specialized training to receive a waiver from the Substance Abuse and Mental Health Services Administration to prescribe buprenorphine for the treatment of OUD (aka the X wavier) and added a training requirement for anyone who has a DEA registration to prescribe Schedule II–IV medications. Per the training requirement, practitioners renewing or newly applying for a registration after June 27, 2023:
   a. Must have a total of 8 hours of training on treating and managing patients with opioid or other substance use disorders
   b. Obtain training from certain accredited organizations, or
   c. Graduate within 5 years from advanced practice nursing or physician assistant school in the United States that included successful completion of an opioid or other substance use disorder curriculum of at least 8 hours.

B. There is constant and everchanging legislative activity in Congress on issues of importance to pain management nurses. Instructions to search for recently enacted and pending legislation can be found in the Resources section (VIII.D.2). It may be beneficial to periodically review the sections of state and federal bills that may have an impact on your practice area.
   1. Examples of enacted legislation:
      a. SUPPORT for Patients and Communities Act (became law in 2018)
      b. Title VIII Nursing Workforce Reauthorization Act of 2019 was included as part of the Coronavirus Aid, Relief, and Economic Security (CARES) Act (became law in 2020).
   2. Examples of pending legislation:
      a. 117th Congress (2021–2022) U.S. House pain-related bills:
         1) H.R.1185 Opioid Patients' Right to Know Act of 2021: Requires the CDC to award grants to states to educate HCPs about opioid-prescribing practices and inform patients about opioid risks
         2) S.586 Non-Opioids Prevent Addiction In the Nation (NOPAIN) Act: Promotes access to non-opioid treatments in the hospital outpatient setting

      b. 117th Congress (2021–2022) U.S. House OUD-related bill, H.R.1384 Mainstreaming Addiction Treatment Act of 2021 eliminates the requirement that practitioners obtain an X waiver to prescribe buprenorphine for OUD treatment
   3. In 2020, with the House Labor, Health and Human Services, and Education Committee Report accompanying the FY 2021 Appropriations Bill, Congress:
      a. Expressed concern over delayed implementation of HHS *Pain Management Best Practices Inter-Agency Task Force Report* recommendations and urged HHS to update pain management policies and educational tools to reflect recommended best practices
      b. Directed the CDC to collect, analyze, and annually publish pain statistics on incidence and prevalence of various pain syndromes differentiated by patient age, comorbidities, socioeconomic status (SES), race, and gender; and encouraged CDC to collect data on cost and effectiveness of non-opioid treatment approaches identified as important by the HHS Pain Management Best Practices Inter-Agency Task Force
      c. Urged HHS to coordinate with VA to launch a public awareness campaign to educate Americans about acute and persistent pain and evidence-based non-opioid treatments, including non-opioid medications, interventional procedures, behavioral health approaches, and complementary and integrative health therapies
      d. Strongly encouraged NIDA to create regional Pain Therapeutics and Opioid Addiction Centers of Excellence to assist states in educating and implementing best practices in opioid prescribing, pain management, and care for individuals with OUD
      e. Much of this work has been static due to other overwhelming issues, but they remain on the agenda until the more pressing issues are addressed.

VI. Social Issues

A. Stigma
   1. Stigma can be defined as a set of negative beliefs a group or society holds about an individual or group of people who demonstrate a particular behavior and can result in prejudice, avoidance, rejection, and discrimination against those who have certain traits or who engage in certain behaviors (e.g., substance use or misuse).
   2. People with persistent pain, especially those treated with opioid analgesics, can experience both subtle and overt stigma from family, friends, coworkers,

HCPs, healthcare systems, and society at large, which can result in barriers to pain care.
  a. Contributing to this stigmatization is the subjective and invisible nature of disease, and societal attitudes that equate acknowledging pain with weakness.
  b. Patients wanting to continue effective opioid analgesic therapy that has maintained or improved function have sometimes been disbelieved, dismissed, or seen as "drug-seeking."
  c. Feelings of guilt, shame, judgment, and embarrassment resulting from stigma can increase risk for behavioral health issues, such as anxiety and depression, which can further contribute to symptom chronicity.
  d. People with painful conditions and comorbidities such as anxiety, depression, or SUD face increased stigma, creating additional barriers to treatment.

3. Reducing barriers to pain care that exist as a consequence of stigmatization is crucial for patient engagement and treatment effectiveness.
  a. To counter attitudes that equate pain with weakness, patient and family education and public awareness campaigns should urge early treatment of pain persisting beyond expected duration for condition or injury.
  b. HCPs should treat patients seeking care with compassion and dignity, without dismissing the need for opioid analgesic therapy.
    1) Because stigmatizing language can negatively influence HCPs' perceptions of people and impact the care they provide, nurses should show leadership by selecting respectful, clear, and accurate language when speaking to or writing/speaking about people with pain, OUD, or SUD (Table 8.1).

Table 8.1

Examples of Language to Reduce Stigma

When ...	Instead of ...	Use ...
Talking about people with persistent pain	• Sufferer • Victim • Patient suffering with persistent pain • Patient afflicted with persistent pain	• Person with persistent pain • Person living with persistent pain • Person with a diagnosis of persistent pain
Talking about treatment of persistent pain	• Patient is treated	• Pain is treated
	• Patient is monitored	• Pain is monitored
	• Narcotic dependent	• Long-term/regular opioid use
Talking about the impact of persistent pain	• Insists pain is "still a 10" • Hopeless • Unbearable • Impossible • Tragic • Devastating	• Reports a pain intensity score of 10/10 • Disabling • Challenging • Life-changing • Stressful
Talking about people with a substance, opioid, or alcohol use disorder	• Addict • User • Substance or drug user/abuser • Junkie • Drug-seeker	• Person with substance use disorder • Person with opioid use disorder • Person with addiction • Patient
	• Former or reformed addict	• Person in recovery/remission • Person with a previous substance use disorder
	• Clean	• In recovery/remission • Abstinent from drugs • Not drinking or taking drugs
	• Alcoholic • Drunk	• Unhealthy or harmful alcohol use • Person with alcohol use disorder
Talking about substance use	• Relapse	• Experienced a recurrence of symptoms • Returned to harmful use
	• Drug abuse	• Drug misuse • Harmful drug use
	• Drug habit	• Substance use disorder • Addiction
	• Compliant	• Adherent
	• Clean drug test	• Tested negative
	• Dirty drug test	• Tested positive

(Data from American Medical Association, 2020; Copeland, 2020; Goddu et al., 2018; National Institute on Drug Abuse, 2021; PainAustralia, 2019.)

a) A study compared medical record notes employing stigmatizing versus neutral language to describe the same hypothetical patient with pain and found HCPs who read notes written with stigmatizing language had more negative attitudes toward the patient and managed pain less aggressively.
b) Because nurses turn to literature to guide their practice, it is also incumbent upon authors, reviewers, and editors to ensure published nursing literature uses respectful, non-stigmatizing language.
2) Recognizing persistent pain as a disease rather than symptom may help shape more positive patient-provider relationships.
c. Interventions that focus on changing individual attitudes, practices, and beliefs are insufficient.
1) A public health response should target stigma at structural level, by identifying—and subsequently eliminating or amending—policies that intensify stigmas against people in pain.
2) Communities can enact policies to inhibit stigma, such as changing or strengthening local health system policies to reflect accurate and respectful language in interacting with and caring for people with pain or OUD.
4. HCPs who treat pain with opioids may experience stigma from colleagues and society that—in addition to fear of scrutiny from state medical boards and the DEA—may dissuade them from using opioids when appropriate. Stigma may also lead to over-referral and patient abandonment.
B. Disparities in healthcare and pain management
1. Stereotyping involves using differences (e.g., race, sex, age, disability) to acquire, process, and recall information about others, resulting in beliefs (stereotypes) and attitudes toward people of that group. Such stereotypes and attitudes may be biased.
a. Explicit biases are attitudes and thoughts people are aware of and consciously endorse.
b. Implicit biases operate unconsciously.
2. Disparities in healthcare
a. It is well documented some HCPs in the United States harbor explicit biases toward minoritized or marginalized people, and yet most well-meaning HCPs wanting to provide equitable care continue patterns of care that perpetuate disparities.
b. Implicit stereotypes and biases operate unconsciously to influence HCPs' behavior toward, communication with, and treatment-related decisions for marginalized patients, which contribute to health disparities. Implicit biases

include using a condescending tone, failing to make eye contact, and recommending treatment options based on assumptions about ability to adhere to treatment.
c. Stereotypes can influence the nature of interactions with patients so they respond in ways that conform to stereotypical expectations. For example, HCPs who believe that "Black patients are less likely to adhere to treatment than White patients" may treat Black patients less optimally.
d. Stereotypes that reflect well-meaning judgments are also harmful. For example, HCPs may be less assertive when recommending certain medical procedures for minority patients out of a heightened (but nonetheless stereotyped) concern that minority patients wish to avoid new technologies.
3. Disparities in pain care
a. More than two decades of research has documented disparities in assessment, management, and outcomes of pain in minoritized and marginalized patients.
b. Given that people with pain are already stigmatized, minority patients with pain are particularly vulnerable to disparities.
c. Minority patients face numerous barriers to quality pain care.
1) Black patients are subjected to increased negative stereotypes and biases and greater scrutiny regarding prescription pain medicine compared with White patients, resulting in fewer opioid prescriptions and less aggressive pain treatment for Black patients.
2) Mistrust of providers and poor patient-provider communication within racially discordant relationships compound disparities in pain care.
a) Many minority patients distrust the healthcare system and HCPs due to historical breaches of trust, as well as more recent perceptions of racial injustice in care. This lack of trust can compromise pain management efforts and make it difficult to establish rapport and gain trust of patients who have been stigmatized or discriminated against.
b) Expression of pain symptoms can differ among cultural and racial groups. Pain assessment is complicated by the personal and subjective nature of pain. This leaves reports of pain open to interpretation by HCPs and can create clinical uncertainty, which is compounded in racially discordant patient-provider relationships.

c) Literacy and language barriers add to miscommunication, further eroding trust and influencing treatment decisions.

d) Many minority patients have difficulty advocating for themselves, and others who do self-advocate are met with suspicion.

3) Economic disadvantage

a) Minority patients may have decreased access to quality pain care due to lack of, inconsistent, or less comprehensive insurance coverage and inability to consistently afford copays and other out-of-pocket expenses for medications, nonpharmacological therapies, primary care provider (PCP) and specialty visits, and interprofessional care.

(1) Despite Medicaid expansion by many states in response to the Patient Protection and Affordable Care Act of 2010 (ACA), healthcare coverage does not ensure affordable access to care.

b) Pharmacies in neighborhoods inhabited predominantly by minority residents have been reported to have insuffcient opioid supplies compared to those in areas inhabited predominantly by White people.

c) Lack of transportation to appointments and pharmacies compounds the problem.

d. Simply raising awareness of disparities in pain care is insufficient. Nurses, who are at the forefront in care of patients with pain, are ethically obligated to act against disparities associated with access to pain management.

1) To minimize these influences, nurses must first identify, acknowledge, understand, and intentionally set aside their own biases.

2) Nurses should talk with patients to gain insight into factors that influence their pain experience and perceived control over pain.

a) Consider individual's unique culture and history when assessing pain to recognize significance in pain coping, the pain experience, and perception of healthcare system. Showing empathy, listening, and allowing patients to voice their concerns can improve pain management outcomes.

b) Consider social, economic, and neighborhood stressors when assessing an individuals' pain experience to aid in development of appropriate interventions for patients.

3) Nurses, as advocates of patient care, play a role across entire patient experience, including advocacy for decreasing pain intensity, increasing function, improved perceived control over pain, better access to healthcare, pain medication, and multimodal intervention.

4) With their emphasis on holistic health, nurses are uniquely positioned to design and participate in research to assess social determinants contributing to pain disparities, develop and assess interventions aimed at reducing disparities, and disseminate this research through publication and presentation.

5) Nurses can play an active role in boardrooms to change institutional practices and policies to advocate for equitable pain care at local, state, and federal levels.

e. ASPMN recognizes the systemic racism that has affected not only patients of color but also colleagues and urges pain management nurses to recognize sources of racial disparities in pain management and find opportunity to address them in their own practice settings. ASPMN has responded to requests from members to examine ways in which ASPMN can begin to address these by forming a Diversity, Equity, Inclusion, and Belonging Committee.

VII. Ethical Challenges Requiring Advocacy

A. Many ethical challenges can arise when caring for people with pain, and nurses must advocate for individualized, patient-centered, and evidence-based care.

1. The provision of medications to relieve pain at end of life is consistent with ethical nursing practice. ASPMN and the Hospice and Palliative Nurses Association (HPNA) hold the position nurses must advocate for effective and safe pain and symptom management for all patients receiving end-of-life care regardless of age, disease, history of SUD, or site of care. Nurses must use evidence-based, effective medication doses prescribed to relieve pain, advocate on behalf of patients when prescribed medication is not managing pain, and advocate for nonpharmacological therapies, when appropriate.

2. Nurses must advocate for a balanced approach to pain management, which includes the use of opioids when appropriate and nonpharmacological therapies.

a. Reports of forced opioid tapers led pain experts and leaders (including nurses) to advocate for urgent action, starting with a review of mandated opioid tapering policies for outpatients at every level of healthcare to minimize harm from aggressive opioid tapering. They asked HHS to:

1) Enact policies that prohibit or minimize rapid, forced opioid tapering in outpatients taking opioid prescriptions who may have been on significant doses for years
2) Provide compassionate, patient-centered systems for opioid tapering, when indicated, that include careful selection, close monitoring, triaging of adverse events (AEs), and evidence-based, realistic end-dose goals derived from applicable data
3) Convene patient advisory boards at all levels of decision-making to ensure patient-centered systems are developed and patient rights are protected
4) Require inclusion of pain management specialists at every level of decision-making about future opioid policies and guidelines

3. Nurses must advocate to stop practice of prescribing and administering opioid doses based solely on pain intensity scores.
   a. Nurses should conduct comprehensive pain assessments and critically consider information garnered from assessments.
   b. The use of as-needed or "PRN" range orders for opioid analgesics that allow nurses to consider multiple patient factors when assessing and managing pain is supported by the ethical principles of beneficence, nonmaleficence, justice, and autonomy.

4. Nurses should advocate for development of policies, processes, and methods of documentation to ensure safe administration of all analgesics.

5. Patient requests for medical aid in dying (MAID), also known as death with dignity, physician-assisted death (PAD), and physician-assisted suicide (PAS), are an ethical dilemma for nurses, and these requests will likely increase as more states consider such legislation.
   a. It is important to note that MAID is not synonymous with euthanasia. Laws that allow MAID permit adult patients with a terminal illness and the capacity for medical decision-making to self-administer oral or enteral medication when certain criteria are met. Euthanasia, which is not legal in the United States, occurs when someone other than the patient administers medication with the intention of hastening the patient's death.
      1) The following U.S. jurisdictions have MAID statutes: California, Colorado, District of Columbia, Hawaii, Maine, Montana, New Jersey, New Mexico, Oregon, Vermont, Washington.

      2) There are currently no federal level laws allowing MAID, and the National Council on Disability recommends that states should not legalize any form of MAID, in part because safeguard provisions in such laws are inadequate, can be readily circumvented, or fail to protect patients from pressure to end their lives.
   b. Guidance for nurses:
      1) Nurses have an ethical duty to be knowledgeable about this evolving issue and have the right to conscientiously object to being involved in the MAID process.
      2) The HPNA has two position statements that provide guidance to nurses. HPNA does not recognize MAID as part of palliative care but emphasizes that all patients are entitled to expert and compassionate palliative care. HPNA guidelines assist nurses on how to respond when hastened death is requested.
      3) The ANA has a position statement on the nurses' role when a patient requests MAID. While nurses are still ethically prohibited from administering aid-in-dying medication, ANA advises nurses to remain objective when patients explore this end-of-life option. ANA does not support or oppose current laws but clarifies the scope of the nursing role in the care of patients who request MAID, with a focus on nurses' ethical obligations and responsibilities.
      4) The International Council of Nurses recognizes the right to die with dignity as a basic human right and views nurses as uniquely prepared to offer compassionate and skilled care for dying patients and their families.

VIII. Resources

A. American Society for Pain Management Nursing
   1. ASPMN's Communications Committee has developed a series of organizational advocacy statements around issues of importance to pain management. These papers are intended to give elected officials, media, and other interested parties a snapshot of ASPMN's expertise on topics of national interest, and to invite them to engage us in more in-depth conversations.
      a. *Statement on the Use of Medical Marijuana*
      b. *Multimodal Therapies to Manage Pain—More than Just Opioids*
      c. *Statement on Abuse Deterrent Formulations*
      d. *Statement on Nurses' Use of Integrative Therapies for Pain*

e. *Statement Regarding the Use of Opioids for Chronic Pain While Preventing Abuse and Diversion*

f. *In Defense of Education (encouraging nurses in the management of pain to become more knowledgeable regarding all facets of the pain area, including those related to pain and addiction)*

2. Organizational position statements (https://aspmn.org/position-statements)

   a. *Acute Perioperative Pain Management Among Adult Patients Undergoing Orthopaedic Surgery*

   b. *Guidelines on Monitoring for Opioid-Induced Advancing Sedation and Respiratory Depression: Revisions*

   c. *Pain Assessment in the Patient Unable to Self-Report*

   d. *"As-Needed" Range Orders for Opioid Analgesics in the Management of Pain: A Consensus Statement of the American Society for Pain Management and the American Pain Society*

   e. *Prescribing and Administering Opioid Doses Based Solely on Pain Intensity*

   f. *Authorized Agent Controlled Analgesia*

   g. *American Society for Pain Management Nursing and Hospice and Palliative Nurses Association Position Statement: Pain Management at the End of Life*

   h. *Monitoring for Opioid-Induced Advancing Sedation and Respiratory*

   i. *Pain Management and Substance Use Disorders*

B. Other organizations involved in pain advocacy

   1. United States Association for the Study of Pain (USASP) (www.usasp.org/)

   2. International Association for the Study of Pain (IASP) (www.iasp-pain.org)

   3. American Society of Regional Anesthesia and Pain Medicine (ASRA) (www.asra.com/)

   4. American Academy of Pain Medicine (AAPM) (www.painmed.org) position statements/consensus reports

   5. The Alliance for Balanced Pain Management (AfBPM) (https://alliancebpm.org/)

   6. American Chronic Pain Association (ACPA) (www.theacpa.org/)

   7. Partners for Understanding Pain (www.theacpa.org/pain-awareness/partners-for-understanding-pain/), spearheaded by the ACPA, is a consortium of organizations interested in the personal, economic, and social impact of pain on our society.

   8. U.S. Pain Foundation (https://uspainfoundation.org/), an organization dedicated to serving those who live with pain conditions and their care providers

   9. Osteoarthritis Action Alliance (https://oaaction.unc.edu/) is a national coalition of concerned organizations mobilized by the Arthritis Foundation and the CDC.

   10. The National Academy of Medicine Action Collaborative on Countering the U.S. Opioid Epidemic (https://nam.edu/programs/action-collaborative-on-countering-the-u-s-opioid-epidemic/) is a public-private partnership comprised of government, communities, health systems, provider groups, payers, industry, nonprofits, and academia committed to sharing knowledge, aligning ongoing initiatives, and advancing collective, multi-sector solutions.

C. State legislation resources

   1. National Conference of State Legislatures (NCSL) (www.ncsl.org/)

      a. Identify and contact your state legislators (House of Representatives Member and Senators) using the State Legislative Websites Directory at www.ncsl.org/aboutus/ncslservice/state-legislative-websites-directory.aspx.

      b. Search the State Legislative Website Directory for information (e.g., bills, statutes, press rooms) from all state legislatures, District of Columbia, and territories.

      c. Searchable databases on legislation introduced or enacted in all states, District of Columbia, and territories

         1) NCSL Injury Prevention Legislation Database/Opioid Abuse Prevention at www.ncsl.org/research/health/injury-prevention-legislation-database.aspx provides up-to-date information on legislation related to prescription opioid abuse prevention in the following categories:

            a) Prescription drug monitoring programs

            b) Prescribing guidelines and limits

            c) Provider education or training

            d) Rescue drugs (e.g., naloxone)

            e) Pain clinics and pain management

            f) Other prescription drug abuse topics

         2) Statewide Prescription Drug Database at www.ncsl.org/research/health/prescription-drug-statenet-database.aspx provides information on legislation introduced or enacted related to prescription drugs in multiple categories.

         3) Scope of Practice Policy Legislative Database at http://scopeofpracticepolicy.org/legislative-search/ provides up-to-date information about scope of practice legislation for health professions.

      d. Visit www.ncsl.org/research/health/state-medical-marijuana-laws.aspx for information on state medical cannabis laws and resources.

D. Federal legislation resources
   1. Identify and contact your federal legislators
      a. United States House of Representatives
         1) Visit www.house.gov/representatives/ find-your-representative and enter your ZIP code to identify your congressional district, with links to your member's website, which contains information about your member and contact details.
            a) Alternatively visit https://clerk.house. gov/Members#MemberProfiles.
            b) Dial (202) 225-3121 to reach House switchboard and operator will connect to Representative's office.
         2) Visit www.house.gov/committees for list of committees, with links to committee websites, which contain information about committee and its activity, subcommittees, contact details, and identifies committee chair and members.
      b. United States Senate
         1) Visit www.senate.gov/senators/senators-contact.htm and click on state to identify U.S. senators, with links to their websites, which contain information about senator and contact details.
            a) Alternatively, dial (202) 224-3121 to reach Capitol switchboard and operator will connect to senators' office.
         2) Visit www.senate.gov/committees/index. htm for list of committees and subcommittees and their members, with links to committee websites, which contain information about committee and its activity and contact details.
   2. Information on legislative activities in House and Senate can be found at www.congress.gov, including bill texts, committee schedules, floor calendars, and bills presented to president.
      a. To search for legislation at www.congress.gov/ advanced-search/legislation
         1) Select current Congress to limit search to recent legislation.
         2) Use key words or phrases such as pain, pain management, opioid, overdose, addiction, or nursing.

Bibliography

Ahmad, F. B., Rossen, L. M., & Sutton, P. (2021). *Provisional Drug Overdose Death Counts*. National Center for Health Statistics. https://www.cdc.gov/nchs/nvss/vsrr/drug-overdose-data.htm.

AMA Pain Care Task Force. (2020). Addressing obstacles to evidence-informed pain care. *AMA Journal of Ethics, 22*(1), E709–E717. https://doi.org/10.1001/amajethics.2020.709.

American Academy of Neurology. (2018). *Position Statement: Use of Medical Cannabis for Neurological Disorders*. https://www. aan.com/siteassets/home-page/policy-and-guidelines/policy/ position-statements/cannabis-position-statement.pdf.

American Academy of Pain Medicine. (2014). *Minimum Insurance Benefits for Patients with Chronic Pain. A Position Statement from the American Academy of Pain Medicine*. https://painmed. org/wp-content/uploads/2019/04/minimum-insurance-benefits-for-patients-with-chronic-pain.pdf.

American Cannabis Nurses Association. (2019). *Scope and Standards of Practice for Cannabis Nurses*. https://www.cannabisnurses.org/assets/docs/2019_RN_APRN%20Cannabis%20 Scope%20and%20Standards%20WEBSITE.pdf.

American Medical Association. (2020). *Stigma. Language Matters to the American Medical Association*. https://end-overdose-epidemic.org/wp-content/uploads/2020/07/Language-Matters_ Template-1.pdf.

American Medical Association. (n.d.). *End the Epidemic. Stigma*. Retrieved April 16, 2021 from https://end-overdose-epidemic. org/awareness/stigma/.

American Nurses Association. (2015). *Code of Ethics for Nurses with Interpretive Statements*. Silver Spring, MD: American Nurses Association.

American Nurses Association. (2016). *Therapeutic Use of Marijuana and Related Cannabinoids. Revised Position Statement*. www.nursingworld.org/~49a8c8/globalassets/ practiceandpolicy/ethics/therapeuticuse-of-marijuana-and-related-cannabinoids-position-statement.pdf.

American Nurses Association. (2018a). *ANA Position Statement: The Ethical Responsibility to Manage Pain and the Suffering It Causes*. www.nursingworld.org/~495e9b/globalassets/docs/ ana/ethics/theethicalresponsibilitytomanagepainandthesufferingitcauses2018.pdf.

American Nurses Association. (2018b). *RNAction. Advocate stories*. American Nurses Association. Retrieved March 22, 2021 from https://ana.aristotle.com/sitepages/YearOfAdvocacy.aspx.

American Nurses Association. (2019). *The Nurse's Role When a Patient Requests Medical Aid in Dying*. Retrieved April 24, 2021 from https://www.nursingworld.org/~49e869/globalassets/ practiceandpolicy/nursing-excellence/ana-position-statements/social-causes-and-health-care/the-nurses-role-when-a-patient-requests-medical-aid-in-dying-web-format.pdf.

American Nurses Association. (n.d.). *Moral Courage/Distress*. American Nurses Association. https://www.nursingworld.org/ practice-policy/nursing-excellence/ethics/ethics-topics-and-articles/.

American Nurses Association, Association of Pain Management Nursing. (2016). *Pain Management Nursing: Scope and Standards of Practice* (2nd ed.). Silver Spring, MD: American Nurses Association.

American Society for Pain Management Nursing. (2012). *Legislative Toolkit*. www.aspmn.org/documents/ ASPMNLegislativeToolkitComplete.pdf.

American Society for Pain Management Nursing. (2015). *Statement on the Use of Medical Marijuana*. http://www.aspmn. org/Documents/Advocacy%20Positions%20Statements/ Statement%20on%20the%20use%20of%20Medical%20 Marijuana%206-17-2015%20final.pdf.

American Society of Regional Anesthesia and Pain Medicine. (2021). *Reducing the Burden of Prior Authorizations to Aid*

Patient Care Delivery. https://www.asra.com/the-asra-family/special-interest-groups/sig-article-item/asra-updates/2021/01/05/reducing-the-burden-of-prior-authorizations-to-aid-patient-care-delivery.

Anderson, A. R., Hyden, K., Failla, M. D., & Carter, M. A. (2021). Policy implications for pain in advanced Alzheimer's disease. *Pain Management Nursing, 22*(1), 3–7. https://doi.org/10.1016/j.pmn.2020.06.005.

Anderson, S. R., Gianola, M., Perry, J. M., & Losin, E. A. R. (2020). Clinician-patient racial/ethnic concordance influences racial/ethnic minority pain: evidence from simulated clinical Interactions. *Pain Medicine, 21*(11), 3109–3125. https://doi.org/10.1093/pm/pnaa258.

Ansari, B., Tote, K. M., Rosenberg, E. S., & Martin, E. G. (2020). A rapid review of the impact of systems-level policies and interventions on population-level outcomes related to the opioid epidemic, United States and Canada, 2014–2018. *Public Health Reports, 135*(1_suppl), 100S–127S. https://doi.org/10.1177/0033354920922975.

Arfken, C. L., & Tutag Lehr, V. (2021). Commercial and public payer opioid analgesic prescribing policies: a case study. *Substance Abuse Treatment, Prevention, and Policy, 16*(1), 4. https://doi.org/10.1186/s13011-020-00340-z.

Bandura, A. (2016). *Moral Disengagement: How People Do Harm and Live With Themselves.* New York, NY: Worth Publishers.

Beauchamp, T. L., & Childress, J. F. (2013). *Principles of Biomedical Ethics* (7th ed.). New York: Oxford University Press.

Becker, W. C., & Tetrault, J. M. (2016). Medical marijuana in patients prescribed opioids: a cloud of uncertainty. *Mayo Clinic Proceedings, 91*(7), 830–832. https://doi.org/10.1016/j.mayocp.2016.04.008.

Bengoechea, I., Gutierrez, S. G., Vrotsou, K., Onaindia, M. J., & Lopez, J. M. (2010). Opioid use at the end of life and survival in a Hospital at Home unit. *Journal of Palliative Medicine, 13*(9), 1079–1083. https://doi.org/10.1089/jpm.2010.0031.

Bonham, V. L. (2001). Race, ethnicity, and pain treatment: striving to understand the causes and solutions to the disparities in pain treatment. *The Journal of Law, Medicine & Ethics, 29*(1), 52–68. https://doi.org/10.1111/j.1748-720x.2001.tb00039.x.

Booker, S., & Herr, K. (2021). Voices of African American older adults on the implications of social and healthcare-related policies for osteoarthritis pain care. *Pain Management Nursing, 22*(1), 50–57. https://doi.org/10.1016/j.pmn.2020.09.001.

Boon, J. T., & Maxwell, C. A. (2021). Policy opportunities to support family caregivers managing pain in people with dementia. *Pain Management Nursing, 22*(1), 8–10. https://doi.org/10.1016/j.pmn.2020.06.008.

Bruckenthal, P. (2020). The role of opioids in the conundrum of care for persons in pain. *Pain Management Nuring, 21*(1), 1–2. https://doi.org/10.1016/j.pmn.2019.12.001.

Carlson, E. S. (2012). How to comment on government regulations. *American Nurse Today, 7*(7), 34–35.

Centers for Disease Control and Prevention. (October 15, 2020). *2019 Opioid Workgroup.* Retrieved April 24, 2021 from https://www.cdc.gov/injury/bsc/opioid-workgroup-2019.html.

Cheon, J., Coyle, N., Wiegand, D. L., & Welsh, S. (2015). Ethical issues experienced by hospice and palliative nurses. *Journal of Hospice & Palliative Nursing, 17*(1), 7–13. https://doi.org/10.1097/NJH.0000000000000129.

Clem, S. N., Bigand, T. L., & Wilson, M. (2020). Cannabis use motivations among adults prescribed opioids for pain versus opioid addiction. *Pain Management Nursing, 21*(1), 43–47. https://doi.org/10.1016/j.pmn.2019.06.009.

Comerci, G., Jr., Katzman, J., & Duhigg, D. (2018). Controlling the swing of the opioid pendulum. *New England Journal of Medicine, 378*(8), 691–693. https://doi.org/10.1056/NEJMp1713159.

Compton, P., & Blacher, S. (2020). Nursing education in the midst of the opioid crisis. *Pain Management Nursing, 21*(1), 35–42. https://doi.org/10.1016/j.pmn.2019.06.006.

Cooney, M. F., Czarnecki, M., Dunwoody, C., Eksterowicz, N., Merkel, S., Oakes, L., et al. (2013). American Society for Pain Management Nursing position statement with clinical practice guidelines: authorized agent controlled analgesia. *Pain Management Nursing, 14*(3), 176–181. https://doi.org/10.1016/j.pmn.2013.07.003.

Copeland, D. (2020). Drug-seeking: a literature review (and an exemplar of stigmatization in nursing). *Nursing Inquiry, 27*(1), e12329. https://doi.org/10.1111/nin.12329.

Coyne, P., Mulvenon, C., & Paice, J. A. (2018). American Society for Pain Management Nursing and Hospice and Palliative Nurses Association Position Statement: Pain Management at the End of Life. *Pain Management Nursing, 19*(1), 3–7. https://doi.org/10.1016/j.pmn.2017.10.019.

Darnall, B. D., Juurlink, D., Kerns, R. D., Mackey, S., Van Dorsten, B., Humphreys, K., et al. (2019). International stakeholder community of pain experts and leaders call for an urgent action on forced opioid tapering. *Pain Medicine, 20*(3), 429–433. https://doi.org/10.1093/pm/pny228.

Death with Dignity. (n.d.). *Death with Dignity Acts.* Retrieved April 7, 2021 from https://www.deathwithdignity.org/learn/death-with-dignity-acts/.

Delk, W., & Quinlan-Colwell, A. (2020). The Journey of the American Society for Pain Management Nursing Into Advocacy and Governmental Affairs. *Pain Management Nursing, 21*(5), 395–398. https://doi.org/10.1016/j.pmn.2020.06.004.

Diamond, D., & Bernstein, L. (January 25, 2021). Biden moving to nix Trump plan on opioid-treatment prescriptions. *The Washinton Post.* https://www.washingtonpost.com/health/2021/01/25/biden-buprenorphine-waiver/.

Donaldson, D. (October 19, 2017). *Health Plans Launch New STOP Initiative to Help Battle Opioid Crisis in America.* https://www.ahip.org/news/press-releases/health-plans-launch-new-stop-initiative-to-help-battle-opioid-crisis-in-america.

Dowell, D., Haegerich, T., & Chou, R. (2019). No shortcuts to safer opioid prescribing. *New England Journal of Medicine, 380*(24), 2285–2287. https://doi.org/10.1056/NEJMp1904190.

Dowell, D., Haegerich, T. M., & Chou, R. (2016). CDC Guideline for Prescribing Opioids for Chronic Pain—United States, 2016. *Morbidity and Mortality Weekly Report (MMWR): Recommendations and Reports, 65*(1), 1–49. https://doi.org/10.15585/mmwr.rr6501e1.

Drew, D. J., Gordon, D. B., Morgan, B., & Manworren, R. C. B. (2018). "As-needed" range orders for opioid analgesics in the management of pain: a consensus statement of the American Society for Pain Management Nursing and the American Pain Society. *Pain Management Nursing, 19*(3), 207–210. https://doi.org/10.1016/j.pmn.2018.03.003.

Duensing, K., Twillman, R., Ziegler, S., Cepeda, M. S., Kern, D., Salas, M., et al. (2020). An examination of state and federal opioid analgesic and continuing education policies: 2016–2018. *Journal of Pain Research, 13*, 2431–2442. https://doi.org/10.2147/JPR.S267448.

Erickson, B. (2017). To carry over or not? *The NCSL Blog.* https://www.ncsl.org/blog/2017/07/24/to-carry-over-or-not.aspx.

Federation of State Medical Boards. (2016). *Model Guidelines for the Recommendation of Marijuana in Patient Care. Report of the FSMB Workgroup on Marijuana and Medical Regulation.* https://www.fsmb.org/Media/Default/PDF/BRD_RPT_16-2_Marijuana_Model_Guidelines.pdf.

Fenton, J. J., Agnoli, A. L., Xing, G., Hang, L., Altan, A. E., Tancredi, D. J., et al. (2019). Trends and rapidity of dose tapering among patients prescribed long-term opioid therapy, 2008–2017. *JAMA Network Open, 2*(11), e1916271. https://doi.org/10.1001/jamanetworkopen.2019.16271.

Fitzcharles, M. A., Niaki, O. Z., Hauser, W., Hazlewood, G., & Canadian Rheumatology, A. (2019). Position statement: a pragmatic approach for medical cannabis and patients with rheumatic diseases. *The Journal of Rheumatology, 46*(5), 532–538. https://doi.org/10.3899/jrheum.181120.

Fowler, M. D. M. (2015). *Guide to the Code of Ethics for Nurses with Interpretive Statements: Development, Interpretation, and Application* (2nd ed.). Silver Spring, MD: American Nurses Association.

Ghoshal, M., Shapiro, H., Todd, K., & Schatman, M. E. (2020). Chronic noncancer pain management and systemic racism: time to move toward equal care standards. *Journal of Pain Research, 13,* 2825–2836. https://doi.org/10.2147/JPR.S287314.

Goddu, A. P., O'Conor, K. J., Lanzkron, S., Saheed, M. O., Saha, S., Peek, M. E., et al. (2018). Do words matter? Stigmatizing language and the transmission of bias in the medical record. *The Journal of General Internal Medicine, 33*(5), 685–691. https://doi.org/10.1007/s11606-017-4289-2.

Goldberg, D. S. (2020). Toward fair and humane pain policy. *The Hastings Center Report, 50*(4), 33–36. https://doi.org/10.1002/hast.1170.

Green, C. R., Anderson, K. O., Baker, T. A., Campbell, L. C., Decker, S., Fillingim, R. B., et al. (2003). The unequal burden of pain: confronting racial and ethnic disparities in pain. *Pain Medicine, 4*(3), 277–294.

Gross, J., & Gordon, D. B. (2019). The strengths and weaknesses of current US policy to address pain. *American Journal of Public Health, 109*(1), 66–72. https://doi.org/10.2105/AJPH.2018.304746.

Hall, W. J., Chapman, M. V., Lee, K. M., Merino, Y. M., Thomas, T. W., Payne, B. K., et al. (2015). Implicit racial/ethnic bias among health care professionals and its influence on health care outcomes: a systematic review. *American Journal of Public Health, 105*(12), e60–e76. https://doi.org/10.2105/AJPH.2015.302903.

Haq, N., McMahan, V. M., Torres, A., Santos, G. M., Knight, K., Kushel, M., et al. (2021). Race, pain, and opioids among patients with chronic pain in a safety-net health system. *Drug and Alcohol Dependence, 222,* 108671. https://doi.org/10.1016/j.drugalcdep.2021.108671.

Herr, K., Coyne, P. J., Ely, E., Gelinas, C., & Manworren, R. C. B. (2019). ASPMN 2019 position statement: pain assessment in the patient unable to self-report. *Pain Management Nursing, 20*(5), 402–403. https://doi.org/10.1016/j.pmn.2019.07.007.

Hospice and Palliative Nurses Association. (2017a). *Guidelines for the Role of the Registered Nurse and Advanced Practice Registered Nurse When Hastened Death is Requested.* https://advancingexpertcare.org/position-statements/.

Hospice and Palliative Nurses Association. (2017b). *HPNA Position Statement: Physician-Assisted Death/Physician-Assisted Suicide.* https://advancingexpertcare.org/position-statements/.

Howes, J. (2015). Nurses' perceptions of medication use at the end of life in an acute care setting. *Journal of Hospice & Palliative Nursing, 17*(6), 508–516. https://doi.org/10.1097/NJH.0000000000000192.

Human Rights Watch. (2018). *"Not Allowed to Be Compassionate" Chronic Pain, the Overdose Crisis, and Unintended Harms in the US.* https://www.hrw.org/sites/default/files/report_pdf/hhr1218_web.pdf.

Institute of Medicine. (2011). *Relieving Pain in America: A Blueprint for Transforming Prevention, Care, and Research.* Washington, DC: The National Academies Press. https://www.ncbi.nlm.nih.gov/books/n/nap13172/pdf/.

International Association for the Study of Pain. (2010). *Declaration of Montréal: Declaration that Access to Pain Management is a Fundamental Human Right.* Retrieved April 22, 2021 from https://www.iasp-pain.org/Advocacy/Content.aspx?ItemNumber=1821&navItemNumber=582.

International Council of Nurses. (2012). *Position Statement: Nurses' role in providing care to dying patients and their families.* https://www.icn.ch/sites/default/files/inline-files/A12_Nurses_Role_Care_Dying_Patients.pdf.

Jungquist, C. R., Quinlan-Colwell, A., Vallerand, A., Carlisle, H. L., Cooney, M., Dempsey, S. J., et al. (2020). American Society for Pain Management Nursing guidelines on monitoring for opioid-induced advancing sedation and respiratory depression: revisions. *Pain Management Nursing, 21*(1), 7–25. https://doi.org/10.1016/j.pmn.2019.06.007.

Kroenke, K., Alford, D. P., Argoff, C., Canlas, B., Covington, E., Frank, J. W., et al. (2019). Challenges with implementing the Centers for Disease Control and Prevention opioid guideline: a consensus panel report. *Pain Medicine, 20*(4), 724–735. https://doi.org/10.1093/pm/pny307.

Lavin, R., & Park, J. (2014). A characterization of pain in racially and ethnically diverse older adults: a review of the literature. *Journal of Applied Gerontology, 33*(3), 258–290. https://doi.org/10.1177/0733464812459372.

Lee, B., Zhao, W., Yang, K. C., Ahn, Y. Y., & Perry, B. L. (2021). Systematic evaluation of state policy interventions targeting the US opioid epidemic, 2007–2018. *JAMA Network Open, 4*(2), e2036687. https://doi.org/10.1001/jamanetworkopen.2020.36687.

Link, B. G., & Phelan, J. C. (2001). Conceptualizing stigma. *Annual Review of Sociology, 27,* 363–385. https://doi.org/10.1146/annurev.soc.27.1.363.

Mallick-Searle, T., & St. Marie, B. (2019). Cannabinoids in pain treatment: an overview. *Pain Management Nursing, 20*(2), 107–112. https://doi.org/10.1016/j.pmn.2018.12.006.

Maly, A., Singh, N., & Vallerand, A. H. (2018). Experiences of urban African Americans with cancer pain. *Pain Management Nursing, 19*(1), 72–78. https://doi.org/10.1016/j.pmn.2017.11.007.

Maly, A., & Vallerand, A. H. (2018). Neighborhood, socioeconomic, and racial influence on chronic pain. *Pain Management Nursing, 19*(1), 14–22. https://doi.org/10.1016/j.pmn.2017.11.004.

Mattson, C. L., Tanz, L. J., Quinn, K., Kariisa, M., Patel, P., & Davis, N. L. (2021). Trends and geographic patterns in drug and synthetic opioid overdose deaths—United States, 2013–2019. *Morbidity and Mortality Weekly Report (MMWR), 70*(6), 202–207. https://doi.org/10.15585/mmwr.mm7006a4.

Part 2

Meacham, M. R. (2021). *Longest's Health Policymaking in the United States* (7th ed.). Washington, DC: Health Administration Press.

Meghani, S. H., Polomano, R. C., Tait, R. C., Vallerand, A. H., Anderson, K. O., et al. (2012). Advancing a national agenda to eliminate disparities in pain care: directions for health policy, education, practice, and research. *Pain Medicine, 13*(1), 5–28. https://doi.org/10.1111/j.1526-4637.2011.01289.x.

Miller, E. (2020). Celebrating our accomplishments and embracing our future. *Pain Management Nursing, 21*(2), 121–122. https://doi.org/10.1016/j.pmn.2020.02.001.

National Academies of Sciences, Engineering, and Medicine. (2017). *The Health Effects of Cannabis and Cannabinoids: The Current State of Evidence and Recommendations for Research.* Washington, DC: The National Academies Press. https://doi.org/doi:10.17226/24625.

National Committee for Quality Assurance. (2021). *HEDIS Measures and Technical Resources.* Retrieved April 24, 2021 from https://www.ncqa.org/hedis/measures/.

National Conference of State Legislatures. (2021a). *Injury Prevention Legislation Database/Opioid Abuse Prevention.* Retrieved April 24, 2021 from www.ncsl.org/research/health/injury-prevention-legislation-database.aspx.

National Conference of State Legislatures. (2021b). *State Medical Marijuana Laws.* Retrieved April 24, 2021 from https://www.ncsl.org/research/health/state-medical-marijuana-laws.aspx.

National Council on Disability. (2019). *The Danger of Assisted Suicide Laws: Part of the Bioethics and Disability Series.* https://ncd.gov/sites/default/files/NCD_Assisted_Suicide_Report_508.pdf.

National Institute on Drug Abuse. (2021). *Words Matter: Terms to Use and Avoid When Talking About Addiction.* https://www.drugabuse.gov/sites/default/files/nidamed_words_matter_508.pdf.

Oliver, J., Coggins, C., Compton, P., Hagan, S., Matteliano, D., & Stanton, M. (2012). American Society for Pain Management nursing position statement: pain management in patients with substance use disorders. *Pain Management Nursing, 13*(3), 169–183. https://doi.org/10.1016/j.pmn.2012.07.001.

Pain News Network. (2017). *2017 CDC Survey Results.* Available at www.painnewsnetwork.org/2017-cdc-survey.

PainAustralia. (2019). *Talking About Pain: Language Guidelines for Chronic Pain.* https://www.painaustralia.org.au/static/uploads/files/talking-about-pain-lgfcp-16-07-2019-wfatiuewwems.pdf.

Palace, Z. J., & Reingold, D. A. (2019). Medical cannabis in the skilled nursing facility: a novel approach to improving symptom management and quality of life. *Journal of the American Medical Directors Association, 20*(1), 94–98. https://doi.org/10.1016/j.jamda.2018.11.013.

Pasero, C., Quinlan-Colwell, A., Rae, D., Broglio, K., & Drew, D. (2016). American Society for Pain Management nursing position statement: prescribing and administering opioid doses based solely on pain intensity. *Pain Management Nursing, 17*(3), 170–180. https://doi.org/10.1016/j.pmn.2016.03.001.

Pergolizzi, J. V., Jr., Rosenblatt, M., & LeQuang, J. A. (2019). Three years down the road: the aftermath of the CDC guideline for prescribing opioids for chronic pain. *Advances in Therapy, 36*(6), 1235–1240. https://doi.org/10.1007/s12325-019-00954-1.

Peterson, A., Berggarden, M., Schaller, A. S., & Larsson, B. (2019). Nurses' advocacy of clinical pain management in hospitals: a qualitative study. *Pain Management Nursing, 20*(2), 133–139. https://doi.org/10.1016/j.pmn.2018.09.003.

Quinlan-Colwell, A. (2013). Making an ethical plan for treating patients in pain. *Nurse Practitioner, 38*(12), 17–21. https://doi.org/10.1097/01.NPR.0000437582.88592.c2.

Rieder, T. N. (2020). Solving the opioid crisis isn't just a public health challenge—it's a bioethics challenge. *The Hastings Center Report, 50*(4), 24–32. https://doi.org/10.1002/hast.1169.

Robinson-Lane, S. G., & Vallerand, A. H. (2018). Pain treatment practices of community-dwelling black older adults. *Pain Management Nursing, 19*(1), 46–53. https://doi.org/10.1016/j.pmn.2017.10.009.

Russell, K., Cahill, M., & Duderstadt, K. G. (2019). Medical marijuana guidelines for practice: health policy implications. *Journal of Pediatric Health Care, 33*(6), 722–726. https://doi.org/10.1016/j.pedhc.2019.07.010.

Saad, L. (2020). *U.S. Ethics Ratings Rise for Medical Workers and Teachers.* Gallup Poll. https://news.gallup.com/poll/328136/ethics-ratings-rise-medical-workers-teachers.aspx.

Silva, M. J., & Kelly, Z. (2020). The escalation of the opioid epidemic due to COVID-19 and resulting lessons about treatment alternatives. *The American Journal of Managed Care, 26*(7), e202–e204. https://doi.org/10.37765/ajmc.2020.43386.

Stanton, M., & McClughen, D. C. (2020). Three steps forward and two steps back: impacts of government action on people with pain and those who treat them. *Pain Management Nursing, 21*(1), 3–6. https://doi.org/10.1016/j.pmn.2019.05.001.

Sutradhar, R., Atzema, C., Seow, H., Earle, C., Porter, J., & Barbera, L. (2014). Repeated assessments of symptom severity improve predictions for risk of death among patients with cancer. *Journal of Pain and Symptom Management, 48*(6), 1041–1049. https://doi.org/10.1016/j.jpainsymman.2014.02.012.

Sykes, N., & Thorns, A. (2003). The use of opioids and sedatives at the end of life. *The Lancet Oncology, 4*(5), 312–318. https://doi.org/10.1016/s1470-2045(03)01079-9.

Tait, R. C., & Chibnall, J. T. (2014). Racial/ethnic disparities in the assessment and treatment of pain: psychosocial perspectives. *American Psychologist, 69*(2), 131–141. https://doi.org/10.1037/a0035204.

The Joint Commission. (n.d.). *Pain Management Standards for Accredited Organizations.* Retrieved April 7, 2021 from https://www.jointcommission.org/resources/patient-safety-topics/pain-management-standards-for-accredited-organizations/.

The NCSBN Medical Marijuana Guidelines Committee. (2018). The NCSBN national nursing guidelines for medical marijuana. *Journal of Nursing Regulation, 9*(2 Supplement), S1–S60. https://www.ncsbn.org/The_NCSBN_National_Nursing_Guidelines_for_Medical_Marijuana_JNR_July_2018.pdf.

Todd, K. H., Deaton, C., D'Adamo, A. P., & Goe, L. (2000). Ethnicity and analgesic practice. *Annals of Emergency Medicine, 35*(1), 11–16. https://doi.org/10.1016/s0196-0644(00)70099-0.

Trainum, B. (2019). ANA works to ensure nurses are equipped to treat their patients' pain effectively. *Capitol Beat from the American Nurses Association.* https://anacapitolbeat.org/2019/04/26/ana-works-to-ensure-nurses-are-equipped-to-treat-their-patients-pain-effectively/.

U.S. Department of Health and Human Services. (2019). *HHS Guide for Clinicians on the Appropriate Dosage Reduction or Discontinuation of Long-Term Opioid Analgesics.* Available at www.hhs.gov/opioids/sites/default/files/2019-10/Dosage_Reduction_Discontinuation.pdf.

U.S. Department of Health and Human Services. (2019). *Pain Management Best Practices Inter-Agency Task Force Report:*

Updates, Gaps, Inconsistencies, and Recommendations. Available at https://www.hhs.gov/sites/default/files/pmtf-final-report-2019-05-23.pdf.

U.S. Department of Health and Human Services. (January 14, 2021). *HHS Expands Access to Treatment for Opioid Use Disorder. Eliminates Certain X-Waiver Requirements for DEA-Registered Physicians,* https://www.hhs.gov/about/news/2021/01/14/hhs-expands-access-to-treatment-for-opioid-use-disorder.html.

U.S. Department of Justice and Drug Enforcement Administration. (2021). *Controlled Substance Schedules.* Retrieved April 7, 2021 from https://www.deadiversion.usdoj.gov/schedules/index.html.

U.S. Department of Transportation. (2009). *Department of Transportation Office of Drug and Alcohol Policy and Compliance Notice: DOT "Medical Marijuana" Notice.* https://www.transportation.gov/odapc/medical-marijuana-notice.

U.S. Department of Veterans Affairs. (2019). *VA and Marijuana—What Veterans need to know.* Retrieved April 7, 2021 from https://www.publichealth.va.gov/marijuana.asp.

U.S. Food and Drug Administration. (2019, October 4, 2019). *Vaping Illness Update: FDA Warns Public to Stop Using Tetrahydrocannabinol (THC)-Containing Vaping Products and Any Vaping Products Obtained Off the Street.* Retrieved April 24, 2021 from https://www.fda.gov/consumers/consumer-updates/vaping-illness-update-fda-warns-public-stop-using-tetrahydrocannabinol-thc-containing-vaping.

U.S. House. Committee on Appropriations. (2020). *Departments of Labor, Health and Human Services, and Education, and Related Agencies Appropriations Bill, 2021. Report of the Committee on Appropriation House of Representatives on H.R. 7614 together with Minority Views.* https://www.congress.gov/116/crpt/hrpt450/CRPT-116hrpt450.pdf.

Vallerand, A. H. (2018). Pain-related disparities: are they something nurses should care about? *Pain Management Nursing, 19*(1), 1–2. https://doi.org/10.1016/j.pmn.2017.11.009.

Whitcomb, B., Lutman, C., Pearl, M., Medlin, E., Prendergast, E., Robison, K., et al. (2020). Use of cannabinoids in cancer patients: a Society of Gynecologic Oncology (SGO) clinical practice statement. *Gynecologic Oncology, 157*(2), 307–311. https://doi.org/10.1016/j.ygyno.2019.12.013.

Williams, H. (2017). The unspoken importance of the nurse in the 2016 National Pain Strategy. *Pain Management Nursing, 18*(3), 123–128. https://doi.org/10.1016/j.pmn.2017.04.007.

Wilson, M., Klein, T., Bindler, R. J., & Kaplan, L. (2021). Shared decision-making for patients using cannabis for pain symptom management in the United States. *Pain Management Nursing, 22*(1), 15–20. https://doi.org/10.1016/j.pmn.2020.09.009.

Zelaya, C. E., Dahlhamer, J. M., Lucas, J. W., & Connor, E. M. (November 2020). *Chronic Pain and High-Impact Chronic Pain Among U.S. Adults, 2019. NCHS Data Brief, no 390.* National Center for Health Statistics. https://www.cdc.gov/nchs/data/databriefs/db390-H.pdf.

CHAPTER 9

Advanced Practice Pain Management Nursing

Teri Reyburn-Orne, MSN, RN-PMGT, PPCNP-BC/CPNP-AC, AP-PMN
Jennifer Kawi, PhD, MSN, APRN, FNP-BC, CNE
Janet A. Pennella-Vaughan, MS, FNP, PMGT-BC
Kimberly Wittmayer, MS, APRN-FPA, PCNS-BC, PMGT-BC, AP-PMN
Ann Schreier, PhD, BSN, MSN, RN*

Introduction

In 2008, the National Council of State Boards of Nursing advanced practice registered nurses (APRNs) Advisory Committee and APRN Consensus Work Group published the *Consensus Model for APRN Regulation: Licensure, Accreditation, Certification, and Education*, which outlined steps for APRNs to become specialized beyond their population focus in areas such as oncology, palliative care, and pain management. Over the last decade, APRNs have become an integral part of care delivery to patients in inpatient and outpatient settings. Use of APRNs in pain management aligns with APRN training and the holistic nursing approach and is cost effective. In this chapter, we will describe roles of the APRN specializing in pain management and identify basic training and competencies recommended for this subspecialty.

I. Advanced Practice Registered Nurses

A. APRNs are educated as independent practitioners who function within scope of practice established by the state in which they are licensed and in alignment with their national certification and organizational policies.
   1. Having APRNs provide pain care can reduce healthcare costs while providing safe, high-quality care.
   2. APRNs continue to face significant barriers related to reimbursement rates and restrictive scopes of practice at state and national levels.
B. APRNs must:
   1. Complete an accredited graduate-level education program preparing them for one of four recognized APRN roles:
      a. Clinical Nurse Specialist (CNS)

      b. Certified Nurse Practitioner (CNP)
      c. Certified Registered Nurse Anesthetist (CRNA)
      d. Certified Nurse Midwife (CNM)
      e. More information on specific APRN roles is available in the 2008 National Council of State Boards consensus statement.
   2. Pass and maintain national certification in their role and population foci
   3. Obtain APRN license per their state regulations
   4. Acquire advanced clinical knowledge and skills preparing them to provide direct and indirect care to patients
   5. Build on Registered Nurses' (RNs) competencies by:
      a. Demonstrating greater depth and breadth of knowledge and clinical expertise
      b. Demonstrating higher levels of data synthesis
      c. Increasing complexity of skills and interventions
      d. Obtaining and maintaining greater role autonomy
   6. Assume responsibility and accountability for health promotion and maintenance, as well as assessment, diagnosis, and pharmacological and nonpharmacological interventions
C. APRN scopes of practice:
   1. Vary between federal and state entities
   2. Vary between states
   3. Range from independent to nonindependent practice requiring a written agreement specifying practice allowed:
      a. With or without supervision
      b. Direct or indirect supervision
      c. With or without prescriptive authority
D. APRN specialty practice
   1. Specialty practice represents a more focused area of practice and requires additional preparation and practice beyond the APRN role/population-focused level (Fig. 9.1).

---

*Section Editor for the chapter.

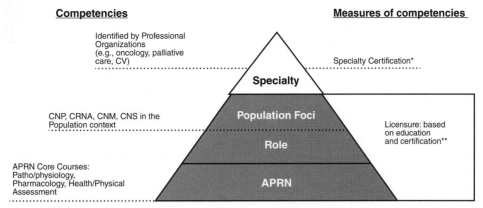

Figure 9.1 Relationship among educational competencies, licensure, and certification in the role/population foci and education and credentialing in a specialty. (© American Nurses Association. Reprinted with permission. All rights reserved.)

2. APRNs cannot expand scope of practice beyond role, population focus, or state-specific scope of practice.
3. Specialty evolves out of population focus and indicates APRN has additional knowledge and expertise in discrete area of practice (e.g., pain management, palliative care).
4. Competence in specialty area may be acquired by educational preparation and skills acquisition and is assessed through professional mechanisms, such as portfolios and examinations.
5. Specialty competencies are developed, recognized, and monitored by the profession.

II. Pain Management APRN Roles in Direct Patient Care

A. Defining acute and persistent pain practice settings and treatment focus
   1. APRNs specializing in pain management can care for patients in various practice settings and across all age groups.
   2. APRN services in acute pain practice settings may be focused on treating underlying cause of pain, interrupting pain signals, and minimizing transition to persistent pain using multimodal analgesia.
   3. APRN services in persistent pain practice settings may include management of persistent or recurrent pain and often involve an interprofessional approach.
   4. Inpatient and outpatient considerations
      a. In inpatient settings, scope of practice is set by hospital medical staff bylaws and cannot exceed scope of practice set by state board of nursing.

         1) May include assessment; diagnosis; and treatment of acute, persistent, or acute on persistent pain and may incorporate interprofessional services
         2) Use of pharmacological and nonpharmacological treatments, including high-risk interventions requiring continuous monitoring
      b. In outpatient setting, scope of practice is set by practice management and cannot exceed scope of practice set by state board of nursing.
         1) Ongoing assessment of persistent pain condition, diagnosis, and treatment
         2) Use of pharmacological and nonpharmacological treatments, including interventional modalities
         3) Coordination of interprofessional services may be more difficult but is often critical in helping patients reach a higher functional state.
         4) Relationship APRN has with patient and family is critical, particularly as it relates to use of medications and follow-up.
         5) Documentation to meet legal and ethical obligations should reflect rationale and standard of care for treatment options as well as safety measures (e.g., documentation of teaching about medications, dispensing naloxone, and opioid management information).
B. Considerations for management strategies
   1. General considerations
      a. Careful history (including patient's underlying health status and comorbidities) and physical assessment are necessary to identify type of

pain (e.g., somatic, neuropathic, acute, acute on persistent, persistent) and its impact on quality of life, and rationale for treatment selection should be clearly documented.

b. Focus on patient as active member of treatment team with defined goals for pain reduction, functional improvement, and improved quality of life.

1) Define specific functional and pain reduction goals to assess efficacy of current treatment, and guide changes if goals not met.

2) Functional goals are particularly important, especially if opioid medications are prescribed, due to potential increased risks.

c. Treatment strategies differ for acute and persistent pain conditions.

1) Maximize use of multimodal therapy to increase efficacy in pain reduction, minimize side effects, and minimize financial burden for patients.

2) Establish pharmacological treatment (if within scope of practice) using evidence-based practices incorporating guidelines as outlined by organizations such as Centers for Disease Control and Prevention, World Health Organization, American Geriatrics Society, American Society for Pain Management Nursing (ASPMN), and International Association for the Study of Pain (IASP), among others.

d. Review treatment plan; reassess patient; and clearly document changes in laboratory values, patient function, pain control, and adverse events at regular intervals.

2. Integrative and complementary therapies

a. Refer to Integrative and Complementary Therapies, chapter 15, as appropriate.

b. Introduce integrative therapies early in treatment planning.

c. Identify nonpharmacological therapies patient has previously used to guide type of therapy to incorporate into current treatment plan.

3. Interventional treatments

a. Maintain awareness and understanding of possible interventional techniques that may be beneficial (see Interventional Pain Management chapter 19, for more information).

1) Medications, dosing, and prescribing considerations for procedural interventions

2) Potential side effects and risks of medications

3) Risks and benefits of procedure

b. If not within APRN scope of practice, refer patient for appropriate procedural intervention.

c. Maintain competency for procedures performed within scope of practice and in

compliance with specific state regulations and institutional privileging.

4. Opioid prescribing

a. APRNs must meet state licensing requirements (e.g., states may require controlled substance permit prior to Drug Enforcement Administration application), as well as continuing education requirements (may vary between states). Topics may include:

1) Prescribing controlled substances (state and federal requirements)

2) Appropriate prescribing

3) Managing acute pain

4) Palliative care

5) Prevention and screening of substance use disorder

6) Responses to misuse and substance abuse disorder

7) End-of-life care

b. Balance patient care with safety measures for patient, family, and community.

1) Review risk mitigation strategies with patients and family (e.g., medication dosing schedule, locked storage, use of naloxone if emergency response needed).

2) Establish functional and pain reduction goals at onset of treatment, and use these goals in regular reassessment visits to demonstrate improvement in function and reduction of pain symptoms without adverse effects or evidence of misuse.

3) Document rationale for use of medications, review of risk-benefit discussion, previous medication or interventional trials, and ongoing assessment of medication use.

c. Use accepted equianalgesic table for dose calculations.

d. A prescription drug monitoring program provides direct access to view controlled substance prescriptions dispensed to patients and is available in all states.

e. Consider use of an objective measure of medication use (e.g., periodic urine or serum toxicology screens).

f. Consider opioid treatment agreements in outpatient settings.

1) May be required by individual state or organizational guidelines

2) May be used as educational tool to:

a) Identify expectations and responsibilities regarding use and management of controlled substances for patient and provider

b) Review and discuss rationale for use of medication with goals of care outlined

c) Review opioid adverse effects, including respiratory depression, sedation, and potential for development of dependence and opioid use disorder

d) While not a legal document, may help protect provider from liability, reflecting appropriate patient teaching has been provided

g. Naloxone

1) Naloxone should be prescribed for outpatients prescribed opioids.

2) Education regarding use should occur with patient, family members, caregivers, or others as appropriate.

3) Many community organizations, state health departments, and select pharmacies have naloxone training and distribution programs.

5. Holistic patient education

a. Be familiar with various change theory models

1) Stages of change model: precontemplation, contemplation, preparation, action, maintenance, relapse

2) Havelock model: establishing relationships, identifying problem, acquiring resources, outlining solution, accepting change, and stabilizing/maintaining

3) Lippit's Seven-Step Theory: Diagnose problem; evaluate motivation/capability for change; assess patient's motivation, resources, experience, and interest; develop strategies; outline expectations of all team members; maintain change once stabilized.

b. When providing education during initial and follow-up visits, RNs and APRNs should:

1) Frame patient's care in conceptual framework to promote healing and improve patient function

2) Use multiple methods to present education to patient and family regarding pain and treatment strategies

3) Coordinate education as appropriate to patient circumstances (e.g., physical, psychosocial, and spiritual)

4) Use teach back/show me method to promote patient engagement and ensure appropriate understanding

c. Develop resource templates and standardized educational materials (attending to health literacy and cognitive or developmental differences) for procedures and medications.

1) Include rationale for use, general risk and benefits, and potential side effects.

2) Provide and review written copy for patient and family.

3) Reinforce information provided at subsequent visits and contacts.

C. Billing considerations

1. APRNs are responsible for understanding billing and financial responsibilities in their employment setting.

a. Billing rules and laws are constantly changing; the following information is to be used only as a guide.

b. APRNs' ability to bill varies between federal and state entities, between states, and sometimes between institutions. APRNs need orientation to billing procedures for their role.

c. APRNs are legally responsible for staying current on billing rules and laws in order to bill accurately.

1) Understanding *International Classification of Diseases* (ICD) diagnostic coding and *Current Procedural Terminology* (CPT) codes is necessary to provide accurate billing.

2) Federal laws covering Medicare fraud and abuse include:

a) False Claims Act

b) Anti-Kickback Statute

c) Physician Self-Referral Law (Stark Law)

d) Social Security Act, which includes the Exclusion Statute and Civil Monetary Penalties law

e) United States Criminal Code

2. APRNs billing for services need National Provider Identifier (NPI) number.

a. Required by Health Insurance Portability and Accountability Act (HIPAA) for electronic transmission of health information to other health entities, including insurance carriers and pharmacies

b. NPI number application is available through Medicare at no charge.

c. NPI numbers are publicly available online.

3. Elements of billing:

a. ICD codes

1) List of codes created by Centers for Medicaid and Medicare Services (CMS) to identify the diagnosis for which patient is being treated. Diagnostic codes are used by all insurance companies and are not limited to patients with Medicare and Medicaid.

2) Codes are based on documentation in health record.

3) Codes are reviewed and updated regularly by CMS.

4) ICD diagnostic codes are same for inpatient and outpatient settings.

5) ARPNs must maintain current knowledge of ICD coding requirements (refer to www.CMS.gov for updates).

b. CPT codes
  1) Standard coding system to identify the level of service and/or procedure performed
  2) Code is determined by several elements.
  3) Procedure CPT codes for interventions (e.g., epidurals, diagnostic interventional injections, trigger points injections)
    a) Need to identify site, laterality, and levels
    b) Need corresponding diagnosis that meets criteria for procedure to be done (e.g., ICD diagnosis of sacroiliac joint dysfunction on left; CPT code of sacroiliac joint injection on left)
    c) CPT procedure codes are same for inpatient and outpatient settings.
  4) Service CPT codes for consult, initial visit, and follow-up visit are determined by documentation. Level of service (complexity) is referred to as evaluation and management level (E/M Level).
    a) Differ by setting of service (inpatient or outpatient)
    b) History that includes:
      (1) Chief complaint
      (2) History of presenting illness/symptoms
      (3) Review of systems
      (4) Past, family, and social history
    c) Examination
      (1) Number of body areas or organ systems examined
    d) Medical decision-making (MDM)
      (1) Number and complexity of problems addressed (e.g., minimal, low, moderate, high)
      (2) Amount and/or complexity of data reviewed/analyzed/ordered (rated as minimal, limited, moderate, extensive)
    e) Tests (e.g., laboratory test, diagnostic imaging)
    f) External documents (e.g., outside health records)
    g) Assessment requiring an independent historian (e.g., spouse of patient with dementia or parent/guardian)
    h) Risk of complications and/or morbidity/mortality (e.g., minimal, low, moderate, high)
      (1) For inpatient: Documentation of history and physical examination combined with MDM defines level of service.
      (2) For outpatient: MDM defines level of service.

      (3) Prolonged service CPT codes can be applied to additional time spent with patient in face-to-face interaction beyond E/M service level (e.g., an E/M level duration is 15 minutes, but counseling extended time to 60 minutes. E/M is based on documentation, not time mentioned for the level).
c. Time-based billing: must occur on calendar date of encounter and includes:
  1) Severity of presenting problem
  2) Counseling and/or coordination of care
    a) Patient and family
    b) Other providers
    c) Additional treatment
  3) Average time
    a) Provider/patient encounter
    b) Inpatient also includes bedside time.
    c) Outpatient is either face-to-face time with patient or add-on time for reviewing pertinent imaging, laboratory test results, and treatment plan with healthcare team and family.
d. Billing qualifiers
  1) Billing charges
    a) 2022–2023 Medicare with new split-shared visit guidelines for facility setting (inpatient, hospital outpatient; Article 28), Emergency Observation, Critical Care, and some skilled nursing facilities (place of service [POS] codes 19, 21, 22, 23):
      (1) Billing of visit should be with provider (e.g., APRN or physician) who performs "substantive portion" of visit met by any of the following elements:
        (a) History
        (b) Physical examination
        (c) Medical decision-making
        (d) Time (more than half of total time spent by practitioner who bills for visit)
      (2) Billing provider must sign note: physician may addend APRN note and sign, though billing remains under APRN license if above criteria met.
      (3) Split-shared fee schedule modifier needed for billing.
    b) If APRN bills independently under their own NPI number, reimbursement is 85% of CPT code allowed charge compared to a physician charge of 100%.
  2) Incident-to-billing
    a) Specific rules by Medicare for services provided by an APRN who is working

under direct supervision of a physician in a private office setting

   b) Plan of care established by physician at initial visit, which APRN follows; allows bill to be submitted using physician NPI number for visit

   c) Billed in an outpatient private setting only (POS 11 for CPT 99221–99215)

   d) Physician must be on site to provide supervision to APRN if any changes to plan of care are required (e.g., physician would need to see patient and document any change in plan of care).

   e) It is recommended physician see patient every third visit to reassess plan of care for ongoing incident-to-billing.

   f) Applies only to Medicare and is not allowed by many other insurance carriers

   g) Although incident-to-billing can increase reimbursement, it limits transparency as to APRN contributions, productivity, quality of care, and outcome measurements.

  e. Telehealth

   1) In 2020, telehealth visits expanded to promote public health and safety during the SARS-CoV-2 (Covid-19) pandemic. CMS approved many new telehealth uses.

   2) Can be performed in inpatient and outpatient settings

   3) All required elements for billing telehealth visits are the same as an in-person office visit, noted previously.

   4) Telehealth visits require addition of qualifying code (G-code) to be identified as telehealth visit.

   5) Some changes made during the pandemic became permanent; check CMS website frequently for updates.

  f. Outpatient time-based code can be an add-on code to high-complexity CPT code consult or follow-up visit code.

   1) Add-on code to high-complexity code can be in 15-minute increments.

   2) Add-on code can be used for all elements of coordinating complex care (e.g., reviewing test results, obtaining outside health records, reviewing care, educating patient and family).

4. Business aspect of billing

  a. Tracking work volume, charges, and receivables is an important part of business of medicine.

  b. This information can help justify new program initiatives and negotiate financial support for individual provider, program, and necessary staffing to provide or expand services.

  c. Intermittent review with APRN billing department and coding specialist will ensure APRN has appropriate coding, charges, and receivables.

  d. APRN should use results of billing information to track contributions to practice (e.g., obtain quarterly reports on CPT coding, review with billing specialist to ensure documentation matches CPT level of service, identify variances needing correction).

III. Pain Management APRN Role in Indirect Patient Care

A. Evidence-based practice

1. Translate scientific research and knowledge to safe and effective care.
2. Be familiar with levels of evidence and have clinical acumen to use evidence-based information.
3. Determine applicability of evidence and use appropriate process improvement strategies to guide practice change.
4. Instrumental in preparation of evidence-based protocols, policies, standards, guidelines, and educational resources

B. Clinical leader

1. May be placed in leadership roles based on their advanced education, training, and strong clinical knowledge
2. Leadership achieves predetermined goals by providing purpose, direction, and motivation.
3. Leadership may be informal or formal.
4. Effective leaders promote an open and caring environment, inspire others, use resources wisely, and role model strong interpersonal communication skills.
5. As leaders, APRNs function as change agents.
  a. Must have knowledge, skills, and ability to analyze organizational variables and enhance quality and safety
  b. Lead with innovative models of healthcare and shared decision-making
6. Frequently involved in organizational compliance efforts with the Joint Commission or Det Norske Veritas standards, analyze current pain management practices, and develop plans to improve practice, if indicated
7. Skills to be effective change agent in pain management:
  a. Expertise in pain management
  b. High-level communication skills

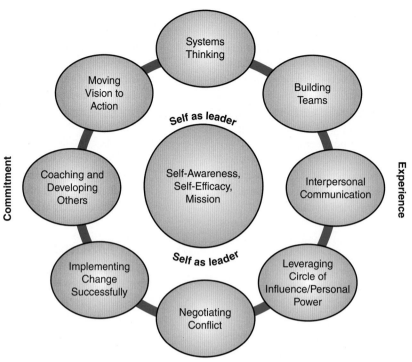

Figure 9.2 Krejci and Malin's leadership model of competencies. (From Jansen M. P. M., Blair K. A. (2015). *Advanced Practice Nursing: Core Concepts for Professional Role Development.* (5th ed). New York, NY: Springer.)

c. Leading collaborative teams to improve pain care delivery and outcomes

d. Leading and promoting evidence-based practice and research

e. Collaboration with interprofessional teams

f. Pedagogical skills for developing educational programs for employees at all levels within an organization

g. Understanding of organization vision and philosophy regarding pain management, ability to influence vision, and skills to strategically design and foster change as needed

h. Understanding of formal and informal organizational structure and decision-making networks within professional organizations to influence healthcare policy

i. Familiarity with various change processes
   1) Grassroots: starts from bottom of system and moves upward
      a) Those identifying need for change develop and submit proposal for change.
      b) Organizational support for proposed change must be solicited to garner success.
   2) Organizational: Change occurs from top down. Change may be supported or motivated by innovators, such as pain management APRN, who incorporate external influences to introduce and facilitate change.

3) Individual: Change occurs through belief there is risk to continue unhealthy or maladaptive behaviors.
   a) Change managed through progression of stages, providing framework to plan interventions based on individual readiness for action.
   b) Individual beliefs influence behavior and are integral factor in group and population behavior modification (Fig. 9.2).

C. Administrator
   1. Coordinating, hiring, evaluating, and scheduling staff to ensure optimal personnel coverage
   2. Developing and understanding reimbursement and billing strategies to ensure appropriate growth and income potential
   3. Evaluating systems, products, and processes to ensure cost containment without decreasing quality of patient care and clinical practices

D. Educator
   1. Lifelong learning
      a. Pain management APRNs gain knowledge through conferences, clinical journals, listserves, and social media, as well as invaluable personal connections within the pain management nursing community.
      b. Certification and recognition
         1) American Nurses Credentialing Center (ANCC) Pain Management Nurse Certification

2) ASPMN Advanced Practice: Pain Management Nurse recognition
2. Serving as content expert for educational materials within and beyond APRN's organization
3. The need to expand pain management education in all healthcare professional curricula is now recognized, yet incorporating these tenets into educational programs lags. APRNs are integral to contributing to this educational goal.
4. Identifying educational needs of staff and facilitating attainment of their educational goals
5. Providing education for clinicians, healthcare professionals, trainees, students, patients, and community at large
6. Promoting learning opportunities for individuals and staff through support of conference attendance
7. Encouraging individuals to share new knowledge
E. Researcher
1. Develops pain research questions by providing unique insight into clinical care and patient outcomes
2. Conducts or participates in pain research based on current issues and questions
3. Identifies relevant gaps in pain practice
4. Reviews literature and shares findings to improve evidence-based practice in pain management
5. Articulates link between nursing, practice, research, and policy
6. Disseminates research findings locally, nationally, and internationally
7. Facilitates implementation of research findings (research utilization) in clinical practice
8. Serves as role model in carrying out research and process improvement and engaging others in these endeavors. For example, APRNs can assist nurses with clear delineation of clinical problems, leading to quality improvement or research projects.
9. Examples of pain management APRN specific research possibilities include (but are not limited to) studies evaluating APRN impact in pain management, assessing care processes, and appraising outcomes of APRN interventions (e.g., cost-effectiveness, access, and clinical outcomes).
F. Advocate
1. Involvement in professional organizations
   a. Provides APRN with resources tailored to their distinct patient population
   b. Provides opportunities for APRN advocacy geared toward pain management and pain management nursing
2. Encourage development of opioid stewardship programs
3. Political involvement (See Advocacy in Pain Management Nursing, chapter 8).
4. Involvement in public health
   a. Cultural transformation in pain management remains a public health imperative.

1) Pain is a public health problem in America, affecting more than one million adults, yet adequate access to evidence-based care remains challenging.
2) More consistent data on pain and pain treatment are needed.
   a) APRNs are equipped with advanced knowledge and education on population health and health disparities.
   b) APRNs can identify barriers for access to expert pain management.
   c) APRNs can monitor incidence and prevalence of pain in general, as well as in specific populations.
   b. APRNs can inform public about nature of pain and use public health strategies (including *Healthy People 2030*) to promote self-management of pain, overall health, prevention, and care to improve pain outcomes for the following leading health indicators:
   1) Drug poisoning deaths
   2) Adolescent health
   3) Obesity
   4) Physical activity
   5) Mental health
   6) Substance abuse
G. Policy expert
1. Having healthcare expertise allows pain management APRNs to guide policy related to pain management.
2. APRNs may be involved at local, regional, and national levels through activities such as:
   a. Involvement in political platforms to influence local, state, or national policy related to pain management and nursing
   b. Legislative processes regulating APRN practice
   c. Grassroots lobbying or choosing a political career focusing on pain issues and healthcare reform
   d. Examples of current policy issues involving APRN practice:
   1) Full independent practice for all APRNs
   2) Equitable reimbursement for APRN services
   3) Insurance companies paying for integrative care and improved access to integrative care
   4) Consistent use of prescription drug monitoring program
   5) Mandatory pain education of healthcare providers
   6) Development of more abuse-deterrent medication formulations
   7) Expanded access to quality palliative care services

IV. Attaining APRN Specialization in Pain Management

A. Entry-level pain management APRN education and training
  1. To have a significant impact and position themselves as experts, pain management APRNs need to receive substantial instruction and training that surpasses entry-level APRN training.
  2. Foundational pain-related education needs to include topics such as:
     a. Pain physiology
     b. Pain theory
     c. Ethics, disparity in pain care, current issues facing pain care (e.g., opioid crisis)
     d. Assessment
     e. Impact of pain
     f. Biopsychosocial model
     g. Nonpharmacological pain management strategies, including integrative and interventional modalities
     h. Pharmacological pain management strategies, including risk-mitigation strategies
     i. Substance use disorder
     j. Research and evidence-based practice
  3. Through education, preceptorship, and mentorship, APRNs learn to:
     a. Collaborate with primary care clinicians to promote evidence-based treatment options
     b. Advocate for appropriate individualized pain management approach for each patient
     c. Ensure patient safety with opioid prescribing
     d. Provide education to people with pain, the public, and healthcare providers by:
        1) Working with regulatory bodies and stakeholders to develop educational programs regarding treatment of pain
        2) Working to enhance healthcare professionals' knowledge, assessment skills, and understanding of treatment options for pain, and to dispel myths related to pain and its treatment
        3) Working with accrediting organizations and health-professional education programs to bridge gaps and enhance curriculums on all aspects of pain management
     e. Contribute to research and evidence-based practice
     f. Participate in advocacy and health policy related to pain management
B. Recommendations for standardized APRN pain management training
  1. Establish APRN scope of practice in state in which practice will occur.
     a. Define APRN role.
        1) Consider certification requirements.
           a) Population (e.g., pediatrics, family, geriatrics, psychiatric)
           b) Acute and primary care
        2) Define expectations for role (e.g., will APRN be expected to function as independently as possible versus under direct supervision of a physician; inpatient versus outpatient setting).
        3) Set expectations for Pain Management Nursing certification and Advanced Practice Pain Management Nursing recognition to be achieved within a reasonable timeframe (discussed later).
     b. Adding new skills to APRN practice
        1) Didactic
           a) Ensure current, rigorous, evidence-based literature for didactic materials.
           b) Attend accredited continuing educational opportunities provided by local and national professional organizations.
           c) Review current guidelines, publications, and evidence-based literature for evaluation and treatment of pain.
        2) Clinical
           a) Shadow APRN specialized in pain management.
              (1) Include all aspects of pain care.
              (2) Duration of shadowing experience is dependent on setting, job expectations, and previous experience.
           b) Increase independence in care of patients over time; duration to do so will vary.
  2. Recommended curriculum
     a. Include both didactic and clinical training.
        1) Recommend broad-based training, including acute and persistent pain, with emphasis on area of practice.
        2) Provide preceptor for orientation with goals to acquire skills in:
           a) Obtaining pain history
           b) Physical examination
           c) Critical thinking of diagnosis and treatment options
           d) Prescribing practices
           e) Interventional procedures
           f) Counseling patients
           g) Appropriate documentation
        3) Provide shadowing experiences with related specialties as appropriate (e.g., surgery, radiology, integrative health, psychiatry).
        4) Time spent in orientation and shadowing:
           a) Should be individualized
           b) Will depend on previous experience
           c) Recommended for a minimum of 3 months

5) Provide a mentor for ongoing professional development (discussed later).
  b. Minimal competencies should include:
    1) Pain physiology (see appropriate chapters for more information)
    2) Current pain theories
    3) Ethics, disparities, and barriers to pain care
    4) Assessment of pain
    5) Treatment of pain
    6) Specific modalities, interventions, treatments expected in specific practice setting
  c. Objective measures of competence should be defined and reassessed on regular basis.
    1) Create and track measurable goals for procedural tasks:
      a) Didactic learning for each skill
      b) Number of exposures required for each skill
      c) Number of times required to perform skill correctly before considered independent
      d) Privileging as needed by practice setting
    2) Create and track measurable goals for process tasks:
      a) Communicating in patient/family meetings
      b) Demonstration of empathetic, supportive interactions attentive to educational literacy and access to treatment options
      c) Establishing patient-driven goals of care, incorporating biopsychosocial model in coordination of care for complex patient issues
3. Professional practice
  a. Strongly encourage participation in professional organizations focused on pain (e.g., ASPMN, IASP, American Academy of Pain Management).
  b. Support relevant conference attendance for continuing education.
    1) Provide funds.
    2) Provide time.
    3) Set expectation for conference attendee to return to organization and present educational content learned.
  c. Require pain management certification/recognition.
    1) ANCC Pain Management Nurse: recommend obtaining within 2 years
    2) ASPMN Advanced Practice Pain Management Nurse recognition: recommend obtaining within 5 years
  d. Include research and process improvement in curriculum, and encourage participation and initiation.
4. Fellowship/residency program considerations
  a. Is program accredited?
  b. Length of program (e.g., 1-year postgraduate training program)

c. Type of training (e.g., structured, intensive)
d. Didactic based on up-to-date literature
e. Clinical experience with increasing autonomy
f. Assigned knowledgeable educator
g. Assigned expert mentor
h. Program outcome measures
  1) Evaluation of participants (e.g. knowledge, competence, and assimilation into practice)
  2) Evaluation of program (e.g., mentor, preceptor, educators).
i. Funding needed for program development
C. Mentoring APRNs in pain management specialty
1. Institute of Medicine report *The Future of Nursing: Leading Change, Advancing Health* (2010) emphasized mentoring as an important part of leadership role for APRNs.
2. Precepting and mentoring
  a. Precepting
    1) Short-term relationship
    2) Defined by length of orientation
    3) Usually assigned, not voluntary
    4) Focus on skill development and organizational practice expectations
  b. Mentoring
    1) Long-term relationship
    2) Requires commitment and willingness by both mentor and mentee
    3) Mentor: teaches, sponsors, encourages, and counsels a less-skilled or less-experienced person for purpose of promoting latter's professional and/or personal development
    4) Starting a mentorship program
      a) Mentor and mentee training is essential. Both parties need to understand and agree to participate.
      b) Phases of mentorship:
        (1) Prepare: Thoughtfully examine what both parties want to get out of relationship.
        (2) Agree
          (a) Lay foundation to relationship and establish trust.
          (b) Complete mentorship partnership agreement.
          (c) Complete confidentiality checklist.
        (3) Cultivate
          (a) Longest phase, which has dual focus on goals/objectives as well as relationship building
          (b) Define meeting model and consider level of interaction (i.e., in person, over phone, via email).

(4) Transition
   (a) Consolidating learning
   (b) Evaluation and reflection
   (c) Redefine relationship: Relationship does not necessarily have to end, but it does signify this is end of mentoring relationship.
3. Benefits
  a. Embraces motivation and is essential to inspiration, innovation, and influence of other APRNs
  b. Shown to increase APRN retention and job satisfaction

Bibliography

American Association of Colleges of Nursing. (2022). *Commission on Collegiate Nursing Education.* https://www.aacnnursing.org/CCNE.

American Nurses Association. (2017). *Recognition of a Nursing Specialty, Approval of a Specialty Nursing Scope of Practice Statement, Acknowledgment of Specialty Nursing Standards of Practice, and Affirmation of Focused Practice Competencies.* https://www.nursingworld.org/~4989de/globalassets/practice-andpolicy/scope-of-practice/3sc-booklet-final-2017-08-17.pdf.

American Nurses Association, Association of Pain Management Nursing. (2016). *Pain Management Nursing: Scope and Standards of Practice* (2nd ed.). Silver Spring, MD: American Nurses Association.

Baheti, D. K., Bakshi, S., Gupta, S., & Gehdoo, R. S. (2016). *Interventional Pain Management: A Practical Approach* (2nd ed.). New Delhi, India: Jaypee Brothers.

Bettinger, J. J., Wegrzyn, E. L., & Fudin, J. (2017). Pain management in the elderly: focus on safe prescribing. *Practical Pain Management, 17*(3). https://www.practicalpainmanagement.com/treatments/pharmacological/opioids/pain-management-elderly-focus-safe-prescribing.

Bickley, L. S., Szilagyi, P. G., Hoffman, R. M., & Soriano, R. P. (2020). *Bates' Guide to Physical Examination and History Taking* (13th ed.). New York, NY: Lippincott Williams & Wilkins.

Blair, K. A. (Ed.). (2018). *Advanced Practice Nursing Roles: Core Concepts for Professional Development* (6th ed.). New York, NY: Springer.

Centers for Medicare and Medicaid Services. (n.d.). *Medicare Benefit Policy Manual. Covered Medical and Other Health Services.* (Publication 100-02, Chapter 15, Section 60). Retrieved February 18, 2021, from https://www.cms.gov/Regulations-and-Guidance/Guidance/Manuals/Downloads/bp102c15.pdf.

Denault, D. L., Wilcox, S. M., Breda, K., Duhamel, K. V., & Eichar, S. (2019). Teach-back: an underutilized tool. *American Nurse.* https://www.myamericannurse.com/teach-back-an-underutilized-tool/.

D'Souza, R. S., Lang, M., & Eldrige, J. S. (2020 September 1). Prescription Drug Monitoring Program. *StatPearls [Internet].* https://www.ncbi.nlm.nih.gov/books/NBK532299/.

Ducharme, J., & Moore, S. (2019). Opioid use disorder assessment tools and drug screening. *Missouri Medicine, 116*(4), 318–324. https://www.ncbi.nlm.nih.gov/pmc/articles/PMC6699803/.

Gast, A., & Mathes, T. (2019). Medication adherence influencing factors—an (updated) overview of systematic reviews. *Systematic Reviews, 8*(1), 112. https://doi.org/10.1186/s13643-019-1014-8.

GraduateNursingEDU.org. (2022). *Nurse Practitioner Residency Programs and Fellowships.* https://www.graduatenursingedu.org/nurse-practitioner-residency-programs/.

Institute of Medicine. (2001). *Crossing the Quality Chasm: A New Health System for the 21st Century.* Washington, DC: National Academies Press.

Kesten, K. S., & El-Banna, M. M. (2021). Facilitators, barriers, benefits, and funding to implement postgraduate nurse practitioner residency/fellowship programs. *Journal of the American Association of Nurse Practitioners, 33*(8), 611–617. https://doi:10.1097/jxx.0000000000000412.

Kesten, K. S., El-Banna, M. M., & Blakely, J. (2021). Educational characteristics and content of postgraduate nurse practitioner residency/fellowship programs. *Journal of the American Association of Nurse Practitioners, 33*(2), 126–132. https://doi.org/10.1097/JXX.0000000000000341.

Klein, C. J., Chan, G. K., Pierce, L., Van Keuren-Parent, K., & Cooling, M. (2020). Development of an advanced practice preceptor evaluation tool. *Journal of the American Association of Nurse Practitioners, 33*(11), 983–990. https://doi.org/10.1097/JXX.0000000000000501.

Krejci, J. W., & Malin, S. (1997). Impact of leadership development on competencies. *Nursing Economics, 15*(5), 235–241.

Martin, J. A., Campbell, A., Killip, T., Kotz, M., Krantz, M. J., Kreek, M. J., et al. (2019). Setting or patient care needs: which defines advanced practice registered nurse scope of practice? *Journal for Nurse Practitioners, 15*(7), 494–495. https://doi.org/10.1016/j.nurpra.2019.03.004.

National Council of State Boards of Nursing. (2008). *Consensus Model for APRN Regulation: Licensure, Accreditation, Certification and Education.* https://www.ncsbn.org/Consensus_Model_for_APRN_Regulation_July_2008.pdf.

National Nurse Practitioner Residency & Fellowship Training Consortium. (2022). *Program Accreditation Standards.* https://www.nppostgradtraining.com/.

National Association for Healthcare Quality, Pelletier, L. R., & Beaudin, C. L. (2017). *HQ Solutions: Resource for the Healthcare Quality Professional* (4th ed.). Riverwoods, IL: Wolters Kluwer Health.

Reuter-Rice, K., Madden, M. A., Gutknecht, S., & Foerster, A. (2016). Acute care pediatric nurse practitioner: the 2014 practice analysis. *Journal of Pediatric Health Care, 30*(3), 241–251. https://doi.org/10.1016/j.pedhc.2016.01.009.

Reville, B., & Foxwell, A. M. (2021). Blueprint for a palliative advanced practice registered nurse fellowship. *Journal of Palliative Medicine, 24*(10), 1436–1442. https://doi.org/10.1089/jpm.2021.0273.

Rumpke, A. (2022 July 8). *New CMS rule on split/shared encounters set to be delayed until 2024.* Medical Group Management Association. https://www.mgma.com/practice-resources/revenue-cycle/new-cms-rule-on-split-shared-encounters-set-to-be.

Sanches, M. B., Poltronieri, M. J., Petronilo, H. B. S., & Pimentel de Siqueira, I. (2017). C2. The core curriculum for pain management nursing: optimizing resources and best health practices. *Pain Management Nursing, 18*(2), 69. https://doi.org/10.1016/j.pmn.2017.02.184.

Skelly, A. C., Chou, R., Dettori, J. R., Turner, J. A., Friedly, J. L., et al. (2020). *Comparative Effectiveness Review Number 227. Noninvasive Nonpharmacological Treatment for Chronic Pain: A Systematic Review Update.* Rockville, MD: Agency for Healthcare Research and Quality. https://effectivehealthcare.ahrq.gov/sites/default/files/pdf/noninvasive-nonpharm-pain-update.pdf.

Substance Abuse and Mental Health Services Administration. (2021 January 27). *Become a Buprenorphine Waivered Practitioner: Statement Regarding X-waiver.* https://www.samhsa.gov/medications-substance-use-disorders/waiver-elimination-mat-act.

Udod, S. A, & Wagner, J. (2018). Common change theories and application to different nursing situations. In J. Wagner (Ed.), *Leadership and Influencing Change in Nursing.* Treaty 4 Territory. Fort Qu'Appelle, Fort Ellice, Canada: University of Regina Press. https://leadershipandinfluencingchangeinnursing.pressbooks.com/chapter/chapter-9-common-change-theories-and-application-to-different-nursing-situations/.

US Department of the Army. (2019). *Army Doctrine Publication 6-22: Army Leadership and the Profession.* https://armypubs.army.mil/epubs/DR_pubs/DR_a/ARN20039-ADP_6-22-001-WEB-0.pdf. https://rdl.train.army.mil/catalog-ws/view/100.ATSC/72D4C9DC-B1F1-45F7-8BB0-148CBA9AF247-1428690957971/adp6_22.pdf.

US Department of Health and Human Services. Office of Disease Prevention and Health Promotion (n.d.). *Healthy People 2030: Leading Health Indicators.* https://health.gov/healthypeople.

US Department of Health and Human Services. (2019). *Pain Management Best Practices Inter-Agency Task Force Report: Updates, Gaps, Inconsistencies, and Recommendations.* https://www.hhs.gov/sites/default/files/pmtf-final-report-2019-05-23.pdf.

Weiner, J., Murphy, S. M., & Behrends, C. (2019 May 29). *Expanding Access to Naloxone: A Review of Distribution Strategies.* Penn Leonard Davis Institute of Health Economics. https://ldi.upenn.edu/brief/expanding-access-naloxone-review-distribution-strategies.

CHAPTER 10

General Principles of Pain Assessment

Jinbing Bai, PhD, RN, FAAN

Introduction

Pain is a multidimensional phenomenon influenced by physical, psychological, social, and spiritual factors. Pain assessment is the crucial first step in the provision of optimal pain care. This chapter will discuss general concepts of comprehensive pain assessment, and pain assessment tools are presented in Chapter 11.

I. Principles of Pain Assessment

A. Every individual has the right to pain care and ongoing comprehensive pain assessment is the foundation of that care.
   1. Pain is an unpleasant sensory and emotional experience. Therefore, assessment should address both physical and psychological aspects of the pain experience.
   2. An individual's self-report of pain is considered most reliable. However, it is essential to use parent/caregiver/significant other's knowledge of an individual's pain behavior for those unable to provide self-report (e.g., infants, toddlers, or those with cognitive impairment).
   3. Behavioral and physiological indicators of pain should not replace self-report unless the individual is unable to self-report their pain experience. Use caution when interpreting physiological indicators (e.g., blood pressure, heart rate), as they may indicate conditions other than pain.
B. As pain is a subjective experience, no uniform pain threshold exists to represent an expected or acceptable pain level. When possible, individuals should be asked to provide a pain intensity goal—a level at which they are able to complete necessary activities (e.g., cough and deep breathe, ambulate, sleep comfortably at night).
C. Biopsychosocial factors influence pain assessment
   1. Individual factors
      a. Age (e.g., infant, young children, elderly), sex, race
      b. Cognitive development

2. Psychological factors (e.g., stress, anxiety, depression, and fear)
3. Behavioral factors (e.g., distraction, relaxation)
4. Social factors (e.g., cultural background, values, housing or living situation, social environment, work, relationships, parental and peer influences)
5. Understanding and meaning of pain
   a. Previous pain experience (e.g., surgeries, cancer pain, persistent pain)
   b. Cause of pain (e.g., postoperative, cancer, injury)
   c. Setting (i.e., hospital setting, outpatient setting, emergency room); Ensure individuals are in a comfortable environment with regard to lighting, noise level, etc. if possible.

II. Components of a Comprehensive Assessment

A. Assess for:
   1. Timing (onset [when does the pain start?], frequency [how often do you experience pain?], duration [how long does the pain last?])
   2. Provoking factors (e.g., movement, anxiety, anger, lack of sleep)
   3. Palliating factors (e.g., rest, positioning, eating, pain medication)
   4. Quality (e.g., aching, dull, stabbing, squeezing, cramping, sharp, burning, tingling)
   5. Intensity (e.g., pain rating)
   6. Location (e.g., use a pain map)
   7. Severity (e.g., no pain, mild, moderate, severe)
   8. Treatment (what type of treatment does the patient receive?)
   9. Overall impact on the patient (e.g., how is pain impacting your quality of life, activities of daily living, work, school?) as well as patient goals for pain management
B. Use appropriate, reliable, and valid pain assessment tools (see Chapter 11).

1. Tools incorporating physical, behavioral, and self-report are preferred.
2. Unidimensional scales:
   a. Have a single underlying element (e.g., intensity) measured using a single measure or test. This type of scale is useful in acute pain when the etiology is clear.
   b. Tend to use words, images, or descriptors to measure pain or pain relief.
   c. Generally used in individuals experiencing acute pain: evaluate any interventions by comparing a person's pain intensity scores at different times (e.g., before and after giving analgesics, before and after ambulation).
   d. Examples of unidimensional assessment tools include:
      1) Visual Analogue Scale
      2) Verbal Rating Scale
      3) Verbal Descriptor Scale
      4) Numeric Rating Scale
      5) Faces Pain Scale
3. Multidimensional scales:
   a. Consist of two or more elements (e.g., intensity and interference in a person's life) and are useful in complex, persistent acute or chronic pain
   b. More descriptive and provide more information about pain than unidimensional assessment
   c. Multidimensional assessment includes:
      1) Intensity
      2) Location
      3) Duration
      4) Description (quality of pain)
      5) Impact on activity and other factors
   d. Examples of multidimensional assessment tools include:
      1) McGill Pain Questionnaire
      2) Brief Pain Inventory
      3) The Comfort Scale
      4) Memorial Pain Assessment Card
      5) Pain Drawing
4. Language may determine the use of unidimensional or multidimensional scales.
5. Consider education and health literacy levels (e.g., patients with lower education or literacy levels may choose to use unidimensional measures)
6. Available time may impact the choice of scale (e.g., time-limited clinical care settings such as emergency room may warrant unidimensional measures).
7. Special populations will have special requirements (e.g., children or adults with cognitive impairment may be better served with unidimensional measures that are easier to understand rather than more complex).
8. Consider requirements of assessment and reassessment frequency.

C. Behavioral indicators
   1. ASPMN position statement recommends a five-step hierarchical pain assessment approach (see Chapter 11).
   2. Behavioral indicators are important for patients who cannot provide pain self-report.
   3. Commonly used for older adults with advanced dementia, infants and preverbal toddlers, critically ill/intubated/unconscious patients, persons with intellectual disabilities, patients at the end of life, or with other assessment challenges (e.g., head trauma/neurological issues, speech or memory deficits, language barriers, delirium)
   4. Behavioral indicators can also be helpful as an *adjunct* to self-report (not in place of) in some situations (e.g., patient reports low pain score but is unwilling to get up to chair).
   5. Behavioral indicators are not unique to pain assessment. For example, a child's crying may be due to anxiety and other discomfort. Therefore, behavioral indicators cannot be used as a measurement for pain independently.
   6. Behavioral indicators of pain can be helpful to determine a person's pain experience in certain circumstances, such as toddlers or a person who is ventilated.
   7. Behavioral indicators may include:
      a. Facial expressions
      b. Verbalizations or vocalizations
      c. Body movements (e.g., rigidity, refusal to move)
      d. Change in interpersonal interactions (e.g., withdrawn)
      e. Change in activity patterns (e.g., unwillingness to participate)
      f. Mental status change
   8. Factors influencing behavioral indicators:
      a. Age, sex, gender identification
      b. Behavioral state (agitation for reasons other than pain [e.g., endotracheal tube] may make assessment more difficult)
      c. Severity of illness
      d. Prior pain experience
      e. Medications
      f. Meaning of pain
      g. Cultural background and considerations
      h. Spirituality or religious belief
D. Physiological indicators
   1. Principles
      a. Physiological indicators cannot be used as a measurement for pain independently, as they may indicate many things other than pain (e.g., heart rate increases in contexts of fever or dehydration).
      b. Pain assessment tool incorporating physical, behavioral, and self-report is preferred when possible.

c. Physiological indicators of pain can be helpful in determining a person's pain experience in certain circumstances such as those who are ventilated or sedated.

d. Of note, people experiencing persistent pain may no longer show alterations in physiologic indicators.

2. Types of physiological indicators
   a. Heart rate (may increase)
   b. Respiratory rate and pattern (may shift from normal to increase, decrease, or change in pattern or depth)
   c. Blood pressure (may increase)
   d. Oxygen saturation (may decrease)

3. Factors influencing physiological indicators:
   a. Age (e.g., infant, young children, older adult)
   b. Behavioral state (e.g., rest, movement, exercise)
   c. Severity of illness (i.e., minor procedures, major surgeries, and with mechanical ventilators)
   d. Prior pain experience (e.g., surgery, painful procedures, fractures)
   e. Medications (e.g., sedative agents, pain medications)
   f. Sex (e.g., female patients reported more cancer pain than male patients)

E. Frequency of pain assessment
   1. Conduct an ongoing and criterion-based pain assessment in relation to the structure, processes, and timeline established in the treatment plan
   2. Should be based on the patient's clinical picture (e.g., assessments often required more often if pain is not yet well controlled) and as directed by hospital or unit policies and procedures
   3. Use ongoing assessment data to revise diagnosis, plan, implementation, and outcome evaluation strategy.
   4. Document relevant data accurately and in a manner accessible to the team that facilitates patient privacy, data retrieval, reassessment, and follow-up.

III. Cultural Considerations in Pain Assessment

A. Culture impacts thoughts, attitudes and beliefs, and behaviors, which in turn shape people's pain experience. Examples include:
   1. Cultural endorsement of stoicism vs. expressivity
   2. Cultural conceptualizations and descriptions of pain
   3. Culturally shaped pain thresholds and pain tolerance levels
   4. Decisions regarding pain management

B. Patient and healthcare provider factors impacting culturally appropriate pain assessment and management
   1. Issues with language and interpretation
   2. Ethnic variation in nonverbal communications
   3. Culturally and linguistically inappropriate pain assessment tools
   4. Underreporting
   5. Reluctance to use pain medications
   6. Access to pain medications
   7. Healthcare providers' fears of drug misuse
   8. Healthcare providers' stereotyping
   9. Healthcare providers' ethnic/racial and/or social class prejudice and discrimination

C. Principles of culturally appropriate pain assessment
   1. Use culturally reliable and valid pain assessment tools
   2. Understand the impact of race/ethnic variations in pain assessment
   3. Do not make stereotypic judgments based on a person's ethnic heritage
   4. Provide culturally oriented pain education
   5. Respect cultural norms of pain assessment

IV. Diversity and Equity in Pain Assessment

A. All patients have the right to effective pain assessment, management, and pain relief when possible. Social determinants of health define conditions in which people are born, grow, live, work, and age; and inequities in power, money, and resources are responsible for disparities in health outcomes (including pain care) within and between countries.

B. Social determinants of health (SDOH) factors influencing pain assessment:
   1. Place of residence (e.g., rural vs. urban)
   2. Race, ethnicity, culture, and language
   3. Occupation
   4. Gender and sex
   5. Religion
   6. Education
   7. Socioeconomic status (especially as it applies to healthcare access)
   8. Social capital

C. Diverse and equitable pain assessment
   1. Collect data based on race and ethnicity, sex and gender, insurance status, and other significant characteristics; identify and address disparities in pain assessment.
   2. Identify our own biases
   3. Establish education programs
   4. Remove as much individual discretion as possible by using clinical guidelines, standardized checklists, and system-wide protocols:
      a. *Centers for Disease Control and Prevention's (CDC's) Guideline for Prescribing Opioids for Chronic Pain*

b. *ASPMN Pain Assessment in the Patient Unable to Self-Report*

c. *ASPMN Procedural Pain Management Position Statement*

Bibliography

American Nurses Association, & American Society for Pain Management, N. (2016). *Pain management nursing: Scope and standards of practice* (2nd ed.). American Nurses Association. https://login.proxy.library.emory.edu/login?url=http://search.ebscohost.com/login.aspx?direct=true&db=nlebk&AN=1355785&site=ehost-live&scope=site.

Flaskerud, J. H. (2015). Pain, culture, assessment, and management. *Issues in Mental Health Nursing, 36*(1), 74–77. https://doi.org/10.3109/01612840.2014.932873.

Herr, K., Coyne, P. J., Ely, E., Gélinas, C., & Manworren, R. C. B. (2019). Pain assessment in the patient unable to self-report: Clinical practice recommendations in support of the ASPMN 2019 Position Statement. *Pain Management Nursing, 20*(5), 404–417. https://doi.org/10.1016/j.pmn.2019.07.005.

Karran, E. L., Grant, A. R., & Moseley, G. L. (2020). Low back pain and the social determinants of health: A systematic review and narrative synthesis. *Pain, 161*(11), 2476–2493. https://doi.org/10.1097/j.pain.0000000000001944.

Orhan, C., Van Looveren, E., Cagnie, B., Mukhtar, N. B., Lenoir, D., & Meeus, M. (2018). Are pain beliefs, cognitions, and behaviors influenced by race, ethnicity, and culture in patients with chronic musculoskeletal pain: A systematic review. *Pain Physician, 21*(6), 541–558.

Part 3

CHAPTER 11

Pain Assessment Tools Across the Lifespan

Staja Q. Booker, PhD, RN
Ann L. Horgas, PhD
Mallory A. Perry-Eady, PhD, RN, CCRN
Kimberly Wittmayer, MS, APRN-FPA, PCNS-BC, PMGT-BC, AP-PMN
Ann Schreier, PhD, BSN, MSN, RN*

Introduction

Pain assessment is an essential nursing and healthcare responsibility. This chapter provides a comprehensive overview of pain assessment tools, including examples, guiding principles, and considerations for patient care and the pain management certification exam. Many scales are available in multiple languages. The use of an interpreter is recommended if needed. This chapter also includes key publications and resources for your pain assessment toolkit.

I. Principles for Selecting, Using, and Documenting Pain Assessment Tools

A. Pain assessment tools provide standardized means to determine presence, intensity, and impact of pain.
   1. Tools vary in application to acute versus persistent (chronic) pain as well as self-report versus behavioral/observational tools for patients unable to self-report reliably.
   2. Self-report and pain behavior tools may be unidimensional, meaning only one dimension of pain is assessed (e.g., intensity/severity), and does not do justice to measuring the complexity of the pain experience.
   3. Other tools may be multidimensional, assessing multiple aspects of the impact of pain on an individual (e.g., intensity, duration, interference, function, social).
   4. There is no universal pain assessment tool applicable to all patients at all times in all settings. Tools must be carefully selected based on individual patient characteristics.
   5. At least 30% reduction or absolute reduction of 2 numeric points is considered clinically meaningful, but patient's baseline pain score and treatment goals should guide what is considered meaningful.

B. One tenet of implementing pain assessment tools in practice is patients' ability to clearly understand how to use self-report tools and nurses knowing how to use, score, and interpret behavioral assessment tools.
C. Pain assessment tools must allow for initial assessment and subsequent reassessments and guide clinical decision-making for treatment planning. *Remember, pain assessment should be considered a continuous improvement process rather than simply a task to be completed.*
D. Regulatory and international guidelines and standards
   1. To foster a patient-centered, team-based, and ethical/legal pain assessment approach, institutions should develop standards or policies for how and when pain is assessed; which tools are selected, used, and documented; and how pain is communicated within the healthcare team.
   2. The Joint Commission (TJC) standards provide guidance for a multilevel approach to individualized pain assessment for a variety of healthcare settings. Pain assessment must be an institutional priority.
      a. Hospital: must have defined criteria and assessment tools to screen, assess, and reassess pain consistent with patient's age, condition, and ability to understand and report
      b. Ambulatory/primary care: Pain assessment tools may differ depending on patient's age; condition; ability to understand and report; and whether pain is acute, persistent, or disease specific. These tools should also be able to identify whether pain is transitioning from acute to persistent.
      c. Home health: Assessment approach should be consistent and evidence based, incorporating tools that assess how pain affects the patient's physical and social functioning. Home health agency must offer flexibility in choosing assessment tool that meets the needs of diverse patients.
      d. Nursing homes/long-term care centers: Facility should have clear protocol and standards to screen, assess, and reassess pain consistent with the resident's age, health condition, pain type,

---

*Section Editor for the chapter.

and ability to understand and report reliably. Tools should assess physical function, quality of life, and pain intensity.

3. The Centers for Medicare and Medicaid Services (CMS) requires patients to have:
   a. Documented pain assessment for presence or absence of pain using standardized tool(s)
      1) Tools must assess multiple characteristics of pain: location, intensity, description, onset, duration, and function.
      2) Examples include: Brief Pain Inventory–Short Form (BPI-SF), McGill Pain Questionnaire (MPQ), and Multidimensional Pain Inventory (MPI)
   b. Documentation of follow-up plan when pain is present
4. Det Norske Veritas Healthcare's National Integrated Accreditation for Healthcare Organizations [DNV]) mandates nursing staff to:
   a. Complete health assessment of patient's condition within 24 hours of admission, including pain history
   b. Give time-critical pain medications
   c. Include patients in developing pain management plan

E. *ANA Scope and Standards for Pain Management:* There are 10 standards for performance of pain management nursing practice. Standard 1 focuses on assessment, including use of scientifically and culturally valid pain assessment tools (see chapter 4 for more detail).

F. Impact of tool characteristics on patient reporting: Characteristics of tool may impact how patients interpret and report their pain. Tools using visuals may not be best for patients with visual or cognitive impairments.
1. Vertical vs. horizontal tools:
   a. Some research shows horizontal orientation produces slightly lower pain scores than vertical alignment.
   b. Some cultures may prefer particular orientation, which may impact results.
2. Faces:
   a. Some tools (e.g., Faces Pain Scale-Revised or Wong-Baker Faces) use a series of animated faces to demonstrate pain severity.
   b. Not all cultures or genders ascribe to demonstrating pain through facial or behavioral expressions (e.g., some people may find crying face to be offensive or sign of weakness).
3. Colors:
   a. Tools, such as Color Analog Scale or Defense and Veterans Pain Rating Scale, use color to signify pain levels.
   b. It is important patients understand what colors mean, as different cultures may associate colors with differing intensities or meanings.

4. Graphics:
   a. Graphical tools may require abstract thinking, which may be difficult for people in pain, people with cognitive deficits, or older adults.
   b. Some pain assessment tools, such as the Iowa Pain Thermometer-revised (IPT-r), use increasing color intensity to indicate increasing pain, which may be confusing to patients who do not think of their pain in terms of metaphorical representations.
5. Anchors:
   a. Not all pain tools include anchors to help patients gauge where their pain falls on a scale.
   b. When present, anchors may be numbers (e.g., 0, 5, 10), words (e.g., no pain, worst pain ever; mild, moderate, severe pain), or tick marks (to signify 0 to 10 on 11-point numeric rating scale).
   c. These anchors or suggested descriptions of pain may be understood differently and, therefore, may result in different responses between patients.
   d. Other tools may have pain example to correspond with a given pain intensity (e.g., paper cut may represent 4/10 while a nail through a finger may represent 10/10). This can be misleading because pain is subjective and no two patients will rate intensity of pain identically for same pain issue.

G. Considerations in selecting appropriate tools (Fig. 11.1):
1. Screen for presence of pain before choosing assessment tool.
2. Adopt validated pain intensity tools to accommodate needs of diverse patient characteristics (e.g., age, culture, language, verbal/nonverbal). These tools should be:
   a. Selected by patient (when appropriate) to enhance congruency with patient's culture of pain expression and communication style
   b. Use accurate language for pain or discomfort
   c. Be available in multiple languages
   d. Easily understood for patient's developmental, intellectual, and cognitive level
   e. Accommodating to patient's sensory impairments (e.g., some tools are available in Braille, audio, or large print)
3. Select tools that can be used across interprofessional team to guide decisional support, treatment planning, and evaluation of treatment, and can allow for consistent documentation in electronic health records (EHR) systems.

H. Using pain assessment tools
1. Tools must be used consistently across patient conditions and across similar conditions (e.g., movement

Part 3

Figure 11.1 **Tips for selecting pain assessment tools.**

activities, at rest, or both) in order to interpret pain scores across time. There is emerging focus on assessing pain during movement as opposed to at rest or during sedentary activities.

2. Use tools appropriate for type of pain: acute, procedural, persistent, or disease specific.

3. Obtaining numeric pain score should not be used or viewed as substitute for talking with patients about their pain.

I. Documentation
1. Consistent and regular documentation of pain assessment is an issue across healthcare settings. Pain terminology and tools may not be standardized within an organization, making it difficult to compare pain ratings during patient's stay.
2. Document tool used, during which condition (e.g., at rest or with movement), time of assessment, patient rating, changes in rating, and progress toward comfort-function-mood goals.

J. Comprehensive approach to pain assessment
1. There is a conceptual and practice shift toward more transactional, patient-centered assessment approaches.
2. One such new tool is Clinically Aligned Pain Assessment (CAPA) tool (Fig. 11.2).
   a. Developed at University of Utah, the tool focuses on five domains: comfort, change in pain, pain control, effect on function, and sleep.
   b. CAPA serves as conversation guide to gather critically important pain information from

patients. A healthcare professional codes and documents conversation.
   c. Strengths:
      1) Can be used for acute or persistent pain assessment
      2) Focuses on pain's effect on function and sleep
      3) Helps guide clinical decision-making with more information than simply pain intensity score
   d. Weaknesses:
      1) Valid in clinical settings but more validation studies are needed to apply tool in research and broader clinical settings
      2) Lacks standardized scoring for how to convert responses to quantitative data
      3) Complete tool may not be pertinent for assessing patient with no need for pain management interventions.
      4) All domains may not be applicable to all patients (e.g., impact on mood may be more important to some patients than sleep).

II. Tools for Pediatric Populations

A. Children are on a wide age spectrum, from infancy to adolescence, with varying range of neurodevelopment. As such, it is imperative to select most chronological age- and developmentally-appropriate scale to assess pain in this population. Children require

Domain/Question	Response
Comfort Note: Ask about pain directly and refrain from general questions such as "How are you feeling?" or "How comfortable are you?"	• Intolerable • Tolerable with discomfort • Comfortably manageable • Negligible pain (Note: patients may not readily know what "negligible pain" is.)
Change in Pain Note: This refers to trajectory of pain severity and perhaps even duration of pain (i.e., Is patient in pain for longer or shorter periods of time?).	• Getting worse • About the same • Getting better
Pain Control	• Inadequate pain control • Partially effective (effective, just about right) • Fully effective (Would like to reduce medication [Why?])
Functioning	• Unable to do anything because of pain • Keeps me from doing most of what I need to do • Can do most things, but pain gets in way of some activities • Can do everything I need (and want) to do
Sleep	• Awake with pain most of night (Note: difficulty getting to and staying asleep) • Awake with occasional pain • Normal sleep

Figure 11.2 Clinically Aligned Pain Assessment (CAPA) Tool. (Topham, D., & Drew, D. [2017].Quality Improvement Project: Replacing the Numeric Rating Scale with a Clinically Aligned Pain Assessment (CAPA) Tool. Pain management nursing : official journal of the American Society of Pain Management Nurses, 18(6), 363–371. https://doi.org/10.1016/j.pmn.2017.07.001.)

age-appropriate explanation on meaning of pain and how to use self-report pain assessment tools (Table 11.1).
B. Guidelines or standards for pediatric pain assessment
   1. Published guidelines
     a. American Academy of Pediatric Dentistry (2020). Pain management in infants, children, adolescents, and individuals with special health care needs. *The Reference Manual of Pediatric Dentistry*. Chicago: American Academy of Pediatric Dentistry, pp. 362–370.
     b. American Academy of Pediatrics, American Pain Society. (2001). The assessment and management of acute pain in infants, children and adolescents. *Pediatrics, 108* (3), 793–797.

     c. Committee on Fetus and Newborn, Section on Anesthesiology and Pain Medicine. (2016). Prevention and management of procedural pain in the neonate. *Pediatrics, 137* (2), e20154271.
C. General principles for assessment in children and adolescents
   1. Children are a vulnerable population, and pediatric pain continues to be underassessed even when children experience a disease process or condition known to cause pain. There is evidence of racial disparities in the assessment and management of pediatric pain.
   2. Children may modify their pain scores based on setting of care, the person asking, whether parent is present, and what they expect to happen because of their answer.

Table 11.1

Self-Report Pain Assessment Tools for Children

Pain Scale and Description	Instructions	Recommended Age and Comments	Validation Studies/ Populations
FACES Pain Rating Scale Scale consists of six cartoon faces ranging from smiling face for "no pain" to tearful face for "worst pain."	*Original Instructions:* Explain to the child that each face is for a person who feels happy because there is no pain (hurt) or sad because there is some or a lot of pain. Face 0 is happy because there is no hurt. Face 1 hurts just a little bit. Face 2 hurts a little more. Face 3 hurts even more. Face 4 hurts a whole lot, but face 5 hurts as much as you can imagine, although you don't have to be crying to feel this bad. Record the number under the chosen face on the pain assessment record. *Brief word instructions:* Point to each face using the words to describe the pain intensity. Ask the child to choose the face that best describes the child's own pain, and record the appropriate number.	Use for children as young as 3 years old. Using original instructions without affected words, such as *happy* or *sad*, or brief words resulted in same pain rating, probably reflecting child's rating of pain intensity. For coding purposes, the numbers 0, 2, 4, 6, 8, and 10 can be substituted for the 0–5 system to accommodate the 0–10 system. FACES system provides three scales in one: facial expressions, numbers, and words. Although not all situations require licensure of Wong-Baker FACES Pain Rating Scale, it is recommended one reviews licensing requirements prior to use: https://wongbakerfaces.org/licensing-dashboard/.	Scale is translated in over 60 languages.
Faces Pain Scale (FPS) and Faces Pain Scale-Revised (FPS-R) Scale consists of six cartoon faces ranging from neutral face (not smiling) for "no pain" to grimacing face (*without tears*) for "worst pain."	In the following instructions, say "Hurt" or "Pain," whichever seems right for particular child: "These faces show how much something can hurt. This face *[point to left-most face]* shows no pain. The faces show more and more pain *[point to each from left to right]* up to this one *[point to right-most face]*. It shows very much pain. Point to the face that shows how much you hurt *[right now]*." Score chosen face 0, 2, 4, 6, 8, or 10, counting left to right, so "0" equals "No pain" and "10" equals "Very much pain." Do not use words like "happy" and "sad." This scale is intended to measure how children feel inside, not how their face looks.	Use for children aged ≥4 years old.	For research use, FPS-R has been recommended on basis of utility and psychometric features. International Association for the Study of Pain (IASP) has the FPS-R translated for free in multiple languages: http://www.iasp-pain.org/FPSR.
Numeric Pain Scale Scale may be verbal or written and is anchored either 0–10 or 0–100.	*Numerical scale:* Point to each section of scale to explain variations in pain intensity: "0 means no hurt. This means little hurts" (pointing to lower part of scale, 1–9). "This means middle hurts" (pointing to middle part of scale 30–69). "This means big hurts" (pointing to upper part of scale 70–99). "100 means the biggest hurt you could ever have". Score is actual number stated by child.	Use for children 3–13 years old. Use numerical scale if child can count to 100 by ones and identify the larger of any two numbers or if child can count by tens.	Tsze et al., showed convergent validity, known-groups validity, and responsivity and reliability of vNRS were strong in children 6–17 years of age. Convergent validity was not strong in 4- and 5-year-olds.
Oucher Scale consists of six photographs of a child's face representing "no hurt" to "biggest hurt you could ever have." It includes a vertical scale with the numbers 0–100.	*Photographic scale:* Point to each photograph on Oucher and explain variations in pain intensity using the following language: "The first picture from the bottom is no hurt, the second is a little hurt, the third is a little more hurt, the fourth is even more hurt than that, the fifth is a lot of hurt, and the sixth is the biggest hurt you could ever have." Score pictures 0–5, with bottom picture scored as 0. *General:* Practice using Oucher by recalling and rating previous pain experiences (e.g., falling off a bike). Child points to number of photograph that describes pain intensity associated with experience. Obtain current pain score from child by asking, "How much hurt do you have right now?"	Determine whether child has cognitive ability to use photographic scale; child should be able to seriate six geometric shapes from largest to smallest. Determine which ethnic version of Oucher to use. Allow child to select version of Oucher or use version that most closely matches physical characteristics of child.	Scales for African American and Hispanic children have been developed (Villarruel & Denyes, 1991).

Table 11.1

Self-Report Pain Assessment Tools for Children—cont'd

Pain Scale and Description	Instructions	Recommended Age and Comments	Validation Studies/ Populations
Pieces of Hurt Tool Tool uses four red poker chips placed horizontally in front of child.	Say to child: "I want to talk with you about the hurt you may be having right now." Align chips horizontally in front of child on bedside table, a clipboard, or other firm surface. Tell child, "These are pieces of hurt." Beginning at chip nearest child's left side and ending at one nearest right side, point to chips and say, "This (point to first chip) is a little bit of hurt, and this (point to fourth chip) is the most hurt you could ever have." For young child or for any child who may not fully comprehend instructions, clarify by saying, "That means this (point to chip 1) is just a little hurt, this (point to chip 2) is a little more hurt, this (point to chip 3) is more yet, and this (point to chip 4) is the most hurt you could ever have." Do not give children option for zero hurt. Research with Poker Chip Tool has verified children without pain will indicate this by responses such as "I don't have any." Ask child, "How many pieces of hurt do you have right now?" After initial use of Poker Chip Tool, some children internalize concept "pieces of hurt." If child gives you a response such as "I have one right now," *before* you ask or lay out poker chips, record the number on pain flow sheet. Clarify child's answer with words such as, "Oh, you have little hurt? Tell me about the hurt."	Use for children as young as 4 years old.	Formerly known as Poker Chip Tool (Hester et al., 1998)
Color Tool Uses crayons or markers for child to construct scale that is used with body outline.	Present eight crayons or markers to child in random order. Ask child to "pick a crayon with a color that reminds you of the most hurt (or pain) that you could possibly have." Once that crayon is selected, separate it from the others. Next, ask child to select crayon with color that "reminds you of pain that is a little less than the pain we just talked about." Once second crayon is selected, separate it from group, and place it with first crayon selected. Ask child to select third crayon with color "that reminds you of only a little pain." Separate crayon and move it to selected group. Finally, ask child to select crayon with color that "reminds you of no hurt (or pain)" and separate fourth color. Show the four crayons selected to child and arrange them in order of "worst hurt (or pain)" to "no hurt (or pain)." Ask child to show on body outline "where the hurt is." If the child offers any verbal comments, note them.	Use for children as young as 4 years old, provided they know their colors, are not color blind, and are able to construct scale if in pain.	
Color Analog Scale (CAS) CAS uses a triangle that increases in width (10–30 mm) and color (from white to dark red).	Scale is anchored with "no pain" at bottom and "most pain" at top. Numbers from 0–10 are on reverse side (not seen by child) and recorded by nurse. Child is asked to slide plastic marker to appropriate color that corresponds to child's amount of pain.	Use with children aged ≥5 years old.	English, Spanish

a. May *underreport* pain if they are concerned high pain rating will result in painful treatment such as analgesic given by intramuscular injection, if they lack knowledge that pain can be treated, if they do not want to upset parents, or if they want be cleared to resume normal activities.

b. May *overreport* pain because parents are present, for increased attention, secondary gains, or to receive higher doses of opioid analgesics. The latter may be particularly true for adolescents and teenagers.

3. QUESTT is a classic strategy to evaluate pain in children using a five-step approach:
   a. **Q**uestion
   b. **U**se pain rating scales
   c. **E**valuate behavior
   d. **S**ecure parents' involvement
   e. **T**ake cause of pain into account
   f. **T**ake action and evaluate

4. Use hierarchy of pain assessment techniques:
   a. Be aware of potential causes of pain including common health conditions and known painful interventions. Assume pain is present, especially in critically ill patients and premature infants.
   b. Attempt self-report. Self-report is the gold standard for 3+ years of age (if developmentally appropriate with appropriate scale).
   c. Observe patient behaviors using pain behavior observational tool for nonverbal children, including intensive care population, children with developmental delays, and children younger than 3 years.
   d. Solicit proxy report of pain and behavior/activity changes.
   e. Attempt analgesic trial and observe for changes in pain behaviors.

5. Use of parent/caregiver assessment with children
   a. Parents know their child best and can be a great asset with assessment and management.
      1) Cultural beliefs and language barriers may make pediatric pain assessment more complex and should be considered during all phases of care.
      2) Assess family's response to illness, pain, and stress because their response can greatly affect the child.
      3) Be aware studies have indicated parents tend to underrate and overrate their child's pain experience.

D. Self-report/verbal-report tools
   1. Unidimensional tools to assess pain intensity
      a. Application
         1) Most pain intensity tools are administered verbally.
         2) Most children who are 3 years old with normal cognitive development can use appropriate self-report scale reliably. However, children must be able to comprehend seriation/rank (i.e., increasing numbers) and order (i.e., worsening facial expression) for Numeric Rating Scale (NRS) and Wong-Baker FACES, respectively.
         3) When introducing child to pain scale, explain that this is one way for child to let others know how much they are hurting. Discussing a simple vignette (e.g., "Imagine you fell down and skinned your knee") can be used to help a child understand how to use scale and establish baseline parameters.
         4) Child should use the same pain scale consistently to avoid confusion and aid in easy interpretation by healthcare team.
         5) For self-report tools, allow ample time for child to respond to pain question(s). For behavioral tools, allow sufficient time to gain global insight into patient's pain (e.g., more than just a glance).
         6) Self-report scale should *not* be switched to observational scale when child is asleep.
            a) Assess pain before going to sleep or awaken child or adolescent to assess for pain on case-by-case basis, if clinically necessary. If no assessment conducted, document "pain assessment was attempted and deferred due to patient sleeping" or "pain assessment deferred due to patient sleeping" if no assessment was attempted.
            b) It is inaccurate to describe child as having "no pain" if child is sleeping.
            c) If child becomes noncommunicative due to declining health (e.g., sedated, comatose), then incorporate an observational/behavioral pain assessment tool.
      b. Advantages
         1) Ease of use
         2) Time efficient
      c. Disadvantages
         1) Unreliable when used in age group that cannot cognitively understand seriation/rank and order for NRS or Wong-Baker FACES
         2) Child may rate how they feel (e.g., sad, angry) as opposed to pain depending upon the scale used.
      d. Commonly used self-report pain intensity tools (Table 11.1)

   2. Multidimensional pain tools include pain intensity, behavior, mood, and function.
      a. Application
         1) Can be used in children 3 years of age and older
         2) Explain each subscale to child.

3) Some children may prefer digital multidimensional tools rather than paper-based tools.
   b. Advantages
      1) Assesses more than pain intensity (and only few pain scales do so)
      2) Consistent with biopsychosocial model, a more comprehensive assessment of pain has been recommended, including pain intensity, satisfaction and treatment response, side effects, pain interference, emotional response, and economic factors.
   c. Disadvantages
      1) Time consuming/lengthy
      2) Not reliable or feasible for children younger than 3 years of age or patients with moderate to severe developmental delay due to potential challenges communicating verbally about their pain and pain outcomes in meaningful, reliable ways.
   d. Commonly used multidimensional self-report pediatric tools are listed in Table 11.2.
E. Behavioral/Observational Tools

1. Observational scales may be considered when child is nonverbal, preverbal, minimally verbal, too distressed to self-report, or physically restricted by medical equipment (e.g., intubated). Pain behavior tools can also be used when "self-report ratings are considered to be exaggerated, minimized, or unrealistic due to cognitive, emotional, or situational factors according to clinical judgment" (Lalloo & Stinson, 2014, p. 322).
2. Most tools include multiple dimensions to assess pain in nonverbal and preverbal children and may include common categories such as vocalizations, facial expressions, sucking, and vital signs/oxygenation status.
3. Application
   a. Should be used when child cannot reliably self-report
   b. Instructions for use must be clear, and observers must know how to score and interpret findings.
4. Advantages

Table 11.2

Multidimensional Self-Report Tools for Pediatrics

Pain Scale and Description	Recommended Age and Comments	Validation Studies and Select Languages Available
Pediatric Pain Questionnaire (PPQ) Includes 10-cm VAS anchored with happy, sad faces, a list of 46 words to describe sensory, affect, and evaluative qualities of pain, as well as location by coloring painful areas on an outline of the body	Children 5–18 years old and takes 10–15 minutes to complete	The PPQ has well-established validity and is available in multiple languages, and offers a parent version.
Pediatric Pain Assessment Tool (PPAT) Includes a 10-cm VAS to rate present and worst pain and includes 32 words to describe sensory, affective, and evaluative qualities of pain	Children 5–16 years old and takes 3–6 minutes to complete	It has good construct validity and is available in both English and Spanish.
Adolescent Pediatric Pain Assessment Tool (APPT) Measures pain intensity using a 0- to 100-mm word rating scale with phrases such as "no pain, little pain, large pain, and worst possible pain," as well as location by coloring painful area on an outline of the body; includes 67 words to describe sensory, affective, and evaluative qualities of pain	Children 5–17 years old and takes 3–6 minutes to complete	The APPT has good construct validity and is available in both English and Spanish.
Bath Adolescent Pain Questionnaire (BAPQ) Designed specifically for use with adolescents who experience persistent pain	Adolescents 11–18 years old	Psychometric evaluation shows both a reliable and valid assessment of the impact of persistent pain on the lives of adolescents. The tool is available in English and offers a parent version (BAPQ-P).
Pediatric American Pain Society-Pain Outcome Questionnaire (Pediatric APS-POQ) (Kaczynski et. al., 2019) Measures pain intensity, functional interference, emotional response, side effects, perceptions of care, and usual pain	Children 3–18 years old and takes <5 minutes to complete	The Pediatric APS-POQ has well established validity, is only available in English, and offers a parent version.

a. Can be used in children who are nonverbal or with developmental delays
b. Ease of use, time efficient
c. Can be used by interprofessional team and family caregivers when provided adequate instruction

5. Disadvantages
   a. Relies on bedside observers' report/observation, which may introduce interrater bias

b. Difficult to differentiate among behaviors specific to pain versus anxiety or opiate withdrawal when using observational tools

6. Commonly used pain behavior observation tools for pediatrics (Table 11.3)

F. Considerations for diverse race, ethnic, and cultural groups
   1. Nonverbal cues and vocalization of pain may differ in diverse racial, ethnic, and cultural groups.

Table 11.3

Pain Behavior Observation Tools for Children

Pain Scale and Description	Instructions	Recommended Age and Comments	Initial Setting of Tool Validation and Select Languages Available
FLACC Behavioral pain scale for those unable to provide self-report of pain intensity	Five domains of evaluation: face, legs, activity, cry, and consolability. Each domain is evaluated from 0–2 with unique descriptors for each domain. Pain can be assessed in patients who are awake or asleep. To assess patients who are awake, rater should observe patient for at least 2–5 minutes, making sure to observe legs and body unobstructed and uncovered. Rater should reposition patient or observe activity, assessing for body's overall tone. Select single choice for each domain. To assess patients who are sleeping, observe for at least 5 minutes. Observe body and legs uncovered. Reposition patient if necessary, taking care not to wake. Gently touch body and assess for tenseness and tone. Sum of each domains is FLACC score. Scores range from 0 (no pain) to 10 (worst pain).	Ideally used in preverbal and nonverbal patients, aged 2-months to 18 years of age	Post anesthesia care, intensive care, acute care • English • Japanese • Thai • Chinese
revised FLACC (rFLACC) Includes behavior specific to children with neurocognitive impairments	See above–scoring is similar to original FLACC, despite specific language for children with cognitive impairment.	Same as original FLACC, though ideal in those with cognitive impairment	Acute care
COMFORT Behavioral scale used to assess pain and sedation in infants, children, and adults. Scale is useful in critically ill individuals, as it includes biometric measures of blood pressure and heart rate in pain assessment.	Evaluates eight domains: alertness, calmness/agitation, respiratory distress, crying, physical movement, muscle tone, facial tension and blood pressure. Each indicator is scored from 1–5 based upon domain and associated behavior descriptor. Similar to FLACC, patients should be observed unbothered for 2 minutes to tabulate score. Total score for each domain can range from 8 (no pain) to 40 (distressed). Score of 17–26 is generally acceptable level of sedation and pain control. To assess domain of blood pressure, rater will review patient's medical record to calculate baseline, upper and lower limits for heart rate (HR), and mean arterial pressure (MAP). Values more than 15% above and below are calculated prior to 2-minute observation. Raters should position themselves where they are able to view physiologic monitors and patient's behavioral pain responses. Every 15–20 seconds, rater will observe HR and MAP and determine if they are within upper and lower limits. Approximately 10 seconds before observation period is due to end, observer rates muscle tone response with rapid and slow flexion of free (no medical devices) extremity. Elbow or knee is ideal, though wrist or ankle may be used if necessary. Most extreme (distressed) behavior observed will be recorded on each variable at end of 2 minutes. Total score is sum of each of eight domains.	Mainly used in critical care settings Useful in children, adults who are cognitively impaired (due to injury and/or medication or illness), or critically ill individuals who are mechanically ventilated and sedated	Intensive care • Dutch • Chinese • English

Table 11.3

Pain Behavior Observation Tools for Children—cont'd

Pain Scale and Description	Instructions	Recommended Age and Comments	Initial Setting of Tool Validation and Select Languages Available
CRIES Observational tool generally used in neonates and infants greater than or equal to 38 weeks gestation; widely used in neonatal intensive care units	Assessed on five domains: crying, oxygenation, vital signs, expression, and sleeplessness. Each domain is scored from 0–2 dependent on domain descriptor. Total sum score ranges from 0 (no pain) to 10 (most pain). Pain score >4 requires additional assessment and possible intervention. To assess each Domain, rater will do as follows: Crying: domain is assessed if infant has high pitched cry. Requires O2 for saturation >95%: assess for changes in oxygenation and if infant needs supplemental oxygen to maintain oxygen saturation >95%; also consider other causes of desaturation such as atelectasis, pneumothorax, over sedation, etc. Increased Vital Signs: assess BP and HR last, as doing so may wake infant and skew CRIES assessment. Use baseline parameters from non-stressed/painful period. CRIES scale uses parameter of >20% as increase in vitals. Multiply baseline HR and MAP by 0.2 then add to baseline for assessment. Expression: facial grimace is often associated with pain in infants. Grimace in presence or absence of crying is evaluated within this domain. Sleepless: domain is assessed for hour preceding CRIES assessment.	Neonates and newborns	Intensive care • English • Thai
Children's Hospital of Eastern Ontario Scale (CHEOPS) Observational scale intended to assess postoperative pain in children, allowing for standardized postoperative pain assessment	Six domains: cry, facial, child verbal, torso, touch, and legs. Each domain has specific scoring scheme with varying ranges. Total score is sum of all domains and ranges from 4 (no pain) to 13 (worst pain). In scores ≥5, analgesia and additional assessment may be considered. Cry: assessed by observing child and measuring their cry intensity Facial: assesses child's expressions, including smiling, composure, or grimacing Verbal: assesses child's complaint, or lack thereof; could be pain related ("I hurt") or non-pain related ("Where are my parents?") Torso: looks directly at child's body position, excluding arm movements Touch: refers to child's behaviors toward surgical site, including reaching, touching, or grabbing at wound Legs: assesses child's extremities and whether they are neutral, squirming/kicking, tense, standing, or if child needs to be restrained.	Pediatric postoperative pain in children <5 years old	Post-anesthesia care unit • English • Thai • Swedish
Individualized Numeric Rating Scale (INRS) Scale uses nurse and/or parent input for pain response in pediatric patients with cognitive impairment. Parent or nurses put in typical pain expressions (verbal and/or nonverbal) of patient, which may characterize pain response.	Rated on 0 (no pain) to 10 (worst possible pain) scale and is individualized to patient. Scale itself is a visual analog scale with equidistant vertical lines at each corresponding whole number. Parent or nurse can use FLACC acronym to populate INRS with patient's typical pain behaviors on corresponding vertical line. To begin, parent or nurse will think about painful events child has experienced prior to painful experiences. How does child generally respond to mild, moderate and severe pain? In INRS diagram, parent or nurse will write in typical pain behavior corresponding with that line. When describing child's pain, think about changes in (adapted from FLACC): Facial expression: squinting eyes, frowning, distorted face, teeth grinding, tongue thrusting Leg or general body movements: tense, gestures (more or less) or touches part of body that hurts Activity or social interaction: not cooperative, cranky, irritable, unhappy; not moving, less active, quiet or more active, fidgety Cry or vocalization: moaning, whimpering, crying, yelling Consolability: less interaction, seeks comfort or physical closeness, difficult to distract/satisfy Other changes: tears, sweating, holding breath, gasping To score, rater will use INRS scale to correlate behavioral response to pain with corresponding number.	Nonverbal children with intellectual disability	Acute care • English

Continued

Table 11.3

Pain Behavior Observation Tools for Children—cont'd

Pain Scale and Description	Instructions	Recommended Age and Comments	Initial Setting of Tool Validation and Select Languages Available
Non-Communicating Children's Pain Checklist (NCCPC) Intended for children aged 3–18 years with cognitive impairments and/or disabilities (though can be used in those without impairment or disability)	Parents and caregivers are able to use NCCPC without prior training in home. There are two versions of the scale: revised and postoperative. Revised version assesses everyday pain in 2-hour observations. Postoperative version includes 5- to 10-minute observations with no eating and sleeping domains. Postoperative version is translatable to most acute situations. Within revised version, raters are instructed to base their observations on last 2 hours of child's behavior, though it is not necessary to watch them continuously. There are seven domains: vocal, social, facial, activity, body/limbs, physiological, and eating/sleeping. Each domain is based on 0 (not at all) to 3 (very often). There is also not an applicable (N/A) option. Postoperative scale has six domains and excludes eating/sleeping domain.	Can be used for everyday pain in home, as well as acute or postoperative pain	Postoperative care • English • Italian • German • French • Swiss
Child Facial Coding System (CFCS) Derived from Facial Coding System (adult) and Neonatal Facial Coding System (NCFS)	Assesses children for 13 facial expressions including brow lowering, squint, eye squeeze, nose wrinkle, nasolabial furrow, cheek raise, lip corner pull, vertical mouth stretch, horizontal mouth stretch, blink, flared nostril, and open lips.	School-aged children	Acute care
Children's and Infants Postoperative Pain Scale (CHIPPS) Behavioral scale for postoperative pain assessment in children	Five categories: crying, facial expression, trunk posture, leg posture, and motor restlessness. Each domain is rated 0–2 dependent on descriptor. Rater should observe child for at least 15 seconds prior to providing score. Scores range from 0 (no pain) to 10 (worst pain). Those scores ≥4 indicate potential need for analgesia.	Best in preterm and term infants, as well as toddlers and older children. It is best used to assess acute pain episodes.	Acute care • English • Thai • Portuguese
Toddler-Preschool Postoperative Pain Scale (TPPPS) Behavioral pain tool used to assess postoperative pain in children 1–5 years old	Made up of seven items, divided into three behavioral pain expression categories: (1) vocal, (2) facial, and (3) bodily. Observation of the child occurs postoperatively once they have to awaken from anesthesia; this scale is not validated in sleeping children.	Best used in toddlers and pre school-aged children for assessment of postoperative pain	Acute care • English • Thai
Neonatal Pain, Agitation & Sedation Scale (N-PASS) Observational pain, agitation, and sedation tool used in premature infants, generally up to 100 days of life	Assesses five domains of crying irritability, behavior state, facial expression, extremities tone, and vital signs (HR, RR, BP, SaO_2). Scales also include gestation/corrected domain, which is scored dependent on neonate's gestational age. Each domain is scored on Likert scale, whereas sedation scores are −2–1 and pain scores are +1/+2 (no pain = 0). Sedation does not need to be assessed/scored with every pain assessment. To assess sedation, observe neonate for 1 minute and then score each individual behavior. Final score should range from 0 (normal) to −10 (sedate). To interpret: – Deep sedation = −10 to −5 – Light sedation = −5 to −2 To assess pain/agitation, observe neonate for 1 minute. Pain/agitation scores are only positive scores. Tabulate each domain for observed behavior. Determine if scoring will need to be adjusted for neonate's gestational/corrected age (premature pain assessment). Range will be from 0 (normal/no pain) to 13 (pain). Any score greater than or equal to 3 should include increased vigilance, as there is possibly pain.	Neonates and newborns; often used in pre- and postoperative/intervention pain assessments, neonatal ICU, pediatric ICU, and home care	Intensive care • English • Indian

Table 11.3

Pain Behavior Observation Tools for Children—cont'd

Pain Scale and Description	Instructions	Recommended Age and Comments	Initial Setting of Tool Validation and Select Languages Available
Neonatal Infant Pain Scale (NIPS) Behavioral observational tool for full term infants to 1-year old	Includes six domains: facial expression, cry, breathing patterns, arms, legs, and state of arousal. Each domain is rated on Likert scale of 0–2 and scored according to appropriate descriptor. Sum score is total NIPS, which will range from 0 (no pain) to 7 (worst pain). Observe neonate for 1 minute prior to selecting score for each domain. Any score greater than 2 indicates potential pain and requires additional vigilance and/or intervention.	Most often used in obstetrics in newborns, pediatric non-ICU areas, including ED, and pre- and postoperative areas	Intensive care • English • Thai
Riley Infant Pain Scale (RIPS) Behavioral pain scale originally developed by two nurses at Riley Children's Hospital; intended to assess pain in preverbal/nonverbal children	Assesses six behavioral categories: facial, body movement, sleep, verbal/vocal, consolability, and response to movement/touch. Each category is rated 0–3 dependent on domain descriptor. Sum scores range from 0 (no pain) to 15 (worst pain).	Best used in term infants and toddlers (<26 months) to assess postoperative pain; has also been validated in children with cerebral palsy	Acute postoperative pain • English
Assume Agitation Present/Assume Pain Present (AAP/APP) There are no validated pain scales to assess pain in children who are muscle relaxed and/or chemically paralyzed. As a proxy, many institutions use AAP/APP to indicate agitation/pain	To assess pain and agitation in muscle relaxed patients (e.g., chemically paralyzed and sedated), rater must search for potential sources of pain and assume pain is present if there is cause for pain (e.g., injury, suctioning via mechanical ventilation, procedure, turning). Mainstay of AAP/APP is to use physiologic variables, which may be indicative of pain and/or agitation (i.e., increased HR, BP). It is important not to rely on these variables exclusively.	Can be used in patients in critical care setting who are muscle relaxed/chemically paralyzed and/or heavily sedated, where behavioral response is not possible to assess	
Nursing Assessment of Pain Intensity Scale (NAPI) Was adapted from CHEOPS scale	Assesses three domains: body movement, facial, and response to touch (specifically to the surgical site). Scores each domain from 0–3 dependent on domain descriptor. Total scores range from 0 (no pain) to 7 (worst pain).	Best used in term infants and toddlers to assess postoperative pain; can be used in children up to 16 years of age	Acute care • English

Ensure individuals are being given comprehensive, holistic, and culturally sensitive pain assessment to verify they are not potentially masking existing pain.

2. Parental report as proxy may be useful in conjunction with child report to help understand whether child is in fact experiencing pain; certain cues may only be noticed by parent.
3. Many scales are available in multiple languages. Use of interpreter is recommended if needed.

III. Tools for Young and Middle-Aged Adult Populations

A. Assessing pain in young and middle-aged adults has primarily focused on obtaining pain intensity rating. Little guidance is provided on best tools or methods for pain assessment.
B. Guidelines or standards for adult pain assessment

1. List of published guidelines:
   a. Institute for Clinical Systems Improvement (ICSI) (September 2019)
   b. Pain: Assessment, Non-Opioid Treatment Approaches and Opioid Management Care for Adults (https://www.icsi.org/wp-content/uploads/2019/10/Pain-Interactive-7th-V2-Ed-8.17.pdf)
2. Self-report is the gold standard for verbal and cognitively intact adults.
3. Behavioral/observational assessment is the gold standard for nonverbal or minimally verbal adults.
C. Self-report/verbal tools
   1. Unidimensional tools assess pain intensity.
      a. Application:
         1) Depending on scale, patients are asked to rate intensity or severity of pain using numbers or words.
         2) Nurses cannot assign pain intensity rating based on patient's physical expressions of pain or body language.
      b. Advantages:
         1) Easy to use and score
         2) Many people are familiar with how to use most numeric pain intensity tools.
      c. Disadvantages:
         1) Only assesses pain intensity, which is only one of several aspects of pain phenomenon
         2) Does not provide complete information for developing and tailoring pain treatment plan
   2. Commonly used uni-dimensional tools for young and middle-aged adults:
      a. 11-point Numeric Rating Scale (NRS)
         1) Most common self-report pain assessment tool used in acute, long-term, and ambulatory settings
         2) Uses numbers to describe pain intensity.
            a) Numbers signifying extremes of pain are presented in increasing order of severity.
            b) Patient selects a whole number (0-10) that best describes their current intensity of pain.
            c) NRS is commonly administered as a verbal tool and may be presented visually as a vertical or horizontal Likert scale when verbal instructions are given to patient.
         3) Most helpful when compared to verbal rating scale, visual analog scale, and Faces Pain Scale-Revised.
         4) Advantages: Easy to score and monitor change over time
         5) Disadvantages
            a) Only measures intensity. Patients may have difficulty describing their pain with a simple whole number. Patients may want to rate in between numbers

(e.g., 6.5). *Know your facility's policy about whole and half ratings.*
            b) Anchors to describe extreme pain are inconsistent (e.g., "worst pain" vs. "worst imaginable pain" vs. "pain as bad as you've ever experienced" vs. "severe pain").
            c) Scores cannot be treated as ratio data, as having equal distance. For example, ratio data can be multiplied and divided because not only is the difference or distance between 1 and 2 the same as 3 and 4, but also 4 is twice as much as 2. Patients, however, may not perceive and use NRS in this manner.
      b. Verbal Descriptor Scale (VDS)
         1) Uses verbal or visual descriptors to describe intensity of pain. Adjectives describe extremes of pain in ranked order. Some scales assign a number to an adjective that reflects pain intensity.
         2) Advantages:
            a) Easy to sue and score.
            b) Some patients prefer words or descriptors over numbers to communicate their pain. However, patients are forced to choose a word that may not accurately describe their experience.
         3) Disadvantages:
            a) Some verbal descriptors may be associated with affective distress.
            b) Less reliable in patients who do not speak English, especially if descriptors take on Westernized description
            c) VDS measures ordinal scale; however, distance between descriptors are not equal but rather categorical.
      c. Visual Analog Scale (VAS)
         1) Uses 100-mm (10-cm) horizontal or vertical line patient marks to indicate pain intensity. Line may be anchored with word descriptors (e.g., no pain, worst possible pain) or numbers (0, 10).
         2) Patient is asked to place a line perpendicular to VAS vertical line at a point that represents pain intensity. Line is measured from beginning of VAS line to patient's mark. For example, a mark at 30-mm point would translate into 3 of 10 (or 30 of 100) for pain intensity.
         3) Administration is visual rather than verbal.
         4) Disadvantages:
            a) Older adults may have difficulty using this scale, so it is not recommended in this population.
            b) Originally designed for use in research and not clinical practice

d. FACES Pain Scale-Revised (FPS-R)
   1) Adapted from Wong-Baker FACES scale to measure pain intensity. This visual tool consists of six oval-shaped faces ranging from neutral/happy face (no pain) to grimacing face with no tears (worst pain). This tool is more acceptable in adults than Wong-Baker FACES.
   2) Disadvantages:
      a) Patients with low visual acuity may have difficulty distinguishing facial expressions.
      b) May measure constructs other than pain intensity (e.g., distress or mood). Clear instructions to rate pain intensity should be given.
      c) Requires some level of abstract thinking
3. Multidimensional tools assessing for intensity, behavior, mood, and function
   a. Application:
      1) Explain importance of assessing and reporting more than intensity.
      2) Tools should be used when adult cannot reliably self-report.
      3) Instructions for use must be clear, and healthcare team must know how to score and interpret findings.
   b. Advantages:
      1) Provides more comprehensive assessment of pain impact in order to set realistic goals
      2) Allows treatment targeting multiple pain dimensions, not just reduction in pain intensity but also improvement in mood and function
      3) Cues involvement of interdisciplinary team members such as physical therapy, arts-in-medicine, or psychology
   c. Disadvantages:
      1) May not be standard practice within organizations
      2) May take longer to administer
   d. Commonly used multidimensional self-report tools for young and middle-aged adults include:
      1) Pain, Enjoyment of Life, General Activity (PEG)
         a) Based on Brief Pain Inventory–Short Form (BPI-SF) and is a short three-item tool to quickly determine pain intensity and interference on enjoyment of life and general activities within the past week.
         b) Can be used in primary care settings
      2) Defense and Veterans Pain Rating Scale (DVPRS)
         a) Developed by Department of Veterans Affairs to assess pain intensity and its corresponding interference with function and activity
         b) Incorporates numeric, word descriptors, graphics, and colors to help patients determine pain level
      3) Brief Pain Inventory–Short Form (BPI-SF)
         a) Has three parts and measures pain intensity, pain interference, and efficacy of pain medications; some forms may include body diagram to mark areas of pain
         b) Assesses current, worse, least, and average pain intensity
         c) Pain interference subscale assesses effect of pain on seven areas of functioning (e.g., normal activities, sleep, social, household chores, etc.).
         d) Translated into multiple languages
         e) Can be used in clinical and research settings and takes approximately 10 to 15 minutes to complete
D. Behavioral/observational tools
   1. These tools are designated for noncommunicative/nonverbal adults, including young, middle-aged, and older.
      a. Application:
         1) When observing for pain, clinicians should be aware certain conditions (e.g., Parkinson's disease or stroke) may impact behaviors like facial expressions and vocalizations.
         2) Nurses or other observers should not assign a pain intensity score based on patient behavior.
         3) Be familiar with tools offered by your organization.
      b. Advantages:
         1) Provides validated approach to identify and assess pain despite lack of verbal communication
         2) Pain behaviors may guide interventions.
      c. Disadvantages:
         1) Requires training to ensure reliability and consistency across disciplines
         2) May be difficult to assess behaviors in critically ill patients who are sedated or comatose
      d. Commonly used tools validated for use in acute and critical care settings are listed in Table 11.4.
E. Considerations for diverse race, ethnic, and cultural groups
   1. Many self-report and pain behavior tools have been translated and tested in multiple countries and languages.
   2. Pain behavior/observational tools may demonstrate varying sensitivity in different cultures.

Table 11.4

Comparison of Pain Behavior Tools For Critically ill Adults

Tool	Description	Advantages	Disadvantages	Select Languages/Countries Available
Critical Care Observation (CPOT)	Assesses pain based on behavior in critically ill and/or mechanically-ventilated patients in intensive care unit. Consists of four domains: 1. Facial expressions 2. Movements 3. Muscle tension 4. Ventilator compliance (this domain can be replaced with vocalizations)	Assesses pain at rest to establish baseline, then assesses during movement, such as turning. Feasible Clinically Useful Sensitive and specific Can be used in patients who are sedated, mechanically ventilated, experiencing delirium, and nonverbal	May have limitations for patients with persistent vs. acute pain Difficulty distinguishing pain behaviors from delirium behaviors	• Portuguese • Polish • English • German • Finnish • Dutch • Korean
Behavioral Pain Scale (BPS)	Determines pain level in sedated, non-verbal adults Consists of three observational items scored from 1–4 for potential total of 12 indicating high levels of pain	Use at rest and during noxious stimulus (e.g., endotracheal suctioning, turning, mobilization). Good interrater reliability in patients under sedation	Interrater agreement varies, particularly after painful procedure	• Swedish • English • Portuguese • Chinese • Spanish • Taiwanese • Dutch • Finnish
Behavioral Pain Assessment Tool (BPAT)	Eight behavior items coded as present or absent: • Four facial expressions derived from facial action coding • Two verbal responses • Two body muscle responses	Valid, reliable, and predicts pain intensity Tested in large sample size	Feasibility and effect on clinical implementation on patient outcomes warrant further study.	Used in 28 different countries
Nonverbal Pain Assessment Tool (NPAT)	Consists of five domains: 1. Emotion 2. Movement 3. Verbal cues/sound expression 4. Facial cues 5. Positioning/guarding	High interrater reliability for verbal adults Validated in various patient populations: intensive care, general surgery, cardiac Easy to use	Additional validation needed	• English • Finnish
Nonverbal Pain Scale (NVPS)	Adapted from FLACC tool Measures behavioral and physiological indications: 1. Facial expression 2. Activity 3. Defense 4. Blood pressure 5. Respiratory rate, SpO2 Each domain is scored from 0–2 with total score ranging from 0 (no pain) to 10 (maximum pain).	Valid and demonstrates high correlation between NVPS and FLACC	Not suitable for patients who are verbal in critical care settings	• English • Iranian • Finnish
Pain Assessment and Intervention Notation (PAIN)	Developed to assess and monitor pain assessment, ability of patient to tolerate opiates, and selection of analgesic treatment. Pain assessment includes six behavioral domains: 1. Motion 2. Posture 3. Facial expression 4. Sound expression 5. Paleness 6. Perspiration As well as increases in three physiological pain indicators: 1. Blood pressure 2. Heart rate 3. Respiratory rate	Algorithm helps provide systematic approach to pain assessment and guides analgesic treatments.	Lacks rigorous validation testing and requires time to complete	• English

IV. Tools for Older and Aging Adult Populations

A. Assessing pain in older adults can be challenging, especially if older person is nonverbal or has limited cognitive abilities. Tools commonly used in younger and middle-aged adults may be used with older adults but with some modification to meet needs associated with aging.

B. Guidelines or standards for pain assessment
   1. Published guidelines
      a. Hadjistavropoulos, T., et al. (2007). An interdisciplinary expert consensus statement on assessment of pain in older persons. *Clinical Journal of Pain, 23*(1 Suppl), S1–43.
      b. Herr, K., Coyne, P.J., Ely, E., Gélinas, C., & Manworren, R.C.B. (2019). Pain assessment in the patient unable to self-report: Clinical practice recommendations in support of the ASPMN 2019 position statement. *Pain Management Nursing, 20*(5), 404–417.
      c. Schofield, P. (2018). The assessment of pain in older people: UK national guidelines. *Age and Ageing, 47*(1 Suppl), i1-i22.

C. Self-report/verbal tools
   1. Unidimensional tools assess pain intensity.
      a. Application:
         1) These tools (e.g., NRS, VDS, VAS, and FPS-R) only measure pain intensity and do not assess other aspects of pain such as functional impact.
         2) Provide clear instructions with visuals to accompany verbal explanation.
         3) Minimize potential bias or influence by providing examples for clarity only when patient asks or appears confused or hesitant to provide clear pain rating.
         4) Standard scales should be printed in large enough font to enhance readability for older adults.
      b. Advantages:
         1) Tools can be easily used by many older adults, although numerical ratings (e.g., which number is high and which number is low) should be clearly explained.
         2) Most older adults are familiar with NRS and can reliably use.
      c. Disadvantages:
         1) Tools do not relate to older adults' level of functioning.
         2) May be difficult for some patients to assign definitive numeric score, especially if multiple types of pain are present in various body locations.
         3) Single dimension scales may have ceiling effect if value of "10" is chosen and patient's perception of pain worsens.
         4) Scales are linear and provide little context such as time of day, activity during assessment (movement or rest), etc.

      d. Commonly used self-report tools for older adults:
         1) Iowa Pain Thermometer-Revised (IPT-R) (Fig. 11.3)
            a) Tool specifically developed for older adults to assess pain intensity. It presents image of thermometer to symbolize "rising" or "lowering" pain.
            b) Modified from vertical VDS, the revised thermometer uses number (0 to 10) along with descriptive anchors (no pain, mild pain, moderate pain, worst pain imaginable). This helps patients gauge what numbers could signify but presupposes a particular number correlates with a severity of pain.
            c) Advantages:
               1) Simple to describe/use
               2) Can be used with patients of varying levels of cognition
               3) Preferred over NRS in older patients
            d) Disadvantage:
               1) It must be presented in printed form (not currently available in digital format)
               2) Patients must have good visual acuity, and must have verbal ability to understand concept of a thermometer to measure pain.

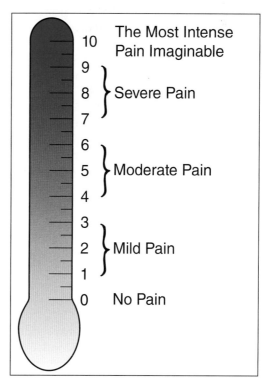

Figure 11.3 Iowa Pain Thermometer-Revised (IPT-R).
(Printed with permission © Keela Herr, The University of Iowa.)

2. Multidimensional pain tools assess pain intensity, interference, and quality of life.
   a. Many multidimensional pain tools have same advantages, disadvantages, and application as those used in young and middle-aged adults.
   b. Application:
      1) Tools provide more comprehensive assessment of pain consistent with biopsychosocial model.
      2) Provide clear instructions and obtain complete information about each dimension.
   c. Advantages:
      1) Multidimensional tools assess pain intensity, satisfaction and treatment response, side effects, pain interference, emotional response, and economic factors.
      2) Allows providers to intervene on multiple pain-related factors
   d. Disadvantages:
      1) More time-consuming/lengthy to complete; may be tiring for some older adults, depending on their clinical status
      2) May not be reliable or feasible for older adults with cognitive decline or visual limitations
   e. Commonly used multidimensional tools for older adults:
      1) Tools include PEG, DVPRS, and BPI-SF.
      2) Geriatric Pain Measure (GPM)
         a) Developed specifically for older adults
         b) Valid and reliable, 24-item questionnaire measures multiple dimensions of pain in older adults, such as intensity, disengagement, pain at ambulation, pain at vigorous activities, and pain during other activities.
         c) Shorter, 12-item questionnaire has been validated in older adults in Europe and US (Geriatric Pain Measure-12).

D. Behavioral/observational tools
   1. Comprehensive pain assessment for older adults includes focus on objective/observable indicators of pain when verbal report of pain is not available.
   2. Behaviors such as guarded movement, bracing, rubbing affected area, grimacing, expressing painful noises or words, and restlessness are considered indicators of pain.
   3. Cognitive impairment due to Alzheimer disease and related dementias impairs older adults' ability to self-report pain. This is often due to impaired memory, judgment, and/or communication skills.
      a. In older adults with dementia, wandering, aggressive, or agitated behaviors may be triggered or exacerbated by pain.
      b. Changes in behavior or affect may signal an underlying condition associated with pain.
   4. ASPMN position statement recommends a hierarchical pain assessment approach with five steps.
      a. Minimize emphasis on vital signs as absolute sign of pain.
      b. Assess regularly, reassess post intervention, and document.
      c. Five steps:
         1) Be aware of potential causes of pain including interventions known to be painful.
         2) Attempt self-report.
         3) Observe patient behaviors.
         4) Solicit proxy report of pain and behavior/activity changes.
         5) Attempt analgesic trial; observe for pain behaviors.
   5. Behavioral pain assessment tools assist in recognition of pain.
      a. Tools thoroughly researched by several authors and with published supporting evidence are recommended.
      b. Use of standardized tools promotes consistency among care providers and facilitates communication and evaluation of pain management practices.
      c. More than 20 behavioral pain tools for older adults have been published.
         1) Tools differ in their content, comprehensiveness, ease of use, and psychometric characteristics (reliability and validity).
         2) Can be helpful to identify presence of pain, monitor for changes, and evaluate effectiveness of pain treatments
      d. Behavioral pain score is not equivalent to self-reported pain intensity rating on numeric rating scale but should trigger comprehensive pain assessment.
      e. Observe for pain indicators at rest, during activity, and during procedures known to be painful.
      f. Observe for changes in behaviors after treatment. Changes in frequency or intensity of observed behaviors suggest changes in pain.
      g. Application: Behavior/observational tools are applicable for older adults with cognitive decline unable to provide verbal report of pain.
      h. Advantages: Tools rely on assessment of recognizable facial and body movements associated with pain. Verbal voices (e.g., moaning and vocalizations) are included.
      i. Disadvantages:
         1) Observational tools vary in type of behaviors assessed, and some are lengthy to administer.
         2) Some tools include assessment of change from usual behavior as a pain indicator. Thus, this would not be feasible to assess in some settings without proxy report (e.g., emergency departments).
      j. Example pain behavior tools for older adults with cognitive impairment, dementia, and other nonverbal conditions. Select validated tools for this population are presented in Table 11.5.
      k. Other tools with more limited psychometric testing include the following:
         1) Abbey Pain Scale (ABBEY)

Table 11.5

Select Behavioral Pain Assessment Tools for Older Adults With Cognitive Impairment, Dementia, and Other Nonverbal Conditions

Nonverbal Pain Behavior Scale	Description	Validity	Reliability	Feasibility and Clinical utility	Languages and Settings	Summary
The Abbey Pain Scale	• Six items including vocalization, facial expression, change in body language, behavioral change, physiological change, and physical change • Items scored on 4-point scale for intensity of behavior with total score for intensity of pain (0–18)	• Good concurrent and construct validity • Differentiates between pre- and postintervention	• Moderate internal consistency • Strong interrater reliability • Sufficient test-retest reliability	• Reported completion 1 minute • Scoring interpretation provided, but relationship with self-report of pain severity questionable • Cut-off of 3.5 for pain/no pain determined using ROC analysis	**Languages:** • English • Japanese • Italian **Settings:** • Australian residential aged care facilities (RACF) • Hong Kong nursing homes • Japanese nursing homes • Italian hospitals	• Clinically usable, brief measure of observable pain behaviors • Evidence of reliability and validity is established. • Issues related to scoring level of pain severity • "Physical change" item may need revision based on consistent problems across studies.
Algoplus	• Five items/categories (facial expressions, look, complaints, body position, atypical behaviors) with 3–6 basic pain behaviors in each category • Items scored yes if one basic behavior observed • Total score 0–5	• Discriminant validity differentiating acute pain and non-acute pain patients • Convergent validity in correlation between Algoplus and pain ratings of cognitively intact patients • Sensitivity to change between rest and movement and before and after analgesia	• Sufficient overall internal consistency, although some items may underestimate pain intensity, particularly in Cambodian patients • Strong interrater reliability overall, but individual item ratings fair to strong	• Training time unclear • Time to administer/score 1 minute • Cut-off of 2 for acute pain recommended based on ROC analysis	**Languages:** • French only—although translated into English **Settings:** • French hospital, emergency departments, rehabilitation units and long-term care facilities • Cambodian emergency department	• Only tool focused on identification of acute pain • Short, reliable tool for rapid evaluation of acute pain • Good preliminary psychometrics, but needs further evaluation in persons with advanced dementia • Testing in other cultures warranted
Checklist of Nonverbal Pain Indicators	• Six items including nonverbal vocalizations, facial grimacing or wincing, bracing, rubbing, restlessness, and vocal complaints • Items scored present or absent at rest and on movement • Total score range 0–12	• Convergent validity with other tools • Discriminates between baseline and pain conditions and between pain at rest vs. on movement	• Moderate internal consistency reliability, although low for observations at rest • Good interrater reliability • Good to very good intrarater reliability • Moderate to good test-retest	• Easy to use • Time to complete not specified, but likely five minutes or less • Scoring instructions provided • No evidence any number of pain behaviors from CNPI corresponds with levels of pain intensity	**Languages:** • English • Norwegian **Settings:** • U.S. nursing homes and hospitals • Canadian nursing homes • Australian RACF • Canadian nursing homes, Australian RACF • Norwegian nursing homes	• Clinically usable, brief measure of observable pain behaviors • One of few tools with testing in hospital setting • Further evaluation of total score use (versus comparison of score at rest and movement) warranted

Continued

Part 3

Part 3

Table 11.5

Select Behavioral Pain Assessment Tools for Older Adults With Cognitive Impairment, Dementia, and Other Nonverbal Conditions —cont'd

Nonverbal Pain Behavior Scale	Description	Validity	Reliability	Feasibility and Clinical utility	Languages and Settings	Summary
CNA Pain Assessment Tool (CPAT)	• Five items including facial expression, behavior, mood, body language, and activity level • Items scored 0 or 1 with different criteria based on item • Total score range 0–5	• Construct validity established with differences before and after painful event; before and after intervention • Criterion validity established with concurrent administration of established research discomfort tool	• Strong interrater reliability • Sufficient internal consistency • Fair test-retest	• Training of 45 minutes required • Observation and scoring requires 1 minute • Score of 1 or greater requires further action by nursing assistant, and high scores are to be evaluated by nursing staff.	**Languages:** • English **Settings:** • U.S. nursing homes	• Clinically usable, brief measure of observable pain behaviors by CNAs • Further evaluation of item scoring criteria and evaluation of tool sensitivity in controlled design recommended • Testing in other cultures and settings warranted
DOLOSHORT	• Five-item, shortened version of Doloplus-2 with items significantly correlated with VAS scores in multiple regression model • Scoring range not provided	• Construct validity established with differences before and after pain intervention • Convergent and discriminant validity established in French-speaking Swiss sample • Moderately high degree of sensitivity and specificity using suggested cut-off scores	• Sufficient internal consistency • Further reliability testing warranted	• Reported to be quick and easy to use • Cut-off score suggested at 3 via ROC analysis • Administration, scoring unclear	**Languages:** • French **Settings:** • Swiss hospital	• High convergent and discriminant validity and strong responsiveness of tool to treatment in preliminary testing • Testing in other cultures and settings warranted
Doloplus-2	• Ten items, three dimensions of somatic (n = 5), psychomotor (n = 2), psychosocial (n = 3) • Scoring range 0–30, reflects progression of experienced pain severity, not current pain experience	• Construct, concurrent, convergent, and discriminant validity established in French and other cultures • Recent construct validity established in English version • Distinguishes between pain/no pain moderately well	• Good or excellent test-retest and interrater reliability in French, English, Italian, Portuguese, and Spanish • Moderate test-retest and interrater reliability in Dutch • Intrarater reliability • Strong internal consistency	• Appears easy to use • Estimated time to complete is 5 minutes • Suggest score of 5 as threshold for pain • Considerable training resource materials available in several languages • Use by health and social care providers, as well as family; however, question regarding training and administration skills • Electronic tool available	**Languages:** • French • Italian • English • Spanish • Dutch • Norwegian • Chinese **Settings:** • Hospitals • Nursing homes • Geriatric clinics • Palliative care	• Clinically useful tool; unclear how score interpreted if some domains not scored • Substantial psychometric support and use in Europe • Limited information on psychometric qualities of English version • Training needs among diverse users not yet clarified • Most translated of nonverbal pain tools • Differences in tool performance (particularly psychosocial domain) may relate to cultural and/or institutional differences

Tool	Description	Validity	Reliability	Administration	Languages & Settings	Limitations
DS-DAT	• Nine items including noisy breathing, negative vocalizations, content facial expression, sad facial expression, frightened facial expression, frown, relaxed body language, tense body language, and fidgeting • Items measured for presence/absence, then for frequency, duration, and intensity during 5-minute observation period • Each item scored 0–3 with scoring range 0–27	• Content validity established in English, Italian, and Dutch • Evidence for discriminant validity moderately strong • Moderate convergent validity with pain tools • Construct validity: no consistency of model identified in confirmatory factor analysis in OA pain sample	• Good internal consistency • Moderately strong interrater reliability • Fair test-retest after 1 hour with independent raters • Strong intrarater reliability	• Complex administration and scoring • Potentially requires extensive training (30+ hours) • Time for completion reported 7–10 minutes	**Languages:** • English • Italian • Dutch **Settings:** • U.S. hospitals and nursing homes • Italian nursing homes • Dutch nursing homes	• Time for training and proper administration may be a barrier to use. • Construct validity issues and complex administration suggest tool refinement may be useful. • Preliminary support for use by clinical users
Elderly Pain Caring Assessment (EPCA-2)	• Eight items divided into two subscales: 1. Signs outside caregiving (facial expression, spontaneous posture adopted at rest, movement of patient out of bed and/or in bed, interaction of all kinds with other people) 2. Signs during caregiving (anxious anticipation of intervention, reactions during caregiver intervention, reactions of patient when painful part nursed, complaints voices in course of caregiving) • Each item scored on 5-point scale (0 = no pain to 4 = extremely intense pain) • Total score 0–20	• Tool developers bring strong evidence for good convergent and discriminant validity and responsiveness of EPCA-2. • Factor analysis confirmed two factors of rest and caregiving pain and explained 56% of variation in EPCA scores.	• Initial reliability tests are favorable. • Internal consistency established for global scale and for each subscale • Good interrater reliability	• Pilot study measured approximate time of 15 minutes to complete, including 5 minutes of observation before, 5 minutes after caregiving, and 5 minutes to score. • Manual explaining rating of each item and precautions for using EPCA2 in day-to-day practice is available from authors.	**Languages:** • French **Settings:** • French hospitals	• High convergent and discriminant validity and strong responsiveness of tool to treatment in preliminary testing • Purports to measure pain severity rather than presence of pain only • Time for proper administration may be a barrier to use. • Not validated in English-speaking populations or in long-term care settings; testing in other cultures and settings warranted

Continued

Part 3

Part 3

Table 11.5

Select Behavioral Pain Assessment Tools for Older Adults With Cognitive Impairment, Dementia, and Other Nonverbal Conditions —cont'd

Nonverbal Pain Behavior Scale	Description	Validity	Reliability	Feasibility and Clinical utility	Languages and Settings	Summary
Mahoney Pain Scale (MPS)	• Four items addressing facial expression, vocalizations, body language, and breathing changes rated on 0–3 scale of minimal pain to severe pain • Four items on agitated behavior, change in activities, physiological state, and current or history of painful conditions • Identifies location of physical pain problems on proxy pain maps • Total score 0–24	• Construct validity established with changes across activities and across groups in MPS score • Concurrent validity between nursing assistants' global pain ratings and nurses' score on MPS, although gold standard questionable	• Good interrater reliability during aversive activity for all tool items, except breathing • Sufficient internal consistency for pain severity items and fair for items differentiating pain and agitation	• Observation of 5 minutes required • Scoring overall is unclear with limited validation of item weighting • Initial study proposes general pain score cut-off of 4.5 for severity of pain and cut-off score on pain vs. agitation of 2.75	**Languages:** • English **Settings:** • Australian nursing homes	• Addresses common pain behaviors and also incorporates aspects of pain assessment beyond direct observation of behaviors • Requires knowledge of normal behavior to rate changes in behavior • Rating schema and assumptions about pain severity ratings need further validation. • Testing in other languages and settings needed
Mobilization-Observation-Behavior-Intensity-Dementia (MOBID and MOBID-2)	• 11-point NRS for three AGS behaviors • MOBID includes three items (pain noises, facial expression, and defense), rating each on pain intensity from 0–10 during guided movement • Includes overall pain intensity rating on 11-point NRS • MOBID-2 adds a second section that includes a body diagram and pain intensity rating of pain behavior related to head, internal organs, and/or skin	• Concurrent validity established with MOBID detecting increased pain with movement but did not connect number of pain behaviors with pain intensity among familiar caregivers • MOBID-2 demonstrates construct validity and concurrent validity associating score with other pain-related variables	• Good internal consistency among external raters • Wide range in interrater reliability for presence of pain behaviors but better interrater reliability for pain intensity • Variable test-retest reliability MOBID-2 • Sufficient internal consistency • Moderate to strong interrater reliability for pain intensity scores • Moderate to strong test-retest	• One to two hours training in reports, however, no information on time to administer/score • No information on scoring cutoff or interpretation • MOBID testing with clinical caregivers with 2 hours training, reported less than 5 minutes average to complete	**Languages:** • Norwegian **Settings:** • Norwegian nursing homes	• Evidence for use in research established and preliminary support for use by clinical users • Further evidence of validity of inferred pain intensity from behavior observation warranted • Testing in other cultures and settings warranted

Continued

Tool	Description	Psychometrics	Features	Languages/Settings	Comments
Non-Communicating Patient's Pain Assessment Instrument (NOPPAIN)	Nursing assistant administered instrument for observing and rating pain in patients with dementia. Four parts: 1. Self-report 2. Observed behavior response to daily activities (i.e., words, pain faces, noises, bracing, rubbing, restlessness) on 6-point Likert scale 3. Pain location 4. VDS pain thermometer for proxy report of global pain intensity	• Construct: specificity moderate to low, sensitivity moderate to strong • Convergent: strong when compared to self-report of presence/absence of pain; moderate when compared to self-report of pain intensity • Discriminant: positive correlations with anger, depression, and anxiety constructs	• Internal consistency: low • Interrater reliability: good to very good across all studies • Test-retest: moderate at 1 week on video sample • Effect size: very large in discriminating pain states vs. baseline	• Provides pictures and text for ease of understanding • Scoring and interpretation unclear, though cut-off of 4.5 for pain-no pain determined using ROC analysis in follow-up study • Reported rating time range: <30"–85.2" by direct care providers • Minimal training required **Languages:** • English • Italian (Ferrari et al., 2009) hospital setting • Brazilian Portuguese (Araujo & Pereira, 2012) translation only; no psychometrics to date **Settings:** • U.S. nursing home • Australian nursing home • Italian hospital	• Internal consistency and discriminant validity findings suggest need for further refinement of tool. • Clinical utility would be enhanced with scoring and interpretation guidelines.
Pain Assessment in the Cognitively Impaired (PACI)	Direct care provider-administered screening tool, seven items in three dimensions: 1. Facial expression (n = 3), verbalizations (n = 2), and body movements (n = 2) • Rate present or absent • Scoring range 0–7	• Construct, concurrent, and convergent validity supported • Able to differentiate between painful states during activity and at rest	• Internal consistency psychometrics are not available. • Moderate interrater reliability during both periods of activity and rest	• Scoring is clear (0–7) with 0 = no pain and 7 = high pain, but debate exists about use of scales to infer pain intensity. • Minimal training required • Definitions of behavioral terms provided **Languages:** • English only **Settings:** • Canadian nursing homes	• Further testing to assess sensitivity and specificity as well as responsiveness to treatment effects needed • Internal consistency data needed • Testing in other cultures and settings warranted
Pain Assessment Scale for Seniors with Severe Dementia (PACSLAC)	60 items in four dimensions: 1. Facial expression (n = 13), 2. Activity/body movements (n = 20), 3. Social/personality/mood (n = 12), 4. Physiological/eating/sleeping/vocal (n = 15) • Rate present or absent • Scoring range 0–60	• Construct, concurrent, and discriminant validity demonstrated • Ability to detect differences in levels of pain • Sensitive to treatment effects	• Good to very good internal consistency • Almost perfect agreement in interrater reliability testing • Interrater reliability strong for both caregivers and qualified nurses • Strong intrarater reliability	• Long list of items • Simple instructions • 5-minute estimated completion time • Preliminary cut-offs for pain presence suggested • Nurses and direct care providers report clinical usefulness. **Languages:** • English primary • French • Portuguese • Japanese • Dutch **Settings:** • Nursing homes	• Substantial psychometric support • Comprehensive in behavioral indicators. • Factor analysis in English-speaking samples with older adults in diverse settings is warranted. • Cultural background and perceptions may affect interpretation of behavioral indicators. • Larger, more diverse samples and settings needed to establish normative values

Table 11.5

Select Behavioral Pain Assessment Tools for Older Adults With Cognitive Impairment, Dementia, and Other Nonverbal Conditions —cont'd

Nonverbal Pain Behavior Scale	Description	Validity	Reliability	Feasibility and Clinical utility	Languages and Settings	Summary
PACSLAC-D	• Modified Dutch version of PACSLAC, direct observation scale with 24 items covering three subscales: facial and vocal expression (n = 10), resistance/defense (n = 6), and social-emotional aspects/mood (n = 8) • Rate present or absent • Scoring range 0–24	• Tool developed with factor analysis-guided refinement of original PACSLAC • Highly correlated with original PACSLAC • High degree of sensitivity and specificity using suggested cut-off scores	• Very good internal consistency for overall tool and subscales • Strong intrarater reliability for whole scale, moderate to strong for subscales	• Minimal training required (30 minutes) • Easy to use • Scoring instructions available to enhance interpretation	**Languages:** • Dutch only (translated to English, but no psychometrics to date) **Settings:** • Dutch nursing homes	• Further testing in larger English-speaking samples with increased diversity needed
PACSLAC 2	• Screening tool for both direct care providers and nurses • 31 dichotomously scored items in six pain behavior categories: facial expressions (n = 11), verbalizations (n = 5), body movements (n = 11), changes in interpersonal interactions (n = 2), changes in activity patterns (n = 1), and mental status changes (n = 1) • Scoring range 0–31	• Construct, convergent, and discriminant established. • Strong effect size • Accounts for unique variance even with contributions of all other tools, including PACSLAC	• Sufficient internal consistency • Moderate interrater reliability	• Clinical usefulness tested in Canadian nursing homes • Used by both direct care providers and nurses who report feasibility • Authors advise individualized scoring rather than population-based scoring.	**Languages:** • English **Settings:** • Canadian nursing homes	• Promising preliminary testing • Easy to use, brief tool • Further testing to establish sensitivity to detect treatment effects needed
Pain Assessment in Dementing Elders (PADE)	• 24 items, three parts: • Part I—13 distinct observed behaviors (rating intensity on semi-VDS scale); Part II—proxy assessment of global pain intensity; and Part III—chart review of 10 activities of daily living including dressing, feeding, and transfers from wheelchair to bed (using 4-point Likert scale rating)	• Construct validity: • As a whole, weakly differentiates between pain and no pain groups; improved differentiation with Part I only • Concurrent validity not yet established; moderate correlation with agitation scale (all parts) and moderate correlation with other pain scales (Part I only) • Discriminant validity supported (Part I only)	• Variable internal consistency range through several studies • Fair/moderate (Part II) to moderate/strong (Parts I, III) interrater reliability • Low/moderate (Part II) to moderate/high (Parts I/III) test-retest reliability	• Long list of items with complex format and different scaling approaches within tool • Authors report 5–10 minutes to complete with practice. • Administration instructions not clear • No score interpretation provided • Unknown training requirements	**Languages:** • English only **Settings:** • U.S. nursing homes	• Addresses common pain behaviors; also incorporates aspects of pain assessment beyond direct observation • Further validation needed if entire tool is to be used and/or refinement of those parts with low reliability • Feasibility and clinical utility issues remain.

Tool	Description	Reliability/Validity	Clinical Utility	Recommendations
The Pain Assessment in Advanced Dementia Scale (PAINAD)	• Five categorical items: breathing, negative vocalizations, facial expression, body language, and consolability • Scoring range 0–10 • 0–2 scale	• Sufficient internal consistency • Good to very good interrater reliability • Strong test-retest reliability • Convergent, concurrent validity established with other pain scales and self-report • Construct validity established with differences before and after pain interventions • Confirmatory factor analysis model with good fit identified only when item "breathing" was removed • Factor analysis explained variance of 61.09% of PAINAD scores in Portuguese version.	• Simple to use • Easy-to-follow definitions of terms provided • Scoring instructions provided • Cut-off of 3.5 for pain/no pain determined using ROC analysis • Time to complete 1–3 minutes • Limited training required • Tested in long-term care and acute care **Languages:** • English • German • Spanish • Dutch • Italian • Portuguese **Settings:** • Acute care nursing home	• "Breathing" item may need revision based on consistent problems across studies. • Reliability and validity established • Further study of tool sensitivity needed to address identification of false positives
Pain Assessment in Noncommunicative Elderly Persons (PAINE)	• Twenty-two items rated for the past week in three dimensions: repetitive physical movements, repetitive vocalizations, physical signs of pain, and changes in behaviors • Items are scored for frequency of occurrence on scale of 1 to 7. • Summary score includes mean of moaning and rigidity ratings and count based on all other variables.	• Sufficient internal consistency • Moderate interrater reliability • Test-retest sufficient after 1 week • Concurrent validity with moderate to good correlations with other informant ratings • Low correlations with self-report and observational measures • Sensitive to treatment effects	• Time to complete unknown • Scoring somewhat complex **Languages:** • English only **Settings:** • Nursing homes	• Preliminary data support need for further evaluation with larger samples • Clinical usefulness undetermined • Testing with direct care providers is needed.
Rotterdam Elderly Pain Observation Scale (REPOS)	• Ten-item tool dichotomously scored after 2-minute observation period • Items cover facial expression, emotional status, physical behavior, and vocalizations. • Scoring range 0 to 10 • Total score of 3 or higher indicative of persistent pain	• Moderate internal consistency • Strong interrater reliability • Moderate intrarater agreement • Construct validity established with good fit in one-dimensional multiple linear regression model • Convergent validity supported with one other pain scale • Observations made during movement • Sensitive to presence of pain in those with advanced dementia	• Easy to use and score • Decision-tree provided to assist with interpretation of score • Optimal cut-off score determined maintaining sufficient sensitivity and specificity • Encourages use of self-report in tandem with REPOS score **Languages:** • Dutch, translated to English **Settings:** • Nursing homes in the Netherlands	• Promising preliminary findings suggest validity, reliability, and clinical utility. • Larger samples in diverse settings and cultures warranted for confirming normative values • Further testing to establish sensitivity to detect treatment effects needed

2) Checklist of Nonverbal Pain Indicators (CNPI)
3) Pain Intensity Measure for Persons with Dementia (PIMD)
4) Algoplus Scale (Algoplus)
5) CPAT (Certified Nurse Assistant Pain Assessment Tool)
6) Discomfort Scale-Dementia of the Alzheimer's Type (DS-DAT)
7) Elderly Pain Caring Assessment (EPCA-2)
8) Mahoney Pain Scale (MPS)
9) Non-Communicating Patient's Pain Assessment Instrument (NOPPAIN)
10) Pain Assessment in the Cognitively Impaired (PACI)
11) Pain Assessment for the Dementing Elderly (PADE)
12) Pain Assessment in Noncommunicative Elderly Persons (PAINE)
13) Rotterdam Elderly Pain Observation Scale (REPOS)
14) Pain Behaviors for Osteoarthritis Instrument for Cognitively Impaired Elders (PBOICIE)

E. Considerations for diverse race, ethnic, and cultural groups
1. Use validated tools available in various languages as appropriate to patient populations/nationalities. If tool is not translated into patient's preferred language, use approved interpreter or interpreter service to assess pain.
2. Some cultures may not have a word equivalent for "pain," or colors on pain scales may have differential meanings than Western connotations.
3. Preferences for tools may vary by race, ethnicity, or culture. For example, older African Americans may prefer DVPRS, IPT-R, or NRS, while Chinese adults may prefer FPS-R and NRS.
4. Cultural expression may influence types and severity of behaviors observed. More research is needed to understand cultural differences in behavior of older adults with dementia.

V. Tools for Adult Populations with Persistent Pain

A. Multidimensional tools assess pain intensity, mood, interference, quality of life, and nature of pain.
1. Application:
   a. May need to evaluate health literacy prior to administering scale
   b. Determine need for provider to administer scale or if scale can be self-completed.
   c. Clearly explain each subscale and how to rate each question.

2. Advantages:
   a. Evaluates complexity of pain experience by assessing sensory, affective, evaluative, and motivational dimensions of pain
   b. Allows for more complete descriptions of pain
   c. Fosters assessment of characteristics and impact of nociceptive, neuropathic, nociplastic, and mixed pain types
3. Disadvantages: may take more time to complete and patients in pain may lack concentration needed to complete long questionnaires
4. Commonly used multidimensional tools for persistent pain:
   a. McGill Pain Questionnaire (MPQ)
      1) Valid and reliable tool used to evaluate effectiveness of pain interventions and identify pain qualities associated with distinct nociceptive and neuropathic pain disorders
      2) Longer version (LF-MPQ) has been translated into more than 25 languages and is widely used.
      3) May be helpful in older adults who have multimorbidity
      4) LF-MPQ consists of 78 items divided into three major subscales evaluating sensory, affective, and evaluative aspects of pain on a 5-point pain intensity scale.
      5) Disadvantages are patients need rich vocabulary to complete and LF-MPQ takes up to 30 minutes to complete. Patients may need assistance with completion.
   b. Shortened version, McGill Pain Questionnaire (SF-MPQ)
      1) Comprised of 15 words with 2 subscales of pain intensity and affect. Includes a body diagram to identify locations of pain.
      2) SF-MPQ takes only 2 to 5 minutes to complete.
      3) Ensure intensity ranking of mild, moderate, or severe is clearly understood by patients.
   c. Graded Chronic Pain Scale (GCPS)
      1) Assesses two dimensions—pain intensity and pain-related disability—by measuring impact of persistent pain on daily, social, and work activities over time
      2) May be used for persistent musculoskeletal conditions, low back pain, and other persistent pain disorders
      3) Easy to use but scoring is complex
      4) Less useful for assessment of pain at point of care; used widely in research.
      5) Can be used as a measure of *high-impact persistent pain*

d. Short Form-36 Bodily Pain (SF-36 Bodily Pain)
   1) One of eight subscales of Medical Outcomes Study Short Form-36 questionnaire
   2) Subscale assesses bodily pain intensity and interference of pain with normal activities.
   3) Translated and used in more than 50 countries
   4) Easy to administer and complete
   5) Useful in making comparisons across populations for research and quality improvement purposes

e. West Haven-Yale Multidimensional Pain Inventory (WHY-MPI)
   1) Available at no charge; paper-and-pencil tool that assesses cognitive, emotional, and behavioral factors associated with experience of pain
   2) Fifty-two items across twelve subscales and three overall domains:
      a) Pain experience
      b) Responses of others to communicated pain
      c) Participation in daily activities
   3) Each item is rated 0 to 6, and higher scores indicate greater intensity in that subscale.
   4) Advantages:
      a) Available in several languages: English, Spanish, German, Dutch, Swedish, Turkish, and Chinese
      b) Comprehension; can be used by adults 18 years of age and older
   5) Disadvantage: takes 15 to 30 minutes to complete; must have cognitive and intellectual ability to complete

B. Condition-specific tools
   1. Numerous tools developed to assess pain in specific health conditions, such as neuropathy and persistent low back pain
   2. Application: Tools can be self-administered or completed with provider depending on complexity of tool and type of information elicited.
   3. Advantages:
      a. Assesses qualities of pain specific to pain condition; allows for greater symptom phenotyping of condition
      b. Can be used to assess changes in disease-symptom trajectory
   4. Disadvantages:
      a. May focus too narrowly on condition and may fail to ask about other general pain characteristics
      b. Some may lack diagnostic sensitivity.
   5. Examples of condition-specific tools:
      a. Self-Administered Leeds Assessment of Neuropathic Symptoms and Signs (S-LANSS) is a self-administered seven-item screening tool to identify pain of neuropathic origin.
      b. painDETECT
         1) Screens for neuropathic symptoms in people with persistent low back pain, various types of arthritis, and fibromyalgia
         2) Simple, patient-reported outcome tool that can determine prevalence of neuropathic pain
      c. Neuropathic Pain Scale
         1) Eleven item scale (using 0 to 10 rating scales) measures intensity of ten pain qualities described by patients with neuropathic pain, including global dimensions of pain intensity, pain unpleasantness, and fluctuation of pain (constant with intermittent increases, intermittent, constant with fluctuation)
         2) Higher scores indicate greater certainty of neuropathic pain mechanisms. However, not all types of neuropathic pain are covered in the 11 items. Further validation is warranted.

Bibliography

Ahn, H., & Horgas, A. (2013). The relationship between pain and disruptive behaviors in nursing home residents with dementia. *BMC Geriatrics, 13,* 14. https://doi.org/10.1186/1471-2318-13-14.

American Academy of Pediatric Dentistry. (2020). Pain management in infants, children, adolescents, and individuals with special health care needs. In *The Reference Manual of Pediatric Dentistry* (pp. 362–370). Chicago: American Academy of Pediatric Dentistry.

American Academy of Pediatrics. Committee on Psychosocial Aspects of Child and Family Health, & Task Force on Pain in Infants, Children, and Adolescents. (2001). The assessment and management of acute pain in infants, children, and adolescents. *Pediatrics, 108*(3), 793–797. https://doi.org/10.1542/peds.108.3.793.

American Nurses Association (ANA) and American Society for Pain Management Nursing (ASPMN). (2016). *Pain Management Nursing: Scope and Standards of Practice* (2nd Ed). Owen Mills, MA: American Nurses Association.

Beyer, J. E., Denyes, M. J., & Villarruel, A. M. (1992). The creation, validation, and continuing development of the Oucher: a measure of pain intensity in children. *Journal of Pediatric Nursing, 7*(5), 335–346.

Beltramini, A., Milojevic, K., & Pateron, D. (2017). Pain assessment in newborns, infants, and children. *Pediatric Annals, 46,* e387–e395. https://dx.doi.org/10.3928/19382359-20170921-03.

Bieri, D., Reeve, R. A., Champion, D. G., Addicoat, L., & Ziegler, J. B. (1990). The faces pain scale for the self-assessment of the severity of pain experienced by children: development, initial validation, and preliminary investigation for ratio scale properties. *Pain, 41*(2), 139–150. https://doi.org/10.1016/0304-3959(90)90018-9.

Blozik, E., Stuck, A. E., Niemann, S., Ferrell, B. A., Harari, D., von Renteln-Kruse, W., Gillmann, G., Beck, J. C., & Clough-Gorr, K. M.

(2007). Geriatric pain measure short form: development and initial evaluation. *Journal of the American Geriatrics Society, 55*(12), 2045–2050. https://doi.org/10.1111/j.1532-5415.2007.01474.x.

Breau, L. M., McGrath, P. J., Camfield, C. S., & Finley, G. A. (2002). Psychometric properties of the non-communicating children's pain checklist-revised. *Pain, 99*(1-2), 349–357. https://doi.org/10.1016/s0304-3959(02)00179-3.

Breau, L. M., McGrath, P. J., Craig, K. D., Santor, D., Cassidy, K. L., & Reid, G. J. (2001). Facial expression of children receiving immunizations: a principal components analysis of the child facial coding system. *Clinical Journal of Pain, 17*(2), 178–186. https://doi.org/10.1097/00002508-200106000-00011.

Breau, L. M., Camfield, C., & Camfield, P. (2010). Development and Initial Validation of the Batten's Observational Pain Scale: A preliminary study. *Journal of Pain Management, 3*, 283–292.

Büttner, W., Finke, W., Hilleke, M., Reckert, S., Vsianska, L., & Brambrink, A. (1998). Entwicklung eines Fremdbeobachtungsbogens zur Beurteilung des postoperativen Schmerzes bei Säuglingen [Development of an observational scale for assessment of postoperative pain in infants]. *Anasthesiologie, Intensivmedizin, Notfallmedizin, Schmerztherapie: AINS, 33*(6), 353–361. https://doi.org/10.1055/s-2007-994263.

Büttner, W., & Finke, W. (2000). Analysis of behavioural and physiological parameters for the assessment of postoperative analgesic demand in newborns, infants and young children: a comprehensive report on seven consecutive studies. *Paediatric Anaesthesia, 10*(3), 303–318. https://doi.org/10.1046/j.1460-9592.2000.00530.x.

Chambers, C. T., Finley, G. A., McGrath, P. J., & Walsh, T. M. (2003). The Parents' Postoperative Pain Measure: Replication and Extension to 2- to 6-Year Old Children. *Pain, 105*(3), 437–443. https://doi.org/10.1016/S0304-3959(03)00256-2.

Chan, S., Hadjistavropoulos, T., Williams, J., & Lints-Martindale, A. (2014). Evidence-based development and initial validation of the pain assessment checklist for seniors with limited ability to communicate-II (PACSLAC-II). *Clinical Journal of Pain, 30*(9), 816–824. https://doi.org/10.1097/AJP.0000000000000039.

Collignon, P., & Giusiano, B. (2001). Validation of a pain evaluation scale for patients with severe cerebral palsy. *European Journal of Pain, 5*(4), 433–442. https://doi.org/10.1053/eujp.2001.0265.

Committee on Fetus and Newborn and Section on Anesthesiology and Pain Medicine (2016). Prevention and Management of Procedural Pain in the Neonate: An Update. Pediatrics, 137(2), e20154271. https://doi.org/10.1542/peds.2015-4271.

Eccleston, C., Jordan, A., McCracken, L. M., Sleed, M., Connell, H., & Clinch, J. (2005). The Bath Adolescent Pain Questionnaire (BAPQ): development and preliminary psychometric evaluation of an instrument to assess the impact of chronic pain on adolescents. *Pain, 118*(1-2), 263–270. https://doi.org/10.1016/j.pain.2005.08.025.

Eccleston, C., McCracken, L. M., Jordan, A., & Sleed, M. (2007). Development and preliminary psychometric evaluation of the parent report version of the Bath Adolescent Pain Questionnaire (BAPQ-P): A multidimensional parent report instrument to assess the impact of chronic pain on adolescents. *Pain, 131*(1-2), 48–56. https://doi.org/10.1016/j.pain.2006.12.010.

Eland, J. A., & Banner, W. (1999). Analgesia, sedation and neuromuscular blockage in pediatric critical care. In Hazinski, M. F. (Ed.), *Manual of pediatric critical care*. St. Louis: Mosby.

Fleegler, E. W., & Schecter, N. L. (2015). Pain and prejudice. *JAMA Pediatrics, 169*(11), 991–993. https://doi.org/10.1001/jamapediatrics.2015.2284.

Gélinas, C. (2010). Nurses' evaluations of the feasibility and the clinical utility of the Critical-Care Pain Observation Tool. *Pain Management Nursing, 11*(2), 115–125. https://doi.org/10.1016/j.pmn.2009.05.002.

Goyal, M. K., Kuppermann, N., Cleary, S. D., Teach, S. J., & Chamberlain, J. M. (2015). Racial Disparities in Pain Management of Children With Appendicitis in Emergency Departments. *JAMA Pediatrics, 169*(11), 996–1002. https://doi.org/10.1001/jamapediatrics.2015.1915.

Hand, I., Noble, L., Geiss, D., Wozniak, L., & Hall, C. (2010). COVERS Neonatal Pain Scale: Development and validation. *International Journal of Pediatrics.* https://doi.org/10.1155/2010/496719.

Herr, K., Coyne, P. J., Ely, E., Gélinas, C., & Manworren, R. (2019). ASPMN 2019 Position Statement: Pain assessment in the patient unable to self-report. *Pain Management Nursing, 20*(5), 402–403. https://doi.org/10.1016/j.pmn.2019.07.007.

Herr, K., Sefcik, J. S., Neradilek, M. B., Hilgeman, M. M., Nash, P., & Ersek, M. (2019). Psychometric evaluation of the MOBID Dementia Pain Scale in US nursing homes. *Pain Management Nursing, 20*(3), 253–260. https://doi.org/10.1016/j.pmn.2018.11.062.

Hester, N. O., Foster, R. L., Jordan-Marsh, M., Ely, E., Vojir, C. P., & Milller, K. L. (1998). Putting pain measurement into clinical practice. In Finley, G. A., & McGrath, P. J. (Eds.), *Measurement of pain in infants and children: Vol. 10.* Seattle: International Association for the Study of Pain Stress.

Hicks, C. L., von Baeyer, C. L., Spafford, P. A., van Korlaar, I., & Goodenough, B. (2001). The Faces Pain Scale-Revised: toward a common metric in pediatric pain measurement. *Pain, 93*(2), 173–183. https://doi.org/10.1016/S0304-3959(01)00314-1.

Horgas, A. L. (2017). Pain assessment in older adults. *The Nursing Clinics of North America, 52*(3), 375–385. https://doi.org/10.1016/j.cnur.2017.04.006.

Hummel, P., Puchalski, M., Creech, S. D., & Weiss, M. G. (2008). Clinical reliability and validity of the N-PASS: neonatal pain, agitation and sedation scale with prolonged pain. *Journal of Perinatology, 28*(1), 55–60. https://doi.org/10.1038/sj.jp.7211861.

Husebo, B. S. (2017). Mobilization-Observation-Behaviour-Intensity-Dementia-2 Pain Scale (MOBID-2). *Journal of Physiotherapy, 63*(4), 261. https://doi.org/10.1016/j.jphys.2017.07.003.

Husebo, B. S., Ostelo, R., & Strand, L. I. (2014). The MOBID-2 pain scale: Reliability and responsiveness to pain in patients with dementia. *European Journal of Pain, 18*(10), 1419–1430. https://doi.org/10.1002/ejp.507.

Husebo, B. S., Strand, L. I., Moe-Nilssen, R., Husebo, S. B., & Ljunggren, A. E. (2010). Pain in older persons with severe dementia. Psychometric properties of the Mobilization-Observation-Behaviour-Intensity-Dementia (MOBID-2) Pain Scale in a clinical setting. *Scandinavian Journal of Caring Sciences, 24*(2), 380–391. https://doi.org/10.1111/j.1471-6712.2009.00710.x.

Jensen, M. P., & Karoly, P. (2011). Self-report scales and procedures for assessing pain in adults. In Turk, D. C., & Melzack, R. (Eds.), *Handbook of pain assessment* (pp. 19–44). New York: The Guilford Press.

Jordan-Marsh, M., Yoder, L., Hall, D., & Watson, R. (1994). Alternate Oucher form testing: gender, ethnicity, and age variations. *Research in Nursing & Health, 17*(2), 111–118. https://doi.org/10.1002/nur.4770170206.

Kaczynski, K., Ely, E., Gordon, D., Vincent, C., Waddell, K., Wittmayer, K., & Bernhofer, E. (2020). The Pediatric American Pain Society Patient Outcomes Questionnaire (Pediatric

APS-POQ): Development and Initial Psychometric Evaluation of a Brief and Comprehensive Measure of Pain and Pain Outcomes in Hospitalized Youth. *Journal of Pain, 21*(5-6), 633–647. https://doi.org/10.1016/j.jpain.2019.10.003.

Krechel, S. W., & Bildner, J. (1995). CRIES: a new neonatal postoperative pain measurement score. Initial testing of validity and reliability. *Paediatric Anaesthesia, 5*(1), 53–61. https://doi.org/10.1111/j.1460-9592.1995.tb00242.x.

Kunz, M., de Waal, M., Achterberg, W. P., Gimenez-Llort, L., Lobbezoo, F., Sampson, E. L., van Dalen-Kok, A. H., Defrin, R., Invitto, S., Konstantinovic, L., Oosterman, J., Petrini, L., van der Steen, J. T., Strand, L. I., de Tommaso, M., Zwakhalen, S., Husebo, B. S., & Lautenbacher, S. (2020). The Pain Assessment in Impaired Cognition scale (PAIC15): A multidisciplinary and international approach to develop and test a meta-tool for pain assessment in impaired cognition, especially dementia. *European Journal of Pain, 24*(1), 192–208. https://doi.org/10.1002/ejp.1477.

Kuttner, L., & LePage, T. (1989). Faces scales for the assessment of pediatric page: A critical review. *Canadian Journal of Behavioral Science, 21*, 198–209.

Lalloo, C., & Stinson, J. N. (2014). Assessment and treatment of pain in children and adolescents. Best practice & research. *Clinical Rheumatology, 28*(2), 315–330. https://doi.org/10.1016/j.berh.2014.05.003.

Lawrence, J., Alcock, D., McGrath, P., Kay, J., MacMurray, S. B., & Dulberg, C. (1993). The development of a tool to assess neonatal pain. *Neonatal Network, 12*(6), 59–66.

Li, L., Herr, K., & Chen, P. (2009). Postoperative pain assessment with three intensity scales in Chinese elders. *Journal of Nursing Scholarship, 41*(3), 241–249. https://doi.org/10.1111/j.1547-5069.2009.01280.x.

Li, L., Liu, X., & Herr, K. (2007). Postoperative pain intensity assessment: a comparison of four scales in Chinese adults. *Pain Medicine, 8*(3), 223–234. https://doi.org/10.1111/j.1526-4637.2007.00296.x.

Malviya, S., Voepel-Lewis, T., Burke, C., Merkel, S., & Tait, A. R. (2006). The revised FLACC observational pain tool: improved reliability and validity for pain assessment in children with cognitive impairment. *Paediatric Anaesthesia, 16*(3), 258–265. https://doi.org/10.1111/j.1460-9592.2005.01773.x.

McGrath, P. J., Johnson, G., Goodman, J. T., et al. (1985). CHEOPS: A behavioral scale for rating postoperative pain in children. In Fields, H.L., Dubner, R., & Cervero, F. (Eds.), *Advances in pain research and therapy*, Vol. 9 (pp. 395–402). New York: Raven Press.

McGrath, P., de Veber, L., & Hearn, M. (1985). Multidimensional pain assessment in children. In Fields, H., Dubner, R., & Cervero, F. (Eds.), *Advances in pain research and therapy*, vol. 9. New York: Raven Press.

Merkel, S. I., Voepel-Lewis, T., Shayevitz, J. R., & Malviya, S. (1997). The FLACC: a behavioral scale for scoring postoperative pain in young children. *Pediatric Nursing, 23*(3), 293–297.

Myrvik, M. P., Drendel, A. L., Brandow, A. M., Yan, K., Hoffmann, R. G., & Panepinto, J. A. (2015). A Comparison of Pain Assessment Measures in Pediatric Sickle Cell Disease: Visual Analog Scale Versus Numeric Rating Scale. *Journal of Pediatric Hematology/Oncology, 37*(3), 190–194. https://doi.org/10.1097/MPH.0000000000000306.

Ruest, M., Bourque, M., Laroche, S., Harvey, M. P., Martel, M., Bergeron-Vézina, K., Apinis, C., Proulx, D., Hadjistavropoulos, T., Tousignant-Laflamme, Y., & Léonard, G. (2017). Can We Quickly and Thoroughly Assess Pain with the PACSLAC-II? A Convergent Validity Study in Long-Term Care Residents Suffering from Dementia. *Pain Management Nursing, 18*(6), 410–417. https://doi.org/10.1016/j.pmn.2017.05.009.

Ruskin, D., Lalloo, C., Amaria, K., Stinson, J. N., Kewley, E., Campbell, F., Brown, S. C., Jeavons, M., & McGrath, P. A. (2014). Assessing pain intensity in children with chronic pain: convergent and discriminant validity of the 0–10 numerical rating scale in clinical practice. *Pain Research & Management, 19*(3), 141–148. https://doi.org/10.1155/2014/856513.

Schade, J. G., Joyce, B. A., Gerkensmeyer, J., & Keck, J. F. (1996). Comparison of three preverbal scales for postoperative pain assessment in a diverse pediatric sample. *Journal of Pain and Symptom Management, 12*(6), 348–359. https://doi.org/10.1016/s0885-3924(96)00182-0.

Schultz, A. A., Murphy, E., Morton, J., Stempel, A., Messenger-Rioux, C., & Bennett, K. (1999). Preverbal, Early Verbal Pediatric Pain Scale (PEPPS): development and early psychometric testing. *Journal of Pediatric Nursing, 14*(1), 19–27. https://doi.org/10.1016/S0882-5963(99)80056-6.

Solodiuk, J., & Curley, M. A. (2003). Pain assessment in nonverbal children with severe cognitive impairments: the Individualized Numeric Rating Scale (INRS). *Journal of Pediatric Nursing, 18*(4), 295–299. https://doi.org/10.1016/s0882-5963(03)00090-3.

Stevens, B. (1990). Development and testing of a pediatric pain management sheet. *Pediatric Nursing, 16*(6), 543–548.

Schuler, M. S., Becker, S., Kaspar, R., Nikolaus, T., Kruse, A., & Basler, H. D. (2007). Psychometric properties of the German "Pain Assessment in Advanced Dementia Scale" (PAINAD-G) in nursing home residents. *Journal of the American Medical Directors Association, 8*(6), 388–395. https://doi.org/10.1016/j.jamda.2007.03.002.

Stevens, B. J., Harrison, D., Rashotte, J., Yamada, J., Abbott, L. K., Coburn, G., Stinson, J., & Le May, S. CIHR Team in Children's Pain. (2012). Pain assessment and intensity in hospitalized children in Canada. *Journal of Pain, 13*(9), 857–865. https://doi.org/10.1016/j.jpain.2012.05.010.

Tarbell, S. E., Cohen, T. I., & Marsh, J. L. (1992). The Toddler-Preschooler Postoperative Pain Scale: an observational scale for measuring postoperative pain in children aged 1-5. Preliminary report. *Pain, 50*(3), 273–280. https://doi.org/10.1016/0304-3959(92)90031-6.

Topham, D., & Drew, D. (2017). Quality Improvement Project: Replacing the Numeric Rating Scale with a Clinically Aligned Pain Assessment (CAPA) Tool. *Pain Management Nursing: Official Journal of the American Society of Pain Management Nurses, 18*(6), 363–371. https://doi.org/10.1016/j.pmn.2017.07.001.

Tsze, D. S., von Baeyer, C. L., Pahalyants, V., & Dayan, P. S. (2018). Validity and reliability of the verbal numerical rating scale for children aged 4–17 years with acute pain. *Annals of Emergency Medicine, 71*(6), 691–702. e3. https://doi.org/10.1016/j.annemergmed.2017.09.009.

Tomlinson, D., von Baeyer, C. L., Stinson, J. N., & Sung, L. (2010). A systematic review of faces scales for the self-report of pain intensity in children. *Pediatrics, 126*(5), e1168–e1198. https://doi.org/10.1542/peds.2010-1609.

van Dijk, M., Peters, J.W., van Deventer, P., & Tibboel, D. (2005). The COMFORT Behavior Scale: a tool for assessing pain and sedation in infants. *American Journal of Nursing, 105*(1), 33–36. https://doi.org/10.1097/00000446-200501000-00019. PMID: 15659992.

Part 3

Varni, J. W., Thompson, K. L., & Hanson, V. (1987). The Varni/Thompson Pediatric Pain Questionnaire. I. Chronic musculoskeletal pain in juvenile rheumatoid arthritis. *Pain, 28*(1), 27–38. https://doi.org/10.1016/0304-3959(87)91056-6.

Villarruel, A. M., & Denyes, M. J. (1991). Pain assessment in children: theoretical and empirical validity. *Advances in Nursing Science, 14*(2), 32–41. https://doi.org/10.1097/00012272-199112000-00005.

Voepel-Lewis, T., Burke, C. N., Jeffreys, N., Malviya, S., & Tait, A. R. (2011). Do 0-10 numeric rating scores translate into clinically meaningful pain measures for children? *Anesthesia and Analgesia, 112*(2), 415–421. https://doi.org/10.1213/ANE.0b013e318203f495.

Warden, V., Hurley, A. C., & Volicer, L. (2003). Development and psychometric evaluation of the Pain Assessment in Advanced Dementia (PAINAD) scale. *Journal of the American Medical Directors Association, 4*(1), 9–15. https://doi.org/10.1097/01.JAM.0000043422.31640.F7.

Ware, L. J., Herr, K., Booker, S. S., Dotson, K., Key, J., Poindexter, N., Pyles, G., Siler, B., & Packard, A. (2015). Psychometric evaluation of the Revised Iowa Pain Thermometer (IPT-R) in a sample of diverse cognitively intact and impaired older adults: A pilot study. *Pain Management Nursing, 16*(4), 475–482. https://doi.org/10.1016/j.pmn.2014.09.004..

Wong, D. L., & Baker, C. M. (1988). Pain in children: comparison of assessment scales. *Pediatric Nursing, 14*(1), 9–17.

Wong, D., & Baker, C. (1999). *Reference manual for the Wong-Baker Faces Rating Scale*. Tulsa, OK: Wong & Baker.

Online Resources

The University of Iowa. Geriatric Pain. (http://www.geriatricpain.org).

#SeePainMoreClearly. https://www.seepainmoreclearly.org/.

SickKids. Pain Management, Research and Education Centre. https://www.sickkids.ca/en/care-services/centres/pain-centre/.

CHAPTER 12

Risk Assessments Related to Pain Management

Theresa J. Di Maggio, MSN, CRNP, PPCNP-BC
Ann Quinlan-Colwell, PhD, MSN
Danielle Dunwoody, BSc, BScN, MS, PhD
Ann Schreier, PhD, BSN, MSN, RN*

Introduction

This chapter describes the concept of risk and the relationship risk has to patient, treatment, and environmental factors. Selection and use of appropriate risk assessment instruments for both adults and children will be described, as well as measures to reduce risk while providing pain management.

I. Risk in Relation to Patient–Treatment–Clinician–Organization

A. Numerous definitions and connotations for "risk" exist. In this chapter, the operational definition for risk is a threat, uncertainty, source of vulnerability or potential for an adverse effect or event.

B. Risk to patient safety can occur as a result of many factors involving patients, treatments, clinicians, and organizations.
1. Across the healthcare spectrum, patients require medications to control pain.
2. Patient safety with risk minimization is paramount to quality pain management nursing. A comprehensive risk assessment should be completed prior to implementing plan of care.
3. Ongoing assessment and appropriate monitoring are essential to providing safe care.

C. Because a primary goal of healthcare personnel and organizations is to minimize risk and optimize patient safety, concepts are closely intertwined among patients, clinicians, and organizations.

*Section Editor for the chapter.

II. Risk Factors Associated With Pain Management

A. Patient-related factors
1. Age
    a. Important risk factor, particularly for those at either end of age spectrum (i.e., pediatrics, geriatrics)
    b. Physical age may affect pharmacokinetics of medications. Distribution, absorption, metabolism, and elimination of medications may be slower in older adults and are variable in children.
    c. Cognitive limitations may range from limited healthcare literacy (understanding healthcare information) to an inability to communicate fully (verbally or nonverbally).
2. Sleep-disordered breathing, such as obstructive sleep apnea (OSA) and patients who score greater than 3 out of 8 on STOP-BANG Questionnaire (Fig. 12.1), are at increased risk for opioid-induced advancing sedation (OIAS) and opioid-induced respiratory depression (OIRD).
3. Weight considerations
    a. Obesity increases risk for adverse events.
    b. Obesity hyperventilation syndrome (OHS), similar to OSA, is highly associated with opioid-induced adverse effects, including OIAS and OIRD (see Box 12.1 for OHS criteria).
    c. Dosing of lipophilic and protein-bound medications needs to be adjusted for patients who are significantly underweight, obese, morbidly obese, or malnourished (see chapter 17 for more information).

STOP-Bang questionnaire

Yes / No		
☐ Yes	☐ No	**Snoring?**
		Do you **snore loudly** (loud enough to be heard through closed doors, or your bed partner elbows you for snoring at night)?
☐ Yes	☐ No	**Tired?**
		Do you often feel **tired, fatigued, or sleepy** during the daytime (such as falling asleep during driving)?
☐ Yes	☐ No	**Observed?**
		Has anyone **observed** you **stop breathing** or **choking/gasping** during your sleep?
☐ Yes	☐ No	**Pressure?**
		Do you have or are you being treated for **high blood pressure**?
☐ Yes	☐ No	**Body mass index more than 35 kg/m²?**
☐ Yes	☐ No	**Age older than 50 years old?**
☐ Yes	☐ No	**Neck size large? (measured around Adam's apple)**
		For male, is your shirt collar 17 inches or larger?
		For female, is your shirt collar 16 inches or larger?
☐ Yes	☐ No	**Gender = Male?**
Scoring criteria:		
Low risk of OSA: Yes to 0 to 2 questions		
Intermediate risk of OSA: Yes to 3 to 4 questions		
High risk of OSA: Yes to 5 to 8 questions		

OSA: obstructive sleep apnea

Figure 12.1 STOP–BANG questionnaire. (Used with permission from Dr. Frances Chung and UHN, http://www.stopbang.ca.)

Box 12.1

Obesity Hyperventilation Syndrome

Criteria for Obesity Hyperventilation Syndrome
- Body mass index (BMI) $\geq$30 kg/m²
- Hypoxemia (SpO$_2$ <90%) during sleep
- Hypercapnia during the day

---

4. Comorbidities
   a. Renal compromise, hepatic failure, and respiratory and cardiac conditions need to be considered when determining safe medication prescribing and administration.
   b. American Society of Anesthesiology (ASA) classification system is based on stratifying patient risk based on comorbidities. Greater ASA scores increase risk for OIAS and OIRD.
   c. Similar to age, comorbidities may affect medication pharmacokinetics.
   d. Many mental health conditions can increase risks associated with pain management (see chapters 3 and 16 for more information).
5. Medications and supplements
   a. Create nonjudgmental environment to facilitate patient accurately sharing information about which products they use.
   b. Identify prescribed medications; over-the-counter (OTC) products; supplements; vitamins; and herbal, botanical, and natural products.
   c. Interactions with analgesics, other medications, botanicals, and food products may cause synergistic or untoward effects.

   d. Substance use or misuse, including tobacco, alcohol, antidepressants, cannabis, opioids, benzodiazepines, or illicit substances, increases risk for adverse events, particularly sedation and OIRD.
6. Genetic considerations
   a. Polymorphisms (particularly cytochrome P450 2D6 [CYP2D6]) are increasingly being researched in relation to pain.
   b. Genetics (specifically OPRM1 gene) may impact opioid doses required, risks, and potential for substance use disorder (SUD).
7. Past experiences with analgesics or procedural sedation
   a. Identify history of allergic reactions to medications and respiratory difficulties or adverse events related to sedation.
   b. Patients with a history of negative experiences may be at increased risk for recurrence.
8. Comfort expectations
   a. Unrealistic comfort expectations can create risk (e.g., higher doses, use of multiple medications, allowing patients to remain inactive) and failure to adhere to plan of care: pharmacological and nonpharmacological regimens.
   b. Discuss reasonable and safe expectations for pain control from functional perspective when developing an individualized pain management plan, regardless of source of pain.
      1) Consider preexisting functional limitations to ensure goals are reasonable and achievable.
      2) Identify baseline pain levels. It is not reasonable for patient with 9 of 10 baseline pain to

have pain goal of 0 out of 10. Amount of medication required to do this would likely be unsafe. Also, inform and remind patients that numeric pain ratings are only one tool used to measure pain and comfort.
3) Helping patients and families to set realistic goals may decrease anger, fear, and anxiety that "something went wrong." As anger and fear can impact pain, realistic expectations may improve comfort (see chapter 13 for discussion of anger and fear).
9. Culture, language and socioeconomic status (SES)
   a. Both culture and SES can influence how each person manages pain, expectations, and proposed plan of care.
   b. Be aware of potential for implicit biases that can skew medical decisions and be barriers to effective treatment.
   c. Language barriers between patients, families, and healthcare team may cause or increase risk.
      1) Language barriers increase risk to not understand or be misunderstood (e.g., the same word in different languages can have different meanings; cultural nuances can lead to incorrect understanding and error).
      2) Medical interpreters are imperative, as terminology of different cultures and languages does not always correspond to medical terminology.
   d. Health literacy
      1) "Personal health literacy is the degree to which individuals have the ability to find, understand, and use information and services to inform health-related decisions and actions for themselves and others" (National Institutes of Health, *Health Literacy*, 2021). Such understanding is not related to intelligence or education.
      2) Anyone is at risk for not understanding healthcare concepts; adverse events and unintended consequences may occur when information is not understood correctly.
      3) Nurses and other clinicians are responsible for assessing person's cognitive function and ensuring concepts are communicated adequately and are understood by patient.
      4) Children are at particular risk for inadequate education. Communication must be adjusted to person's developmental level, knowledge base, and ability to understand healthcare information.
      5) People (adults and children) with developmental delays are at risk for receiving information based on chronological age that is not customized to their cognitive and emotional level.

a) Increased vigilance is needed when developing care plans for this population.
b) Family or support system should be included during educational sessions.
B. Treatment-related factors
1. Any treatment has potential to contribute to an adverse event or untoward effect.
2. Components of surgery (e.g., anesthetic type, surgical site, time in operating room) affect risk.
   a. General anesthesia is associated with higher risk for untoward effects compared to regional anesthesia.
   b. Greater risk for OIAS and OIRD is present during first 12 to 24 postoperative hours.
3. Select medication classes pose increased risk
   a. Acetaminophen
      1) Generally safe when taken in therapeutic doses
      2) Sometimes prescribed in combination with other medications; important to consider amount of acetaminophen from all sources in 24-hour time period and educate patients accordingly
      3) Acetaminophen is metabolized and converted into hepatotoxic metabolite (*N*-acetyl-*p*-benzoquinone imine) that can cause liver damage when taken in excessive doses or when ingested with alcohol.
   b. Nonsteroidal anti-inflammatory drugs (NSAIDs)
      1) Use limited by serious adverse effects, including gastrointestinal bleeding, gastric ulceration, renal toxicity, platelet aggregation inhibition, and cardiac events
      2) Listed in American Geriatrics Society (AGS) Beers Criteria as medication to be limited or avoided with older adults
      3) Considered teratogenic when taken during pregnancy and when taken late in pregnancy; have been associated with premature closure of ductus arteriosus
   c. Opioids
      1) Pure *mu*-agonist opioids (e.g., morphine, fentanyl, hydromorphone) pose increased risk of central nervous system (CNS) depression, OIAS, and OIRD.
      2) Pharmacokinetics (movement of medication in body) and pharmacodynamics (medication's power, action, or effect) vary by route (see chapter 17).
      3) Dosing and administering opioids based solely on pain intensity scores with no consideration for other patient related-factors poses increased risk for OIAS and OIRD.
      4) Opioid-delivery systems may pose added risks and necessitate assessment of patient's

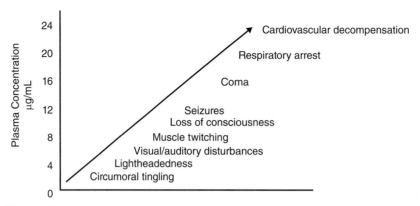

Figure 12.2 Assess patients for signs of local anesthetic systemic toxicity.

cognitive and physical ability to safely use device.
5) With higher risk of dependency or misuse, newer findings reflect incorporating an opioid-sparing approach for many types of pain, including postoperative pain.
6) Patient agreements: Documentation in electronic health record stating that risks of opioids have been discussed and agreed upon with patient (or parent if age-appropriate) is starting to be mandated in some states prior to prescribing opioids for outpatient use.
d. Local anesthetics
1) Side effects can include drowsiness, dizziness, and nausea and vomiting that can progress to toxicity.
2) Local anesthetic systemic toxicity (LAST)
a) Serious adverse effects can range from temporary neurological symptoms to cauda equina syndrome (loss of neurological function in lower extremities).
b) Occurs with high plasma concentrations of local anesthetic, which can occur with accumulation over time, or from unintentional intravascular injection.
c) Signs of LAST include:
(1) Drowsiness
(2) Anxiety/agitation
(3) Confusion
(4) Diplopia
(5) Ringing in ears
(6) Metallic taste in mouth
(7) Circumoral numbness or tingling
(8) Dizziness
(9) Twitching or seizures
(10) Changes in speech (slurred or slow)
(11) Reduced consciousness
(12) Cardiac dysrhythmias
d) Patients must be regularly assessed and local anesthetic treatment stopped with signs of toxicity (see Fig. 12.2). Treatment

may also include ACLS and IV lipid emulsion administration depending upon the severity of LAST.
e. Co-analgesics
1) Potential side effects and interactions with other medications, foods, and botanicals
2) Nurses need to be aware of intended and unintended medication effects.
3) Medication considerations presented in Beers Criteria need to be taken into consideration when working with older adults.
4) Medications with sedating effects compound OIAS and OIRD risks.
C. Clinician-related factors
1. Joint Commission and Institute for Healthcare Improvement strongly recommend clinicians:
a. Assess patient and environmental risk factors
b. Incorporate evidence-based practice and use outcome measures (including adverse events) to support safe care
2. Nurses and healthcare providers (HCPs) must maintain accurate current knowledge as pain management evolves.
3. Careful medication verification and administration improve patient care.
4. Thorough nursing assessment can detect medication side effects, thereby decreasing risk of adverse events (e.g., a full respiratory assessment can decrease risk of OIRD by detecting trends of reduced or labored breathing and intervening early).
5. Prescribers should use principle of "lowest effective dose," minimize risks associated with polypharmacy, and revise pharmacological pain regimens as indicated by patient status and progression.
D. Organization-related factors
1. Evidenced-based guidelines and procedures are necessary within healthcare as appropriate to specific patient populations.
2. Barcoding and "smart pump" technology have shown to decrease medication errors and are strongly recommended.

3. Organizations need to ensure HCPs receive education, including current information, standards, and protocols.
4. Adequate staffing improves patient care and decreases overall risk of adverse events, including OIAS and OIRD.
5. "Alarm fatigue" (decreased attention or desensitization to alarms as a result of high exposure, overuse, and "false" alarms) and call-light fatigue are environmental hazards that can adversely affect patients.
   a. Organizations should promote use of monitors when necessary, patient-appropriate alarm settings, and realistic expectations for nurses to attend to alarms in a timely manner.
   b. Factors such as inadequate staffing, increased acuity, and nursing burnout compound likelihood of nurses developing alarm fatigue and critical distinctions in patient assessment being missed.
   c. Currently, there are no identified countermeasures for alarm fatigue; however, awareness and supporting nurses and other healthcare team members are important.
6. Timely and effective communication among clinicians with changes in patient condition and shift "handoff" promotes patient safety. Organizations promoting collaborative, respectful relationships among HCPs can help ensure appropriate communication occurs.

III. Risk Assessment

A. Nursing assessment is critical to decreasing risk.
   1. Early identification of changes in patient's status can be captured more frequently with increased patient assessment and interactions (see Table 12.1 for sample observations associated with sedation).
   2. Threshold versus trend monitoring
      a. *Threshold* monitoring will alert nurses to patient status outside what is defined as "within normal limits."
      b. *Trend* monitoring is more complex and requires additional insight and analysis of information. For example, a decrease in oxygen saturation in presence of opioids often presents as a progressive decrease as opposed to a single event. While pulse oximetry readings in the low 90s may still be considered within normal limits,

Table 12.1

Identifying the Picture of Sedation

Patient Who Is Arousable Is…	Patient Who Is Somnolent Is…	Patient Who Is Over-Sedated Or Heading Toward Respiratory Compromise Territory Is…
• Waking up to voice, spontaneously • Able to follow commands • Able to open eyes, focuses on you • Able to cough and protect their own airway • Breathing and responsiveness within normal limits • Has good color • Able to move spontaneously • Able to know where they are • Able to follow a conversation, answering simple questions, engaging in interaction • Able to push the call bell for help if needed	• Difficult to wake up (doesn't respond to voice) • Waking up to physical stimuli • Not able to stay awake • Possibly not maintaining an oxygen saturation while awake • Demonstrating slowed breathing, increased calmness, shallow breathing • Possibly requiring oxygen • Demonstrating pinpoint pupils • Not focusing on you • Foggy, "snowed" looking • Not cognitively alert, not engaging in conversation or responding completely to questions • Demonstrating delayed movement or lack of movement, lack of eye contact, glassy eyes • Can't reliably push the call button or express their needs	• Requiring you hold their airway open for an hour • Demonstrating low BP, HR, RR • Asleep, obstructing their airway • Unable to arouse or arouses with great difficulty to painful stimuli for short periods • Slurring their speech • Not following conversation, not focused, demonstrating pinpoint pupils, glassy eyes • Floppy, limp, or showing lack of muscle tone • Showing dusky color, lips a little blue • Not reliably protecting their airway • Requiring oxygen • Unable to push the call button or express their needs

BP, Blood pressure; *HR*, heart rate; *RR*, respiratory rate

(From Dunwoody, D., Jungquist, C., Chang, Y., & Dickerson, S. [2018]. The common meanings and shared practices of sedation assessment in the context of managing patients with an opioid: a phenomenological study. *Journal of Clinical Nursing, 28*, 104–115.)

the slow decrease from high to mid to low 90s over a few hours should be alarming.

   c. Practice has shifted to trend monitoring to increase sensitivity and specificity in assessment of pain, OIAS, and OIRD.

B. Delirium

1. Considered a mental state consisting of confusion, disorientation, and unclear thinking; tends to start suddenly, is temporary, and treatable

2. May be caused by multiple etiologies: symptoms are not explained by other causes (e.g., preexisting condition, related to intoxication or withdrawal)

3. Multiple types exist:
   a. Hypoactive: decreased activity, sleepiness
   b. Hyperactive: restlessness, agitation
   c. Mixed: combines periods of hypo- and hyperactive delirium

4. Risk factors include:
   a. Hospitalization or care in long-term care facility
   b. Multiple serious illnesses
   c. Receiving multiple medications that impact cognition or behavior, including pain medication (e.g., opioids)

5. Symptoms may include:
   a. Rapid change in attention and awareness to environment
   b. Change from baseline attention that fluctuates in severity throughout day and night
   c. Disturbance in cognition, such as memory deficit, disorientation, language, visuospatial ability, or perception

6. Delirium can result in prolonged stays and increased healthcare costs.

7. Early identification with appropriate treatment may decrease long-term sequalae.

8. Pediatric considerations
   a. Prevalence rates in critically ill children range from 4% to 56%.
   b. Non-iatrogenic, nonpharmacological risk factors for acute pediatric delirium include:
      1) Sex (males at greater risk)
      2) Developmental delay
      3) Mechanical ventilation
      4) Anxiety, associated with mixed delirium
   c. Most common characteristics of pediatric delirium include agitation, disorientation, hallucinations, inattention, and sleep-wake cycle disturbances.
   d. Children should be screened for delirium if they present with:
      1) Acute change or fluctuation in baseline mental status
      2) Inattention
      3) Altered level of consciousness
      4) Disorganized thinking

9. Delirium assessment tools (select examples included; more exist)
   a. Delirium Observation Screening Scale
      1) Scale with 15 items based on the *Diagnostic and Statistical Manual of Mental Disorders,* 4th Edition (DSM-IV) criteria
      2) Designed for use by nurses for early identification of delirium
   b. Sour Seven Questionnaire
      1) Used to assess patients in acute care
      2) Seven items using an 18-point scale, with higher scores indicating delirium
   c. Informant Assessment of Geriatric Delirium (I-AGeD)
      1) Validated 10-item scale
      2) Sensitivity reportedly decreases with dementia
   d. Neelon and Champagne Confusion Scale (NEECHAM)
      1) Validated for use in intensive care units (ICUs)
      2) Identifies patients as being with delirium, confused, at risk for delirium, or not with delirium
   e. Cornell Assessment of Pediatric Delirium (CAP-D) (Fig. 12.3)
      1) Rapid, valid, and sensitive screening tool for delirium in pediatric ICUs.
      2) Questions, based on DSM-IV criteria for pediatric delirium, assess for eye contact with caregiver, purposeful actions, awareness of surroundings, communication of needs and wants, restlessness, inconsolability, underactivity (very little movement when awake), and taking a long time to respond to interactions.
      3) Assess children every 12 hours. Scores ≥ 9 suggest presence of delirium. Assess sedation using Richmond Agitation-Sedation Scale (RASS) every 4 hours; cannot be used in presence of RASS scores ≤-4.
      4) Do not adjust for baseline behavior in children with developmental delays. Score what you see. A CAPD score ≥9 in children with developmental delays is not definitively delirium. Trend score over time and use best judgment.
   f. Sophia Observation Withdrawal Symptoms Scale–Pediatric Delirium (SOS-PD) (Fig. 12.4)
      1) A portion of Sophia Observation Withdrawal Symptoms scale is used to assess delirium in children experiencing iatrogenic withdrawal symptoms (see below).
      2) Good reliability and validity for early screening and identification of pediatric delirium in critically ill children

RASS Score___(if -4 or -5 do not proceed) Please answer the following questions based on your interactions with the patient over the course of your shift:	Never 4	Rarely 3	Sometimes 2	Often 1	Always 0	Score
1. Does the child make eye contact with the caregiver?						
2. Are the child's actions purposeful?						
3. Is the child aware of his/her surroundings?						
4. Does the child communicate needs and wants?						
	Never 0	Rarely 1	Sometimes 2	Often 3	Always 4	
5. Is the child restless?						
6. Is the child inconsolable?						
7. Is the child underactive—very little movement while awake?						
8. Does it take the child a long time to respond to interactions?						
					TOTAL	

Figure 12.3 **Cornell Assessment of Pediatric Delirium (CAP-D).** (From Silver G., Kearney J., Traube C., & Hertzig M. [2015]. Delirium screening anchored in child development: the Cornell Assessment for Pediatric Delirium. *Palliative Support Care, 13*[4]:1005–1011.)

g. Pediatric Confusion Assessment Method for the Intensive Care Unit (pCAM-ICU) (Fig. 12.5)
1) Identifies delirium in children 5 years of age and older; adapted from adult Confusion Method for the ICU (CAM-ICU)
2) Requires assessment of patient's arousal or level of consciousness using a sedation scale such as RASS or State Behavioral Scale (SBS).
3) Child who is not responsive to voice or light touch (RASS −4 or −5 and SBS −2 or −3) is considered comatose, and level of consciousness therefore does not allow for an accurate delirium assessment.
4) Please note there are varieties of CAM-ICU for various age groups (e.g., preschool, pediatric) and should be used based on developmental level.
h. Preschool Confusion Assessment Method for the ICU (psCAM-ICU) identifies delirium in

critically ill infants and children less than 5 years of age (Fig. 12.6).
C. Opioid-induced advancing sedation and opioid-induced respiratory depression
1. Sedation assessment is first line in preventing OIAS and OIRD.
a. OIAS precedes OIRD and highlights importance of early identification of advancing sedation and vigilance needed to prevent progression to OIRD.
b. Although many tools are used to assess sedation, most sedation scales were constructed for assessing intentional sedation, such as in operating room (OR) or ICU setting. The Pasero Opioid-Induced Sedation Scale was developed specifically to assess unintended sedation following opioid administration.
2. Assessment tools to assess unintended sedation
a. Pasero Opioid-Induced Sedation Scale (Fig. 12.7)

Part 3

Comfort assessment

SOS-PD scale
Sophia Observation withdrawal Symptoms-scale and Delirium

Date/time 1   Date/time 2

Observer   Observer

Sticker with patient's name

Step 1a Withdrawal	1	2	Explanation
Heart rate	..... /min	..... /min	Enter highest rate in past 4 hours if available (electronic patient data management system), otherwise read the monitor or feel pulse.
Breathing rate	..... /min	..... /min	Enter highest rate in past 4 hours if available (electronic patient data management system), otherwise read the monitor or count breathing.
Baseline heart rate	..... /min	..... /min	Baseline is the mean value over the past 24 hours.
Baseline breathing rate	..... /min	..... /min	Baseline value is the mean value over the past 24 hours.

Step 1b Delirium*	1	2	Tick if yes
Parents do not recognize their child's behavior	☐*	☐*	Parents perceive their child's behavior as very different or unrecognizable in comparison with what they are accustomed to when the child is ill or in hospital; "this is not my child".

Step 2	Withdrawal 1 2	Delirium 1 2	
Tachycardia	☐ ☐		Heart rate exceeds baseline by ≥ 15%.
Tachypnea	☐ ☐		Breathing rate exceeds baseline by ≥ 15%.
Fever	☐ ☐		Body temperature exceeded 38.4° C now or in past 4 hours.
Sweating	☐ ☐	☐ ☐	Without apparent reason.
Agitation	☐ ☐	☐ ☐	E.g.: irritable, restless, agitated, fumbling (trying to pull out catheters, venous lines, gastric tubes etc.).
Anxiety	☐ ☐	☐ ☐	Child shows anxious facial expression (eyes wide open, raised and tensed eyebrows). Behavior varies from panicky to introvert.
Tremors	☐ ☐	☐ ☐	Trembling, involuntary sustained rhythmic movements of hands and/or feet.
Motor disturbance	☐ ☐	☐ ☐	Involuntary movements of arm and/or legs; little muscle twitches.
Muscle tension	☐ ☐	☐ ☐	Clenching wrists and toes and/or hunched shoulders. Or: abnormal tensed position of head, arm and/or legs caused by muscle tension.
Attentiveness		☐ ☐	If you (nurses) or parents fail to attract or hold the child's attention. Child is not aware of surroundings; living in "his own world"; Apathy.
Purposeful acting		☐ ☐	If child has difficulty in doing things that normally are no problem; e.g. cannot grab pacifier or cuddly toy
Lack of eye contact		☐ ☐	No or little eye contact with caregiver or parents.
Inconsolable crying	☐ ☐	☐ ☐	Inconsolable (shown by refusing food, pacifier or not wanting to play). Score silent crying in ventilated children as inconsolable crying.
Grimacing	☐ ☐	☐ ☐	Eyebrows contracted and lowered, nasolabial fold visible.
Sleeplessness	☐ ☐	☐ ☐	Child doesn't sleep more than one hour at a stretch; catnaps.
Hallucinations	☐ ☐	☐ ☐*	Child seems to see, hear of feel things that were not there.
Disorientation		☐ ☐	Only for children >5 years. Child doesn't know whether it is morning, afternoon or evening, is not aware where it is, does not recognize family or friends.
Speech		☐ ☐	If speech is incomprehensible, unclear or child cannot tell a coherent story (not age appropriate).
Acute onset of symptoms		☐ ☐	Acute change of symptoms compared to before hospital admission.
Fluctuations		☐ ☐	The occurrence of symptoms strongly varies over the past 24 hours.
Vomiting	☐ ☐		At least once in past 4 hours.
Diarrhea	☐ ☐		At least once in past 4 hours.

Total score

SOS score* ☐ ☐   Withdrawal score (max. is 15) Count ticked boxes
PD score* ☐ ☐   Delirium score (max. is 16/17) Count ticked boxes

* Consult child-psychiatrist if: Step 1b is positive AND/OR Step 2 score is ≥ 4 or symptom with * is positive.

Please turn over for further instructions

Figure 12.4 Sophia Observation Withdrawal Symptoms Scale (SOS-PD). (From Ista E., Te Beest H., van Rosmalen J., de Hoog M., Tibboel D., van Beusekom B., et al. [2018]. Sophia Observation withdrawal Symptoms-Paediatric Delirium scale: a tool for early screening of delirium in the PICU. *Australian Critical Care, 31*[5], 266–273.)

1) Widely used and supported by expert consensus for use in preventing OIAS and OIRD
2) Developed specifically to assess unintended sedation resulting from opioids using standardized descriptors and to provide guidance when nursing intervention is required
3) Demonstrated utility for assessing pediatric patients in acute care.

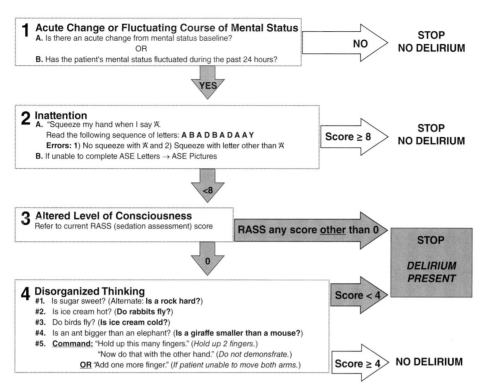

Figure 12.5 Pediatric Confusion Assessment Method for the Intensive Care Unit (pCAM-ICU). (Copyright © 2011, Heidi, A. B., Smith, M. D. MSCI and Monroe Carrell Jr. Children's Hospital at Vanderbilt, all rights reserved.)

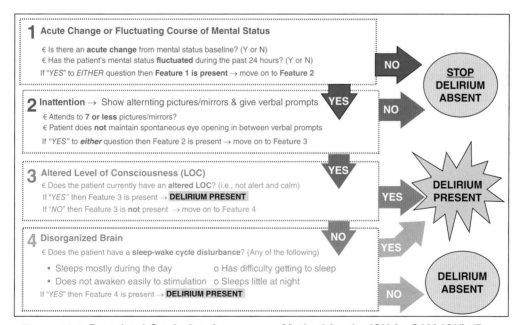

Figure 12.6 Preschool Confusion Assessment Method for the ICU (psCAM-ICU). (From Smith H. A., Gangopadhyay M., Goben C. M., Jacobowski N. L., Chestnut M. H., Savage S., et al. [2016]. The Preschool Confusion Assessment Method for the ICU: valid and reliable delirium monitoring for critically ill infants and children. *Critical Care Medicine, 44*[3], 592–600.)

PASERO OPIOID-INDUCED SEDATION SCALE (POSS)*

S = Sleep, easy to arouse
   Acceptable; no action necessary; may increase opioid dose if needed
1 = Awake and alert
   Acceptable; no action necessary; may increase opioid dose if needed
2 = Slightly drowsy, easily aroused
   Acceptable; no action necessary; may increase opioid dose if needed
3 = Frequently drowsy, arousable, drifts off to sleep during conversation
   Unacceptable; monitor respiratory status and sedation level closely until sedation level is stable at less than 3 and respiratory status is satisfactory; decrease opioid dose 25% to 50%[1] or notify primary[2] or anesthesia provider for orders; consider administering a non-sedating, opioid-sparing nonopioid, such as acetaminophen or a NSAID, if not contraindicated; ask patient to take deep breaths every 15-30 minutes.
4 = Somnolent, minimal or no response to verbal and physical stimulation
   Unacceptable; stop opioid; consider administering naloxone[3,4]; stay with patient, stimulate, and support respiration as indicated by patient status; call Rapid Response Team (Code Blue) if indicated; notify primary[2] or anesthesia provider; monitor respiratory status and sedation level closely until sedation level is stable at less than 3 and respiratory status is satisfactory.

---

*Appropriate action is given in italics at each level of sedation.
[1] If opioid analgesic orders or hospital protocol do not include the expectation that the opioid dose will be decreased if a patient is excessively sedated, such orders should be promptly obtained.
[2] For example, the physician, nurse practitioner, advanced practice nurse, or physician assistant responsible for the pain management prescription.
[3] For adults experiencing respiratory depression give intravenous naloxone very slowly while observing patient response ("titrate to effect"). If sedation and respiratory depression occurs during administration of transdermal fentanyl, remove the patch; if naloxone is necessary, treatment will be needed for a prolonged period, and the typical approach involves a naloxone infusion. Patient must be monitored closely for at least 24 hours after discontinuation of the transdermal fentanyl.
[4] Hospital protocols should include the expectation that a nurse will administer naloxone to any patient suspected of having life-threatening opioid-induced sedation and respiratory depression.

Figure 12.7 Pasero Opioid-Induced Sedation Scale. (© 1994, Pasero C. Used with permission. As cited in Pasero C., McCaffery M. *Pain Assessment and Pharmacologic Management*, p. 510. St. Louis, Mosby/Elsevier, 2011.)

Value	Patient state
0	Awake and alert
1	Minimally sedated: tired/sleepy, appropriate response to verbal conversation, and/or sound
2	Moderately sedated: somnolent/sleeping, easily aroused with light tactile stimulation or a simple verbal command
3	Deeply sedated: deep sleep, aroused only with significant physical stimulation
4	Unarousable

Figure 12.8 University of Michigan Sedation Scale. (From Malviya, S., et al. [2002]. Depth of sedation in children undergoing computed tomography: Validity and reliability of the University of Michigan Sedation Scale (UMSS). *British Journal of Anaesthesia*, 88(2), 241–245.)

b. University of Michigan Sedation Scale (UMSS) (Fig. 12.8)
   1) Includes five indicators looking at behavior ranging from awake and alert to unarousable
   2) Valid and reliable for rapid assessment of sedation in children
   3) Provides guidance for titration of medication and improves communication among providers
   4) Does not address agitation

RAMSAY SEDATION SCALE

Score	Level of Sedation
1	Patient is anxious and agitated or restless, or both
2	Patient is co-operative, oriented, and tranquil
3	Patient responds to commands only
4	Patient exhibits brisk response to light tactile stimuli or loud auditory stimulus
5	Patient exhibits sluggish response to light tactile stimuli or loud auditory stimulus
6	Patient exhibits no response

Figure 12.9 **Ramsay Sedation Scale.** (From Sessler, C. N., Grap, M. J., Ramsay, M. A. [2008]. Evaluating and monitoring analgesia and sedation in the intensive care unit. *Crit Care. 12* (suppl 3): S2.)

Richmond Agitation and Sedation Scale (RASS)		
+4	Combative	Violent, immediate danger to staff
+3	Very agitated	Pulls or removes tube(s) or catheter(s): aggressive
+2	Agitated	Frequent non-purposeful movement, fights ventilator
+1	Restless	Anxious, apprehensive but movements not aggressive of vigorous
0	Alert & calm	
-1	Drowsy	Not fully alert, but has sustained awakening to *voice* (eye opening & contact ≥ 10 sec)
-2	Light sedation	Briefly awakens to *voice* (eye opening & contact < 10 sec)
-3	Moderate sedation	Movement or eye-opening to *voice* (but no eye contact)
-4	Deep sedation	No response to voice, but movement or eye opening to *physical* stimulation
-5	Unarousable	No response to *voice or physical* stimulation

Figure 12.10 **Richmond Agitation Scale.** (From Sessler, C. N., Grap, M. J., Brophy, G. M. [2001]. Multidisciplinary management of sedation and analgesia in critical care. *Seminars in Respiratory Critical Care Medicine, 22*, 211–225.)

3. Assessment tools designed to assess intended sedation
   a. Ramsay Sedation Scale (RSS) (Fig. 12.9)
      1) Originally developed to assess intentional sedation in the operating room and focuses specifically on arousability and reflex responses
      2) Well validated in adults in OR setting but lacks specificity for use in assessment of unintended sedation
      3) Includes six indicators rating behaviors ranging from anxiety and/or agitation to exhibiting no response
   b. Richmond Agitation and Sedation Scale (RASS) (Fig. 12.10)
      1) Used and psychometrically validated in ventilated and non-ventilated populations in ICU
      2) Concise, simple, intuitive tool combining both sedation and agitation into one scale
      3) Although *not* originally developed for use in pediatric patients, RASS has since been validated in children.
   c. Riker Sedation-Agitation Scale
      1) Concise, simple, intuitive tool combining sedation and agitation to one scale
      2) Determines level of stimulation necessary to elicit patient response and evaluate sedation
      3) Not originally developed to monitor for opioid induced sedation
   d. State Behavioral Scale (Fig. 12.11)
      1) Validated in critically ill intubated children
      2) Identifies six behaviors that describe state behavior on scale of −3 to +2
         a) More negative scores reflect sedated state, and more positive scores reflect more agitated state.
         b) Zero is most reflective of patient who is awake and able to be calmed.
      3) Observes respiratory drive/response to ventilation, coughing, best response to stimulation, attentiveness to care provider, tolerance to care, ability to be consoled, and movement after consoled

	State Behavioral Scale (SBS)	
	Score as patient's response to voice then gentle touch then noxious stimuli (planned endotracheal suctioning or <5 seconds of nail bed pressure)	
Score	**Description**	**Definition**
−3	Unresponsive	• No spontaneous respiratory effort • No cough or coughs only with suctioning • No response to noxious stimuli • Unable to pay attention to care provider • Does not distress with any procedure (including noxious) • Does not move
−2	Responsive to noxious stimuli	• Spontaneous yet supported breathing • Coughs with suctioning/repositioning • Responds to noxious stimuli • Unable to pay attention to care provider • Will distress with a noxious procedure • Does not move/occasional movement of extremities or shifting of position
−1	Responsive to gentle touch or voice	• Spontaneous but ineffective nonsupported breaths • Coughs with suctioning/repositioning • Responds to touch/voice • Able to pay attention but drifts off after stimulation • Distresses with procedures • Able to calm with comforting touch or voice when stimulus removed • Occasional movement of extremities or shifting of position
0	Awake and able to calm	• Spontaneous and effective breathing • Coughs when repositioned/Occasional spontaneous cough • Responds to voice/No external stimulus is required to elicit response • Spontaneously pays attention to care provider • Distresses with procedures • Able to calm with comforting touch or voice when stimulus removed • Occasional movement of extremities or shifting of position/increased movement (restless, squirming)
+1	Restless and difficult to calm	• Spontaneous effective breathing/Having difficulty breathing with ventilator • Occasional spontaneous cough • Responds to voice/No external stimulus is required to elicit response • Drifts off/Spontaneously pays attention to care provider • Intermittently unsafe • Does not consistently calm despite 5 minute attempt/unable to console • Increased movement (restless, squirming)
+2	Agitated	• May have difficulty breathing with ventilator • Coughing spontaneously • No external stimulus required to elicit response • Spontaneously pays attention to care provider • Unsafe (biting ETT, pulling at lines, cannot be left alone) • Unable to console • Increased movement (restless, squirming or thrashing side-to-side, kicking legs)

Figure 12.11 **State Behavioral Scale (SBS).**

4) SBS assessment in preverbal or nonverbal children is challenging.

5) Includes both pain and sedation but does not differentiate cause of discomfort; clinical judgment required to differentiate between behavioral distress and pain

6) Limited value guiding interventions if used alone

4. Respiratory assessment
   a. Respiratory rate, quality, and depth have increased sensitivity in identifying OIAS and OIRD and are essential for prevention.

b. Respiratory function assessment includes:
1) Respiratory rate counted for 30 to 60 seconds
2) Evaluate rise and fall of chest during respiration.
3) Concern is for:
   a) Shallow breathing
   b) Irregular breathing
   c) Ventilatory effort (e.g., labored breathing)
   d) Noisy breathing (e.g., stridor, snoring)
c. Nurses can detect signs and symptoms of opioid or other sedating medication complications and thereby decrease risks.
d. Monitors to detect respiratory depression
1) Continuous pulse oximetry
   a) Supported in clinical practice for patient monitoring and risk mitigation
   b) Recent reports and recommendations support use of monitoring but provide clear caution that decreasing pulse oximetry is a late indicator of OIAS and OIRD.
   c) Supplemental oxygen decreases effectiveness of oxygen saturation monitoring as readings drop more slowly for patients receiving supplemental oxygen.
2) Capnography or end-tidal CO_2 (ETCO$_2$) monitoring
   a) Measures exhaled end-tidal CO_2 levels via nasal cannula
   b) Research supports efficacy and use in preventing adverse events regarding OIAS and OIRD.
      (1) Sensor positioning, changes in respiratory patterns, and changes in oxygen supplementation affect ETCO$_2$ monitoring in non-ventilated patients.
      (2) Only reliable if cannula is not mispositioned, which can produce artificially low reading
      (3) Young children may attempt to remove device.
      (4) Patient who is agitated due to elevated CO_2 level may also attempt to remove device.
      (5) Skilled nursing assessment is required to differentiate causes of agitation.
      (6) Insufficient research to determine which pediatric patients should be monitored with ETCO$_2$
   c) Increased cost, often limited availability, challenges with patient adherence, and necessary training contribute to slow incorporation into clinical practice.

3) Minute volume monitoring
   a) Transcutaneous monitoring using tidal volume and respiration rate to calculate minute volume
   b) Technology is still quite new to practice and considered costly
D. Opioid–benzodiazepine withdrawal assessment
1. General concepts of withdrawal
   a. Nurses must be aware of risk factors for development of withdrawal symptoms.
   1) Infants exposed to substances (e.g., opioids, benzodiazepines, nicotine, methamphetamine) in utero are at risk for neonatal abstinence syndrome (NAS).
   2) Generally, patients receiving opioids or benzodiazepines for more than 5 days with abrupt discontinuation are at risk for withdrawal syndrome.
   3) Withdrawal should be diagnosis of exclusion, meaning symptoms cannot be attributed to other causes (e.g., feeding intolerance, infection).
      a) Abrupt and drastic reductions in medication doses (e.g., 50%) are generally required to cause withdrawal syndrome.
      b) As most tapers (weans) are much more gradual, withdrawal is not expected.
   b. Obtain baseline assessment prior to beginning medication tapers.
   c. Monitor patient for signs and symptoms of pain throughout weaning process (if pain is suspected).
   d. Signs of withdrawal syndrome include:
   1) Autonomic dysfunction (e.g., tachycardia, tachypnea, fever, sweating)
   2) CNS irritability (e.g., agitation, anxiety, tremors, motor disturbance such as muscle jerks or uncontrolled robust movements)
   3) Increased muscle tension, inconsolable crying, grimacing, sleeplessness, hallucinations
   4) Gastrointestinal dysfunction (e.g., vomiting, diarrhea)
2. Specific withdrawal syndromes
   a. Neonatal abstinence syndrome
   1) Constellation of clinical findings occurring in newborns exposed to opioids or other substances in utero
   2) Symptoms include but are not limited to tremors, seizures, overactive reflexes, fussiness, excessive or high-pitched crying, and poor feeding.
   3) When caring for newborns, review history for presence of maternal substance use and, if appropriate, assess for signs of NAS.
   4) While Finnegan Neonatal Abstinence Scoring Tool (FNAST) has traditionally

been used for assessment, the Eat, Sleep, Console (ESC) assessment approach may result in less morphine for treatment of withdrawal and shorter lengths of stay (see tools below). Large well-designed randomized controlled studies are needed to further validate the ESC assessment and evaluate long-term outcomes of infants managed with the ESC assessment.

   b. Iatrogenic withdrawal syndrome (IWS)
      1) Occurs following abrupt cessation of opioids or other sedating medications during hospitalization and most commonly following care in ICU setting
      2) May also occur when enteral opioids are used consistently for several days and there is alteration in gastric absorption and corresponding decrease in medication plasma levels
      3) Generalized symptoms of IWS involve overstimulation of CNS, autonomic dysregulation, and gastrointestinal symptoms.
      4) Most literature describing IWS involves pediatric patients, but there is some evidence to support occurrence in adults.

3. Withdrawal assessment tools
   a. Clinical Opioid Withdrawal Scale (COWS)
      1) Psychometric validity; popular among acute care clinicians
      2) Used to assess severity and progression of withdrawal symptoms
   b. Clinical Institute Withdrawal Assessment for Alcohol–Revised (CIWA-Ar) (Fig. 12.12)
      1) Used to assess suspected alcohol withdrawal by assessing and stratifying severity
      2) Ten indicators, scored from 0 to 7: agitation, anxiety, auditory disturbances, clouding of sensorium, headache, nausea/vomiting, paroxysmal sweats, tactile disturbances, tremors, and visual disturbances
      3) Three indicators can be visually observed, and the remaining indicators require patient discussion.
      4) Assessment stratification:
         a) Mild withdrawal = cumulative score of 8 to 10
         b) Moderate withdrawal = cumulative score of 8 to 15
         c) Severe withdrawal = cumulative score ≥15
   c. Withdrawal Assessment Tool (WAT-1) (Fig. 12.13)
      1) Standardizes identification of iatrogenic-acquired withdrawal symptoms with demonstrated validity from 2 weeks (full-term infants) to 18 years of age
      2) Assessment is to be done every 12 hours (ideally at start of a shift) to identify

changes from baseline. More frequent assessment may result in serial bias.
      3) Assesses for tremor, temperature >37.8°C, loose/watery stools, vomiting/retching/gagging, sweating, uncoordinated or repetitive movement, startle to touch, muscle tone, yawning/sneezing, and time to gain calm state following stimulation
      4) Increased risk for withdrawal defined as score ≥3. Higher scores indicate more distress.
      5) Treatment (pharmacological or nonpharmacological) of elevated scores should be followed with reassessment within an hour to ensure symptoms have improved or resolved.

   d. Sophia Observation Withdrawal Symptoms Scale (See Fig. 12.4)
      1) Designed to identify benzodiazepine and opioid withdrawal syndrome in pediatric critical care patients up to 16 years of age
      2) After determining baseline heart and respiratory rates, assessment is done evaluating behavior during past 4 hours, scoring most extreme or worst moment during prior 4 hours.
      3) Assessment is once per shift, at suspicion of withdrawal syndrome, and 2 hours after an intervention for treatment of withdrawal symptoms.
   e. Finnegan Neonatal Abstinence Scoring Tool (FNAST)
      1) Contains 21 signs and symptoms and was developed for newborns experiencing opioid withdrawal syndrome
      2) Modified versions have been developed over time.
      3) Several studies have documented longer lengths of stay when used for management of opioid withdrawal in infants.
   f. Eat, Sleep, Console
      1) Focuses on how baby is functioning
         E = Is baby eating at least an ounce, breast feeding well, or tolerating tube feeds?
         S = Is baby sleeping at least an hour at a time?
         C = Can baby be consoled within 10 minutes of crying?
      2) Assessment using ESC combined with reinforcement of nonpharmacological modalities and use of as-needed morphine has resulted in decreased length of stay and less opioid administration.

E. Assessing and managing opioid use
   1. General concepts
      a. Using standardized assessment tools to identify patients at high risk for SUD and specifically opioid use disorder (OUD) helps determine level of monitoring required when opioid therapy is required.

Addiction Research Foundation Clinical Institute Withdrawal Assessment for Alcohol (CIWA-Ar)

Patient _____ Date |__|__|__| Time ____:____
y m d (24 hour clock, midnight = 00:00)

Pulse or heart rate, taken for one minute: _____ Blood pressure:_____/_____

NAUSEA AND VOMITING—As "Do you feel sick to your stomach? Have you vomited?" Observation.
0 no nausea and no vomiting
1 mild nausea with no vomiting
2
3
4 intermittent nausea with dry heaves
5
6
7 constant nausea, frequent dry heaves and vomiting

TREMOR—Arms extended and fingers spread apart. Observation.
0 no tremor
1 not visible, but can be felt fingertip to fingertip
2
3
4 moderate, with patient's arms extended
5
6
7 severe, even with arms not extended

PAROXYSMAL SWEATS—Observation.
0 no sweat visible
1 barely perceptible sweating, palms moist
2
3
4 beads of sweat obvious on forehead
5
6
7 drenching sweats

ANXIETY—Ask "Do you feel nervous?" Observation.
0 no anxiety, at ease
1 mildly anxious
2
3
4 moderately anxious, or guarded, so anxiety is inferred
5
6
7 equivalent to acute panic states as seen in severe delirium or acute schizophrenic reactions

AGITATION— Observation.
0 normal activity
1 somewhat more than normal activity
2
3
4 moderately fidgety and restless
5
6
7 paces back and forth during most of the interview, or constantly thrashes about

TACTILE DISTURBANCES—Ask "Have you any itching, pins and needles sensations, any burning, any numbness or do you feel bugs crawling on or under your skin?" Observation.
0 none
1 very mild itching, pins and needles, burning or numbness
2 mild itching, pins and needles, burning or numbness
3 moderate itching, pins and needles, burning or numbness
4 moderately severe hallucinations
5 severe hallucinations
6 extremely severe hallucinations
7 continuous hallucinations

AUDITORY DISTURBANCES—Ask "Are you more aware of sounds around you? Are they harsh? Do they frighten you? Are you hearing anything that is disturbing to you? Are you hearing things you know are not there?" Observation.
0 not present
1 very mild harshness or ability to frighten
2 mild harshness or ability to frighten
3 moderate harshness or ability to frighten
4 moderately severe hallucinations
5 severe hallucinations
6 extremely severe hallucinations
7 continuous hallucinations

VISUAL DISTURBANCES—Ask "Does the light appear to be too bright? Is its colour different? Does it hurt your eyes? Are you seeing anything that is disturbing to you? Are you seeing things you know are not there?" Observation.
0 not present
1 very mild sensitivity
2 mild sensitivity
3 moderate sensitivity
4 moderately severe hallucinations
5 severe hallucinations
6 extremely severe hallucinations
7 continuous hallucinations

HEADACHE, FULLNESS IN HEAD—Ask "Does your head feel different? Does it feel like there is a band around your head?" Do not rate for dizziness or lightheadedness. Otherwise, rate severity.
0 not present
1 very mild
2 mild
3 moderate
4 moderately severe
5 severe
6 very severe
7 extremely severe

ORIENTATION AND CLOUDING OF SENSORIUM—Ask "What day is this? Where are you? Who am I?"
0 oriented and can do serial additions
1 cannot do serial additions or is uncertain about date
2 disoriented for date by no more than 2 calendar days
3 disoriented for date by more than 2 calendar days
4 disoriented for place and/or person

Total CIWA-A Score _____
Rater's Initials _____
Maximum Possible Score 67

This scale is not copyrighted and may be used freely.

Figure 12.12 Clinical Institute Withdrawal Assessment for Alcohol, Revised. (From Sullivan J. T., Sykora K., Schneiderman J., Naranjo C. A., Sellers E. M. [1989]. Assessment of alcohol withdrawal: the revised Clinical Institute Withdrawal Assessment for Alcohol Scale [CIWA-Ar]. *Br J Addict, 84*[11], 1353–1357.)

1) Information obtained through assessment of drug use is protected by Federal Confidentiality of Alcohol and Drug Abuse patient record rules.
2) Disclosure of this information requires specific written consent from patient.
3) Records may be shared in certain circumstances. Refer to Tip 42: Substance Abuse and Mental Health Services Administration

(SAMHSA) *Code of Federal Regulation*, Title 42, and your individual state law.

b. Reviewing the prescription drug monitoring program has become an expectation and even standard of care in most states.

c. Urine drug testing is not an adequate screening tool by itself because many substances are present in body for only 2 to 3 days, and it does not address frequency of use.

Part 3

WITHDRAWAL ASSESSMENT TOOL VERSION 1 (WAT-1)

Patient Identifier		Date:													
		Time:													
Information from patient record, previous 12 hours															
Any loose/watery stools	No = 0 / Yes = 1														
Any vomiting/wretching/gagging	No = 0 / Yes = 1														
Temperature > 37.8°C	No = 0 / Yes = 1														
2 minute pre-stimulus observation															
State	SBS[1] ≤ 0 or asleep/awake/calm = 0 / SBS[1] ≥ +1 or awake/distressed = 1														
Tremor	None/mild = 0 / Moderate/severe = 1														
Any sweating	No = 0 / Yes = 1														
Uncoordinated/repetitive movement	None/mild = 0 / Moderate/severe = 1														
Yawning or sneezing	None or 1 = 0 / ≥2 = 1														
1 minute stimulus observation															
Startle to touch	None/mild = 0 / Moderate/severe = 1														
Muscle tone	Normal = 0 / Increased = 1														
Post-stimulus recovery															
Time to gain calm state (SBS[1] ≤ 0)	< 2 min = 0 / 2 - 5 min = 1 / > 5 min = 2														
Total Score (0-12)															

WITHDRAWAL ASSESSMENT TOOL VERSION 1 (WAT-1) INSTRUCTIONS

- Start WAT-1 scoring from the **first day of weaning** in patients who have received opioids +/or benzodiazepines by infusion or regular dosing for prolonged periods (e.g., > 5 days). Continue twice daily scoring until 72 hours after the last dose.
- The Withdrawal Assessment Tool (WAT-1) should be completed along with the SBS[1] at least once per 12 hour shift (e.g., at 08:00 and 20:00 ± 2 hours). The progressive stimulus used in the SBS[1] assessment provides a standard stimulus for observing signs of withdrawal.

Obtain information from patient record (this can be done before or after the stimulus):
- ✓ **Loose/watery stools**: Score 1 if any loose or watery stools were documented in the past 12 hours; score 0 if none were noted.
- ✓ **Vomiting/wretching/gagging**: Score 1 if any vomiting or spontaneous wretching or gagging were documented in the past 12 hours; score 0 if none were noted
- ✓ **Temperature > 37.8°C**: Score 1 if the modal (most frequently occurring) temperature documented was greater than 37.8°C in the past 12 hours; score 0 if this was not the case.

2 minute pre-stimulus observation:
- ✓ **State**: Score 1 if awake and distress (SBS[1]: ≥ + 1) observed during the 2 minutes prior to the stimulus; score 0 if asleep or awake and calm/cooperative (SBS[1] ≤ 0).
- ✓ **Tremor**: Score 1 if moderate to severe tremor observed during the 2 minutes prior to the stimulus; score 0 if no tremor (or only minor, intermittent tremor).
- ✓ **Sweating**: Score 1 if any sweating during the 2 minutes prior to the stimulus; score 0 if no sweating noted.
- ✓ **Uncoordinated/repetitive movements**: Score 1 if moderate to severe uncoordinated or repetitive movements such as head turning, leg or arm flailing or torso arching observed during the 2 minutes prior to the stimulus; score 0 if no (or only mild) uncoordinated or repetitive movements.
- ✓ **Yawning or sneezing > 1**: Score 1 if more than 1 yawn or sneeze observed during the 2 minutes prior to the stimulus; score 0 if 0to 1 yawn or sneeze.

1 minute stimulus observation:
- ✓ **Startle to touch**: Score 1 if moderate to severe startle occurs when touched during the stimulus; score 0 if none (or mild).
- ✓ **Muscle tone**: Score 1 if tone increased during the stimulus; score 0 if normal.

Post stimulus recovery:
- ✓ **Time to gain calm state** (SBS[1] ≤ 0): Score 2 if it takes greater than 5 minutes following stimulus; score 1 if achieved within 2 to 5 minutes; score 0 if achieved in less than 2 minutes.

Sum the 11 numbers in the column for the total WAT-1 score (0-12).

[1]Curley et al. State behavioral scale: A sedation assessment instrument for instants and young children supported on mechanical ventilation. Pediatr Crit Care Med 2006;7(2): 107-114.

Figure 12.13 Withdrawal Assessment Tool (WAT-1). (From Franck, L. S., Harris, S. K., Soetenga, D. J., Amling, J. K., & Curley, M. A. Q. [2008]. *Pediatric Critical Care Medicine, 9*[6], 573–580.)

d. Educate patients and families about both safe controlled substance storage and timely and safe disposal (e.g., use safe, at-home disposal systems, police station or pharmacy drop boxes, not in trash).

e. Help families assess their risk:
   1) Where is medication going to be stored?
   2) Who will have access to it?
   3) Who is aware of medication in house?
   4) How can medication be secured?

2. Pediatric opioid use risk
   a. Risk assessment in pediatrics is as important as it is in adult populations.
   b. Adolescents are at higher risk given the developing adolescent brain and social environment.
   c. Legitimate opioid exposure (e.g., prescribed following surgery) in children and young adults is associated with an increased lifetime risk of SUD both in children with little previous drug experience and in those who disapprove of illegal drug use at baseline (those least expected to misuse opioids).
   d. Leftover prescription opioids from previous prescriptions have been shown to account for substantial source of nonmedical use of prescription opioids in high school seniors.
   e. Situational awareness is needed to decrease a child's risk when opioids, benzodiazepines, or other medications at risk of misuse are needed (Box 12.2).
3. Substance Use Disorder Assessment Tools
   a. For additional information, see chapter 22.
   b. Opioid risk tool (ORT) (Fig. 12.14)
      1) Evidence-based screening tool recommended by National Institute on Drug Abuse and the American Academy of Pediatrics Committee on Substance Abuse
      2) Brief, self-report screening tool validated in adults to assess level of risk (low, moderate, or high) for opioid misuse; to be completed prior to initiating therapy
   c. Opioid risk tool for OUD (ORT-OUD) (Fig. 12.15)
      1) Derived from the original ORT, tool has excellent predictive ability; ORT-OUD score classifies patients as either "at risk" or "not at risk" of developing OUD.
   d. CAGE (cut down, annoyed, guilty, eye-opener)
      1) A self-report screening tool (which necessitates that the individual recognizes they have a problem)
         a) Have you ever felt you should cut down on your drinking?
         b) Have people annoyed you by criticizing your drinking?
         c) Have you ever felt bad or guilty about your drinking?
         d) Have you ever had a drink first thing in the morning to steady your nerves or to get rid of a hangover ("eye-opener")?
      2) Validated only for alcohol use
      3) Not validated for use among children; some questions (e.g., term "eye opener") are not developmentally appropriate for children
      4) CAGE-AID (adapted to include drugs) adds "or drug use" to each question found in CAGE tool. May be used with adolescents.

Box 12.2

Situational Awareness

A. Situational awareness is needed to decrease a patient's risk when opioids/benzodiazepines are being administered.
   1. Is patient receiving a continuous opioid infusion?
      a. Knowledge that patient who appears sleepy or sedated 1 or 2 hours into opioid infusion will likely become more sedated as infusion continues
   2. Is this the first 24 hours receiving opioids, or is it nighttime?
      a. Monitor patient more frequently during first 24 hours and at night, when hypoventilation and nocturnal hypoxia is high risk.
   3. Is patient receiving authorized agent-controlled analgesia?
      a. A parent, spouse, or caregiver who believes it is best for patient to rest or sleep through pain may be more likely to push pain button even if patient is sleeping.
      b. More frequent assessments and interrogation of pump history and additional education may be needed.
   4. Is pulse oximetry the only monitor?
      a. Knowledge that a decrease in pulse oximetry is late indicator of respiratory depression
   5. What are institution's capabilities?
      a. When reading literature or participating in Listserv discussions, be knowledgeable of similarities and differences between your organization and other organizations. For example, if you would like to administer ketamine infusions on your pediatric medical/surgical floor similar to the way other organizations having published on this practice, you need to explore whether your institution has similar safeguards in place (e.g., central monitoring) to alert registered nurse to a problem, and/or appropriate nurse: patient ratio to allow for timely reassessment and intervention.
      b. Exercise caution when trying to generalize information about adult patients cared for in adult organizations through either published literature or Listserv discussions. Children are not little adults. Practices that may be more common in pediatrics differ from adult practices.
   6. Is this an infant or young child with no parent/caregiver at the bedside?
      a. A young child cannot function as their own advocate. They may even answer to the wrong name.

From T. DiMaggio

Opioid Risk Tool

This tool should be administered to patients upon an initial visit prior to beginning opioid therapy for pain management. A score of 3 or lower indicates low risk for future opioid abuse, a score of 4 to 7 indicates moderate risk for opioid abuse, and a score of 8 or higher indicates a high risk for opioid abuse.

Mark each box that applies	Female	Male
Family history of substance abuse		
Alcohol	1	3
Illegal drugs	2	3
Rx drugs	4	4
Personal history of substance abuse		
Alcohol	3	3
Illegal drugs	4	4
Rx drugs	5	5
Age between 16—45 years	1	1
History of preadolescent sexual abuse	3	0
Psychological disease		
ADD, OCD, bipolar, schizophrenia	2	2
Depression	1	1
Scoring totals		

Figure 12.14 Opioid Risk Tool. (From Webster L. R., & Webster R. [2005]. Predicting aberrant behaviors in opioid-treated patients: preliminary validation of the Opioid Risk Tool. *Pain Medicine, 6*[6], 432–442.)

Opioid Risk Tool for OUD (ORT-OUD)

This tool should be administered to patients upon an initial visit prior to beginning or continuing opioid therapy for pain management. A score of 2 or lower indicates low risk for future opioid use disorder; a score of >= 3 indicates high risk for opioid use disorder.

Mark each box that applies	YES	NO
Family history of substance abuse		
Alcohol	1	0
Illegal drugs	1	0
Rx drugs	1	0
Personal history of substance abuse		
Alcohol	1	0
Illegal drugs	1	0
Rx drugs	1	0
Age between 16-45 years	1	0
Psychological disease		
ADD, OCD, bipolar, schizophrenia	1	0
Depression	1	0
Scoring totals		

Figure 12.15 Opioid Risk Tool for Opioid Use Disorder (ORT-OUT). (From Cheatle, M. Compton, P. A., Dhingra, L., Wasser R., & O'Brien C. [2019]. Development of the Revised Opioid Risk Tool to predict opioid use disorder in patients with chronic non-malignant pain. *Journal of Pain, 20*[7], 842–851.)

e. CRAFFT (car, relax, alone, forget, friends, trouble)
   1) Brief behavioral health screening (not diagnostic) tool developed and validated for screening adolescents and young adults (12 to 21 years of age) for SUD
   2) Designed to determine whether further assessment and conversation around substance use and risks is needed
   3) Recommended by American Academy of Pediatrics' Committee on Substance Abuse and is the most well-studied adolescent substance use screening tool; has been validated in adolescents from diverse socioeconomic, racial, and ethnic backgrounds
   4) Available in clinician interview and self-administered versions
   5) CRAFFT 2.1 + N (Fig. 12.16) is updated version, includes vaping and marijuana edibles, and is available in many languages.
   6) Tool available from John R. Knight, MD, Boston Children's Hospital, 2020. Obtain permission from the Center for Adolescent Behavioral Research (CABHRe), Boston Children's Hospital. crafft@children's.harvard.edu, https://crafft.org.

The CRAFFT+N Questionnaire
To be completed by patient

Please answer all questions **honestly**; your answers will be kept **confidential**.

During the PAST 12 MONTHS, on how many days did you:

1. Drink more than a few sips of beer, wine, or any drink containing **alcohol**? Put "0" if none. *# of days*

2. Use any **marijuana** (cannabis, weed, oil, wax, or hash by smoking, vaping, dabbing, or in edibles) or "**synthetic marijuana**" (like "K2," "Spice")? Put "0" if none. *# of days*

3. Use **anything else to get high** (like other illegal drugs, pills, prescription or over-the-counter medications, and things that you sniff, huff, vape, or inject)? Put "0" if none. *# of days*

4. Use a **vaping device* containing nicotine and/or flavors**, or use any **tobacco products†**? Put "0" if none. *# of days*
   *Such as e-cigs, mods, pod devices like JUUL, disposable vapes like Puff Bar, vape pens, or e-hookahs. †Cigarettes, cigars, cigarillos, hookahs, chewing tobacco, snuff, snus, dissolvables, or nicotine pouches.

READ THESE INSTRUCTIONS BEFORE CONTINUING:
- **If you put "0" in ALL of the boxes above, ANSWER QUESTION 5 BELOW, THEN STOP.**
- **If you put "1" or more for** Questions 1, 2, or 3 **above, ANSWER QUESTIONS 5-10 BELOW.**
- **If you put "1" or more for** Question 4 **above, ANSWER ALL QUESTIONS ON BACK PAGE.**

Circle one

5. Have you ever ridden in a CAR driven by someone (including yourself) who was "high" or had been using alcohol or drugs? **No Yes**

6. Do you ever use alcohol or drugs to RELAX, feel better about yourself, or fit in? **No Yes**

7. Do you ever use alcohol or drugs while you are by yourself, or ALONE? **No Yes**

8. Do you ever FORGET things you did while using alcohol or drugs? **No Yes**

9. Do your FAMILY or FRIENDS ever tell you that you should cut down on your drinking or drug use? **No Yes**

10. Have you ever gotten into TROUBLE while you were using alcohol or drugs? **No Yes**

NOTICE TO CLINIC STAFF AND MEDICAL RECORDS:
The information on this page is protected by special federal confidentiality rules (42 CFR Part 2), which prohibit disclosure of this information unless authorized by specific written consent.

Figure 12.16 Craft 2.1+N Questionnaire. (From John R. Knight, MD, Boston Children's Hospital, 2020. Center for Adolescent Behavioral Research (CABHRe), Boston Children's Hospital, Boston, MA. crafft@children's.harvard.edu, https://crafft.org.)

   f. Screening, brief intervention, and referral to treatment (SBIRT)
     1) Recommended by U.S. Substance Abuse and Mental Health Services (SAMHSA) as option for screening for SUD in adolescents
     2) American Academy of Pediatrics (AAP) Committee on Substance Use and Prevention promotes use of SBIRT in primary care setting during routine medical appointments or when concerns arise:
       a) Wellness visit
       b) Hospital admission
       c) Emergency department visit
       d) Change in behavior, behavior different from that of baseline
       e) Unexplained behavior
       f) Altered mental status
       g) New-onset seizures
       h) Weight loss
       i) Prior to opioid/benzodiazepine/stimulant prescription
       j) Family history of substance abuse
       k) Skin abscesses
       l) Bacteremia

Bibliography

Abou Hammoud, H., Simon, N., Urien, S., Riou, B., Lechat, P., & Aubrun, F. (2009). Intravenous morphine titration in immediate postoperative pain management: Population kinetic-pharmacodynamic and logistic regression analysis. *Pain, 144*(1–2), 139–146. https://doi.org/10.1016/j.pain.2009.03.029.

American Academy of Pediatrics. (2014). Clinical Report: Recognition and management of iatrogenically induced opioid dependence and withdrawal in children. *Pediatrics, 133*(1), 152–155.

American Geriatrics Society Beers Criteria Update Expert Panel. (2019). American Geriatrics Society 2019 Updated AGS Beers Criteria for Potentially Inappropriate Medication Use in Older Adults. *Journal of the American Geriatrics Society, 67*(4), 674–694. https://doi.org/10.1111/jgs.15767.

American Psychiatric Association. (2013). *Diagnostic and Statistical Manual of Mental Disorders* (5th ed.). American Psychiatric Association.

Arroyo-Novoa, C., Figueroa-Ramos, M., & Puntillo, K. A. (2019). Opioid and Benzodiazepine Iatrogenic Withdrawal Syndrome in Patients in the Intensive Care Unit. *AACN Advances in Critical Care, 30*(4), 353–364. https://doi.org/10.4037/aacnacc2019267.

Baker, K., & Rodger, J. (2020). Assessing causes of alarm fatigue in long-term acute care and its impact on identifying clinical changes in patient conditions. *Informatics in Medicine Unlocked, 18*, 100300.

Blount, T., Painter, A., Freeman, E., Grossman, M., & Sutton, A. G. (2019). Reduction in length of stay and morphine use for NAS with the "Eat, Sleep, Console" method. *Hospital Pediatrics, 9*(8), 615–623. doi:10.1542/hpeds.2018–0238.

Booker, S. Q., Baker, T. A., Epps, F., Herr, K. A., Young, H. M., & Fishman, S. (2022). Interrupting biases in the experience and management of pan. *American Journal of Nursing, 122*(9), 48–54.

Burchum, J. R., & Rosenthal, L. D. (2019). *Lehne's Pharmacology for Nursing Care* (10th Ed.). St. Louis, MO: Elsevier.

Burchum, J. (2021). *Lehne's Pharmacology for Nursing Care* (10th Ed.). Elsevier.

Canter, M. O., Tanguturi, Y. C., Wilson, J. E., Williams, S. R., Exum, S. A., Umrania, H. M., Betters, K. A., Raman, R., Ely, E. W., Pandharipande, P. P., Fuchs, D. C., & Smith, H. A. B. Prospective validation of the preschool confusion assessment method for the ICU to screen for delirium in infants less than 6 months old. *Critical Care Medicine 49*(10):e902–e909.

Chua, K. P., Brummett, C. M., Conti, R. M., & Bohnert, A. S. (2021). Opioid prescribing to US children and young adults in 2019. *Pediatrics, 148*(3), e2021051539.

Chung, F., Yang, Y., & Liao, P. (2013). Predictive performance of the STOP-BANG score for identifying obstructive sleep apnea in obese patients. *Obes Surg, 23*(12), 2050–2057. doi:10.1007/s11695-013-1006-z.

Cooney, M., & Quinlan-Colwell, A. (2021). *Assessment and Multimodal Management of Pain: An Integrative Approach.* St. Louis: Elsevier.

Curley, M. A., Harris, S. K., Fraser, K. A., Johnson, R. A., & Arnold, J. H. (2006). State Behavioral Scale: A sedation assessment instrument for infants and young children supported on mechanical ventilation. *Pediatric Critical Care Medicine, 7*(2), 107–114.

Davis, C., Geik, C., Arthur, K., Fuller, J., Johnston, E., Levitt, F., Leung, E., McCart, G., McMichael, D., Painter, J., Staublin, T., & Walroth, T. (2017). A multisite retrospective study evaluating the implementation of the Pasero opioid-induced sedation scale (poss) and its effect on patient safety outcomes. *Pain Management Nursing, 18*, 193–201. https://dx.doi.org/10.1016/j.pmn.2017.03.006.

Duceppe, M. A., Perreault, M. M., Frenette, A. J., Burry, L. D., Rico, P., Lavoie, A., Gelinas, C., Mehta, S., Dagenais, M., & Williamson, D. R. (2019). Frequency, risk factors and symptomatology of iatrogenic withdrawal from opioids and benzodiazepines in critically ill neonates, children and adults: a systematic review of clinical studies. *Journal of Clinical Pharmacy & Therapeutics, 44*, 148–156. https://dx.doi.org/10.1111/jcpt.12787.

Dunwoody, D. R., & Jungquist, C. R. (2018). Sedation Scales: Do they capture the concept of opioid induced sedation? *Nursing Forum, 53*(4), 399–405.

Dunwoody, D., Jungquist, C., Chang, Y., & Dickerson, S. (2018). The common meanings and shared practices of sedation assessment in the context of managing patients with an opioid: A phenomenological study. *Journal of Clinical Nursing, 28*, 104–115. https://doi.org/10.1111/jocn.14672.

Dunwoody, D. R., & Jungquist, C. R. (2020). Opioid-induced sedation and respiratory depression: Are sedation scales enough to prevent adverse drug events post-operatively? *Pain Management Nursing.* doi:10.1016/j.pmn.2018.09.009.

ECRI Institute. (2020). Evaluation background: Monitors for detecting respiratory depression-recommended for patients on opioids. https://www.ecri.org/search-results/member-preview/hdjournal/pages/eval-background-monitors-respiratory-depression. Accessed May 11, 2022.

ECRI Institute. (2017). *ECRI Institute PSO Deep Dive Opioid Use in Acute Care.* Plymouth Meeting, PA: ECRI Institute.

Food and Drug Administration. (2017). FDA restricts use of prescription codeine pain and cough medicines and tramadol pain medicines in children; recommends against use in breastfeeding women. Available at: https://www.fda.gov/downloads/Drugs/DrugSafety/UCM553814.pdf. Accessed January 2, 2021.

Franck, S. L., Harris, K. S, Soetenga, J. D., Amling, K. J., & Curley, M. (2008). The Withdrawal Assessment Tool -Version 1 (WAT-1): An assessment instrument for monitoring opioid and benzodiazepine withdrawal symptoms in pediatric patients. *Pediatric Critical Care Medicine, 9*(6), 573–580. (Classic reference).

Franck, S. L., Scoppettuolo, L. A., Wypij, D., & Curley, M. (2012). Validity and generalizability of the Withdrawal Assessment Tool-1 (WAT-1) for monitoring iatrogenic withdrawal syndrome in pediatric patients. *International Association for the Study of Pain, 153*(1), 142–148.

Galinkin, J., & Koh, J. L. Committee on Drugs, Section on Anesthesiology and Pain Medicine, American Academy of Pediatrics. (2014). Recognition and management of iatrogenically induced opioid dependence and withdrawal in children. *Pediatrics, 133*, 152–155. https://dx.doi.org/10.1542/peds.2013-3398.

Garcia, M. G., & McMullan, T. W. (2019). Pasero opioid-induced sedation scale in a pediatric surgical ward: a quality improvement project. *Journal of Pediatric Surgical Nursing, 8*(2), 29.

Glicksman, A., DeMaria, R., Mauer, E., Joyce, C., Gerber, L., Greenwald, B., Silver, G., & Traube, C. (2016). Validity of the Richmond Agitation-Sedation Scale (RASS) in critically ill children. *Journal of Intensive Care, 4*(65), 1–6. doi:10.1186/s40560-016-0189-5.

Grossman, M. R., Lipshaw, M. J., Osborn, R. R., & Berkwitt, A. K. (2018). A novel approach to assessing infants with neonatal abstinence syndrome. *Hosp. Pediatrics, 8*(1), 1–6. doi:10.1542/hpeds.2017–2018.

Holly, C., Porter, S., Echevarria, M., Dreker, M., & Ruzehaji, S. (2018). Recognizing delirium in hospitalized children: A systematic review of the evidence on risk factors and characteristics. *American Journal of Nursing, 118*(4), 24–37.

Institute for Healthcare Improvement (IHI). (2019). Advancing the safety of acute pain management. Boston, Massachusetts: Available on ihi.org.

Ista, E., van Beusekom, B., van Rosmalen, J., Kneyber, M. C., Lemson, J., Brouwers, A., Dieleman, G. C., Dierckx, B., de Hoog, M., Tibboel, & van Dijk, M. (2018). Validation of the SOS-PD scale for assessment of pediatric delirium: A multicenter study. *Critical Care, 22*(1), 1–11. doi:10.1186/s13054-018-2238-z.

Jungquist, C. R., Correll, D. J., Fleisher, L. A., Gross, J., Gupta, R., Pasero, C., Stoelting, R., & Polomano, R. (2016). Avoiding adverse events secondary to opioid-induced respiratory depression: implications for nurse executives and patient safety. *Journal of Nursing Administration, 46*, 87–94. https://dx.doi.org/10.1097/NNA.0000000000000301.

Jungquist, C. R., Pasero, C., Tripoli, N. M., Gorodetsky, R., Metersky, M., & Polomano, R. C. (2014). Instituting best practice for monitoring for opioid-induced advancing sedation in hospitalized patients. *Worldviews Evid Based Nurs, 11*(6), 350–360. doi:10.1111/wvn.12061.

Junquist, C. R., Quinlan-Colwell, A., Vallerand, A., Carlisle, H. L., Cooney, M., Dempsey, S. J., Dunwoody, D., Maly, A., Meloche,

K., Meyers, A., Sawyer, J., Singh, N., Sullivan, D., Watson, C., & Polomano, R. (2020). American Society for Pain Management Nursing guidelines on monitoring for opioid-induced sedation and respiratory depression: Revisions. *Pain Management Nursing, 21*(1), 7–25.

Jungquist, C. R., Smith, K., Nicely, K. L., & Polomano, R. C. (2017). Monitoring hospitalized adult patients for opioid-induced sedation and respiratory depression. *American Journal of Nursing, 117*(3 Suppl 1), S27–S35. doi:10.1097/01.NAJ.0000513528.79557.33.

Jungquist, C. R., Willens, J. S., Dunwoody, D. R., Klingman, K. J., & Polomano, R. C. (2014). Monitoring for opioid-induced advancing sedation and respiratory depression: ASPMN membership survey of current practice. *Pain Management Nursing, 15*(3), 682–693. doi:10.1016/j.pmn.2013.12.001.

Kaur, S., Silver, G., Samuels, S., Rosen, A. H., Weiss, M., Mauer, E. A., Gerber, L. M., Greenwald, B. M., & Traube, C. (2020). *Pediatric Critical Care Medicine, 21*(5), 409–414. doi:10.1097/PCC.0000000000002248.

Knight, J. R., Shier, L. A., Bravender, T. D., Farrell, M., Vander Bilt, J., & Shaffer, H. J. (1999). A new brief screen for adolescents substance abuse. *Arch Pediatrics & Adolescent Medicine, 153*(6), 591–596.

LaRosa, J. M., & Aponte-Patel, L. (2019). Iatrogenic Withdrawal Syndrome: A Review of Pathophysiology, Prevention, and Treatment. *Current Pediatrics Reports, 7*, 12–19. https://doi.org/10.1007/s40124-019-00187-4.

Lewandowska, K., Weisbrot, M., Cieloszyk, A., Mędrzycka-Dąbrowska, W., Krupa, S., & Ozga, D. (2020). Impact of alarm fatigue on the work of nurses in an intensive care Environment: A systematic review. *International Journal of Environmental Research and Public Health, 17*(22), 8409.

Malviya, S., Voepel-Lewis, T., Tait, A. R., Merkel, S., Tremper, K., & Naughton, N. (2002). Depth of sedation in children undergoing computed tomography: Validity and reliability of the University of Michigan Sedation Scale (UMSS). *British Journal of Anaesthesia, 88*(2), 241–245.

McCabe, S. E., West, B. T., & Boyd, C. J. (2013). Leftover prescription opioids and nonmedical use among high school seniors: A multi-cohort national study. *Journal of Adolescent Health, 52*(4), 480–485.

Mehta, J. H., Harvey, B. C., Grewal, N. K., & George, E. E. (2017). The relationship between minute ventilation and end tidal CO_2 in intubated and spontaneously breathing patients undergoing procedural sedation. *PloS One, 12*(6), e0180187. doi:10.1371/journal.pone.0180187.

Miech, R., Johnston, L., O'Malley, P. M., Keyes, K. M., & Heard, K. (2015). Prescription opioids in adolescence and future opioid misuse. *Pediatrics, 136*(5), e1169–e1177. doi:10.1542/peds.2015–1364.

Mulkey, M. A., Roberson, D. W., Everhart, D. E., & Hardin, S. R. (2018). Choosing the right delirium assessment tool. *Journal of Neuroscience Nursing, 50*(6), 343–348.

National Institute on Drug Abuse (NIDA). (2021). Drug overdoses in youth. Retrieved from https://teens.drugabuse.gov/drug-facts/drug-overdoses-youth on 2022, January 5 https://nida.nih.gov/drug-topics.

National Institutes of Health (NIH). (2021). Health Literacy. https://www.nih.gov/institutes-nih/nih-office-director/office-communications-public-liaison/clear-communication/health-literacy. Accessed May 14, 2022.

Paul, A. K., Smith, C. M., Rahmatullah, M., Nissapatorn, V., Wilairatana, P., Spetea, M., Gueven, N., & Dietis, N. (2021).

Opioid analgesia and opioid-induced adverse effects: a review. *Pharmaceuticals, 14*(11), 1091. https://dx.doi.org/10.3390/ph14111091.

Quinlan-Colwell, A., Rae, D., & Drew, D. (2022). Prescribing and Administering Opioid Doses Based Solely on Pain Intensity: Update of A Position Statement by the American Society for Pain Management Nursing. *Pain Management Nursing, 23*(1), 68–75.

Quinlan-Colwell, A., Thear, G., Miller-Baldwin, E., & Smith, A. (2017). Use of the Pasero opioid-induced sedation scale (POSS) in pediatric patients. *Journal of Pediatric Nursing, 33*(3), 83–87. doi:10.1016/j.pedn.2017.01.006.

Quinn, P. D., Fine, K. L., Rickert, M. E., et al. (2020). Association of opioid prescription initiation during adolescence and young adulthood with subsequent substance-related morbidity. *JAMA Pediatrics, 174*(11), 1048–1055.

Ramachandran, S. K., Pandit, J., Devine, S., Thompson, A., & Shanks, A. (2017). Postoperative Respiratory Complications in Patients at Risk for Obstructive Sleep Apnea: A Single-Institution Cohort Study. *Anesthesia and Analgesia, 125*(1), 272–279. doi:10.1213/ANE.0000000000002132.

Redeimeier, D., Ruff, C. C., & Tobler, P. N. (2016). Cognitive biases associated with medical decisions: A systematic review. *BMC Medical Informatics and Decision Making, 16*, 138. doi:10.1186/S12911-016-0377-1.

Schondelmeyer, A. C., Brady, P. W., Goel, V. V., Cvach, M., Blake, N., Mangeot, C., & Bonafide, C. P. (2018). Physiologic monitor alarm rates at 5 children's hospitals. *Journal of Hospital Medicine, 13*(6), 396–398.

Sessler, C. N., Gosnell, M. S., Grap, M. J., Brophy, G. M., O'Neal, P. V., & Keane, K. A. (2002). The Richmond Agitation Sedation Scale: Validity and reliability in adult intensive care patients. *American Journal of Respiratory and Clinical Care Medicine, 166*(10), 1338–1344.

Smith, H. A., Williams, S., Griffith, K., & Fuchs, C. (2021). *Critical Illness, Brain Dysfunction, and Survivorship Center.* Vanderbilt University Medical Center. Retrieved December 5, 2021 from https://www.icudelirium.org/medical-professionals/pediatric-care.

Smith, H. A. B., Besunder, J. B., Betters, K. A., Johnson, P. N., Srinivasan, V., Stormorken, A., Farrington, E., Golianu, B., Godshall, A. J., Acinelli, L., Almgren, C., Bailey, C. H., Boyd, J. M., Cisco, M. J., Damian, M., deAlmeida, M. L., Fehr, J., Fenton, K. E., Gilliland, F., Grant, M. J. C., Howell, J., Ruggles, C. A., Simone, S., Su, F., Sullivan, J. E., Tegtmeyer, K., Traube, C., Williams, S., & Berkenbosch, J. W. (2022). 2022 society of critical care medicine clinical practice guidelines on prevention and management of pain, agitation, neuromuscular blockade, and delirium in critically Ill pediatric patients with consideration of the ICU environment and early mobility.

Pediatric Critical Care Medicine: A Journal of the Society of Critical Care Medicine and the World Federation of Pediatric Intensive and Critical Care Societies, 23(2):e74–e110.

Smith, H. A. B., Gangopadhyay, M., Goben, C. M., Jacobowski, N. L., Chestnut, M. H., Savage, S., Rutherford, M. T., Denton, D., Thompson, J. L., Chandrasekhar, R., Acton, M., Newman, J., Noori, H. P., Terrell, M. K., Williams, S. R., Griffith, K., Cooper, T. J., Ely, E. W., Fuchs, D. C., & Pandharipande, P. P. (2016). The preschool confusion assessment method for the ICU: valid and reliable delirium monitoring for critically Ill infants and children. *Critical Care Medicine, 44*(3):592–600. PMID: 26565631 PMCID: PMC4764386.

Smith, H. A. B., Gangopadhyay, M., Goben, C. M., Jacobowski, N. L., Chestnut, M. H., Thompson, J. L., Chandrasekhar, R., Williams, S. R., Griffith, K, Ely, E. W., Fuchs, D. C., & Pandharipande, P. P. (2017). Delirium and benzodiazepines associated with prolonged ICU stay in critically Ill infants and young children. *Critical Care Medicine, 45*(9):1427–1435.

Substance Abuse and Mental Health Services Administration. (2020). *Key substance use and mental health indicators in the United States: Results from the 2019 National Survey on Drug Use and Health.* Rockville, MD: Center for Behavioral Health Statistics and Quality.

Substance Abuse and Mental Health Services Administration. (2019). *Substance misuse prevention for young adults. Publication No PEP19-PL-Guide-1.* Rockville, MD: National Mental Health and Substance Use Policy Laboratory. Substance Abuse and Mental Health Services Administration.

Sullivan, J. T., Sykora, K., Schneiderman, J., Naranjo, C. A., & Sellers, E. M. (1989). Assessment of alcohol withdrawal: The revised Clinical Institute Withdrawal Assessment for alcohol scale (CIWA-Ar). *British Journal of Addiction, 84*, 1353–1357.

Traube, C., Silver, G., Kearney, J., Patel, A., Atkinson, T. M., Yoon, M. J., Halpert, S., Augenstein, J., Sickles, L. E., Li, C., & Greenwald, B. (2014). Cornell Assessment of Pediatric Delirium: A valid, rapid, observational tool for screening delirium in the PICU. *Pediatric Critical Care Medicine, 42*(3), 656–663. doi:10.1097/CCM.0b013e3182a66b76.

Weeks, K., Timalonis, J., & Donovan, L. (2021). Does alarm fatigue start in nursing school? *Nursing, 51*(5), 59–63.

Weingarten, T. N., Warner, L. L., & Sprung, J. (2017). Timing of postoperative respiratory emergencies: when do they really occur? *Curr Opin Anaesthesiol, 30*(1), 156–162. doi:10.1097/ACO.0000000000000401.

Williams, M., McKeown, A., Dexter, F., Miner, J. R., Sessler, D. L., & Vargo, J. (2016). Efficacy outcome measures for procedural sedation clinical trials in adults: An ACTTION systematic review. *Anesthesia & Analgesia, 122*(1), 152–170.

CHAPTER 13

Intrapersonal Relationships/Influences of Emotions, Sleep, Fatigue, Nutrition, Obesity, and Eating Disorders With Pain

Ann Quinlan-Colwell, PhD MSN
Ann Schreier, PhD, BSN, MSN, RN*

Introduction

The intrapersonal influences of emotions, fatigue, sleep, nutrition, obesity, and eating disorders affect the perception, experience, and management of pain. They contribute to pain being the unique experience that is whatever the experiencing person says it is. Considering these factors in a holistic multimodal pain management plan is important to individualized care. Since patients do not commonly consider these influences as being related to their pain experience, it is important for clinicians to be aware of relationships with pain and to assess for various influences. A sampling of recognized tools to assess each situation is offered. Several studies are discussed with references provided at the end of the chapter; however, many involve small numbers of subjects, and more work is needed.

I. Terminology/Definitions

A. **Anger:** "emotional reaction characterized by extreme displeasure, rage, indignation, or hostility… vary widely among individuals and cultures" (O'Toole, p. 97)

B. **Body mass index (BMI):** calculation of height and body mass in which mass in kilograms is divided by height in meters squared and reported as kg/m^2

C. **Eating disorders:** "group of behaviors often fueled by unresolved emotional conflicts symptomized by altered food consumption" (O'Toole, p. 279) and include anorexia nervosa, binge eating, bulimia nervosa, compulsive eating, and dysorexia

D. **Emotion:** "outward expression or display of mood or feeling states" (O'Toole, p. 279)

E. **Emotional intelligence:** "ability to monitor one's own and others' feelings and emotions, to discriminate among them and use this information to guide one's thinking and actions" (Salovey & Mayer, p. 189)

F. **Emotion regulation:** process (automatic and controlled) through which experience, strength, and duration of emotions are initiated, maintained, influenced, modified, and controlled

G. **Emotional stability:** ability to address and cope with negativity including fear, anger, sadness, stress, and anxiety; strongly correlated with positive mental health

H. **Fatigue:** "state of exhaustion or loss of strength or endurance such as may follow strenuous exercise; emotional state associated with extreme or extended exposure to psychic pressure" (O'Toole, p. 279)

I. **Fear:** unpleasant feeling stimulated in response to perceived threats of harm or of impending danger

J. **Fear avoidance model:** within a psychosocial context, fear of pain is addressed either through confrontation or avoidance

K. **Fear conditioning:** through repeated association of noxious stimulus (e.g., electrical shock) with neutral stimulus (e.g., red light) resulting in conditioned neutral stimulus (e.g., red light) alone eliciting fear

L. **Fear extinction:** when conditioned stimulus is continually produced alone with eventual extinction of associated fear response (see fear conditioning above)

M. **Fear generalization:** adaptive capacity to use information from one negative, harmful, painful experience and then attribute and use it with other experiences perceived to be hostile; is an adaptive quality unless applied to situations that are in fact safe

N. **Glymphatic system:** glial-dependent brain pathway that clears and drains waste through system including cerebrospinal fluid to meningeal lymphatic system

O. **Happiness:** considered from most general perspective, refers to totality of various valuations made in relation to environment, life circumstances, individual self, or combination; shares constructs with *subjective well-being* and *quality of life*

P. **High-impact chronic (persistent) pain:** relatively new concept and integrates pain duration with degree of

---

disability to describe pain that more dramatically impacts the experiencing person cognitively, with functionality and quality of life

Q. **Interoception:** process through which internal body sensations continually flow in map-like form with delivery to nervous system where they are recognized, interpreted, and processed with influence upon feelings, urges, and other emotional responses; involvement of process has been identified with emotions, pain, and eating disorders

R. **Interoceptive sensitivity:** sensitivity to internal states with great variability among people; impacts variety of processes including emotions and is associated with psychological disorders including eating disorders

S. **Joy:** considered distinct positive emotion or emotional state correlated with personal perception of well-being and response to something good

T. **Modulation:** process by which pain intensity is either increased or decreased; pain perception can be decreased when neurotransmitters are released in descending pain pathway

U. **Negative emotionality:** proclivity to be easily and rapidly aroused (opposite of emotional stability)

V. **Nutrition:** aggregate of processes comprising intake, assimilation, and utilization of nourishing food to maintain body function and health

W. **Operant conditioning:** method of changing behaviors through use of rewards (for desired behaviors) and punishments (for undesired behaviors)

X. **Optimism:** trait of having positive expectations regarding what will occur

Y. **Pessimism:** negative outlook or propensity in which unwanted, bad, or worst consequences are expected to result with no hope for improvement

Z. **Physiology:** scientific focus on interactions, functions, and regulations within body that contribute to ability of body to regulate internal environment

AA. **Positive affect:** umbrella term that includes positive moods and emotions that facilitate positive behaviors and feelings of relaxation, happiness, and joy but not future focused optimism

BB. **Sadness:** an emotion that reflects feeling in response to loss or grief

CC. **Sleep:** "state marked by reduced consciousness, diminished activity of the skeletal muscles and depressed metabolism" (O'Toole, p. 279)

DD. **Social pain:** an unlikable experience connected with actual or perceived rejection, loss, negative assessment, and exclusion leading to social disconnection

EE. **State:** from psychological perspective, refers to transient way of responding to particular situation; used with anger, anxiety, joy, gratitude, and other emotions

FF. **Trait:** from psychological perspective, refers to dispositional characteristic and inclination to

generally feel, think, and respond in a particular way in variety of different situations; used with anger, anxiety, joy, gratitude, and other emotions

GG. **Well-being:** positive psychological resources in combination with absence of any mental disorder

II. Emotions

A. Emotion as concept
  1. Although emotions have been identified and studied for centuries, specific understanding of what they are and how they function remains speculative.
    a. Traditionally, emotions are intricate, multidimensional, dynamic, affective appraisals of or adaptive responses to either internal or external situations, processes, or phenomena experienced in a conscious, subjective manner. More recently, the idea that emotions can be experienced in unconscious states is being considered and studied.
    b. With each emotion, there are numerous manifestations including physiological, neural, conscious, cognitive, behavioral, and/or expressive. There is also attention to personal well-being.
    c. As with pain, emotions are influenced by culture, past experiences, beliefs, and expectations.
  2. Emotions can be considered from two facets.
    a. *Valence:* either negative or positive
    b. *Intensity:* reflects potency or forcefulness with which emotion is experienced
  3. It has been suggested that to qualify as an emotion, the following four elements are necessary:
    a. Evolutionary or phylogenetic function such as alerting to prevent danger as occurs with fear
    b. Antecedent conditions initiating emotion as occurs when expectations are not met and anger ensues
    c. Consequent conditions are quantifiable actions that satisfy antecedent condition, such as removing oneself from perceived danger when sensing fear.
    d. Circuitry in brain is specific and able to reconcile antecedent and consequent conditions, as seen in four classic emotions of anger, fear, joy, and sadness.
  4. Distinguishing emotions from moods
    a. Emotions are distinguished from moods (see Chapter 3) in that emotions are characterized by defining characteristics noted above and result from recognizable antecedent or cognition.
    b. Although emotions can exist as either a state experience or trait within a person, compared

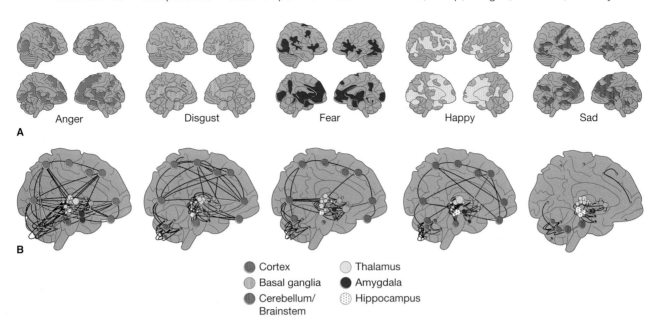

Figure 13.1 Neurocircuitry of basic emotions. (A) Lateral and medial views of the unique and prototypical representation of sadness in comparison to other basic emotions across multiple brain regions, including those associated to Salience (e.g., anterior cingulate and insula), Default Mode (e.g., medial prefrontal and hippocampus), Frontoparietal (e.g., lateral prefrontal and dorsal anterior cingulate), and Visceromotor (e.g., cerebellum/brainstem) systems. (B) Connectional profiles associated to each emotion category in anatomical space of the brain. The nodes (circles) are regions or networks, color-coded by anatomical system. The edges (lines) reflect co-activation between pairs of regions or networks. The size of each circle reflects its betweenness-centrality, a measure of how strongly it connects disparate networks. One location is depicted for each cortical network for visualization purposes, though the networks were distributed across regions (see A). Compared to other emotions, sadness involves largely isolated brain networks, with large-scale connectivity among major systems essentially lacking. Specifically, sadness includes dramatically reduced connectivity within the cortex, and between cortical and subcortical systems, while connectivity within cerebellar/brainstem systems seems rather exaggerated. These network functional patterns seemingly link sadness to a neurocognitive profile inclined/biased towards interoceptive and homeostatic information processing. (Reprinted from PLoS Publishing: *PLoS Computational Biology.*)

to moods, they exhibit as more episodic and transient rather than the persistent and pervasive nature of moods.

5. Emotions are similar to pain in a number of ways.
   a. Emotional experience is always unique and dependent upon understanding what is felt within distinct perceptual construct of each person.
   b. Emotional response to an event is dependent upon perception, evaluation, and subsequent meaning of event by experiencing person.
   c. Gold standard for assessing and measuring emotions is self-report by person.
   d. Emotions are strongly impacted by cultural influences affecting person. These qualities are seen in circumstances eliciting emotion, emotional behavior, and intensity of emotional response.

B. Classifications of emotions
   1. Emotions can be classified as either dimensions or categories, or a mix of the two.
   2. Dimensions of emotions
      a. Valence is inkling to sentiment or feeling being either positive or negative.
      b. Arousal is degree or intensity of provocation or excitement regarding sensation or feeling.
      c. Dominance is degree of control or mediation exerted upon feeling or sentiment.
   3. Categories of emotions
      a. Joy or happiness
      b. Sadness
      c. Fear
      d. Anger
C. Emotion physiology (Fig. 13.1)
   1. Interconnectedness of emotion and physical manifestations have long history of investigation, yet

body of scientific research in physiology of emotions is relatively meager.

2. From somatic perspective, each of six common emotions (anger, disgust, fear, happiness, sadness, and surprise) is associated with particular and universal facial expressions.

3. Use of functional magnetic resonance imaging (fMRI) to investigate human emotion is increasing. However, a potential confounder is the emotions (e.g., fear) possibly elicited by undergoing the scanning experience itself, thus confounding results.

4. Even though regions of the brain where emotions are processed are known, there is no specific process identified for emotions akin to nociception with pain.

5. Circumstances stimulating an emotion are processed by amygdala, parahippocampal gyrus, and ventromedial prefrontal cortex. Together, they form an *emotional generative network,* with prefrontal cortex being site of emotion regulation.
   a. Independent of higher brain structures, amygdala is associated with perception and housing of emotions and associated responses.
   b. Limbic system, neocortical hippocampus, and amygdala also have been identified in emotional processing.

6. There is no evidence specific to autonomic nervous system changes (e.g., pulse, respirations, blood pressure) occurring consistently when any particular emotion is experienced. Of note, however, respiratory patterns are generally affected by emotional experiences.

D. Relationship between emotion and pain
1. Emotions, particularly negative emotions, are part of affective component of pain experiences. Emotions and pain are bidirectional and impact each other.

2. Since pain tends to provoke negative emotions, it is suggested promoting positive emotions can be analgesic and using positive interventions can be beneficial in managing pain.

3. Emotions and pain are both coded in several cerebral areas including insula, limbic structures, cortical sites, amygdala, and cingulate cortices of brain. These regions are also involved with interoceptive processing.

4. Eisenberger described neurological association involving anterior insula and dorsal anterior cingulate cortex with both physical and social pain experiences

5. Universal facial expressions associated with core or basic emotions are closely aligned with most behavioral assessment tools used to assess pain in patients who are unable to self-report pain.

E. Emotional intelligence
1. During early part of 20th century, emotional intelligence (EI) was originally discussed as a subsection of social intelligence, which is understanding and interacting with other people in relationships. Subsequently, EI was defined as a separate concept (see Fig. 13.2).

2. EI includes being aware of, monitoring, understanding, and managing emotional experiences; controlling emotional impulses; having empathy; and being persistent, motivated, and socially deft.

3. High EI levels are associated with stronger physical and psychological health.

4. Investigation into relationship between EI and pain is in preliminary stages with associations involving:
   a. Relationship between EI among people experiencing variety of persistent pain conditions including fibromyalgia, osteoarthritis (OA), adolescents, and those with comorbid alcohol dependence
   b. Greater EI as predictor of lower reports of acute pain
   c. EI possibly having mediating effect on acute and persistent pain
   d. Relationship of EI with perception and management of emotions

5. Implications for pain management
   a. *Measurement*: could be included in pain assessment to potentially understand and predict pain experiences better
   b. *Research*: needed to further explore potential benefits of improving EI among people living with persistent pain
   c. *Interventions*: from perspective that EI is an ability that can be refined, techniques to hone and improve it can be taught as part of multimodal pain management care

F. Emotion regulation (ER)
1. Although considered separate concept from EI, ER is also discussed as strategy for modifying emotions and improving EI.

2. Specific guidelines for using ER are determined by individual goals of ER.

3. Among other factors is some evidence that adverse childhood experiences (ACEs) may limit ability to regulate negative emotions. Recent study reported ACEs were correlated with impaired ability to regulate negative emotions among women with persistent pain leading to increased opioid use disorder.

4. Process to improve ER and consequently EI involves strategies including:
   a. Situation selection: identifying and/or avoiding potentially negative situations (e.g., avoiding congested routes)
   b. Situation modification: modifying what is occurring (e.g., changing topic of conversation)
   c. Attentional deployment: intentionally changing focus to modify emotion such as through

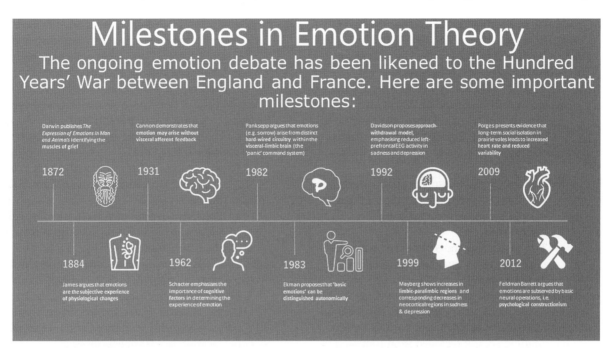

Figure 13.2 A brief history of emotion theory with implications for sadness. (From Arias, J. A., Williams, C., Raghvani, R., Aghajani, M., Baez, S., Belzung, C., et al. (2020). The neuroscience of sadness: A multidisciplinary synthesis and collaborative review. Neuroscience & Biobehavioral Reviews, 111, 199–228.)

distraction (e.g., redirecting focus to background music)

  d. Cognitive change or reappraisal: reframing what a situation means (e.g., perceiving being terminated as opportunity for new adventure)

  e. Response modulation: regulating response to emotion experienced (e.g., suppressing nervous laughter)

5. Relationship between ER and pain is an area in which research is needed; however, preliminary research indicates patients living with persistent pain who learn ER techniques may be able to lessen some negative aspects of their persistent pain. Cognitive-behavioral therapy (CBT) and self-hypnosis have been used successfully to assist people living with persistent pain who are learning emotional restructuring.

G. Emotional intelligence assessment tools

1. *Mayer-Salovey-Caruso Emotional Intelligence Test (MSCEIT):* measures EI as an ability

2. *Trait Meta-Mood Scale (TMMS):* measures subjective attitudes and beliefs about emotional experience of individual

3. *Emotional Intelligence Questionnaire (TEIQue-SF):* measures EI as personality trait through self-report

4. *Bar-On Emotional Intelligence Inventory (EQ-i):* self-report of emotional and social behavior providing estimate of emotional-social intelligence

H. Happiness, joyfulness, gratitude, and optimism

1. Concept description

  a. Since happiness and joy are often used interchangeably, they will each be explored as positive emotion in relation to pain.

  b. Because dispositional gratitude and optimism are qualities related to both happiness and joy, they will also be explored in relation to pain.

2. **Joy** is considered a distinct positive emotion or emotional state correlated with personal perception of well-being and response to something good.

  a. Not all pleasurable experiences elicit joy, rather, joy is generally experienced when something desired is achieved or fulfilled. Joy is likely to be experienced when a diagnosis is given that "no cancer was detected."

  b. Since appraisal of experience is subjective within conceptual framework of an individual, not everyone responds to the same experience with joy.

  c. Related to discussion of joy as an emotion are concepts of happiness, dispositional gratitude, and optimism

  d. Like anxiety and anger, joy can be perceived as either state joy or trait joy.

    1) Joy can be experienced solely in response to a particular event (state joy).

    2) Joy can be experienced as a basic tenet when a person experiences life joyfully (trait joy).

3. **Happiness,** considered from the most general perspective, refers to totality of various valuations made

in relation to environment, life circumstances, self, or a combination dependent on subjective cognitive and emotional criteria determined by an individual.

   a. A positive affect that is not specific

   b. Concept of happiness shares constructs with subjective well-being and quality of life.

     1) Throughout history, humans have strived to achieve health, financial status, and human connection as paths to happiness—their optimal goal.

     2) Ancient Greek philosophers conceptualized happiness as a person satisfying their particular human needs and realizing their capabilities.

     3) Two personality traits associated with happiness are optimism and having an internal locus of control.

4. **Dispositional gratitude** is global propensity to acknowledge, focus on, appreciate, and be thankful for positive actions of others and positive aspects of life. Gratitude is also regarded from trait- and state-specific perspectives.

5. **Optimism** is considered an important coping factor during stressful situations when used to positively interpret situations and have positive expectations.

   a. Generally associated with good physical health, enhanced immunity, and low all-cause mortality

   b. Likely correlated to buffering effect resulting from addressing health challenges and other adversities using positive coping and problem-solving

   c. Correlated with lower pain sensitivity and ability to cope with persistent pain

   d. As with other emotions, optimism can be either state or trait. When trait, it is often referred to as *dispositional optimism*.

   e. Authors of a 15-study meta-analysis reported significant association between optimism and lower risk for cardiovascular events and all-cause mortality. Authors noted optimism is associated with healthy lifestyles, including quality dietary choices and consistent physical exercise, which are important components of multimodal approach to managing pain.

6. Physiological aspects of joy, happiness, gratitude, and optimism are not well understood because there is little research.

   a. Electroencephalogram (EEG) peaks noted with happiness, compared with anger, have been correlated with improved cardiac function.

   b. Joy is associated with enhanced visual perception and easier body movement.

   c. Optimism is reported to be inversely related to cortisol levels (high optimism correlating with lower cortisol levels). Also reported to have important positive effect with hypothalamic-pituitary-adrenal axis, autonomic nervous system, immune system, and circadian rhythm regulation.

7. Relationship of these positive emotions and constructs to pain is not well researched.

   a. Often, relationship between joy and pain is considered reciprocal.

     1) Most common link seen between them is joy is experienced when pain or threat of pain is removed.

     2) Possible correlation between trait joy with perception and pain self-management warrants investigation.

   b. Some neuroimaging indicated positive affect on pain has physiologic basis in central pain modulation network including anterior cingulate cortex, bilateral insula, and left orbital frontal cortex along with spinal mediation. From this perspective, it is feasible positive affect not only contributes to positive adaptation to persistent pain but to actually modulating pain experiences.

   c. Dispositional gratitude is positively correlated with increased well-being (both physical and psychological), self-efficacy, happiness, quality of sleep, and reduced pain. Conversely, dispositional gratitude is negatively correlated with depression and general anxiety.

   d. Dispositional optimism is associated with lower pain sensitivity.

     1) As with relationship between optimism and general health, optimism is considered protective with both acute and persistent pain.

     2) In part, this is likely related to having positive expectations about what will occur next.

     3) Another effect of optimism is it is protective against pain catastrophizing and hypervigilance of negative messages.

   e. Authors of a systematic review assessing how optimism is related to pain experiences reported positive correlation between optimism and pain in majority (70%) of studies with participants experiencing variety of clinical and experimental pain situations. One experimental study involved university students who performed a cold pressor task with half participating in optimism-inducing exercise ("best possible self"). Students who participated in optimism-inducing exercise reported less pain unrelated to their pain expectations.

8. Assessment tools

   a. Happiness assessment tools

     1) Oxford Happiness Questionnaire (OHQ)

2) World Health Organization Quality of Life Questionnaire
3) Satisfaction with Life Scale
4) Positive and Negative Affect Scale
5) State Optimism Measure
   b. Joy assessment tools
1) State Joy Scale (SJS)
2) Dispositional Joy Scale (DJS)
3) Assessment of facial expressions using computer software
   c. Optimism
1) Life Orientation Test-Revised (LOT-R)
2) Minnesota Multiphasic Personality Inventory
3) Questionnaire for Future Expectations (FEX)
4) State Optimism Measure (SOM)
   d. Gratitude assessment tools
1) Gratitude Questionnaire 6 (GQ-6)
2) The Multi-Component Gratitude Measure
9. Implications for pain management
   a. Researchers compared effect on pain levels of people living with chronic spinal cord injury pain when individualized personal positive psychology exercises with mindful writing about life occurrences were completed. In randomized parallel-group controlled study, participants in positive exercise group were noted to have statistically significant less pain at 3-month follow-up.
   b. Research is needed to explore potential benefits of using positive emotions and affect to improve management of persistent pain.
10. Interventions
   a. Neither pharmacological nor nonpharmacological interventions are needed as treatment for joy, happiness, dispositional gratitude, or optimism. However, therapies to achieve or enhance these positive emotions may be prescribed as treatment for persistent pain that interferes with being able to experience them.
   b. CBT can be used to reframe perception of situations to increase optimism and gratitude, ideally leading to greater happiness and joy.
   c. Mindfulness has been used as a positive psychology intervention to improve happiness and vanquish suffering.
   d. Spending time in nature is gaining increased attention for improving happiness and quality of life.
   e. Yoga is traditionally considered a practice and philosophy through which ultimate joy can be attained.
   f. A consistently successful intervention for inducing optimism is "best possible self" exercise that can be practiced daily. Although there

are variations of intervention, one example consists of focusing on best possible self for 1 minute; then writing about this for 15 minutes; then imagining what was written for 5 minutes.
   g. CBT, meditation, mindfulness, guided or Internet interventions, and psychodrama have been used to enhance optimism and gratitude.
I. Sadness (Fig. 13.2)
   1. Concept description
      a. Sadness is difficult to define because of the intricate psychobiological nature.
1) As with pain and joy, it is purely subjective and best defined by the experiencing person.
2) It is a common, universal, transient feeling of lowness, heaviness, or feeling "down" associated with reaction to setback, defeat, or loss.
3) Adjectives of heaviness or lowness are consistent with physical behaviors associated with sadness.
      b. *Negative emotionality* and other innate qualities such as *pessimism* are associated with predisposition to sadness.
      c. There is some evidence individuals who are depressed may be more inclined or motivated toward feeling sadness and using negative emotional regulation strategies such as rumination.
      d. Sadness is frequently discussed as occurring on a continuum.
1) At one extreme, it borders on clinical depression, with elements of anguish and psychological pain.
2) On other extreme, sadness can be considered as positive emotion in that it allocates time for person to absorb and process loss or disappointment.
      e. Sadness is often confused with depression, which is a serious mental health disorder, but they are different in many ways, particularly in intensity and duration.
1) In contrast to depression, sadness resolves in a brief time.
2) With sadness, it is still possible to be happy regarding other aspects of life even while sad about particular aspect or situation (e.g., feeling happiness about birth of child, while feeling sadness about death of parent).
   2. Physiological aspects of sadness
      a. Sadness involves group of cerebral neural patterns correlated with activity of subgenual anterior cingulate, hippocampus, lateral prefrontal cortex, and insular and somatosensory nodes of Salience network. It is also associated with diminished cortical activation.
      b. EEG changes vary with experience of pain, but in one study, peaks were less for sadness than for either fear or anger.

c. Recent research results suggest there may be differences in how sadness is experienced and recognized based on sex.

d. Physical behaviors associated with sadness include downcast appearance with drooping eyelids, lowered corners of the mouth, heavy or slow ambulation, flat vocalization, stooped or slumped posture, and lowered heart rate if not crying (often heart rate is increased while crying).

e. Further research is needed regarding possible genetic basis or predisposition to sadness.

3. Relationship to pain

a. Sadness is at times considered a type of psychological pain.

b. Neurological association involving anterior insula and dorsal anterior cingulate cortex with both physical and social pain experiences has been described.

c. Increased perception of pain has been reported in presence of sadness. In some people, perceptions were greater with sadness than with major depressive disorder. Although research in this area is scarce, this is important to consider when caring for patients with pain who are also experiencing sadness.

d. This area needs more research.

4. Assessment factors

a. It is crucial to assess sadness in order to rule out depression. Beck Depression Inventory, Patient Health Questionnaire (PHQ-9), and other validated tools to assess depression can be used to differentiate sadness from depression.

b. Sadness is difficult to measure due to highly subjective nature but can be assessed using 5-point Likert scale to assess low versus high mood and frequency of low mood experience.

c. Two tools were designed to assess factors involved with children coping with a sad experience:
   1) Childrens' Sadness Management Scale
   2) Childrens' Emotion Management Scales for Anger and Sadness Coping (CEMS)

5. Implications for pain management

a. It is important to rule out depression when working with patients with pain who report being sad because depression frequently coexists with persistent pain; both issues need to be addressed.

b. Sadness and depression may be seen in people who have recently experienced trauma or loss or both.

6. Interventions

a No pharmacological interventions were identified for sadness. As a situational, temporary experience, sadness is expected to resolve with expression and time. However, if sadness persists and depression is diagnosed, antidepressant therapy including medications may be beneficial.

b No nonpharmacological interventions were identified for sadness, most likely because sadness is considered a short-term, transient emotion that resolves with expression and time.

J. Fear

1. Concept description

a. Fear, like pain, is essentially a primal emotion that alerts a person of impending harm. Fear can be lifesaving by preventing one from getting too close to edge of cliff and falling. Fear of COVID-19 infection led many people to modify their daily behaviors and lifestyles to avoid infection.

b. Power of fear as an overwhelming emotion is based in fear being strong in both personal and species preservation. Preservation may be enhanced by alerting for defense not only of self but of overall species as seen during COVID-19 pandemic.

c. However, in maladaptive ways, fear can interfere with quality of life and peace of mind. It can negatively affect potentially pleasurable activities, such as when fear of heights prevents someone from riding a Ferris wheel. Fear may become paralyzing when extreme, as seen with agoraphobia.

d. Fear exists on continuum with anxiety, panic, and phobias.

e. Fear has been described as response to an immediate threat while panic at one extreme occurs in response to escalating threats and anxiety occurs in response to less impending threats. Fear can also be learned or conditioned with associated learned or conditioned behaviors.

2. Physiological aspects of fear (Fig. 13.3)

a. Fear is based in neurophysiological interactive processes engaging various subnuclei of central amygdala in fear learning, conditioning, and extinction.

b. Neuromodulators and other input are transmitted to central amygdala from cerebral areas including cortex, auditory thalamus, and regions of brainstem.

c. There is evidence, in addition to amygdala role, of a circadian mechanism involving medial prefrontal cortex and hippocampus in neural plasticity of fear memories and retrieval of those memories.

d. Research in rodents is promising for learning more about physiology of fear.

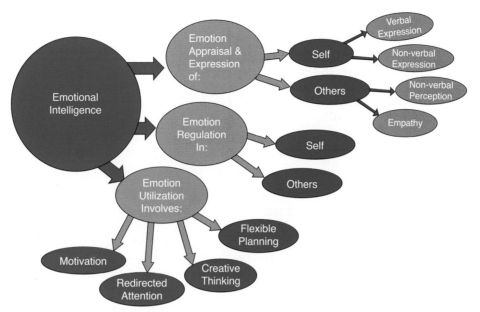

Figure 13.3 Emotional Intelligence Schemata. (From A. Quinlan-Colwell, 2022. Based on Sallovey, P., & Mayer, J.D. (1990) Emotional Intelligence. *Imagination, Cognition and Personality*, *9*(3), 185-211.)

3. Relationship to pain
   a. There are similarities between fear and acute pain. Both fear and pain:
      1) Alert organism or person of harm or threat
      2) Trigger defensive behaviors
      3) Strongly motivate learning
      4) Are used in classic conditioning
      5) In acute phase, both are important and life-saving interventions. However, both can evolve into maladaptive situations, with fear leading to anxiety disorder and acute pain evolving to persistent pain.
   b. Pain is robust source of fear with long history of being used in operant conditioning as stimulus to modify behavior.
   c. Fear of pain can also have strong operant conditioning effect. When intrinsically nonpainful activities are construed as painful or potentially painful, fear of pain or of increasing pain develops regarding those activities. Such fear, then, results in avoiding movements or actions that are intrinsically not painful (see fear avoidance below). Avoiding activity not only prevents potential pain but also alleviates fear and associated anxiety. A fear-and-avoidance behavior cycle is perpetuated, resulting in functional disability.
   d. Researchers in Turkey studying people surviving COVID-19 infection reported fear of pain was higher and quality of life was lower among people who experienced intense pain during their illness.
   e. Fear is associated with actual pain modulation or minimizing pain experience.

      1) Fear is such an overwhelming emotion, it actually overpowers the sensation of pain.
      2) Following research with rodents, *fear-induced analgesia* was described as an analgesic effect resulting from release of endorphins in response to fear, and analgesic effect could be reversed with naltrexone.
4. Fear-avoidance model (FAM) (Fig 13.4)
   a. Fear-avoidance (FA) describes response to pain when movements and activities are averted or rejected because of fear they will cause or intensify pain.
   b. It is presumed FA is one factor contributing to progression from acute to persistent pain with an overgeneralization of fear of pain to situations or activities that are not themselves painful.
   c. FA is considered an important factor in deconditioning and functional impairment.
   d. Meta-analysis and systematic review reported positive associations were found among FA, pain perception, and pain intensity.
   e. *Interpersonal Fear Avoidance Model of Pain* expounds on FAM with hypothesis there is bidirectional association between child and parent with response to pain and fear of pain.
5. FA tools
   a. Fear of Pain Questionnaire-9
   b. Fear of Pain Questionnaire, child report (FOPQ-C). FOPQ-C has subscales, including one for Fear of Pain and one for Avoidance of Activities.
   c. Pediatric Pain Fear Questionnaire (PPFQ)

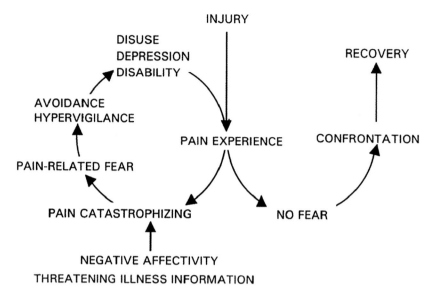

Figure 13.4 **Fear-avoidance model.** (From Vlaeyen, J. W., & Linton, S. J. (2012). Fear-avoidance model of chronic musculoskeletal pain: 12 years on. *Pain*, 153(6), 1144–1147.)

  d. Scale of Self-assessment of Fear Faces in Children 4–12 years old
  e. McMutry Children's Fear Scale
  f. Rapid Screener for the Assessment of Fear of Progression (for people who have survived cancer)
  g. Brief Fear of Negative Evaluation Scale revised (BFNE-II)
  h. Fear-Avoidance Beliefs Questionnaire (FABQ)
  i. Tampa Scale for Kinesiophobia (TSK)
6. Implications for pain management
  a. Since pain is both an unpleasant sensation and innate warning to protect the body, it is not surprising fear of pain develops.
  b. When fear of pain becomes conditioned response akin to persistent pain, it does not serve as protection but rather becomes pathological. When this happens, fear of pain triggers excessively cautionary behaviors limiting movement and participation in recovery activities, resulting in limited functioning, impaired quality of life, and debility.
  c. Pharmacological interventions are not identified as specific to treat fear; however, anxiolytic medications may be prescribed to assist with fear in association with anxiety management.
  d. Nonpharmacological interventions
    1) CBT interventions are used to address fear, pain, and fear of pain. Psychologists and mental health advanced practice registered nurses (APRNs) use extinction, exposure treatment, and counterconditioning to interrupt and replace conditioned fear association.
    2) Internet CBT including modules over 10 weeks for children with functional

abdominal pain and their parents was used to effectively reduce fear related to pain. Modules were designed to reduce fear and avoidance by gradually exposing child to stimuli that could elicit untoward symptoms.
    3) Recently, researchers reported using computer-generated conditioning exercises to successfully extinguish pain-related fear. Although additional research is needed, this study is encouraging for helping patients with fear of pain and fear avoidance to amend those fears and become more active and engaged in life.
    4) Virtual reality (VR) is being used successfully to help children and adults manage fear and pain during painful procedures.
      a) When VR was used for pain and fear among children who were being vaccinated, children who used VR responded with less fear and significantly less pain.
      b) When VR was used with children and teens with cancer undergoing venous port needle insertions, pain and fear were significantly reduced.
    5) Use of kaleidoscope was effective in reducing postoperative fear and pain following circumcision among children 7 to 11 years old.
    6) Authors of one systematic review reported manual therapy (e.g., joint mobilization, myofascial release, deep pressure massage) was not shown to be more effective than no intervention or comparative interventions for treatment of pain-related fear. They did

qualify the evidence as being of low quality, and additional research is needed.

K. Anger
  1. Concept description
     a. Many definitions of anger abound in the literature. Anger is a complex emotion that involves objecting to actions of a culpable source (e.g., another person) perceived as reproachable, leading to an adverse event or consequence perceived as distressing. The result of this cognitive appraisal then leads to aggression and antagonism in an effort to regain control and/or seek reparation.
     b. Anger can be understood as affective response occurring when expectations are not met.
        1) This definition is particularly poignant with regard to pain management when there is an expectation of no pain or mild pain but pain is actually experienced moderately or severely.
        2) Anger can occur when patients are told they will have no pain or "we'll manage your pain after surgery," but they do experience pain and their pain is not managed to their expectations.
     c. Anger can be aroused through physical experiences perceived as being distasteful or offensive (i.e., certain odors, temperature extremes, listening to snoring, and pain).
     d. Anger is considered from both trait and state perspectives.
        1) *State anger:* temporary, subjective, emotional experience rooted in a particular situation and expecting it to likely alter with change of situation
        2) *Trait anger:* relatively consistent and observable attitudes, behaviors, and personality attributes likened to hostility
     e. Anger also is considered as *anger-in* and *anger-out.*
        1) *Anger-in:* anger or angry feelings that are repressed
        2) *Anger-out:* outward manifestation of anger exhibited in aggressive behavior
     f. Related concepts are aggression, hate, frustration, impulsivity, irritation, passive-aggression, and rumination.
  2. Perceived injustice or injustice appraisal
     a. Perceived injustice or injustice appraisal related to anger and pain can be understood as the person with pain perceiving judgment, unfairness, fault, gravity, and irretrievability of losses related to pain experience.
     b. Perceived injustice in children was assessed, and results suggest direct relationship between perceived injustice with increased pain and impaired function.
     c. Negative impact with children was also correlated with perceived injustice, anger of their parents, and how parents respond to perception of injustice in child. Outcomes were most negative when children perceived their pain as greatly unjust and parents did not share that perspective.
     d. *Measurement tools:* Injustice Experience Questionnaire (IEQ) is used to measure perceived injustice.
  3. Relationship to pain
     a. Although anxiety is often correlated with and discussed in relation to pain, many researchers believe bidirectional relationship between pain and anger is greater than that seen with other emotions considered as negative (i.e., anxiety or sadness).
     b. In addition to resulting from pain, anger can affect pain as a predisposing, aggravating, or perpetuating factor. These are not mutually exclusive and can interplay as sole factor or in combination.
     c. Anger-in (i.e., inhibition of anger) is particularly linked with greater pain intensity, which may be related to less ability to modulate emotions or greater sense of negative affect.
     d. Anger is correlated with increased pain intensity and greater functional disability.
     e. Important antecedent of anger is *perceived injustice,* which is also strongly associated with poor pain-related outcomes (e.g., intensity, function, and opioid use). Negative impact of appraisal of pain-related injustice upon pain-related function was also seen in pediatric patients.
     f. Researchers who explored relationship of pain and anger among a group of individuals who sought help with problematic anger reported pain intensity was correlated with trait anger and other anger-related constructs including not being able to forgive. These researchers reported pain was correlated with hostile ideation among women, not men.
  4. Assessment factors
     a. Considering intricacy and potentially exacerbating effects of anger with persistent pain, assessment of anger is an important consideration for pain management.
     b. Tools to measure anger include:
        1) Anger Control Inventory (ACI)
        2) Anger Discomfort Scale (ADS)
        3) State-Trait Anger Expression (STAXI)
        4) Anger Expression Inventory (AEI)
        5) Anger Expression Scale (AES)
        6) Anger Situation Questionnaire (ASQ)
        7) Pediatric Anger Expression Scale (PAES-III)

8) Children's Emotion Management Scales for Anger and Sadness Coping
9) Clinical Anger Scale (CAS)
10) Multidimensional Anger Inventory (MAI)
11) Minnesota Multiphasic Personality Inventory–2 Anger Scale (MMPI-2-ANG)
12) Novaco Anger Scale (NAS)
13) State-Trait Anger Scale (STAS)
14) State-Trait Anger Expression (STAXI)
15) Targets of Anger Scale (TAS)
16) Targets and Reasons for Anger in Pain Sufferers (TRAPS)
17) Patient-Reported Outcomes Measurement Information System (PROMISE*, 2007): Anger Scale

5. Implications for pain management
   a. Relationship between anger and pain is complex and at times circular.
   b. Internalized or suppressed anger is more frequently associated with greater intensity of pain and persistent pain.
   c. Anger is associated with patients *not feeling heard*. During consultations to assess patients with advanced cancer for possible palliative care, those who endorsed anger reported not feeling heard during the 72 hours preceding consultation.
      1) Patients who endorsed anger also reported improvement of symptoms when they perceived consulting clinician listened to and understood them.
      2) Feeling heard can ease at least some feelings of anger and can be generalized and applied when working with patients who experience or live with pain.
   d. An area in need of exploration is benefit of interventions to modify pain-related injustice appraisals in effort to modify anger, alleviate pain, and improve function.

6. Pharmacological interventions are not identified as specific for anger management, but antidepressants, antipsychotic medications, and atypical antipsychotics may be prescribed to assist with anger management.

7. Nonpharmacological interventions are most frequently and effectively based on CBT.
   a. One CBT anger management intervention is Selection Menus for Anger Reduction Treatment (SMART) based on a person understanding their anger and how it affects their lives, clinician-guided skill development in response to anger triggers, and learning acceptance.
   b. "Window of Tolerance" model can be used to help patients identify their tolerance for

stressors and anger triggers and then work to increase their abilities to manage them.
   c. Group therapy anger management courses have been effective in teaching techniques to identify and control anger.
   d. Relaxation group interventions and family therapy have been positive interventions.
   e. Virtual reality is being used with increased frequency as intervention for both pain and anger.
   f. Compassion and forgiveness work are suggested as interventions for anger management. Loving kindness meditation is positive; compassionate emotion-focused meditation based in Buddhist tradition has been used successfully in management of anger and pain.

III. Sleep

A. Concept description
1. Sleep is understood as an essential restorative state during which there is decreased consciousness, a slowing down of bodily activities with reduced metabolism, and a reduction of skeletal muscle activity.
   a. Despite intimate relationship among all living beings with sleep, physiology of sleep is still not well understood.
   b. As with pain and emotion, sleep is complex, involving factors such as genetics, past experiences, emotional input, age, functioning, body temperature, and respiratory and cardiovascular input.
2. Optimal amount of sleep required is unique for each person. Duration of adequate sleep varies across lifespan and progressively decreases with age (see Table 13.1).
   a. As with food intake, it is possible to have too much or too little, with either extreme resulting in negative consequences.
   b. Extremes in length of sleep are correlated with both circadian rhythms and hormone levels.
3. Sleep is often categorized as combination of non-rapid eye movement (NREM) characterized by slow activity and rapid eye movement (REM) characterized by episodes of high activity.
4. Five sleep stages are:
   a. Sleep stages 1 and 2 are shallow, slow activity, with progressive lack of awareness of environment.
   b. Sleep stages 3 and 4 are slow activity, deep sleep stages when metabolic activity is at minimum. These stages are associated with rest, recuperation, and healing.
   c. The fifth stage is REM sleep during which there are increased levels of activity; critical process comprises approximately 20% to 25% of sleep,

Table 13.1	
Recommended Sleep Duration by Age	
Age	**Recommended Sleep Time in Hours**
Newborns	14–17
Infants	12–15
Toddler	11–14
Preschoolers	10–13
School-aged children	9–11
Teenagers	8–10
Young adults and adults	7–9
Older adults	7–8

Data from Hirshkowitz, M., Whiton, K., Albert, S. M., Alessi, C., Bruni, O., DonCarlos, L., Hazen, N., Herman, J., Katz, E.S., Kheirandish-Gozal, L., Neubauer, D.N., & Hillard, P. J. A. (2015). National Sleep Foundation's sleep time duration recommendations: methodology and results summary. *Sleep Health, 1*(1), 40–43.

is when dreams occur, and is considered important in how person manages stress.

5. Glymphatic system is cerebral perivascular spaces network and macroscopic clearance system for removing metabolic waste from parenchyma.
   a. Only functions during sleep when norepinephrine levels are reduced
   b. Through this system, CNS metabolites, soluble proteins, β-amyloid, and other neurotoxic wastes are removed.
   c. In addition to waste removal, there is distribution through CNS of compounds including amino acids, glucose, and neuromodulators.
   d. Malfunction of this system has been implicated with some neurodegenerative conditions.
6. Similar to relationship between pain and sleep, there is bidirectional relationship between diet and duration and quality of sleep.
   a. Although impaired sleep has been associated with low fiber, high carbohydrate, and high saturated fat diets, shorter duration of sleep is associated with deficiencies in both protein and carbohydrates.
   b. Deficiencies in micronutrients (vitamins and minerals) have also been associated with sleep disturbances. Most studies focused on relationship between sleep and diet are small, and further research is needed.
   c. Current information indicates Mediterranean diet discussed in section below may be an excellent choice to improve both sleep and pain management.
B. "Sleep disturbances" is a broad term referring to a number of conditions.
   1. Common types of sleep disturbances include:
      a. *Sleep deprivation:* Restriction or insufficiency occurs when person does not sleep long enough to be awake and alert; can be accompanied by increased musculoskeletal pain and hyperalgesia
      b. *Insomnia:* Characterized by difficulty getting to sleep and/or sustaining restorative sleep with difficulties functioning the next day; it is estimated as much as 30% of general adult population struggle with insomnia
      c. *Sleep bruxism:* Repetitive, painful clenching and/or grinding of teeth and/or similar movements of mandible while sleeping; associated with facial pain and headaches
      d. *Narcolepsy:* Results from abnormal REM sleep with disproportionate daytime drowsiness and sleeping
      e. *Obstructive sleep apnea (OSA):* Sleep disorder (i.e., intermittent cessation of breathing during sleep) is of concern in safe pain management and discussed in Chapter 12.
C. Physiology of sleep
   1. Sleep–awake cycle is regulated physiologically by neurons in brainstem, either L-glutamate (excitatory amino acid) or GABA (inhibitory amino acid), which are regulated by other brainstem and hypothalamic neurons including melanin-concentrating hormone neurons.
   2. Growth hormone and melatonin are released while sleeping. *Melatonin* is natural hormone critical to sleep, but natural production declines with aging.
D. Relationship to pain
   1. There is bidirectional association between sleep disturbances and persistent pain.
      a. Not only does pain interfere with and reduce quality of sleep, but also poor sleep leads to increased pain. There is potentially a greater impact of sleep on pain than the reverse.
      b. With inadequate stage 3 and stage 4 sleep, fatigue results and exacerbation of pain can occur.

c. Efforts to improve insomnia have also been beneficial in reducing pain.

2. It is possible there is impaired healing in presence of inadequate deep sleep and greater pain sensitivity with impaired CNS chemical cleaning with impaired glymphatic system activation that is sleep dependent.

   a. Information regarding glymphatic system is relatively new, and further investigation is needed.

   b. Two implications for pain management have to do with relationship with cerebral neurologic function and distribution of intrathecal medications.

   c. Relationship of malfunction of this system with some neurodegenerative conditions is of interest, as many people who live with persistent neuropathic pain also experience sleep disturbances.

3. Researchers using functional MRI (fMRI) guardedly reported there was increased activity in right executive control network of brain and functional activity following disruption of sleep with subsequent increased sensitivity to pain (sleep loss–induced hyperalgesia). This is early work, and it is noted neither actual existence nor pathophysiology supporting this concept has been determined to corroborate existence of *sleep-induced hyperalgesia*.

4. Considering significant role of opioids in pain management, particularly role of progressive sedation in assessment of opioid-induced respiratory depression (OIRD), the relationship between sleep and opioids must be considered (see Chapter 12).

E. Assessment considerations

1. Sleep among patients who are experiencing pain is essential for number of reasons.

   a. Sleep is crucial for replenishing body and supporting quality of life; thus, with adequate sleep, people experiencing pain are better able to manage pain.

   b. Conversely, disturbed and inadequate sleep can lead to increased pain.

   c. OSA is significant risk factor for development of OIRD.

2. Behavioral sleep assessment includes determining/identifying:

   a. Usual sleep pattern

   b. Current medications with sedative side effects or used to induce sleep

   c. Current use of supplements and herbal preparations used to assist with sleep

   d. Relationship with current medications and sleep

   e. Frequency of alcohol use

   f. Frequency of cannabidiol (CBD) use

   g. Current stressors including significance and intensity

h. Comorbid conditions including anxiety, depression, and PTSD

i. Interactions with significant others (e.g., relationships, sleeping patterns)

3. There are many assessment tools used to assess sleep (both clinical and research perspectives) including:

   a. Pittsburgh Sleep Quality Index (PSQI) is a 19-item self-assessment tool.

   b. Global Sleep Assessment Questionnaire (GSAQ)

   c. Epworth Sleepiness Scale

   d. Attitude Toward Sleep Questionnaire

   e. Leeds Sleep Evaluation Questionnaire

   f. Pittsburgh Sleep Quality Index

   g. Karolinska Sleepiness Scale

   h. PRIMIS–SD

   i. Pediatric Daytime Sleepiness Scale is an 8-item self-report tool designed for children between 11 and 15 years of age.

   j. Modified Epworth Sleepiness Scale–pediatric specific

   k. Cleveland Adolescent Sleepiness Questionnaire is a 16-item tool designed for teenagers (11–17 years).

   l. Neurophysiological Assessment of Sleepiness
      1) Multiple Sleep Latency Test
      2) Maintenance of Wakefulness Test

4. Implications for pain management are related to reciprocal relationship between improvement of quality of sleep and sensitivity to pain.

   a. Important but often overlooked aspect of managing persistent pain is to optimize quality of sleep.

   b. Treating insomnia can help with reducing pain severity and increasing pain tolerance.

5. Pharmacological interventions for the treatment of sleep disturbance abound (both prescription and over-the-counter)

   a. Numerous pharmaceuticals are available for treating sleep disturbances, many of which focus on specific signaling pathways and stimulate alterations in sleep structure.

   b. Medications and other substances commonly used to address sleep disturbances include antidepressants, antihistamines, hypnotics, and benzodiazepines, which induce sleep but inhibit sleep in stages 3 and 4, leading to increased pain. Long-term use of benzodiazepines can lead to cognitive disorders, impaired driving, and dementia.

   c. Melatonin is an easily synthesized hormone crucial for sleep. There is lack of research supporting benefit, appropriate doses, and specific formulations.

6. Nonpharmacological interventions for sleep disturbances include acupuncture, massage, and energetic therapies (see Chapter 15). However, majority of and most successful interventions are based in CBT for insomnia (CBTi), which has been assessed to be at least as effective as medications. In their 2021 clinical practice guidelines, the American Academy of Sleep Medicine gave a strong recommendation for CBTi. Examples of some specific forms of CBTi follow.
   a. Sleep education including:
      1) Basics of sleep stages, circadian rhythms, and physiology
      2) Dispel myths and misconceptions including minimum need for sleep
      3) Environmental considerations
      4) Control room temperature and humidity
      5) Sound therapy, modification, and control
      6) Light modification including device lights and visual alarms
      7) Bedroom activities: avoid reading, watching television, using electronic devices
      8) Sleepwear choices: select for comfort and avoid overheating
      9) Avoid focusing on or "working" to go to sleep, which may be counterproductive.
      10) If not sleeping in 30 minutes, rise and pursue boring activity.
      11) Relaxation therapy
      12) Titrate off medications used to induce sleep
      13) Control caffeine intake (e.g., in coffee, tea, chocolate); may interfere with falling asleep
      14) Alcohol may interfere with deep sleep and after 5–6 hours acts as a stimulant.
   b. Stimulus control is intervention for adults with chronic insomnia intended to stop association of being awake in bed and replace it with being asleep in bed. Process involves:
      1) Only go to bed when feeling sleepy.
      2) If unable to sleep, get up.
      3) Limit bedroom activities to sleep and sexual activities.
      4) Rise at same time each day.
      5) Avoid any napping during day.
   c. Sleep restriction is intervention used to treat insomnia. Process includes:
      1) Determine average number of hours slept per night.
      2) Establish standard wake time.
      3) Set sleep schedule to begin at least 5 hours before usual wake-up time
      4) Every 5 days, increase sleep by 30 minutes until sleep is at desired level.
      5) **Not advised** with people living with bipolar disorder or experiencing seizures

   d. Sleep readiness involves feeling fatigued and reduction in core body temperature, which is controlled by autonomic nervous system (ANS) and circadian rhythm.
      1) Sleep will not occur when sympathetic nervous system is active (e.g., with anger, agitation, anxiety, fear).
      2) Circadian rhythm is extremely sensitive to sunlight and occurs on a clock that takes 5 days to set.
      3) Consider warm bath or shower.
   e. Presleep relaxation includes variety of interventions to induce feelings of relaxation, such as progressive muscle relaxation, guided imagery, medication, and relaxation breathing.
   f. *Bright light therapy*: use of morning bright light to treat circadian rhythm dysregulation issues to coordinate circadian rhythms with sleep-wake cycle
   g. Telephone-supported CBT was effective in reducing insomnia in older adults with painful osteoarthritis in one study. More than half of participants stayed in remission from insomnia symptoms at 1 year.
   h. Technological CBTi includes following commercially available apps:
      1) My Sleep Coach
      2) DrLullabyl
      3) Sleepio
      4) Somryst
      5) BetterNight Insomnia

IV. Fatigue

A. Concept description
   1. Fatigue is complex and can include physiological weariness, low energy, and feeling weakened with diminished physical and mental capability resulting from disruption of circadian rhythm and/or lack of sleep or increased activity.
      a. Classic understanding of fatigue is the experience of tiredness not lessened with rest.
      b. It is associated with mental as well as physical energy expenditure and is impacted by environmental and socioeconomic influences.
      c. As with pain, fatigue is subjective and uniquely manifested by each experiencing person.
   2. Three types of fatigue:
      a. *Acute fatigue* occurs after being awake for 16 or more hours.
      b. *Cumulative fatigue* ensues from poor or inadequate sleep occurring over days or weeks.
      c. *Circadian fatigue*, also known as *chronodisruption*, develops following changes in sleep-wake cycles.

3. There is circular or dual relationship between fatigue and cognition.
   a. Fatigue can negatively impact cognition including judgment, interpersonal interactions, insight, mood, risk assessment, perspective, and ability to recall information and learn new information.
   b. Origin of fatigue can also be considered from purely cognitive or mental perspective.
   c. Early in fatigue process, cerebral areas associated with executive function, including morality and impulse control, are impacted.

B. Physiology of fatigue
   1. At least in part based on physiology of sleep (discussed previously)
   2. Physically, fatigue is also affected by general health, metabolism, nutrition, body habitus, comorbidities (e.g., myofascial pain syndrome, fibromyalgia, cancer), age, stress, and lifestyle choices. It is difficult to generalize physiological information regarding fatigue since research studies tend to focus on fatigue among individuals with particular condition (e.g., stroke, multiple sclerosis, cancer, HIV, or COVID-19).
   3. There is some evidence to support relationship between fatigue and inflammatory markers.
      a. In recent study of people who survived stroke, cytokines interleukin-6 (IL-6) and high sensitivity C-reactive protein (hsCRP) (peripheral proinflammatory markers) were not only statistically greater than among control cohort, but participants who reported greater fatigue had higher levels of IL-6 and hsCRP. These findings are noteworthy, as those biomarkers are involved in nociceptive processes.
      b. In another study, people who continued to experience fatigue following recovery from acute COVID-19 underwent testing with transcranial magnetic stimulation of the primary motor cortex; serum levels of IL-6 were elevated among participants during acute phase of COVID-19, and it was reported fatigue possibly was result of corresponding damage of GABAergic neurotransmission. Again, noteworthy since these substances are involved with nociception.
   4. Authors of a secondary analysis of 2007–2010 National Health and Nutrition Examination Survey (NHANES) reported participants with osteoarthritis who reported fatigue had CRP and white blood cell levels significantly higher than those participants with osteoarthritis but no report of fatigue.

C. Relationship to pain
   1. Fatigue is frequently seen as coexisting symptom with pain in variety of chronic situations including fibromyalgia syndrome, poststroke, and post–COVID-19 infection.
   2. Although research in physiology of fatigue and pain is scarce, levels of IL-6 are reported to be elevated in people with fatigue and in those with pain.
   3. Fatigue is more frequently experienced daily by individuals with high-impact persistent pain.

D. Assessment factors
   1. Fatigue can be a symptom of depression and anxiety, so ruling out depression and anxiety is an important first step in assessment.
   2. Similarly, it is important to rule out side effects of medications (e.g., antidepressants, anxiolytics, opioids) as source of fatigue.
   3. Fatigue Assessment Tools include:
      a. Fatigue Assessment Scale (FAS)—10 items on 5-point Likert scale
      b. Fatigue Severity Scale (FSS)—9 items with a 7-point Likert scale
      c. Fatigue Rating Scale (FRS)—0-to-10 numeric rating scale
      d. Modified Fatigue Impact Scale
      e. Modified Fatigue Impact Scale–5 item (MFIS-5)
      f. Multidimensional Fatigue Inventory (MFI)
      g. Sleepiness-Wakefulness Inability and Fatigue test—12-item scale

E. Pharmacological interventions for fatigue include:
   1. Stimulant medications can be used (e.g., modafinil or armodafinil) but need to be individually considered for each person.
   2. Supplements including beta-carotene, magnesium, zinc, and adrenal extract can be used after evaluation by clinician.
   3. Caffeine ingested through variety of sources is commonly used to counteract fatigue.

F. Nonpharmacological interventions
   1. Basic intervention for fatigue management is to improve sleep habits to attain regular adequate sleep and reconcile circadian rhythms as discussed previously.
   2. Regular exercise can be helpful in managing fatigue. Authors of systematic review of studies focusing on fatigue among men with prostate cancer reported resistance training appears to be effective in reducing fatigue and improving quality of life.
   3. Physical therapy with focus on therapeutic ergonomics, posture, and gait is beneficial in conservation of energy and important for regaining function and preventing further injury.
   4. Cognitive-behavioral interventions
      a. Stress management and self-care education including:
         1) Time management
         2) Setting healthy boundaries
         3) Mindfulness

  b. Acceptance and Commitment Therapy (ACT) was used by researchers in Sweden.
    1) Fatigue was assessed among patients with persistent pain who were participating in ACT therapy to manage their pain.
    2) Participants demonstrated less pain, less fatigue, and improvement in fatigue interference with life.
    3) Improvements in fatigue were correlated with improvement in pain acceptance rather than changes in pain intensity.
  c. Internet-based applications of CBT are an evolving option for fatigue and persistent pain for those individuals with access to care challenges.
 5. In a Turkish study, reflexology and progressive muscle relaxation (PMR) were compared with exercise and no intervention among women with cancer; both pain and fatigue lessened with reflexology and PMR.
 6. Reiki and guided imagery were used with people with cancer in another Turkish study. Those who received Reiki and those who participated in guided imagery had reductions in pain and fatigue compared to control group.
 7. Study using physiotherapy tape to modify slumped posture of people with depression reported increasing upright posture was associated with less depression and less fatigue.
 8. Nutritional therapy and improvements in nutrition are generally discussed and researched with fatigue specific to underlying pathology.
  a. In cancer-related fatigue, there is insufficient evidence to support specific nutritional recommendations.
  b. It is reasonable to recommend well-balanced nutrition that supports immune system and any underlying conditions.

V. Nutrition

A. Concept description
 1. Nutrition consists of cumulative processes involving intake, assimilation, and utilization of food to maintain body function and health, including providing energy for activities and warding off disease.
 2. Nearly 20 years ago, World Health Organization (WHO) identified nutrition as a crucial contributing factor in the development and trajectory of noncommunicable chronic diseases.
  a. Critical to health and well-being is the fact that nutrition is almost entirely modifiable.
  b. While physiologic barriers such as food intolerances or gastrointestinal disorders are important,

major barriers to modification are education, cultural, and socioeconomic limitations.
 3. As with fatigue and sleep, nutrition, in particular food intake, is affected or even guided by emotions; conversely, food impacts emotions.
  a. Food and emotions are involved with celebrating, calming, energizing, and comforting.
  b. Caffeine and sources of protein tend to be stimulating or energizing, and carbohydrates tend to have calming effect.
B. Physiology
 1. Nutrition is intricately involved with all physiological functions of living organisms. This is true not only when diet and thus nutrition of body are healthy, but also when it is lacking critical components when challenged by unhealthy foods.
 2. An ideal situation is for there to be physiological homeostasis; however, nutrition involves intricate biochemical processes affected by numerous factors such as appetite, activity, swallowing, medication effects, and medication side effects.
C. Relationship with pain
 1. Historically, little attention was given to interaction between pain and nutrition.
 2. Recently, this relationship has been considered in variety of persistent pain conditions including migraine headaches, neuropathy, musculoskeletal and visceral pain, fibromyalgia, low back pain, myofascial pain syndrome, and postcancer pain.
 3. Microglial cells are involved in neuropathic pain and hypothesized to be involved in transition from acute to persistent pain.
 4. In a rodent study, glial cell activation, neuroinflammation, phosphorylation of NMDA subunits, and pain behaviors were reduced when animals were limited to 40% of their daily calorie intake.
 5. One theory of the relationship between pain and nutrition involves diet-induced neuroinflammation model, which illustrates the connection between diet-induced neuroinflammation and central sensitization experienced by some patients with persistent pain and nutritional neurobiology.
  a. Authors propose poor nutrition leads to oxidative stress, cell necrosis with tissue damage, peripheral inflammation, and vagus nerve afferent activation, which all lead to activation of CNS glial cells and subsequent CNS sensitization.
  b. Peripheral proinflammatory cytokines resulting from poor nutrition can transfer to CNS by crossing blood-brain barrier.
D. Assessment factors
 1. Physical examination appropriate for age and known health status of individual
 2. Comorbid conditions may affect sense of taste or appetite such as long-term COVID-19.

3. Laboratory biochemical analysis including hematology values, lipid profile, renal and liver function tests, electrolytes, and trace elements and vitamins
4. Anthropometric measures
   a. Body mass index: calculated using person's height and weight; many electronic medical records generate this value
   b. Skinfold measurements: using circumference of limbs
   c. Bioelectrical impedance analysis: noninvasive technique of measuring body mass as current transmits through tissue; should be avoided with older patients and those with fluid overload, in intensive care, and with either extremely low or extremely high BMI
   d. Creatinine height index (CHI): measure of body weight and lean body mass; CHI is calculated: 24-hour urinary creatinine × 100/normal 24-hour urinary creatinine = CHI%
   e. Dual energy x-ray absorptiometry: radiological density analysis; considered gold standard for measuring body composition
   f. Computed tomography and magnetic resonance tomography
5. Clinicians use food diaries to assess what foods and nutrients are being consumed.
   a. Can be used by clinicians as educational tools to guide patients about how to make desired changes in areas needing improvement
   b. Food diaries vary from being simple 24-hour recall record of what has been consumed throughout day to detailed, in-time listing of exactly measured quantities of substances consumed.
   c. Applications for smartphones and other electronic devices have facilitated recording.
6. Nutrition assessment tools include:
   a. Subjective Global Assessment
   b. Nutritional Risk Screening 2002 (NRS-2002)
   c. Malnutrition Universal Screening Tool (MUST)
   d. Malnutrition Universal Screening Tool short form (MUST-SF)
   e. Mini Nutritional Assessment (MNA)
E. Implications for pain management
1. Recent research provided information encouraging further exploration into role of nutrition in pain management.
   a. Authors of 2018 systematic review of effects of nutritional interventions among people living with persistent noncancer pain concluded pain was significantly reduced with variety of nutritional interventions (e.g., specific nutrient changes, total diet modification, supplement-based interventions, fasting therapies).
   b. Recent multinational team reviewed studies related to role of nutrition in pain experienced with fibromyalgia and concluded a variety of

nutritional factors influence fibromyalgia pain, with pain lessening when nutrition is optimized.
2. Dietary factors and choices with relation to pain management are receiving increasing attention.
   a. High-fat, high-sugar diet common in the U.S. and some other Western countries not only leads to obesity but also has been implicated with decreased prefrontal cortex synaptic plasticity and diminished function in amygdala, both of which are involved with processing and assessing pain.
   b. Anti-inflammatory diet focuses on high fibers, omega-3 fatty acids rather than omega-6 fatty acids, deep water fish, full-fat dairy products, lean poultry, fruits, and vegetables with anti-inflammatory effects.
      1) Similar to Mediterranean Diet
      2) Spices including turmeric (curcumin), ginger, basil, rosemary, oregano, and thyme are also considered anti-inflammatory.
      3) Authors of large international study assessing Mediterranean Diet reported patients with OA of knees who more strictly followed Mediterranean Diet had less risk of pain worsening at 4-year follow-up. It was also reported that among people who did not have OA, those who more strictly followed Mediterranean Diet were less likely to develop OA.
F. Pharmacological interventions to improve nutrition need to be patient specific and consistent with individual status of person and any comorbid conditions.
G. Nonpharmacological interventions
1. Educate patients about role of diet choices in pain control.
2. Encourage patients who are experiencing or living with pain to make healthy dietary choices.
   a. Not only is there potential benefit for alleviating pain but also for improving underlying pathologies, promoting optimal health, and controlling weight.
   b. Since diets high in sugar and fat are associated with contributing to or exacerbating pain, it is reasonable to minimize dietary sugar and fat intake.
3. Consultation with nutritionist for educational counseling

VI. Obesity

A. Concept description
1. Obesity
   a. Is now considered chronic condition and generally involves consumption of more calories than expended, resulting in energy imbalance and excessive fat storage
   b. Related to nutrition and exercise

c. Obesity can be closely related to EI when person is not able to differentiate hunger from emotions such as fear or anger.

2. Demographics
   a. Prevalence of obesity as well as severe or morbid obesity has steadily increased during last two decades in the U.S.
   b. Obesity among adults has increased from 30.5% in 2000 to 42.4% in 2018.
   c. Severe obesity among adults has more than doubled from 4.7% in 2000 to 9.2% in 2018.
   d. In 2019, Centers for Disease Control and Prevention (CDC) estimated at least 72 million Americans are obese, and their per capita annual health care costs $1429 more than for their nonobese counterparts.

3. Numerous factors may contribute to obesity, including genetic susceptibility, cultural influences, behavior, medications, education, and socioeconomic factors.
   a. Dietary behaviors involved with obesity include:
      1) Intaking more food/calories than needed to sustain body
      2) Consuming foods with high caloric content and low nutritional value
      3) Disproportionately consuming most calories later in the day
   b. Current obesity epidemic correlates with obesogenic environment that fosters obesity through great availability of inexpensive and convenient high-calorie foods.
      1) There has been a paradigm shift since end of 20th century with obesogenic environment being predominant in many developed countries, resulting in need for public health prevention efforts to alter this trend.
      2) Nurses can be instrumental in reversing this trend.

B. Physiology of obesity
   1. Physiology of obesity is complex due to influence of genetic, behavioral, psychological, circadian rhythm, and environmental factors.
   2. Hypothalamus and brainstem are both linked to appetite, and other CNS structures interact with endocrine system.
   3. Increasingly, obesity is being viewed as state of chronic, low-grade inflammation. Inflammatory cytokines (e.g., IL-6 and CRP, tumor necrosis factor-alpha), adiponectin, and hormone leptin are implicated in obesity.

C. Relationship to pain
   1. Many patients living with persistent pain are comorbidly obese, and the relationship is circular, with pain leading to inactivity, which leads to greater obesity and thus to more inactivity and more pain.

2. Obesity is associated with many painful conditions including OA, persistent low back pain (especially with enlarged abdominal girth), headaches, and diabetic neuropathy.

3. Relationship is seen in adults, children, and teens.

4. Pain is not only comorbid factor among people living with persistent pain, but it is now considered risk factor for developing persistent pain.
   a. People who are obese are at greater risk of suffering with persistent pain, with estimates ranging from two to four times as likely.
   b. Investigators of two studies involving obesity among people with persistent pain reported risks of developing both persistent low back pain and persistent knee pain that limited function was increased among those who are obese as young adults.
      1) In addition, pain sensitivity seems to be affected by obesity. In one research study with veterans who were overweight or obese, correlations were found with greater pain intensity and pain interference with increased obesity.
      2) However, research findings have been inconsistent both in rodent and human studies.
      3) This is an area where more research is needed.

D. Assessment factors
   1. Obesity is determined by BMI.
      a. BMI of 18.5–24.9 kg/m^2 indicates normal weight.
      b. BMI of 25–29.9 kg/m^2 indicates overweight status.
      c. BMI of ≥30 kg/m^2 signifies obesity.
      d. BMI of ≥40 kg/m^2 signifies morbid obesity.
   2. Visceral adiposity index is considered more specific to obesity than BMI.
   3. Assessment of portion control behavior can be done using one of the following:
      a. Portion Control Self-Efficacy Tool
      b. Portion Control Strategies Questionnaire using 5-point scale
      c. Portion Control Practices Survey
   4. Food diaries, as discussed above, can be helpful in assessing patients who are obese.

E. Implications for pain management
   1. Since weight reduction is effective in reducing pain and increasing function, it is key component of multimodal analgesia in persons with obesity.
   2. Weight reduction can help prevent the development of some painful conditions like OA, and even a small amount of weight loss can relieve stress on painful joints. This supports belief there may be an association between degree of obesity and degree of pain.
   3. Obesity is associated with reduced activity, which can contribute to disuse and increased pain.

4. There is information obesity increases nociceptive sensitivity and inflammatory responses.
5. There are pharmacological agents and surgical procedures to help patients manage obesity. These options need to be individualized for each person in collaboration with prescriber or surgeon.
6. Nonpharmacological interventions
   a. Weight loss programs
   b. Lifestyle modifications including:
      1) Dietary education and modification
      2) Physical activity education and adherence
      3) CBT interventions: Authors of systematic review and meta-analysis reported type of CBT or behavioral therapy is most effective when targeted to particular subtype of obesity:
         a) Simple obesity disorder
         b) Obesity with binge-eating disorder
         c) Obesity with depression
      4) Education to interrupt/reverse obesogenic environment include:
         a) Understand current dietary guidelines.
         b) Improve timing of food consumption including need to avoid skipping meals and disproportionally consuming more calories later in day/evening,
         c) Eliminate or minimize between meal snacking.
         d) Improve food choices to include nutrient-dense lower-calorie foods.
         e) Limit portion sizes, which have increased during past 40 years.
         f) Use smaller plates; plate size has also increased in recent decades.
         g) Improve culinary skills, thereby decreasing reliance on prepared foods.
      5) Pre-meal planning
         a) Pre-meal planning involves selection of portion size in preparation of eating. This can involve identifying amount of each type of food, plating that food once, and avoiding second helpings. When eating out, this can be accomplished by requesting half of meal be placed in a to-go container.
         b) Research evaluating intentional pre-meal choosing of portion sizes noted when choice was made based on health, increased activity was seen in prefrontal cortex, but when choices were made based on pleasure, there was increased activity in left orbitofrontal cortex.
      6) Motivational interviewing: explores past experiences, changing behaviors, and motivations to reduce weight
      7) Behavior modification: focuses on goal setting, stimulus control, self-monitoring behavior, and reinforcement of positive efforts
      8) Behavioral weight loss treatment (BWLT): focuses on behavior with diet and exercise
      9) Acceptance and Commitment Therapy (ACT)
      10) Mindfulness-based interventions
      11) Technology options through telehealth and other technologies are promising options.
      12) Hypnosis: Authors reviewing two meta-analyses assessing effectiveness of hypnosis in combination with CBT for obesity indicated hypnosis has promise, particularly when used in combination with CBT and advised additional research is needed, specifically with longitudinal studies.

VII. Eating Disorders

A. Concept of eating disorder or disordered eating is one of several psychological conditions portrayed by unhealthy habits of taking in food.
   1. Eating disorders include anorexia nervosa (AN), bulimia nervosa (BN), binge-eating disorder (BED), pica, and avoidant/restrictive food intake disorder.
   2. The most common disorders (AN, BN, and BED) will be discussed in greater detail.
B. Concept descriptions
   1. AN is serious psychiatric illness characterized by distorted body image, intense fear of gaining weight, and limited food consumption.
      a. Subtypes include:
         1) Restrictive
         2) Binge-eating/purging type
      b. Although there is no causative link between substance use disorders (SUDs) and AN, they often occur comorbidly.
   2. BN is serious psychiatric and multisystem disorder involving emotional dysregulation manifested in binge eating (excessive quick food intake) with compensatory activities of purging through induced vomiting, medicating (laxatives, diuretics, and diet preparations), and excessive exercising.
      a. Subtypes of BN include:
         1) Purging
         2) Nonpurging
      b. Common comorbidities include affective, attention, and SUDs.
      c. Food insecurity or limited access to food can be predisposing factor. Authors of one study reported BN was correlated with food

insecurity, but this relationship was not found with BED.

3. BED is characterized by eating larger than usual amount of food in brief period of time without having control over doing so.
   a. Considered most prevalent of all eating disorders
   b. Associated characteristics are eating rapidly, eating until overfull, overeating when not feeling hungry, and experiencing guilt or embarrassment concerning the behavior. For diagnostic purposes, at least three of these characteristics must be present.
   c. Unlike AN and BN, with BED, behaviors that counteract binging to avoid weight gain are not present. This disorder is frequently associated with obesity.
   d. Common comorbidities are attention deficit disorder, hyperactivity, anxiety, mood and personality disorders, and SUDs.

4. Pica is eating or mouthing items not considered edible, including dirt, stones, metal, feces, material, and foam. It is considered a serious eating disorder occurring most commonly among people with behavioral disorders.

5. Avoidant/restrictive food intake disorder involves not satisfying nutritional requirements due to restricting and/or avoiding food. This can result in nutritional deficits, being underweight, possible need for artificial nutrition, and psychosocial issues.

C. General physiology of AN, BN, and BED
   1. Most people with eating disorders are female; however, among males, BED is more prevalent than AN and BN.
   2. Relationship of dopamine and serotonin with eating disorders has been investigated. Dopamine is important with both food consumption and emotion. Serotonin has key roles in regulation of appetite, sleep, and aggression related to anger.
   3. Evolving research indicates neurological actions may involve immune system overreaction resulting in neuropeptide signal abnormality. Dysfunction of serotonergic system is thought to be very involved in eating disorders.
   4. Twin studies clearly demonstrated there are inheritable factors involved in AN (28%–74%), BN (28%–83%), and BED (39%–45%). However, it is not clear whether those are family environment or genetic relationships. To date, no clear genetic link has been identified.
   5. Physiology of AN
      a. Changes occur in somatosensory systems of people with AN. Tactile perception, interoception, and nociception are thought to be affected.

1) Neurotransmitter function is different than in other people.
2) Neural activation is not what is usually expected.
3) People with AN also have difficulties with multisensory integration of somatosensory stimuli.
   b. Levels of circulating oxytocin have been noted to be altered with AN.
   c. Circulating levels of leptin (satiety hormone) were lower than normal in some people with AN.
   d. There is some evidence to suggest that when people with AN were shown a distortion of their own body image, there was activity in right amygdala and prefrontal cortex. Since amygdala and prefrontal cortex are involved with pain, these are areas in need of greater research.

6. Physiology of BN
   a. Similar to AN, there is abnormal neurotransmitter function with BN.
   b. Circulating leptin levels were also noted to be reduced in some people with BN.
   c. Brain gut peptide glucagon, like peptide-1, was noted to be reduced in patients with BN. GLP-1 has a hormone-neurotransmitter action involved with insulin levels and impeding food intake.
   d. Although additional research using neuroimaging is needed, authors of one systematic review reported there were some repeated findings, including:
      1) Reduced activity in frontostriatal areas
      2) Atypical activity in insula, amygdala, and occipital cortex
      3) Intensity of BN (and BED) was correlated with more significant neural variations.

7. Physiology of BED
   a. BED is believed to evolve from neurocognitive dysfunction, particularly involving inhibition control and reward processes.
   b. In research using fMRI, low activity was noted in prefrontal cortex with increased activity in medial orbitofrontal cortex. Decreased activity in anterior insula and ventrolateral prefrontal cortex was noted in other studies.
   c. BED was correlated with inadequate sleep, but more research is needed.

D. Relationship to pain
   1. Pain, hunger, taste, and satiety are interoceptive senses signaled by C-fiber and A-delta afferent nerves.
   2. Researchers in Czech Republic study reported not only do people with eating disorders have increased sensitivity to pain, but the greater the desire for thinness, the greater is the sensitivity to pain.

3. In a U.S. study with teenagers who had comorbid persistent pain and eating disorder, researchers reported 41% of participants' persistent pain preceded the eating disorder, and in 35%, the eating disorder preceded persistent pain. They also reported when persistent pain and eating disorders were comorbid, the eating disorder went undiagnosed for longer period of time.
4. AN and relationship to pain
    a. Authors of a recent scoping review noted people living with AN demonstrated elevated thermal pain threshold (i.e., needing greater stimulation for pain to be perceived), possibly the result of malnutrition-related endocrine and cardiovascular changes. Since thermal pain threshold returns to normal range with recovery from AN, it is believed this is manifestation of AN state rather than global trait. This increase in pain threshold was not observed in testing with mechanical pain; this was also true in one group in which thermal pain threshold was elevated.
    Another study found no relationship between patients with AN compared to controls with response to cold pain stimuli.
    b. Since people with AN have abnormal multisensory processing and integration, it is possible there may be abnormality in pain perception, interpretation, and modulation. These are areas in which additional research is needed.
    c. A novel explanation of AN proposed aversive memory of early gastrointestinal pain actually is basis for developing AN.
5. BN and relationship to pain
    a. There is very little information regarding this relationship; this is area for further research.
    b. According to authors of one systematic review, patients with BN may have increased tolerance for pain (heat, cold, mechanical) threshold and intensity due to pain-processing impairment. Increased pain tolerance persisting after recovery from BN was also reported.
6. BED: Authors of study with female veterans reported among women with BED, persistent pain was most common coexisting medical condition and was cited as first treatment priority for participants.
E. Assessment factors
    1. Assessment of AN
        a. Comprehensive history including all childhood gastrointestinal experiences
        b. BMI of ≤18.5 is considered underweight.
        c. Assessment–Screening tools include:
            1) Eating Attitudes Test (EAT-12)
            2) SCOFF (acronym for Sick, Control, One stone, Fat Food)
            3) Eating Disorder Examination Questionnaire (EDE-Q)
            4) Yale-Brown-Cornell Eating Disorder Scale
            5) Somatoform Dissociation Questionnaire
            6) Body Attitude Test (BAT) consists of 20 items on 5-point Likert score and measures disturbance in body image.
            7) Patient Health Questionnaire 15-Item Somatic Symptom Severity Scale
            8) Eating Disorder Examination (EDE)
            9) Tools are available for assessing portion control behavior.
    2. Assessment of BED
        a. Diagnosis based on DSM-5 criteria
        b. Underrecognized and thus undertreated, BED needs to be considered as an underlying cause of obesity.
        c. Since eating behaviors (excessive consumption, increased snacking/nibbling, and less consistency of meals) are characteristic, interviews in safe environment and food diaries may be helpful for assessment.
        d. Assessment tools include:
            1) Binge Eating Disorder Screen for Primary Care (ESP)
            2) Eating Disorder module of the Patient Health Questionnaire
            3) Binge Eating Disorder Screener-7
            4) Binge Eating Scale (BES)
            5) Eating Disorder Examination-Questionnaire
            6) Eating Loss of Control Scale (ELOCS)
            7) Seven-Item Binge-Eating Disorder Screener (BEDS-7)
F. Implications for pain management
    1. From available but scant research, some evidence exists suggesting people living with AN and BN have either increased tolerance, less perception, or higher thresholds for pain. This is important considering focus of quantifying pain intensity as single measure of pain.
    2. Since pain is often the presenting factor for many conditions, it is important to understand pain intensity may not be reported as expected by people with AN and particularly those with BN.
    3. People with BED may have high likelihood for coexisting persistent pain conditions.
    4. Additional research is needed to understand relationships between various eating disorders and pain.
G. Pharmacological interventions:
    1. AN:
        a. Off-label use of olanzapine and lanzapine has shown some benefit. Earlier antipsychotic preparations are not indicated.

  b. Antidepressant medications have not been successful treatments for AN.
2. BN:
  a. Fluoxetine was FDA approved in 1997.
  b. All types of antidepressants have been used off label in treatment of BN, but selective serotonin reuptake inhibitors (SSRIs) and serotonin-norepinephrine reuptake inhibitors (SNRIs) are more commonly prescribed to avoid untoward side effects.
  c. Topiramate has been used off label with some success in treating binge and purge behaviors. Side effects must be considered prior to prescribing.
  d. In at least two adult cases of BN (one male and one female), neural therapy involving injections of local anesthetic (procaine) was effective in controlling BN symptoms for up to 2 years.
3. BED:
  a. Lisdexamfetamine dimesylate (CNS stimulant) received FDA approval in 2015 for treatment of BED in adults. It is important to note significant cardiovascular effects of this medication.
  b. Off-label second-generation antidepressants and topiramate were used in some studies.
H. Nonpharmacological interventions
1. AN:
  a. Requires psychotherapeutic intervention but is very resistant to treatment, with as many as 50% of people relapsing during first year following hospitalization; relapse and remission are significant concerns.
  b. Mindfulness meditation was effective in reducing symptoms among women with both restrictive and binge-purge types of AN in one study.
  c. Interoceptive remapping with focus on understanding visceral messages and assisting with differentiating between harmless and ominous sensations may be helpful.
2. BN:
  a. Requires psychotherapeutic intervention
  b. Eye movement desensitization and reprocessing (EMDR) are used in treatment of BN.
  c. CBT can be helpful, particularly in normalizing patterns of eating and behaviors.
  d. Virtual reality has been used less frequently but is a potentially effective way to use CBT in this population.
3. BED:
  a. Psychotherapy is hallmark of interventions for BED.
  b. Self-help groups using variety of CBT interventions are effective for some people.

  c. Applications for electronic and mobile devices are available to support treatment and self-help.

VIII. Nursing Implications

Since nursing implications are similar for all issues discussed in this chapter, they are discussed from a global perspective.
A. Clinical implications include:
1. Awareness of how emotions, sleep, fatigue, nutrition, obesity, and eating disorders are involved with experiencing and managing pain is important to help people better manage pain from holistic perspective.
2. Understand relationship of these concepts with pain and apply these concepts when collaborating with patients.
3. Assess for trait emotions, emotional intelligence, sleep patterns, fatigue, obesity, and eating disorders.
4. Learn interventions to use and teach patients and families.
5. Educate patients and families regarding these concepts in relation to pain and how to modify them to better manage pain.
6. Encourage patients to make lifestyle changes to better manage pain and increase quality of life.
B. Research is clearly needed with all concepts presented, with focus on:
1. Physiology of emotion or concept
2. Relationship of these factors to pain
3. Interventions to alleviate pain
4. Exploring benefit of evaluating emotional intelligence of clinicians and educating them to increase emotional intelligence
5. Gaining better understanding of relationships between nutrition, diet, body mass, and eating behaviors with nociception and pain management
6. Gaining better understanding of physiology of all areas discussed as well as their interactions with pain experience
7. Assessing effect and benefit of nonpharmacological interventions to improve health, quality of life, and pain management

Bibliography

Althumairi, A., Sahwan, M., Alsaleh, S., Alabduljobar, Z., & Aljabri, D. (2021). Virtual reality: is it helping children cope with fear and pain during vaccination? *Journal of Multidisciplinary Healthcare, 14*, 2625–2632. https://doi:10.2147/JMDH.S327349.

Arias, J. A., Williams, C., Raghvani, R., Aghajani, M., Baez, S., Belzung, C., Booij, L., Busatto, G., Chiarella, J., Fu, C. H. Y.,

Ibanez, A., Liddell, B. J., Lowe, L., Penninx, B. W. J. H., Rosa, P., & Kemp, A. H. (2020). The neuroscience of sadness: A multidisciplinary synthesis and collaborative review. *Neuroscience & Biobehavioral Reviews, 111*, 199–228. https://doi.org/10.1016/j.neubiorev.2020.01.006.

Astin, R. (2020). Neurophysiology. In K. M. Spyer, G. L. Ackland, & A. V. Gurine. (Eds.), *Encyclopedia of Respiratory Medicine* (2nd Ed). Elsevier, Inc. https://doi.org/10.1016/B978-0-12-801238-3.11616-2.

Baguley, B. J., Skinner, T. L., & Wright, O. R. (2019). Nutrition therapy for the management of cancer-related fatigue and quality of life: a systematic review and meta-analysis. *British Journal of Nutrition, 122*(5), 527–541. https://doi.org/10.1017/S000711451800363X.

Basten-Günther, J., Peters, M., & Lautenbacher, S. (2019). Optimism and the experience of pain: A systematic review. *Behavioral Medicine, 45*(4), 323–339. https://doi.org/10.1080/08964289.2018.1517242.

Baumgartner, J. N., Schneider, T. R., & Capiola, A. (2018). Investigating the relationship between optimism and stress responses: A biopsychosocial perspective. *Personality and Individual Differences, 129*, 114–118. https://doi.org/10.1016/j.paid.2018.03.021.

Benarroch, E. E. (2018). Brainstem integration of arousal, sleep, cardiovascular, and respiratory control. *Neurology, 91*(21), 958–966. https://doi.org/10.1212/WNL.0000000000006537.

Benveniste, H., Liu, X., Koundal, S., Sanggaard, S., Lee, H., & Wardlaw, J. (2019). The glymphatic system and waste clearance with brain aging: a review. *Gerontology, 65*(2), 106–119. https://doi.org/10.1159/000490349.

Berboth, S., & Morawetz, C. (2021). Amygdala-prefrontal connectivity during emotion regulation: A meta-analysis of psychophysiological interactions. *Neuropsychologia*, 107767. https://doi.org/10.1159/000490349.

Bjørklund, G., Dadar, M., Chirumbolo, S., & Aaseth, J. (2018). Fibromyalgia and nutrition: Therapeutic possibilities? *Biomedicine & Pharmacotherapy, 103*, 531–538. https://doi.org/10.1016/j.biopha.2018.04.056.

Blume, M., Schmidt, R., & Hilbert, A. (2019). Abnormalities in the EEG power spectrum in bulimia nervosa, binge-eating disorder, and obesity: A systematic review. *European Eating Disorders Review, 27*(2), 124–136. https://doi.org/10.1002/erv.2654.

Boselie, J. J. L. M., Vancleef, L. M. G., & Peters, M. L. (2018). Filling the glass: Effects of a positive psychology intervention on executive task performance in chronic pain patients. *European Journal of Pain, 22*(7), 1268–1280. https://doi.org/10.1002/ejp.1214.

Brasure, M., MacDonald, R., Fuchs, E., Olson, C. M., Carlyle, M., Diem, S., Carlyle, M., Witt, T. J., Ouellette, J., Butler, M., & Kane, R. L. (2016). Psychological and behavioral interventions for managing insomnia disorder: an evidence report for a clinical practice guideline by the American College of Physicians. *Annals of Internal Medicine, 165*(2), 113–124. https://doi.org/10.7326/M15-1782.

Brain, K., Burrows, T. L., Rollo, M. E., Chai, L. K., Clarke, E. D., Hayes, C., Hodson, F. J., & Collins, C. E. (2019). A systematic review and meta-analysis of nutrition interventions for chronic noncancer pain. *Journal of Human Nutrition and Dietetics, 32*(2), 198–225. https://doi.org/10.1111/jhn.1260.

Brockman, R., Ciarrochi, J., Parker, P., & Kashdan, T. (2017). Emotion regulation strategies in daily life: Mindfulness, cognitive reappraisal and emotion suppression. *Cognitive Behaviour Therapy, 46*(2), 91–113. https://doi.org/10.1080/16506073.2016.1218926.

Bulut, M., Alemdar, D. K., Bulut, A., & Şalcı, G. (2020). The effect of music therapy, hand massage, and kaleidoscope usage on postoperative nausea and vomiting, pain, fear, and stress in children: A randomized controlled trial. *Journal of PeriAnesthesia Nursing, 35*(6), 649–657. https://doi.org/10.1016/j.jopan.2020.03.013.

Burns, J. W., Bruehl, S., France, C. R., Schuster, E., Orlowska, D., Chont, M., Gupta, R. K., & Buvanendran, A. (2017). Endogenous opioid function and responses to morphine: the moderating effects of anger expressiveness. *The Journal of Pain, 18*(8), 923–932. https://doi.org/10.1016/j.jpain.2017.02.439.

Buyukbayram, Z., & Saritas, S. C. (2021). The effect of Reiki and guided imagery intervention on pain and fatigue in oncology patients: A non-randomized controlled study. *EXPLORE, 17*(1), 22–26. https://doi.org/10.1016/j.explore.2020.07.009.

Carriere, J. S., Sturgeon, J. A., Yakobov, E., Kao, M. C., Mackey, S. C., & Darnall, B. D. (2018). The impact of perceived injustice on pain-related outcomes: A combined model examining the mediating roles of pain acceptance and anger in a chronic pain sample. *The Clinical Journal of Pain, 34*(8), 739–747. https://doi:10.1097/AJP.0000000000000602.

Casioppo, D. (2020). The cultivation of joy: practices from the Buddhist tradition, positive psychology, and yogic philosophy. *The Journal of Positive Psychology, 15*(1), 67–73. https://doi:10.1080/17439760.2019.1685577.

Castelnuovo, G., Pietrabissa, G., Manzoni, G. M., Cattivelli, R., Rossi, A., Novelli, M., Varallo, G., & Molinari, E. (2017). Cognitive behavioral therapy to aid weight loss in obese patients: current perspectives. *Psychology Research and Behavior Management, 10*. Article 165-173. https://doi.org/10.2147/PRBM.S113278.

Centers for Disease Control and Prevention (CDC). (2019). Disability and Obesity. *Disability and Health Promotion*. Retrieved 3/14/2021 from https://www.cdc.gov/ncbddd/disabilityandhealth/obesity.html.

Cha, J. Y., Kim, S. Y., Shin, I. S., Park, Y. B., & Lim, Y. W. (2020). Comparison of the Effects of Cognitive Behavioral Therapy and Behavioral Treatment on Obesity Treatment by Patient Subtypes: A Systematic Review and Meta-analysis. *Journal of Korean Medicine for Obesity Research, 20*(2), 178–192. https://doi.org/10.15429/jkomor.2020.20.2.178.

Cooney, M., & Quinlan-Colwell, A. (2020). *Assessment and Multimodal Management of Pain: An Integrative Approach*. St. Louis, MO: Elsevier.

Cuesto, G., Everaerts, C., León, L. G., & Acebes, A. (2017). Molecular bases of anorexia nervosa, bulimia nervosa and binge eating disorder: shedding light on the darkness. *Journal of Neurogenetics, 31*(4), 266–287. https://doi:10.1080/01677063.2017.1353092.

Daenen, F., McParland, J., Baert, F., Miller, M. M., Hirsh, A. T., & Vervoort, T. (2020). Child pain-related injustice appraisals mediate the relationship between just-world beliefs and pain-related functioning. *European Journal of Pain, 25*(4), 757–773. https://doi.org/10.1002/ejp.1707.

Darwin, C. (1872). *The Expression of Emotion in Man and Animals*. Oxford University Press.

Dijk, D. J., & Landolt, H. P. (2019). Sleep Physiology, circadian rhythms, waking performance and the development of sleep-wake therapeutics. In *Sleep-Wake Neurobiology and Pharmacology* (pp. 441–481). Cham: Springer.

Dikmen, H. A., & Terzioglu, F. (2019). Effects of reflexology and progressive muscle relaxation on pain, fatigue, and quality of life during chemotherapy in gynecologic cancer patients. *Pain Management Nursing, 20*(1), 47–53. https://doi.org/10.1016/j.pmn.2018.03.001.

Donnelly, B., Touyz, S., Hay, P., Burton, A., Russell, J., & Caterson, I. (2018). Neuroimaging in bulimia nervosa and binge eating disorder: a systematic review. *Journal of Eating Disorders, 6*(1), 1–24. https://doi:10.1186/s40337-018-0187-1.

Dunne, J. P., Shindul-Rothschild, J., White, L., Lee, C. S., & Wolfe, B. E. (2021). Mindfulness in persons with anorexia nervosa and the relationships between eating disorder symptomology, anxiety and pain. *Eating Disorders, 29*(5), 497–508. https://doi.org/10.1080/10640266.2019.1688009.

Edinger, J. D., Arnedt, J. T., Bertisch, S. M., Carney, C. E., Harrington, J. J., Lichstein, K. L., Sateia, M. J., Troxel, W. M., Zhou, E. S., Kazmi, U., Heald, J. L., & Martin, J. L. (2021). Behavioral and psychological treatments for chronic insomnia disorder in adults: an American Academy of Sleep Medicine clinical practice guideline. *Journal of Clinical Sleep Medicine, 17*(2), 255–262. https://doi.org/10.5664/jcsm.8986.

Eisenberger, N. I. (2012). The pain of social disconnection: examining the shared neural underpinnings of physical and social pain. *Nature Reviews Neuroscience, 13*(6), 421–434.

Elma, Ö., Yilmaz, S. T., Deliens, T., Coppieters, I., Clarys, P., Nijs, J., & Malfliet, A. (2020). Do nutritional factors interact with chronic musculoskeletal pain? A systematic review. *Journal of Clinical Medicine, 9*(3), 702. https://doi.org/10.3390/jcm9030702.

Engin, A. (2017). The pathogenesis of obesity-associated adipose tissue inflammation. In A. B, Engin, & A. Engin (Eds.), *Obesity and Lipotoxicity*, 221–245. https://doi:10.1007/978-3-319-48382-5_9.

Fanselow, M. S. (2018). Emotion, motivation and function. *Current Opinion in Behavioral Sciences, 19*, 105–109. https://doi.org/10.1016/j.cobeha.2017.12.013.

Fanselow, M. S., & Baackes, M. P. (1982). Conditioned fear-induced opiate analgesia on the formalin test: Evidence for two aversive motivational systems. *Learning and Motivation, 13*(2), 200–221. (CLASSIC).

Finan, P. H., & Garland, E. L. (2015). The role of positive affect in pain and its treatment. *The Clinical Journal of Pain, 31*(2), 177–187. https://doi:10.1097/AJP.0000000000000092.

Flor, H., & Birbaumer, N. (2015). Fear conditioning: overview. In *International Encyclopedia of Social and Behavioral Sciences*. Oxford: Elsevier (pp. 849–853).

Fox, A. S., & Shackman, A. J. (2019). The central extended amygdala in fear and anxiety: Closing the gap between mechanistic and neuroimaging research. *Neuroscience Letters, 693*, 58–67. https://doi.org/10.1016/j.neulet.2017.11.056.

Frilander, H., Solovieva, S., Mutanen, P., Pihlajamäki, H., Heliövaara, M., & Viikari-Juntura, E. (2015). Role of overweight and obesity in low back disorders among men: a longitudinal study with a life course approach. *British Medical Journal Open, 5*(8). http://dx.doi.org/10.1136/bmjopen-2015-007805.

Frilander, H., Viikari-Juntura, E., Heliövaara, M., Mutanen, P., Mattila, V. M., & Solovieva, S. (2016). Obesity in early adulthood predicts knee pain and walking difficulties among men:

a life course study. *European Journal of Pain, 20*(8), 1278–1287. https://doi.org/10.1002/ejp.852.

Garland, E. L., Reese, S. E., Bedford, C. E., & Baker, A. K. (2019). Adverse childhood experiences predict autonomic indices of emotion dysregulation and negative emotional cue-elicited craving among female opioid-treated chronic pain patients. *Development and Psychopathology, 31*(3), 1101–1110. doi:10.1017/S095457941900062.

Gerçeker, G.Ö., Bektaş, M., Aydınok, Y., Ören, H., Ellidokuz, H., & Olgun, N. (2021). The effect of virtual reality on pain, fear, and anxiety during access of a port with huber needle in pediatric hematology-oncology patients: Randomized controlled trial. *European Journal of Oncology Nursing, 50*, 101886. https://doi.org/10.1016/j.ejon.2020.101886.

Gilam, G., Gross, J. J., Wager, T. D., Keefe, F. J., & Mackey, S. C. (2020). What is the relationship between pain and emotion? Bridging constructs and communities. *Neuron, 107*(1), 17–21. https://doi.org/10.1016/j.neuron.2020.05.024.

Glogan, E., van Vliet, C., Roelandt, R., & Meulders, A. (2019). Generalization and Extinction of Concept-Based Pain-Related Fear. *The Journal of Pain, 20*(3), 325–338. https://doi.org/10.1016/j.jpain.2018.09.010.

Goldman, N., Hablitz, L. M., Mori, Y., & Nedergaard, M. (2020). The Glymphatic System and Pain. *Medical Acupuncture, 32*(6), 373–376. https://doi.org/10.1089/acu.2020.1489.

Godfrey, K. M., Bullock, A. J., Dorflinger, L. M., Min, K. M., Ruser, C. B., & Masheb, R. M. (2018). Pain and modifiable risk factors among weight loss seeking Veterans with overweight. *Appetite, 128*, 100–105. https://doi.org/10.1016/j.appet.2018.06.010.

Gramling, R., Straton, J., Ingersoll, L. T., Clarfeld, L. A., Hirsch, L., Gramling, C. J., Durieux, B. N., Rizzo, D. M., Epstein, M. J., & Alexander, S. C. (2021). Epidemiology of Fear, Sadness, and Anger Expression in Palliative Care Conversations. *Journal of Pain and Symptom Management, 61*(2), 246–253. e1. https://doi.org/10.1016/j.jpainsymman.2020.08.017.

Gross, J. J. (2014). *Emotion Regulation: Conceptual and Empirical Foundations*. NY, NY: Guilford Publications. Inc.

Gunzelmann, G., James, S. M., & Caldwell, J. L. (2019). Basic and applied science interactions in fatigue understanding and risk mitigation. *Progress in Brain Research, 246*, 177–204. https://doi.org/10.1016/bs.pbr.2019.03.022.

Guerdjikova, A. I., Mori, N., Casuto, L. S., & McElroy, S. L. (2019). Update on binge eating disorder. *Medical Clinics, 103*(4), 669–680. http://dx.doi.org/10.1016/j.mcna.2019.02.003.

Gurevich, M. I., Chung, M. K., & LaRiccia, P. J. (2018). Resolving bulimia nervosa using an innovative neural therapy approach: two case reports. *Clinical Case Reports, 6*(2), 278–282. https://doi:10.1002/ccr3.1326.

Gyawali, P., Hinwood, M., Chow, W. Z., Kluge, M., Ong, L. K., Nilsson, M., & Walker, F. R. (2020). Exploring the relationship between fatigue and circulating levels of the pro-inflammatory biomarkers interleukin-6 and C-reactive protein in the chronic stage of stroke recovery: A cross-sectional study. *Brain, Behavior, & Immunity-Health, 9*, 100157. https://doi.org/10.1016/j.bbih.2020.100157.

Hackney, A. J., Klinedinst, N. J., Resnick, B., & Johantgen, M. (2019). Association of Systemic Inflammation and Fatigue in Osteoarthritis: 2007–2010 National Health and Nutrition Examination Survey. *Biological Research for Nursing, 21*(5), 532–543. https://doi.org/10.1177/1099800419859091.

Part 3

Hales, C. M., Carroll, M. D., Fryar, C. D., & Ogden, C. L. (2020). *Prevalence of Obesity and Severe Obesity Among Adults: United States, 2017–2018. NCHS Data Brief, no 360.* Hyattsville, MD: National Center for Health Statistics.

Hanssen, M. M., Peters, M. L., Vlaeyen, J. W., Meevissen, Y. M., & Vancleef, L. M. (2013). Optimism lowers pain: evidence of the causal status and underlying mechanisms. *Pain, 154*(1), 53–58. https://doi.org/10.1016/j.pain.2012.08.006.

Haynes, J., Talbert, M., Fox, S., & Close, E. (2018). Cognitive Behavioral Therapy in the Treatment of Insomnia. *Southern Medical Journal, 111*(2), 75–80. https://doi:10.14423/smj.0000000000000769.

Hege, M. A., Veit, R., Krumsiek, J., Kullmann, S., Heni, M., Rogers, P. J., Brunstrom, J. M., Fritsche, A., Preissl, H., & Preissl, H. (2018). Eating less or more–Mindset induced changes in neural correlates of pre-meal planning. *Appetite, 125*, 492–501. https://doi.org/10.1016/j.appet.2018.03.006.

Hershler, A. (2021). Window of Tolerance. In P. Nguyen, & S. Wall (Eds.), *Looking at Trauma: A Tool Kit for Clinicians* (pp. 23–29). University Park, PA: The Pennsylvania State University Press.

Hilbert, A. (2019). Binge-eating disorder. *Psychiatric Clinics, 42*(1), 33–43. https://doi.org/10.1016/j.psc.2018.10.011.

Jessen, N. A., Munk, A. S. F., Lundgaard, I., & Nedergaard, M. (2015). The glymphatic system: a beginner's guide. *Neurochemical Research, 40*(12), 2583–2599. https://doi.org/10.1007/s11064-015-1581-6.

Kamonseki, D. H., Christenson, P., Rezvanifar, S. C., & Calixtre, L. B. (2020). Effects of manual therapy on fear avoidance, kinesiophobia and pain catastrophizing in individuals with chronic musculoskeletal pain: Systematic review and meta-analysis. *Musculoskeletal Science and Practice*, 102311. https://doi.org/10.1016/j.msksp.2020.102311.

Kassinove, H., & Tafrate, R. C. (2019). *The Practitioner's Guide to Anger Management: Customizable Interventions, Treatments, and Tools for Clients with Problem Anger.* New Harbinger Publications.

Keifer, P. O. Jr., Hurt, R. C., Ressler, K. J., & Marvar, P. J. (2015). The physiology of fear: reconceptualizing the role of the central amygdala in fear learning. *Physiology, 30*(5), 389–401. https://doi.org/10.1152/physiol.00058.2014.

Khalsa, S. S., Adolphs, R., Cameron, O. G., Critchley, H. D., Davenport, P. W., Feinstein, J. S., Feusner, J. D., Garfinkel, S. N., Lane, R. D., Mehling, W. E., Meuret, A. E., Nemeroff, C. B., Oppenheimer, S., Petzchner, F. H., Pollatos, O., Rhudy, J. L., Schramm, L. P., Simmons, W. K., … Zucker, N. (2018). Interoception and mental health: a roadmap. *Biological Psychiatry: Cognitive Neuroscience and Neuroimaging, 3*(6), 501–513. https://doi.org/10.1016/j.bpsc.2017.12.004.

Klabunde, M., Collado, D., & Bohon, C. (2017). An interoceptive model of bulimia nervosa: A neurobiological systematic review. *Journal of Psychiatric Research, 94*, 36–46. https://doi:10.1016/j.jpsychires.2017.06.009.

Koechlin, H., Coakley, R., Schechter, N., Werner, C., & Kossowsky, J. (2018). The role of emotion regulation in chronic pain: A systematic literature review. *Journal of Psychosomatic Research, 107*, 38–45. https://doi.org/10.1016/j.jpsychores.2018.02.002.

Korkut, S., & Ülker, T. (2021). The Effect of Pain Experienced During the COVID-19 Infection on the Fear of Pain and Quality of Life. *Pain Management Nursing.* On line 20 August 2021. https://doi:10.1016/j.pmn.2021.08.007.

Kornstein, S. G. (2017). Epidemiology and recognition of binge-eating disorder in psychiatry and primary care. *The Journal of Clinical Psychiatry, 78*(suppl 1), 3–8. https://doi.org/10.4088/JCP.sh16003su1c.01.

Kotsou, I., Mikolajczak, M., Heeren, A., Grégoire, J., & Leys, C. (2019). Improving emotional intelligence: A systematic review of existing work and future challenges. *Emotion Review, 11*(2), 151–165. https://doi.org/10.1177/1754073917735902.

Lalouni, M., Hesser, H., Bonnert, M., Hedman-Lagerlöf, E., Serlachius, E., Olén, O., & Ljótsson, B. (2021). Breaking the vicious circle of fear and avoidance in children with abdominal pain: A mediation analysis. *Journal of Psychosomatic Research, 140*, 110287. https://doi.org/10.1016/j.jpsychores.2020.110287.

Lapidus, R. C., Puhl, M., Kuplicki, R., Stewart, J. L., Paulus, M. P., & Rhudy, J. L., … Tulsa 1000 Investigators. (2020). Heightened affective response to perturbation of respiratory but not pain signals in eating, mood, and anxiety disorders. *PLoS One, 15*(7), e0235346. https://doi.org/10.1371/journal.pone.0235346.

Lea, R. G., Davis, S. K., Mahoney, B., & Qualter, P. (2019). Does emotional intelligence buffer the effects of acute stress? A systematic review. *Frontiers in Psychology, 10*, 810. https://doi.org/10.3389/fpsyg.2019.00810.

Lee, L. O., James, P., Zevon, E. S., Kim, E. S., Trudel-Fitzgerald, C., Spiro, A., Goldstein, F., & Kubzansky, L. D. (2019). Optimism is associated with exceptional longevity in 2 epidemiologic cohorts of men and women. *Proceedings of the National Academy of Sciences, 116*(37), 18357–18362. https://doi.org/10.1073/pnas.1900712116.

Legler, S. R., Beale, E. E., Celano, C. M., Beach, S. R., Healy, B. C., & Huffman, J. C. (2019). State gratitude for one's life and health after an acute coronary syndrome: Prospective associations with physical activity, medical adherence and re-hospitalizations. *The Journal of Positive Psychology, 14*(3), 283–291. https://doi.org/10.1080/17439760.2017.1414295.

Letzen, J. E., Remeniuk, B., Smith, M. T., Irwin, M. R., Finan, P. H., & Seminowicz, D. A. (2020). Individual differences in pain sensitivity are associated with cognitive network functional connectivity following one night of experimental sleep disruption. *Human Brain Mapping, 41*(3), 581–593. https://doi.org/10.1002/hbm.24824.

Linardon, J., Wade, T. D., De la Piedad Garcia, X., & Brennan, L. (2017). The efficacy of cognitive-behavioral therapy for eating disorders: A systematic review and meta-analysis. *Journal of Consulting and Clinical Psychology, 85*(11), 1080. https://doi.org/10.1037/ccp0000245.

Liu, F., You, J., Li, Q., Fang, T., Chen, M., Tang, N., & Yan, X. (2019). Acupuncture for Chronic Pain-Related Insomnia: A Systematic Review and Meta-Analysis. *Evidence-Based Complementary and Alternative Medicine, 2019.* https://doi.org/10.1155/2019/5381028.

Lock, A. M., Bonetti, D. L., & Campbell, A. D. K. (2018). The psychological and physiological health effects of fatigue. *Occupational Medicine, 68*(8), 502–511. https://doi:10.1093/occmed/kqy109.

Luo, P., Wang, J., Jin, Y., Huang, S., Xie, M., Deng, L., Fang, J., Zheng, X., Chen, X., Li, Y., Jiang, Y., & Zheng, X. (2015). Gender differences in affective sharing and self–other distinction during empathic neural responses to others' sadness. *Brain Imaging and Behavior, 9*(2), 312–322. https://doi.org/10.1007/s11682-014-9308-.

Lydecker, J. A., & Grilo, C. M. (2019). Food insecurity and bulimia nervosa in the United States. *International Journal of Eating Disorders, 52*(6), 735–739. https://doi:10.1002/eat.23074.

Markfelder, T., & Pauli, P. (2020). Fear of pain and pain intensity: Meta-analysis and systematic review. *Psychological Bulletin, 146*(5), 411–450. https://doi.org/10.1037/bul0000228.

Martinez-Calderon, J., Flores-Cortes, M., Morales-Asencio, J. M., & Luque-Suarez, A. (2020). Conservative interventions reduce fear in individuals with chronic low back pain: a systematic review. *Archives of Physical Medicine and Rehabilitation, 101*(2), 329–358. https://doi.org/10.1016/j.apmr.2019.08.470.

McCuen-Wurst, C., Ruggieri, M., & Allison, K. C. (2018). Disordered eating and obesity: associations between binge eating-disorder, night-eating syndrome, and weight-related co-morbidities. *Annals of the New York Academy of Sciences, 1411*(1), 96–105. https://doi:10.1111/nyas.13467.

McCurry, S. M., Zhu, W., Von Korff, M., Wellman, R., Morin, C. M., Thakral, M., Yeimg., K., & Vitiello, M. V. (2021). Effect of Telephone Cognitive Behavioral Therapy for Insomnia in Older Adults With Osteoarthritis Pain: A Randomized Clinical Trial. *JAMA Internal Medicine, 181*(4), 530–538. https://doi:10.1001/jamainternmed.2020.9049.

McDermott, K. A., Smith, H. L., Matheny, N. L., & Cougle, J. R. (2017). Pain and multiple facets of anger and hostility in a sample seeking treatment for problematic anger. *Psychiatry Research, 253*, 311–317. http://dx.doi.org/10.1016/j.psychres.2017.04.006.

Meevissen, Y., Peters, M., & Alberts, H. (2011). Become more optimistic by imagining a best possible self: effects of a two week intervention. *Journal of Behavior Therapy and Experimental Psychiatry, 42*(3), 371–378. https://doi:10.1016/j.jbtep.2011.02.012.

Mestre, H., Mori, Y., & Nedergaard, M. (2020). The brain's glymphatic system: current controversies. *Trends in Neurosciences, 43*(7), 458–466. https://doi.org/10.1016/j.tins.2020.04.003.

Meulders, A. (2019). From fear of movement-related pain and avoidance to chronic pain disability: A state-of-the-art review. *Current Opinion in Behavioral Sciences, 26*, 130–136. https://doi.org/10.1016/j.cobeha.2018.12.007.

Miao, C., Humphrey, R. H., & Qian, S. (2018). The relationship between emotional intelligence and trait mindfulness: A meta-analytic review. *Personality and Individual Differences, 135*, 101–107. https://doi.org/10.1016/j.paid.2018.06.051.

Miller, M. M., Scott, E. L., Trost, Z., & Hirsh, A. T. (2016). Perceived injustice is associated with pain and functional outcomes in children and adolescents with chronic pain: A preliminary examination. *The Journal of Pain, 17*(11), 1217–1226. https://doi.org/10.1016/j.jpain.2016.08.002.

Miller, M. M., Wuest, D., Williams, A. E., Scott, E. L., Trost, Z., & Hirsh, A. T. (2018). Injustice perceptions about pain: Parent–child discordance is associated with worse functional outcomes. *Pain, 159*(6), 1083–1089. https://doi.org/10.1097/j.pain.0000000000001192.

Miller, M. M., Williams, A. E., Scott, E. L., Trost, Z., & Hirsh, A. T. (2021). Anger as a mechanism of injustice appraisals in pediatric chronic pain. *The Journal of Pain*. https://doi.org/10.1016/j.jpain.2021.07.005.

Milling, L. S., Gover, M. C., & Moriarty, C. L. (2018). The effectiveness of hypnosis as an intervention for obesity: A meta-analytic review. *Psychology of Consciousness: Theory, Research, and Practice, 5*(1), 29–45. https://doi.org/10.1037/cns0000139.

Morgan, B., Gulliford, L., & Kristjánsson, K. (2017). A new approach to measuring moral virtues: the multi-component gratitude measure. *Personality and Individual Differences, 107*, 179–189. https://doi.org/10.1016/j.paid.2016.11.044.

Müller, R., Segerer, W., Ronca, E., Gemperli, A., Stirnimann, D., Scheel-Sailer, A., & Jensen, M. P. (2020). Inducing positive emotions to reduce chronic pain: a randomized controlled trial of positive psychology exercises. *Disability and Rehabilitation*, 1–14. doi:10.1080/09638288.2020.1850888. (published online).

Munn-Chernoff, M. A., & Baker, J. H. (2016). A primer on the genetics of comorbid eating disorders and substance use disorders. *European Eating Disorders Review, 24*, 91–100. https://doi:10.1002/erv.2424.

Neville, A., Kopala-Sibley, D. C., Soltani, S., Asmundson, G. J., Jordan, A., Carleton, R. N., Nichols, R., Yeates, K. O., Schulte, F., & Noel, M. (2021). A longitudinal examination of the interpersonal fear avoidance model of pain: the role of intolerance of uncertainty. *Pain, 162*(1), 152–160. https://doi.org/10.1097/j.pain.0000000000002009.

Nijs, J., Elma, Ö., Yilmaz, S. T., Mullie, P., Vanderweeën, L., Clarys, P., Deliens, T., Coppieters, I., Weltens, N., Van Oudenhove, L., & Malfliet, A. (2019). Nutritional neurobiology and central nervous system sensitisation: missing link in a comprehensive treatment for chronic pain? *British Journal of Anaesthesia, 123*(5), 539–543. https://doi:10.1016/j.bja.2019.07.016.

Ortelli, P., Ferrazzoli, D., Sebastianelli, L., Engl, M., Romanello, R., Nardone, R., Bonini, I., Koch, G., Saltuari, L., Quartarone, A., Oliviero, A., Kofler, M., & Versace, V. (2020). Neuropsychological and neurophysiological correlates of fatigue in post-acute patients with neurological manifestations of COVID-19: Insights into a challenging symptom. *Journal of the Neurological Sciences, 420*, 117271. https://doi.org/10.1016/j.jns.2020.117271.

O'Toole, M. T. (Ed.). (2022). *Mosby's Medical Dictionary - e book* (11ᵗʰ Ed.). St. Louis, MO: Elsevier ISBN 978-0-323-63915-6.

Parmelee, P. A., Scicolone, M. A., Cox, B. S., DeCaro, J. A., Keefe, F. J., & Smith, D. M. (2018). Global versus momentary osteoarthritis pain and emotional distress: emotional intelligence as moderator. *Annals of Behavioral Medicine, 52*(8), 713–723. https://doi.org/10.1093/abm/kax044.

Paul, E. S., Sher, S., Tamietto, M., Winkielman, P., & Mendl, M. T. (2020). Towards a comparative science of emotion: affect and consciousness in humans and animals. *Neuroscience & Biobehavioral Reviews, 108*, 749–770. https://doi.org/10.1016/j.neubiorev.2019.11.014.

Peters, M., Smeets, E., Feijge, M., et al. (2017). Happy despite pain: a randomized controlled trial of an 8-week internet-delivered positive psychology intervention for enhancing well-being in patients with chronic pain. *The Clinical Journal of Pain, 33*(11), 962–975. https://doi:10.1097/AJP.0000000000000494.

Portocarrero, F. F., Gonzalez, K., & Ekema-Agbaw, M. (2020). A meta-analytic review of the relationship between dispositional gratitude and well-being. *Personality and Individual Differences, 164*, 110101. https://doi.org/10.1016/j.paid.2020.110101.

Poza, J. J., Pujol, M., Ortega-Albás, J. J., & Romero, O. (2021). Melatonin in sleep disorders. *Neurología (English Edition)*. IN PRESS.

Prefit, A. B., Cândea, D. M., & Szentagotai-Tătar, A. (2019). Emotion regulation across eating pathology: A meta-analysis. *Appetite, 143*, 104438.

Rosenbaum, D. L., Kimerling, R., Pomernacki, A., Goldstein, K. M., Yano, E. M., Sadler, A. G., Carney, D., Bastian, L. A.,

Bean-Mayberry, B. A., & Frayne, S. M. (2016). Binge eating among women veterans in primary care: Comorbidities and treatment priorities. *Women's Health Issues, 26*(4), 420–428. https://doi.org/10.1016/j.whi.2016.02.004.

Rozanski, A., Bavishi, C., Kubzansky, L. D., & Cohen, R. (2019). Association of optimism with cardiovascular events and all-cause mortality: a systematic review and meta-analysis. *JAMA Network Open, 2*(9), e1912200. https://doi:10.1001/jamanetworkopen.2019.12200.

Salovey, P., & Mayer, J. D. (1990). Emotional intelligence. *Imagination. Cognition and Personality, 9*(3), 185–211. https://doi.org/10.2190/DUGG-P24E-52WK-6CDG.

Sarrionandia, A., & Mikolajczak, M. (2020). A meta-analysis of the possible behavioural and biological variables linking trait emotional intelligence to health. *Health Psychology Review, 14*(2), 220–244. https://doi.org/10.1080/17437199.2019.1641423.

Scheier, M. F., & Carver, C. S. (2018). Dispositional optimism and physical health: A long look back, a quick look forward. *American Psychologist, 73*(9), 1082–1094. https://doi.org/10.1037/amp0000384.

Shaygan, M., & Karami, Z. (2020). Chronic Pain in Adolescents: The Predictive Role of Emotional Intelligence, Self-Esteem, and Parenting Style. *International Journal of Community Based Nursing and Midwifery, 8*(3), 253–263. doi:10.30476/ijcbnm.2020.83153.1129.

Sim, L. A., Lebow, J., Weiss, K., Harrison, T., & Bruce, B. (2017). Eating disorders in adolescents with chronic pain. *Journal of Pediatric Health Care, 31*(1), 67–74. https://doi.org/10.1016/j.pedhc.2016.03.001.

Smith, M. T., McCrae, C. S., Cheung, J., Martin, J. L., Harrod, C. G., Heald, J. L., & Carden, K. A. (2018). Use of actigraphy for the evaluation of sleep disorders and circadian rhythm sleep-wake disorders: an American Academy of Sleep Medicine systematic review, meta-analysis, and GRADE assessment. *Journal of Clinical Sleep Medicine, 14*(7), 1209–1230. https://doi.org/10.5664/jcsm.7228.

Sommer, I., Lukic, N., Rössler, W., & Ettlin, D. A. (2019). Measuring anger in patients experiencing chronic pain-A systematic review. *Journal of Psychosomatic Research, 125*, 109778. https://doi.org/10.1016/j.jpsychores.2019.109778.

Stefan, S. I., & Hofmann, S. G. (2019). Integrating metta into CBT: how loving kindness and compassion meditation can enhance CBT for treating anxiety and depression. *Clinical Psychology in Europe, 1*(3), 1–15. https://doi.org/10.32872/cpe.v1i3.32941.

Teaford, M., McMurray, M. S., Billock, V., Filipkowski, M., & Smart, L. J., Jr. (2021). The somatosensory system in anorexia nervosa: A scoping review. *Journal of Experimental Psychopathology, 12*(1), 2043808720987346. https://doi.org/10.1177/2043808720987346.

Thomas, J. J., Lawson, E. A., Micali, N., Misra, M., Deckersbach, T., & Eddy, K. T. (2017). Avoidant/restrictive food intake disorder: a three-dimensional model of neurobiology with implications for etiology and treatment. *Current Psychiatry Reports, 19*(8), 1–9. https://doi:10.1007/s11920-017-0795-5.

Toledo, T. A., Hellman, N., Lannon, E. W., Sturycz, C. A., Kuhn, B. L., Payne, M. F., Palit, S., G€uereca, M., Shadlow, J. O., & Rhudy, J. L. (2019a). Anger inhibition and pain modulation. *Annals of Behavioral Medicine, 53*(12), 1055–1068. https://doi.org/10.1093/abm/kaz016.

Toledo, T., Hellman, N., Lannon, E., Sturycz, C., Kuhn, B., Payne, M., Palit, S., Guereca, J., & Rhudy, J. (2019b). Does Anger Inhibition Alter Pain Modulation? *The Journal of Pain, 20*(4), S39–S40. https://doi.org/10.1016/j.jpain.2019.01.183.

Troynikov, O., Watson, C. G., & Nawaz, N. (2018). Sleep environments and sleep physiology: a review. *Journal of Thermal Biology, 78*, 192–203. https://doi.org/10.1016/j.jtherbio.2018.09.012.

Valikhani, A., Ahmadnia, F., Karimi, A., & Mills, P. J. (2019). The relationship between dispositional gratitude and quality of life: The mediating role of perceived stress and mental health. *Personality and Individual Differences, 141*, 40–46. https://doi.org/10.1016/j.paid.2018.12.014.

Veenhoven, Ruut. (2015). *Happiness: History of the concept (2nd ed.)* In *International Encyclopedia of Social and Behavioral Sciences* 10 (pp. 521–525). Oxford: Elsevier.

Veronese, N., Koyanagi, A., Stubbs, B., Cooper, C., Guglielmi, G., Rizzoli, R., Punzi, L., Ragoli, D., Caruso, M. G., Rotolo, O., Notarnicola, M., Al-Daghri, N., Smith, L., Reginster, J. Y., & Maggi, S. (2019). Mediterranean diet and knee osteoarthritis outcomes: a longitudinal cohort study. *Clinical Nutrition, 38*(6), 2735–2739. https://doi:10.1016/j.clnu.2018.11.032.

Watkins, P. C., Emmons, R. A., Greaves, M. R., & Bell, J. (2018). Joy is a distinct positive emotion: Assessment of joy and relationship to gratitude and well-being. *The Journal of Positive Psychology, 13*(5), 522–539. https://doi.org/10.1080/17439760.2017.1414298.

Wilkes, C., Kydd, R., Sagar, M., & Broadbent, E. (2017). Upright posture improves affect and fatigue in people with depressive symptoms. *Journal of Behavior Therapy and Experimental Psychiatry, 54*, 143–149. http://dx.doi.org/10.1016/j.jbtep.2016.07.015.

Yamamotova, A., Bulant, J., Bocek, V., & Papezova, H. (2017). Dissatisfaction with own body makes patients with eating disorders more sensitive to pain. *Journal of Pain Research, 10*, 1667–1675. https://doi:10.2147/JPR.S133425.

Yu, L., Scott, W., & McCracken, L. M. (2019). Change in fatigue in acceptance and commitment therapy-based treatment for chronic pain and its association with enhanced psychological flexibility. *European Journal of Pain, 24*(1), 234–247. https://doi:10.1002/ejp.1480.

Zhou, P., Critchley, H., Garfinkel, S., & Gao, Y. (2021). The Conceptualization of Emotions across Cultures: A Model Based on Interoceptive Neuroscience. *Neuroscience & Biobehavioral Reviews, 125*(6), 314–327. https://doi.org/10.1016/j.neubiorev.2021.02.023.

Zucker, N. L., & Bulik, C. M. (2020). On bells, saliva, and abdominal pain or discomfort: Early aversive visceral conditioning and vulnerability for anorexia nervosa. *International Journal of Eating Disorders, 5*. https://doi.org/10.1002/eat.23255.

CHAPTER 14

Overview of Pain Assessment, Management, and Select Clinical Practice Guidelines

Karen P. Hall, MSN, MSHSA, RN-BC
Maureen F. Cooney, DNP, FNP-BC, ACHPN, AP-PMN*

Introduction

This chapter explains ways in which pain management has evolved over the past several decades. Pain assessment and interventions, as well as impact of the opioid crisis, are briefly reviewed, as are select pain management guidelines.

I. Evolution of Pain Assessment and Management

A. 1990: Dr. Mitchell Max (President of American Pain Society) raised issue of poorly assessed and treated pain, believing pain assessment and treatment should be made "visible."

B. 1991: American Pain Society created pain standards.
1. Use simple and valid pain intensity measures.
2. Document pain assessment, interventions, and pain relief.
3. Use pain ratings to review patient's current pain care.

C. Early 1990s: Acute pain services started to appear in hospitals.
1. Determined patients were often undertreated for pain following surgery, other medical procedures, and trauma
2. Goals of these services included effective pain treatment, patient education, and reduction of postoperative complications.
3. Acute pain services were most often led by anesthesiologists, and some were interprofessional, including nurses, pharmacists, and surgeons. Over time, these services have evolved and may be successfully led by nurses or nurse practitioners.

D. 1995: Approval and support for sustained-release oxycodone (OxyContin)
1. Promoted as a less addictive medication
2. Unethical marketing practices involving the way prescribers were approached and informed about the medication, expectations of outcomes, and potential for misuse/abuse
3. 2001: Unsubstantiated claims about the medication were required to be removed from labels; however, studies refuting original claims were not published until years later.

E. 1999: California legislature joined the effort, passing Assembly Bill 791, requiring pain to be assessed with vital signs.

F. 2000: United States Congress passed H.R. 3244, title VI, Sec. 1603, establishing "Decade of Pain Control and Research."

G. 2001: The Joint Commission on Accreditation of Healthcare Organizations (TJC) published its first Patient Pain Assessment and Management pain standards, with the support of Robert Wood Johnson Foundation in collaboration with University of Wisconsin-Madison School of Medicine and other experts.
1. TJC pain standards are updated regularly and apply to:
   a. Ambulatory care
   b. Behavioral healthcare
   c. Critical access hospitals
   d. Hospitals
   e. Nursing care centers
   f. Office-based surgeries
   g. Home health services
2. Examples of ways to implement standards were included and caused confusion when some considered these examples to be standards rather than examples.
3. 2002: Standards requiring use of pain scales in post-anesthesia care units (PACUs) were implemented.
   a. Amount of opioid used per patient increased on average from 40.4 mg (morphine equivalents) in 2000 to 46.6 mg in 2002, with largest increase occurring in PACUs.
   b. Length of stay, use of an antagonist (e.g., naloxone), and frequency of nausea and vomiting did not increase.

*Section Editor for the chapter.

c. Nurses, other healthcare professionals, and parents were found to often underestimate pain in comparison to patients' self-report.

d. Some overzealousness in treatment of pain caused issues related to patients' rights, as needed (PRN) range orders, pain as "fifth vital sign" and policy implementation including algorithms in relation to numeric pain scores. These practices may have contributed to over sedation and death.

4. 2009: Requirement that all patients must be assessed for pain was controversial and removed from standards.

5. 2011: TJC recognized role of both pharmacological and nonpharmacological strategies in pain management.

6. 2017: Pain-related questions were permanently removed from TJC survey in response to concerns related to hospitals incentivized for excellent pain satisfaction scores, leading to opioid overprescribing.

7. Since 2018: TJC pain standards increased focus on safe opioid prescribing, patient education, and multimodal pharmacological and nonpharmacological approaches.

H. 2002: Patient Satisfaction/Hospital Consumer Assessment of Healthcare Providers and Systems Survey (HCAHPS), added pain questions regarding pain management.

a. Pain survey results became connected with financial incentives for hospitals.

b. Evidence supports some providers felt pressured to prescribe opioids to ensure patient satisfaction with pain care.

c. Satisfaction with pain care did not necessarily correlate with well-managed pain.

d. Evidence also showed no difference in satisfaction scores with opioid administration.

I. 2016: Centers for Disease Control and Prevention (CDC) published guidelines for primary care prescribers to improve communication about benefits and risks of opioid treatment for persistent pain, improve safety and efficacy of pain management, and reduce risks related to long-term opioid use.

II. Key Considerations in Today's Pain Management

A. Revised definition of pain from International Association for the Study of Pain after four decades went from "An unpleasant sensory and emotional experience associated with actual or potential tissue damage or described in terms of such damage" to "An unpleasant sensory and emotional experience associated with, *or resembling* that associated with, actual or potential tissue damage" (Raja et al., 2020, p. 1).

B. Need to assess, intervene, and reassess if pain continues

C. Effect of psychosocial factors must be considered. Stepped Care to Optimize Pain Care Effectiveness trial recently studied effects of depression, anxiety, and pain catastrophizing on pain outcomes. Patients were screened for five common anxiety disorders (i.e., generalized anxiety disorders, panic, social anxiety, posttraumatic stress, and obsessive-compulsive disorder). This study recognized detection and treatment of anxiety as an important component of pain management.

D. Effects of opioid epidemic have brought about many changes related to pain management (multiple chapters provide more information on this topic).

1. An increase in use of multimodal analgesia (MMA) (discussed later)

a. Multimodal analgesia involves concurrent use of primarily non-opioid analgesics to take advantage of additive, if not synergistic, effects producing superior analgesia while decreasing opioid use and opioid-related side effects.

b. Integrative and complementary therapies (see chapter 15) are no longer considered "complementary" by some and, in many locations, now fall within prescribing guidelines.

2. May play large part in management of patients with persistent pain

3. Changes in using opioids as first-line treatment

4. Increased patient education

5. Improved assessment tools

6. Increased nurse education

7. Use of enhanced recovery after surgery (ERAS) methodology has increased.

a. Originally developed for colon resections; now included in management of many other surgical approaches

b. Comprehensive system using an interprofessional team and evidence-based approach, allowing patients to recover more quickly, spend less time in hospital, and minimize use of opioids

c. Includes care before, during, and after surgical procedure to decrease physiological stress on body and results in decreased pain, increased mobility, decreased length of stay, decreased complications, and decreased readmissions

d. Primary elements of ERAS include:
   1) Preoperative counseling
   2) Optimization of nutrition
   3) Standardized MMA plans (discussed later)
   4) Early mobilization

E. Social determinants of health, hindering access to optimal pain care (more information available in other chapters)

III. Key Concepts in Comprehensive/ Multidimensional Pain Assessment and Management

A. Assess regularly, before and after interventions, and document.
B. Inclusion of all elements and dimensions of pain is essential for optimal treatment and thorough understanding of patients' pain experience.
  1. Developmental factors (including parent or caregiver involvement)
  2. Physiological and sensory factors
    a. Location
    b. Intensity
    c. Duration
    d. Quality
    e. Aggravating and alleviating factors
    f. One mnemonic, OLDCARTS, may aid nurses in remembering key elements (Onset, Location/ radiation, Duration, Character, Aggravating factors, Relieving factors, Timing, and Severity).
  3. Affect
  4. Cognitive factors
  5. Sociocultural influence
  6. Environmental factors
  7. Patient-defined goals
  8. Impact of pain (e.g., on function, socialization, work/school)
  9. Pertinent medical history
  10. Opioid-induced sedation and respiratory depression
C. Assess for adverse responses to therapy (chapter 12).
D. Multimodal pharmacological and nonpharmacological interventions
  1. MMA uses individual analgesics from different medication classes with varying mechanisms of action to provide effective pain treatment and minimize adverse effects while allowing for opioid sparing. Medications may include:
    a. Non-opioids
      1) Acetaminophen
      2) Local anesthetics
      3) Regional anesthetics
      4) Gabapentinoids
      5) Nonsteroidal anti-inflammatory drugs (NSAIDs)
      6) N-methyl-D-aspartate (NMDA) receptor antagonists
      7) Corticosteroids
      8) Central alpha-2 agonists
      9) Topical agents [e.g., lidocaine, capsaicin]
      10) Musculoskeletal agents
      11) Anti-anxiety medication
      12) Other adjuvants developed for different indications and found to have pain-relieving properties (e.g., antidepressants, anticonvulsants)
    b. Opioids, many of which can be administered by various routes (chapter 17)
    c. Regional anesthetic interventions (chapter 19)
    d. Rehabilitative/physical therapies
      1) Heat/cold
      2) Massage
      3) Exercise
    e. Integrative and complementary therapies (chapter 15), such as:
      1) Yoga
      2) Acupuncture
      3) Acupressure
      4) Guided imagery
      5) Art therapy
      6) Music therapy
      7) Animal-assisted therapy
      8) Biofeedback
    f. Psychological support (chapters 3 and 16):
      1) Mindfulness-based approach
      2) Cognitive behavioral therapy
      3) Relaxation techniques
      4) Somatic anchoring
      5) Hypnosis
      6) Acceptance and commitment therapy
    g. Surgical interventions can overlap with regional interventional techniques and may be indicated when other pain management techniques fail.

IV. Key Pain Management Guidelines

A. Nurses are advised to remain aware of current guidelines and recommendations as they apply to their specific practice.
B. CDC (2022) updated recommendations aimed at provision of safe and effective treatment of pain (https:// www.cdc.gov/mmwr/volumes/71/rr/rr7103a1.htm).
  1. Importantly, CDC clearly states: Persons with pain should receive appropriate pain treatment, with consideration to benefits and risks of treatment options in context of individual patient's circumstances and the guidelines not be applied as inflexible standards across all patient populations.
  2. Guideline was expanded to include acute and persistent (chronic) pain for adults and does not apply to pain secondary to sickle cell disease, cancer, palliative care, or end-of-life care.
  3. Guideline addresses:
    a. Determining whether or not to initiate opioids
    b. Assistance with selection of opioid medication, dose, duration, and follow-up
    c. Assessing risk and addressing such risks
    d. Improved communication between providers and patients

4. Guideline included 12 recommendations with levels of evidence for their support.

C. United States Health and Human Services (2019) guidelines provide direction for an effective pain management plan.
   1. Acute pain as a result of trauma, burns, musculoskeletal injury, neural injury, as well as surgical intervention or procedural pain
      a. Multimodal approach
      b. Nerve blocks
      c. Physical therapy
      d. Other modalities, such as complementary and integrative health, including acupuncture, massage, yoga, tai chi, and spirituality
   2. Persistent pain treatments may include:
      a. Non-opioid therapies as first-line therapies
      b. Opioids only when benefits exceed risks
      c. Buprenorphine
      d. Restorative therapies
      e. Interventional procedures
      f. Behavioral health approaches
      g. Complementary and integrative health
D. World Health Organization (WHO)
   1. WHO analgesic ladder originally proposed in 1986 to provide adequate relief for cancer patients (Fig. 14.1), updated in 2023
      a. First step: mild pain: non-opioid analgesics such as NSAIDS or acetaminophen, with or without adjuvants
      b. Second step: moderate pain: weak opioids with or without non-opioid analgesics and with or without adjuvants
      c. Third step: severe and persistent pain: potent opioids with or without non-opioid analgesics and with or without adjuvants
   2. Some scholars recommend adaptations eliminating weak opioids (offer little advantage over low-dose stronger opioids and have less evidence available) and including a fourth step to include invasive and minimally invasive treatment.
   3. *WHO Guidelines for the Pharmacological and Radiotherapeutic Management of Cancer Pain in Adults and Adolescents* (2018)
      a. Initiation of pain relief
      b. Maintenance of pain relief with opioids
      c. Adjuvant medications for cancer pain
      d. Management of pain related to bone metastases
      e. Radiotherapy
   4. *WHO Guidelines on the Management of Chronic Pain in Children* (2021) provides recommended physical, psychological, and pharmacological interventions for pain relief in children 0 to 19 years of age.
E. Several specialty organizations have offered additional pain guidelines.
   1. National Comprehensive Cancer Network guidelines for cancer pain
   2. American College of Surgeons *Best Practices Guidelines for Acute Pain Management in Trauma Patients*
   3. American Academy of Pain Management has consensus guidelines (Enhanced Recovery after Spine Surgery; *Migraine Diagnosis, Prevention and Treatment; Opioid Discontinuation*) in development at time of this publication.

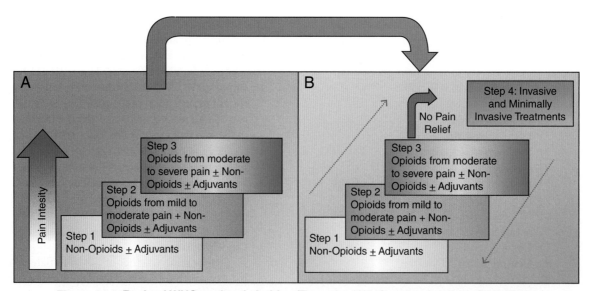

Figure 14.1 Revised WHO analgesic ladder. (The revised WHO analgesic ladder. Contributed by Marco Cascella, MD.) WHO Analgesic Ladder. Treasure Island, FL: StatPearls [Internet] Publishing. 2023.

V. Continued Evolution of Pain Management

A. Pain management is and will continue to become more integrated and collaborative, leading to improved understanding of complexity of pain and new therapeutic possibilities.

B. The following areas will need continued attention in evolution of pain management:

1. Understanding pain experience
   a. Refine understanding of interaction with physiological, psychological, and societal influences
   b. Applying individual treatments to patients experiencing same injury/event
   c. Genetic factors may apply.
   d. Sex and gender differences

2. Pain psychology as part of biopsychosocial model for pain treatment covering topics including:
   a. Fear avoidance
   b. Shared mechanisms between pain, distress, and disability
   c. Cognitive behavioral therapy

3. Accurate and early understanding of cause of pain prevents advancement of damage (e.g., rheumatoid arthritis, diabetic neuropathy).

4. Safe use of opioid therapy when indicated
   a. White paper: *Introduction to FDA's Opioid Systems Model*
   b. Awareness of opioid crisis and ease of access to unsafe illicit medications
   c. Biopsychosocial assessment before and while on opioid treatment

5. Appropriate use of non-opioid medications
   a. There are a number of side effects to be aware of when using non-opioid medications.
   b. There continues to be need for development of new non-opioid analgesic options.

6. Expansion of interventional pain treatments (chapter 19)
   a. Commonly used for pain not responsive to first-line treatments
   b. Interventional pain procedures are not considered first-line treatments given their invasive nature.
   c. Medications commonly used for invasive pain procedures include local anesthetics and glucocorticoids.
   d. Contraindications include existing infection, anticoagulation, hypersensitivity to glucocorticoids, contrast dye, anesthetic medications, local malignancy, or implanted cardiac devices.

7. Expansion of integrative approaches to pain management
   a. Shown to be effective in treatment of fibromyalgia-related pain in adults
   b. Being incorporated into other treatment plans

8. Multidisciplinary pain management programs
   a. Effective for persistent pain conditions
   b. All clinicians have expertise in pain management
   c. Different specialties work together to establish policies, procedures, and therapies

9. Increased focus on importance of function in pain assessment and inclusion of restorative therapies in preventing and treating persistent pain

Bibliography

Abeles, A., Kwasnicki, R. M., & Darzi, A. (2017). Enhanced recovery after surgery: current research insights and future direction. *World Journal of Gastrointestinal Surgery, 9*(2), 37–45. https://doi.org/10.4240/wjgs.v9.i2.37.

Anand, K. J. S., Roue, J. M., Rovnaghi, C. R., Marx, W., & Bornmann, L. (2020). Historical roots of pain management in infants: a bibliometric analysis using reference publication year spectroscopy. *Paediatric & Neonatal Pain, 2*, 22–32. https://dx.doi.org/10.1002/pne2.12035.

Andrews-Cooper, I. N., & Kozachik, S. L. (2020). How patient education influences utilization of nonpharmacological modalities for persistent pain management: an integrative review. *Pain Management Nursing, 21*, 157–164. https://dx.doi.org/10.1016/j.pmn.2019.06.016.

Anekar, A. A., & Cascella, M. (2023). WHO Analgesic Ladder. [Updated April 23, 2023]. In: *StatPearls [Internet]*. Treasure Island, FL: StatPearls Publishing. [Figure, The revised WHO analgesic ladder. Contributed by Marco Cascella, MD.] https://www.ncbi.nlm.nih.gov/books/NBK554435/figure/article-31358.image.f1/

Arnstein, P., Gentile, D., & Wilson, M. (2019). Validating the functional pain scale for hospitalized adults. *Pain Management Nursing, 20*, 418–424. https://dx.doi.org/10.1016/j.pmn.2019.03.006.

Arnstein, P., Herr, K. A., & Butcher, H. K. (2017). Evidence-based practice guideline: persistent pain management in older adults. *Journal of Gerontological Nursing, 43*, 20–31. https://dx.doi.org/10.3928/00989134-20170419-01.

Baker, D. W. (2017). History of The Joint Commission's pain standards: lessons for today's prescription opioid epidemic. *JAMA, 317*(11), 1117–1118. https://doi.org/10.1001/jama.2017.0935.

Becker, W. C., Bair, M. J., Picchioni, M., Starrels, J. L., & Frank, J. W. (2018). Pain management for primary care providers: a narrative review of high-impact studies, 2014–2016. *Pain Medicine, 19*, 40–49. https://dx.doi.org/10.1093/pm/pnx146.

Flink, I., Reme, S., Jacobsen, H., Glombiewski, J., Vlaeyen, J., Nicholas, M., et al. (2020). Pain psychology in the 21st century: lessons learned and moving forward. *Scandinavian Journal of Pain, 20*(2), 229–238. https://doi.org/10.1515/sjpain-2019-0180.

Hall, S., & Belgrade, M. (2021). CAM therapies are no longer complementary or alternative: yoga, acupuncture, and mind-body medicine. *Pain Management Nursing, 22*, 233.

Halm, M., Bailey, C., St Pierre, J., Boutin, N., Rojo, S., Shortt, M., et al. (2019). Pilot evaluation of a functional pain assessment scale. *Clinical Nurse Specialist, 33*, 12–21. https://dx.doi.org/10.1097/NUR.0000000000000416.

Herr, K., Coyne, P. J., Ely, E., Gelinas, C., & Manworren, R. C. B. (2019). ASPMN 2019 position statement: pain assessment in the patient unable to self-report. *Pain Management Nursing, 20*, 402–403. https://dx.doi.org/10.1016/j.pmn.2019.07.007.

Joint Commission on Accreditation of Healthcare Organizations, The. https://www.jointcommission.org/.

Jungquist, C. R., Quinlan-Colwell, A., Vallerand, A., Carlisle, H. L., Cooney, M., Dempsey, S. J., et al. (2020). American Society for Pain Management nursing guidelines on monitoring for opioid-induced advancing sedation and respiratory depression: revisions. *Pain Management Nursing, 21*, 7–25. https://dx.doi.org/10.1016/j.pmn.2019.06.007.

Marchand, S. (2020). Mechanisms challenges of the pain phenomenon. *Frontiers in Pain Research, 1*, 574370. https://dx.doi.org/10.3389/fpain.2020.574370.

Mohabbat, A. B., Mahapatra, S., Jenkins, S. M., Bauer, B. A., Vincent, A., & Wahner-Roedler, D. L. (2019). Use of complementary and integrative therapies by fibromyalgia patients: a 14-year follow-up study. *Mayo Clinic Proceedings: Innovations, Quality & Outcomes, 3*(4), 418–428. https://doi.org/10.1016/j.mayocpiqo.2019.07.003.

Narouze, S., & Stengel, A. (2022). ASRA is now ASRA Pain Medicine: your home for acute and chronic pain. *ASA Monitor, 86*, 34. https://doi.org/10.1097/01.ASM.0000806060.67077.c0.

NEJM Knowledge+ Team (2019). Non-opioid analgesics role in pain management. https://knowledgeplus.nejm.org/blog/non-opioid-analgesics-role-in-pain-management/.

International Association for the Study of Pain. (n.d.). Pain Treatment Services. https://www.iasp-pain.org/resources/guidelines/pain-treatment-services/.

Raja, S. N., Carr, D. B., Cohen, M., Finnerup, N. B., Flor, H., Gibson, S., et al. (2020). The revised International Association for the Study of Pain definition of pain: concepts, challenges, and compromises. *Pain, 161*(9), 1976–1982. https://doi.org/10.1097/j.pain.0000000000001939.

Scher, C., Meador, L., Van Cleave, J. H., & Reid, M. C. (2018). Moving beyond pain as the fifth vital sign and patient satisfaction scores to improve pain care in the 21st century. *Pain Management Nursing, 19*, 125–129. https://dx.doi.org/10.1016/j.pmn.2017.10.010.

U.S. Department of Health and Human Services (2019). Pain Management Best Practices Inter-Agency Task Force Report: Updates, Gaps, Inconsistencies, and Recommendations. https://www.hhs.gov/sites/default/files/pmtf-final-report-2019-05-23.pdf.

Wardhan, R., & Chelly, J. (2017). Recent advances in acute pain management: understanding the mechanisms of acute pain, the prescription of opioids, and the role of multimodal pain therapy. *F1000Research, 6*, 2065. https://dx.doi.org/10.12688/f1000research.12286.1.

Warren, C., Jaisankar, P., Saneski, E., Tenberg, A., & Scala, E. (2020). Understanding barriers and facilitators to nonpharmacological pain management on adult inpatient units. *Pain Management Nursing, 21*(6), 480–487. https://doi.org/10.1016/j.pmn.2020.06.006.

World Health Organization. (2020). *WHO Guidelines on the Management of Chronic Pain in Children*. Geneva, Switzerland: World Health Organization. https://iris.who.int/bitstream/handle/10665/337999/9789240017870-eng.pdf.

World Health Organization. (2018). *WHO Guidelines for the Pharmacological and Radiotherapeutic Management of Cancer Pain in Adults and Adolescents*. Geneva, Switzerland: World Health Organization. https://www.ncbi.nlm.nih.gov/books/NBK537492/.

CHAPTER 15

Integrative and Complementary Therapies for Pain Management

Susan Kathleen O'Conner-Von, PhD, RN-BC, CNE, FNAP
Marilyn Ann Bazinski, DNP, AGCNS, RN, PMGT-BC
Ann Quinlan-Colwell, PhD, MSN
Maureen F. Cooney, DNP, FNP-BC, ACHPN, AP-PMN*

Introduction

Terminology regarding nonpharmacological techniques—alternative, complementary, and integrative care—has evolved over the years. For the purpose of this chapter, terms may be used interchangeably. More information on nonpharmacological techniques can be found in other chapters. This chapter will explore the multitude of integrative and complementary therapies for pain management as a key element to a pain management multimodal approach. The context, education, and logistical support necessary to provide patient-centered pain management interventions in healthcare settings will be explored.

I. Background

A. Key concepts surrounding integrative and complementary therapies
1. Pain is a complex and multifaceted problem requiring a thorough biopsychosocial assessment. Evaluation of all aspects of health and lifestyle, including diet, sleep, activity, stress, relationships, and spirituality, may be considered (see Chapter 13).
2. Providing comfort is the essence of standard nursing care, and nurses sometimes provide comfort measures without formal instruction about their mechanisms, indications, and contraindications.
3. Interventions may include nonpharmacological, noninvasive methods that target cognitive, emotional, and behavioral function.
4. Complementary and integrative therapies can be an essential part of pain management because medical interventions often do not entirely resolve pain, especially persistent (chronic) pain.
5. Use of complementary or integrative therapies prior to medication administration is currently the accepted and optimal standard of care for persistent pain.

6. Components of complementary and integrative therapies
   a. Patient-centered, whole-person care emphasizing the self-healing capabilities and importance of lifestyle to optimize health
   b. Evidence-based
   c. Focused on health and healing; may be prevention-oriented
   d. Incorporates conventional medicine with complementary healthcare
   e. Therapeutic patient-practitioner relationships optimize nonpharmacological interventions
   f. Can include use of nutrition, movement, and mind-body strategies
   g. Can help manage emotional and mental stressors associated with pain
7. Barriers
   a. Knowledge: Patients and clinicians may not be aware of the health benefits.
   b. Perception:
      1) Holding a belief that specialized education is required for any nonpharmacological strategy.
      2) Patient perception that nonpharmacological treatments are ineffective for treatment of moderate to severe pain
   c. Cost:
      1) Reimbursement: may be prohibitive if paying out of pocket
      2) Insurance coverage is increasing for some interventions, especially for pediatric patients.
   d. Stigma
      1) Both patients and healthcare providers may be skeptical about integrative and complementary therapies, particularly psychological therapies.
      2) When making a referral, validate patient's pain is real; reassure patient that pain is not "all in their head" and what you're recommending may be helpful.

---

*Section Editor for the chapter.

e. Research: lack of unequivocal evidence

f. Communication: often not considered standard intervention in patient pain management care plans

8. Facilitators

a. Patient/caregiver endorsement

b. Can be used at home

c. Individuals request complementary therapies in clinical settings

d. Increasing evidence to support specific interventions

e. Known impact and effectiveness on pain experiences, with few negative side effects

f. Patient-centered approach to holistic care

B. Context

1. Complementary and integrative therapies are recognized as an optimal, inclusive, and responsive approach to address patient's diverse and evolving needs.

2. Renewed interest in integrative health therapies relates to changes in opioid prescribing practices in response to ongoing opioid crisis.

3. Both medical and public policies are reconsidering how pain is managed.

a. Integrative and complementary therapies may provide adequate relief of persistent pain and avoid need for pharmacological approaches.

b. Combining various pain-relieving methods, including multimodal therapy, provides more significant relief with fewer adverse effects and substance misuse risk than use of opioids alone. Evidence supports short-term efficacy for use of opioids, yet few studies have been conducted to assess long-term benefits of opioids for persistent pain.

4. State and federal agencies endorse inclusion of nonpharmacological therapies.

a. Federal entities (Centers for Disease Control, The Joint Commission, Centers for Medicare and Medicaid, Federal Drug Administration, World Health Organization, Veterans Health Administration) advocate for use of non-pharmacological measures, including integrative and complementary therapies and nonopioid medications, as first-line approaches for pain in an effort to provide more holistic, patient-centered care.

b. Integrative and complementary measures can attend to a variety of mechanisms along peripheral and central pain pathways and reduce overall amount of opioids prescribed.

c. Nurses and other healthcare providers and patients/caregivers demonstrate growing interest and enthusiasm for these therapies.

C. Prevalence

1. According to an older National Center for Health Statistics survey, 33.2% of adults and 11.6% of children in the United States used some form of complementary health approach in prior 12 months.

2. Out-of-pocket spending for these interventions was estimated at $30.2 billion for adults and $1.9 billion for children.

D. Supportive theories

1. Engel's biopsychosocial model acknowledges impact of mood (e.g., depression, anxiety, or fear) on increased pain perceptions, compared to positive mindsets and decreased pain.

2. Bandura's self-efficacy theory describes person's belief in their abilities to control their circumstances and functioning, such as believing one's ability to control pain.

3. Melzak and Wall's gate control theory

a. Provides physiological explanation for how psychological phenomena such as attention, learning, past experiences, and emotions are incorporated into experience of pain

b. Explains how traditional treatments, such as acupuncture, modulate pain, and spawned novel treatments (e.g., transcutaneous electrical nerve stimulation [TENS] and spinal cord stimulation) may be effective

4. Kolcaba's comfort theory

a. Developed as patient/family-centered theory recognizing comfort is central to nursing

b. Defined as three types of comfort:
   1) Relief: state of having specific comfort needs met
   2) Ease: state of calm or contentment
   3) Transcendence: state in which one can rise above problems or pain

5. Roger's diffusion of innovations

a. Middle-range theory useful to nursing when studying adaption of healthcare innovations by individuals or groups

b. Requires a change agent and adopter who will help communicate information across an organization and establish the practice as key element of complementary pain management

E. Mechanisms of action/rationale supporting integrative therapies

1. Intention is to target brain and body through various physiological mechanisms, including:

a. Neurological changes in prefrontal cortex, limbic system, and cerebral cortex

b. Alteration of hypothalamic-pituitary-adrenal axis and sympathetic and parasympathetic nervous systems

c. Stimulation of endogenous opioid release (e.g., endorphins)

d. Reduction of physical and emotional tension that exacerbates pain; reduction of stress hormones that amplify pain (e.g., adrenaline, cortisol)

    e. Competing for attention and limiting cognitive capacity to attend to painful stimuli

    f. Helping patients change maladaptive coping behaviors (e.g., inactivity, isolation) and replaces with healthier adaptive behaviors

  2. Purpose/aims:

    a. Help individuals reinterpret the meaning of pain

    b. Diminish thoughts that exacerbate pain

    c. Enhance perceptions of personal control over pain and make pain less bothersome or upsetting

    d. Alleviate pain

    e. Restore function

    f. Promote health and well-being

    g. Promote self-efficacy

    h. Reduce opioid requirements

    i. Minimize opioid-related side effects

F. Nurse's role

  1. When incorporating complementary and integrative therapies to promote patients' well-being, nurses should consider the following points (additional considerations for specific types of therapies will be covered in each section below as appropriate):

    a. Assess for current use of complementary and integrative therapies, explore patient's understanding and beliefs of interventions not yet considered, and advocate for patients who are interested.

    b. Advise patients seeking complementary and integrative therapies to inquire about practitioner's qualifications and credentials.

    c. Encourage patients to inquire about their health insurance coverage for treatments.

    d. Assist patients to locate experienced practitioners who work with people with pain and conditions similar to their own.

    e. Share information about community and educational resources with interested patients.

  2. Practice setting considerations

    a. Feasibility of clinical applications (e.g., equipment, supplies, availability of certified practitioners)

    b. Regulatory compliance with state boards of nursing

    c. Interprofessional education

    d. Collaborative integration of pain assessments and treatment recommendations

  3. Research considerations

    a. Remain up to date on current research for complementary and integrative therapies.

    b. Advocate and support future research in integrative and complementary therapies.

G. Institutional support for integrative and complementary therapies

  1. Hospital and clinic administrators, key stakeholders, end users

  2. Budgetary considerations

    a. Availability and delivery of services

    b. Measurement of efficacy

    c. Provision of equipment and materials

  3. Role of technology (e.g., cell phone apps, tablets, virtual reality)

  4. Institutional policies and procedures

    a. Integrative and complementary care should be considered an integral approach to multimodal pain management.

    b. Transforming systems of care toward a more responsive and comprehensive model necessitates increasing access to integrative and complementary treatments within collaborative, interprofessional care.

  5. Safety

    a. Evidence-based integrative and complementary therapies are generally safe and effective components of comprehensive pain care.

    b. Secure input from patients and caregivers about nonpharmacological preferences.

    c. Offer a variety of options in your clinical setting.

    d. It is important for clinicians to review evidence-based practices to familiarize themselves with integrative care therapies before they are used and assess their effectiveness and any negative side effects.

II. Integrative and Complementary Therapies

A. Manipulative and body-based practices

  1. Acupuncture/acupressure

    a. Introduction: Acupuncture and acupressure have been practiced in Asian countries for thousands of years. Millions of people in the United States use acupuncture for pain every year. It is considered safe, and most patients tolerate it well.

    b. Description: Acupuncture is an ancient therapeutic technique that involves insertion of needles into body to promote health and treat various symptoms.

    c. Theory: Acupressure is ancient healing art based on Traditional Chinese Medicine (TCM) practice of acupuncture. Using similar points on body, acupressure (Shiatzu) uses fingertips to apply gentle pressure on acupoints to stimulate body's healing ability. Pressing these points can help release muscle tension and promote blood circulation.

Part 4

Patterns of energy (qi [pronounced "chee"]) flow through the body and are essential for health. Disruption of qi is thought to be responsible for disease. Acupuncture corrects imbalances of qi by using meridian system. According to theory underlying practice of acupressure, applying pressure allows energy to flow.

d. Indication: Acupuncture can be used for variety of pain issues, such as fibromyalgia, headache, menstrual cramps, osteoarthritis, musculoskeletal pain, low back pain, and carpal tunnel. Goal of Shiatzu is to maintain health, whereas acupuncture is more often used to treat imbalances.

e. Biological effect: Acupuncture is based on belief qi flows through body on 12 main and 8 extraordinary pathways known as meridians. Located on meridians are specific points designated for insertion of acupuncture needles, or finger or hand pressure applied during acupressure. There are numerous explanations for biological effect of acupuncture, such as enhancing activation of body's opioid systems or changes in brain chemistry during stimulation of acupuncture points.

f. Efficacy: Studies involving use of acupuncture in treatment of musculoskeletal pain and chronic headache have shown efficacy and sustained effects over time. Other studies have examined benefits of acupuncture for treatment of pain and associated symptoms in those with sickle cell disease, active duty veterans with posttraumatic stress disorder, and other patient populations. Additional research is needed.

2. Chiropractic/spinal manipulation
   a. Introduction: Chiropractors and osteopathic physicians use technique called spinal manipulation. Term *chiropractic* combines Greek words "chair" (hand) and "praxis" (practice) to describe hands-on treatment. Chiropractic care is based on belief health is affected by relationship between spine and its function through nervous system.
   b. Description: Chiropractic care is a healthcare discipline emphasizing inherent recuperative power of body to heal itself without use of drugs or surgery. Development of chiropractic and osteopathy professions was an important early influence on use of complementary therapies in healthcare.
   c. Theory: theoretical underpinnings of chiropractic care include:
      1) Structure and function exist in intimate relation to each other.
      2) Structural distortions can cause functional abnormalities.

   3) Nervous system occupies preeminent role in restoration and maintenance of proper bodily function.
   4) Vertebral subluxation influences bodily function primarily through neurological means.

   d. Indication: Major focus of chiropractic care is adjustment of spinal column, which is proposed to improve health, arrest disease and pain, or both. Chiropractors may also use heat or ice, relaxation techniques, dietary supplements, and counseling on diet and exercise. Purpose of spinal manipulation or adjustment is to improve motion and function of joints, relieve pain, and improve health. Of patients who seek chiropractic care, a majority do so for musculoskeletal pain such as low back pain, neck ache, or headache.
   e. Biological effect: Research is in early stages of establishing biological effects of spinal manipulation therapy.
   f. Efficacy: Although evidence is limited, use of manual therapies, including spinal manipulation for pain-related conditions such as low back pain, appears to provide benefit.

3. Massage therapy
   a. Introduction: Massage is healing therapy with ancient roots in China, Japan, India, and Greece. It is widely used complementary intervention particularly to manage stress and for musculoskeletal types of pain. In 2017, it was estimated therapeutic massages were received by 15.4 million adults in the United States. Different schools of massage therapy evolved from the culture in which they were originally used, including Swedish, Thai, and Japanese (Shaitsu), among others. There are a variety of techniques used in most therapeutic massages, including stroking, kneading, moving, and applying directed pressure. Additional information is available through American Massage Therapy Association at https://www.amtamassage.org.
   b. Description: Consistent with linguistic Greek origin *msssein*, meaning to knead, massage therapy involves manual manipulation of soft tissues with intention to ease discomfort and pain.
   c. Theoretical support: Although specific theory supporting massage was not identified, philosophy and focus on body's ability to heal are basic in most massage education programs. Gate control theory, as outlined by Melzack and Wall, has been used to support analgesic effect of massage on pain, hypothesizing pressure exerted during massage has

competing and modulating effect on pain stimuli.

   d. Indication: Massage is used to alleviate symptoms of stress, increase mobility, increase range of motion, improve function, ease pain, and support preterm infants. It has been used effectively to ease pain in variety of painful conditions including postsurgical pain, low back pain, fibromyalgia, cancer, multiple sclerosis, pelvic and carpal tunnel syndrome, and a variety of musculoskeletal conditions, both acute and persistent. Internationally, massage is used to ease both pain and duration of labor during childbirth. Massage is successfully used with children during procedures, burn care, and sickle cell crises.

   e. Biological effect: Effects are believed to be related to relaxation of tissues, changes in blood flow, improving muscle tone, and releasing tense adhesions. Results of microneurography research demonstrated low-threshold, slow-conducting C fibers, which are involved with nociception, are very sensitive to human touch, with degree of response related to intensity and cadence of touch. It is suggested serotonin levels are amplified during stimulation of pressure receptors, and substance P (a pro-nociceptive substance) is decreased.

   f. Efficacy: Studies support massage as effective for postoperative pain, people living with cancer as intervention to manage pain, fatigue, and anxiety, as well as for other conditions. However, recommendations for using massage compared to other complementary interventions are weak.

   g. Nurse's role: Remind patients of appropriate touch boundaries and how to intervene if there is perceived violation. Although massage is generally considered safe, it should not be used in presence of fever, open wounds, burns, rashes, fractures, hematomas, tumors, or bone metastases, and should be used with caution in any lymphatic malignancies and bleeding disorders.

4. Reflexology

   a. Introduction: Reflexology has roots in ancient cultures, particularly Chinese and Egyptian. Today, in many countries, reflexology is considered an aspect of massage, but in the United States, it is often considered a unique therapy independent of massage. For additional information, the reader is referred to the Reflexology Association of America at https://reflexology-usa.org.

   b. Description: Most commonly, reflexology is understood to be noninvasive therapy in which practitioner systematically applies specific movements, generally to feet or hands, with intention of optimizing function in body. Most frequent movements are circular in nature with some long movements using or not using pressure. A technique unique to reflexology is thumb walking, in which distal thumb joint is placed on sole of foot and is moved forward with a caterpillar-like motion with varying degrees of pressure.

   c. Theory: Underlying concept supporting reflexology is particular areas of feet correspond with particular areas of body in what is known as homuncular map. A number of theories are used to support reflexology, including:

     1) Hemodynamic theory posits this technique improves circulation to body parts correlated with foot regions.

     2) Nerve impulse theory suggests reflexology improves neural networks to body part correlated with foot regions.

     3) Energy theory hypothesizes there are communication linkages within the electromagnetic field, and reflexology can improve action among them.

     4) Lactic acid theory postulates lactic acid crystals accumulate in plantar surfaces of feet and impede circulation, but reflexology works to restore optimal energy flow and circulation.

   d. Indication: General effect of reflexology is promotion of relaxation. Foot reflexology has been utilized with people who live with pain etiologies, including rheumatoid arthritis, fibromyalgia, back pain, migraine headaches, cancer, and those undergoing procedures, including vaccinating infants. Reflexology is known to be effective in managing anxiety and sleep disturbances.

   e. Biological effect: There is little information regarding biological effect of reflexology. One study reported improved cerebral oxygen saturation in a group of people following myocardial infarction. When polysomnography (a technique exploring physiology of sleep) was used to assess patients during reflexology sessions, alterations in brain wave activity were recorded. Additional research is needed to ascertain physiological effects of reflexology.

   f. Efficacy: One study found reflexology to be as effective as hypnosis and more effective than music therapy in reducing anxiety. A second study reported pain and anxiety were significantly reduced following reflexology among children living with persistent pain.

Part 4

g. Nurse's role: Nurses interested in learning and providing reflexology need to be aware of state board of nursing regulations and state licensure requirements.

B. Movement therapies

1. Tai chi

   a. Introduction: Tai chi (pronounced "tie chee") is complex multicomponent intervention integrating physical, psychosocial, emotional, spiritual, and behavioral elements to promote mind-body interaction. Tai chi is mind-body therapy based on TCM and martial arts, which incorporates slow, gentle, connected movements combined with meditation and deep breathing. Over 2.5 million individuals practice tai chi for health reasons; in the United States, tai chi is known to offer a multitude of physical and psychological benefits.

   b. Description: There are five major styles of tai chi varying in postures, forms, pace, and order of movements. Tai chi can be practiced indoors or outdoors, alone or in groups, and no special equipment is required. Tai chi is often performed in groups multiple times a week, contributing to social benefits. Despite gentle pace, tai chi is performed with mild to moderate intensity, allowing for adequate workout. Metabolic equivalent of task (MET) for tai chi is considered to range from 2.5 to 6.5. Comparatively, moderate intensity exercise (brisk walking) ranges from 3 to 6 MET. Variances are accounted for in duration, pace, and experience of participant.

   c. Theory: Tai chi is based on Taoist and Confucian Chinese philosophies that view tai chi as driving force of universe. Tai chi is a symbol representing two opposing forces, yin and yang. The philosophies maintain life consists of conflicts, and harmony is achieved through balancing conflicts. Symbol reflects movement and changing direction, much like tai chi exercises reflect transfer of body weight, separation, and merging of opposing forces. Taoist and Confucian philosophies behind tai chi also assert balancing flow of energy (qi) will enhance healing.

   d. Indication: Tai chi is indicated for those who require rehabilitation from physical or psychological injury or illness, fall prevention, balance and flexibility improvements, and improved endurance. Tai chi has been studied in people experiencing persistent musculoskeletal pain, headaches, rheumatoid arthritis, osteoarthritis, and cancer pain.

   e. Biological effect: Biological effects are based on neurocognitive model. Tai chi is believed to inhibit attention paid to pain signals. The mind (referred to as yi) provokes movement of energy (qi) that leads to physical movement. Focused attention through meditative practices allows for organized movement and balance of mind and body. Body movements and postures in Tai chi are named in metaphors, which add to visual imagery known to positively impact pain and immune and autonomic nervous systems. Psychological improvements are attributed to directive to focus mind and direct inner energy. The mind is therefore peaceful and coordinated with relaxed breathing, consequently decreasing anxiety often associated with pain. Physical activity of tai chi offers improvements consistent with established benefits to other forms of exercise.

   f. Efficacy: Qualitative research findings have revealed five themes of tai chi effects, including pain reduction/pain relief, functional improvement, psychospiritual benefits, improved social support, and integration of tai chi into daily activities. More specifically, several studies support use of tai chi for improving pain, joint stiffness, aerobic capacity, musculoskeletal strength, balance, sleep, depression, quality of life, psychological well-being, stress, mood disturbance, self-esteem, anxiety, and disability in patients with multiple conditions, including fibromyalgia, osteoarthritis, rheumatoid arthritis, persistent low back pain, cancer, and headaches. Although tai chi is most often associated with community participation, it is possible to modify instructions for people in acute care settings who are able only to sit or remain in bed.

   g. Nurse's role: Assess which patients may benefit and safely participate in tai chi considering any mobility and balance contraindications.

2. Yoga

   a. Introduction: The word *yoga* stems from root word *yui,* which means to unite. Yoga is practice used for mind and body balance and dates back to 200 BC. Popularity of yoga has grown at rapid pace and is estimated over 15 million people in the United States use yoga. Although yoga therapy is not a licensed profession, there are established regulating entities working to formalize yoga therapy research, education, and credentialing, such as the International Association of Yoga Therapy.

   b. Description: Yoga is described as meditative movement practice with origins in ancient Indian philosophy. Yoga focuses on breathing techniques, physical movement or postures, meditation, relaxation, and lifestyle adjustment. Although there is a variety of forms, most commonly used form in the United States is Hatha yoga. Like other types of exercise, yoga has health benefits, such as improving overall well-being and reducing stress.

c. Theory: Through practice of physical movement, breath control, meditation, and disciplined lifestyle, yoga is hypothesized to reduce stress and restore homeostasis in body.

d. Indication: Many health benefits are linked to yoga, such as treatment of anxiety, depression, and insomnia; however, most studied area is management of persistent pain (e.g., low back pain and migraines), stress, and arthritis.

e. Biological effect: It is speculated yoga emphasizes mental focus and breathing along with physical movement, thereby connecting body and mind. Additional benefits of yoga are improved sleep quality and decreased anxiety and depressive symptoms, which most likely contribute to pain reduction.

f. Efficacy: Research on effectiveness of yoga for pain management is an emerging field of study. Cheung and colleagues conducted a focused review of 12 studies (589 participants) of patients with osteoarthritis. A variety of types, frequencies, and durations of yoga interventions were reported, and frequency of intervention ranged from once a week to 6 days a week. Duration of interventions ranged from 45 to 90 minutes per session for 6 to 12 weeks. Yoga interventions resulted in significant reductions in pain, stiffness, and swelling. As with tai chi, yoga is most often associated with community participation, yet it is possible to modify instructions for patients in acute care settings who are able only to sit or must remain in bed.

g. Nurse's role:
   1) Majority of patients who practice yoga do so without risk, but it is important to instruct them to start program with proper instruction from qualified instructor and at patient's own pace.
   2) Nurses can encourage patients to minimize risk of injury and avoid any pose that is hurtful or unnatural.

C. Mind-body therapies
   1. Breathing
      a. Introduction: Practice of attending to one's breath is fundamental to many integrative therapies, such as mindfulness, meditation, yoga, relaxation therapy, and aromatherapy. All evolve around importance of breath. Breathing can help patients better manage pain and associated symptoms and has advantages including being easy to learn and not needing special tools or equipment. Breathing during pain (veresus holding breath) results in longer exhalations, which can induce a calmer state.
      b. Description of breathing techniques:
         1) Diaphragmatic breathing involves intentionally slowing inhalation and exhalation by expanding descent of diaphragm while inhaling and expanding ascent of diaphragm while exhaling.
         2) Abdominal breathing increases attention on abdomen and attentively inhaling air while expanding abdomen without expanding chest. During exhalation, attention is focused on contracting abdomen.
         3) Square breathing is controlled breathing with inhaling to count of 4, then holding breath for count of 4, exhaling for count of 4, and then waiting for count of 4. This is similar to Pranayama yoga breathing (Fig. 15.1).
         4) Alternate nostril breathing involves a cycle of fully exhaling, then breathing in through right nostril with left nostril closed, then holding breath with both nostrils closed, then fully exhaling. The cycle is repeated alternately with each nostril.
         5) Lamaze breathing is often used during childbirth with a partner/coach. It involves individualized quick breathing progressing to a slower cadence of breathing.
      c. Theory: Bandura's theory of self-efficacy and Kolcaba's theory of comfort help explain comfort as fundamental need of all human beings. Technique encourages individuals to ease reaction to stressful stimuli.
      d. Indication: Intentionally controlled breathing may be used to minimize breath holding and hyperventilation that may occur with pain, fear, or anxiety.

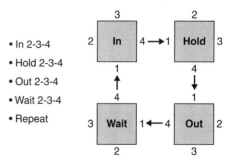

Figure 15.1 Square breathing diagram. Courtesy ©2008 Ann Quinlan-Colwell.

e. Biological effects:
1) Sympathetic nervous system controls our fight-or-flight response. In contrast, deep breathing triggers parasympathetic nervous system to slow heartbeat, relax muscles, neutralize stress, and elicit calming feeling.
2) Deep breaths oxygenate blood, which causes brain to release endorphins, which in turn helps reduce stress in body and decrease pain levels.
3) Breathing induces a range of psychophysiological effects on respiratory, cardiovascular, autonomic, and emotional systems.
f. Efficacy: Although research is limited and results are variable, breathing techniques have been found to be effective during labor, with chest tube removal, and with burn care.
g. Nurse's role:
1) Educate and guide patients with age-appropriate methods to experience benefits of slow, deep breaths.
   a) For pediatrics, blowing through a straw onto wet paint or water helps teach younger individuals how technique might work for them. Young children may benefit engaging imagination while blowing on objects (e.g., blowing two or more colors of wet paint across a paper).
   b) For adults or older children, four-square breathing or 4-7-8 breathing techniques are helpful tools. Cater cadence, depth, and length of breaths to individual. Some patients may not have capacity to exhale for a long (4-to-7 count) duration.

2. Distraction techniques
   a. Introduction: A wide variety of age-appropriate activities can be included for distraction from pain experience. Examples of distraction techniques include journaling, social interactions with family/friends, coloring, watching an engaging program or movie, singing, or playing a musical instrument.
   b. Description: Distraction involves use of engaging stimuli to direct attention away from pain, either actively or passively.
      1) Active distraction: Patient is fully and attentively involved in activity such as coloring, playing a game, journaling, cooking, or gardening.
      2) Passive distraction: Patient's attention is directed to event or activity such as watching bubbles or a movie.
   c. Theory: Neurocognitive processing limits amount of information we can process at any one time. With distraction, attention is diverted from painful stimuli. The more mentally demanding a distractive task is, the less attention is available to notice pain.
   d. Indication: Distraction may be a component of multimodal analgesic plans and beneficial for short, procedural pain instances. Distraction may be less effective for individuals suffering from intense, acute pain. It may also be helpful when trying to taper to lower analgesic doses.
   e. Biological effect: When individuals with mild pain focus on distractive activity, it may reduce perception of pain. In addition to reducing perception of pain, endogenous opioids and other physiologic effects are believed to contribute to analgesic effect. Distraction can also be beneficial when anxiety and nausea exacerbate painful experience.
   f. Efficacy:
      1) Traditionally, distraction was evaluated among children with procedural pain, such as needle sticks, bone marrow biopsy, lumbar puncture, and dressing changes.
      2) Also shown to be effective as adjunct during acute postoperative pain, resulting in less analgesic use.
      3) With various virtual reality programs now available, it is expected there will be greater research.
   g. Nurse's role: Try a variety of distraction methods appealing to patient.

3. Music
   a. Introduction: Listening to music as part of pain management can involve all aspects of person: physical, emotional, cognitive, spiritual, and social. Important to know listening to music both live and recorded can be beneficial but is very different from professional music therapy provided by professional music therapist. Music therapists are specially trained to use specific musical components, (e.g., melody, rhythm, tempo, dynamics, pitch, volume) therapeutically and align with patient's treatment goals. During music therapy sessions, therapists adjust method of music-making in response to patient's needs (https://www.musictherapy.org/).
   b. Description: Goals of music interventions may include reduction of stress and anxiety, pain, depression, hopelessness, and helplessness.
   c. Theory: Research suggests analgesic effects of music are aroused in brain and act through top-down regulations via modulating effects of descending pain pathways. Additionally, mechanisms described in gate control theory and pain neuromatrix theories may also apply. Both cognitive and emotional processes are

stimulated when musical stimuli are used to engage participant.

d. Indication: Relaxing and distracting effects of music may be effective in helping patients to better manage both acute pain (procedural, perioperative) and persistent pain (cancer, arthritis) and during procedures.

e. Biological effect: Music may provoke calming influence or pleasurable memory that improves mood and state of mind. It may evoke relaxation and calmness, reduce stress, and enhance well-being of clients across variety of clinical populations. Music interventions may provide temporary distraction from pain, stimulate relaxation, and positively alter mood and thoughts.

f. Efficacy: Recent publications suggest music is advantageous for improving quality of life and reducing anxiety, depression, pain, and fatigue in patient-care settings. Music interventions of 20 to 30 minutes have been associated with larger decreases in pain scores. Recent research has demonstrated value of music in cognitively impaired older adults.

g. Nurse's role needs to be based upon understanding:

1) Preferences for music style genre, tempo, and tone must be accommodated.

2) Headphones allow personal control and focused listening experience.

3) Engagement in musical experiences can also be promoted by drumming rhythms, singing, humming, or dancing.

4) Suggesting musical interventions can be convenient, safe, and inexpensive.

5) Many musical interventions can be accommodated to most locations.

6) While musical therapists may not be available to provide direct patient care in all settings, research can help guide institutions toward independent musical interactions without special equipment or advanced education.

4. Relaxation

a. Introduction: There is direct correlation between anxiety, stress, and increased pain perception. Use of relaxation techniques triggers release of physical and emotional tension and results in calming of mind and body. Relaxation techniques can help reduce anticipatory pain, fear, and anxiety.

b. Description: Physical and mental relaxation can be used to manage pain by reducing reactions to stressful situations, fear, and anxiety. Examples of relaxation techniques include breathing exercises, progressive muscle

relaxation, meditation, guided imagery, and meditation.

c. Theory: Roger's diffusion of innovation theory can be used to guide implementation of relaxation and other therapies within a social (healthcare) system. This middle-range theory provides a framework for studying adoption of innovations by individuals or groups.

d. Indication: Physical and mental relaxation may rely upon a variety of techniques and can promote analgesia by reducing stress to neutral or even positive experiences. Patients with significant cognitive impairments may benefit from modified relaxation techniques, especially those centered on physical comforting.

e. Biological effect: Relaxation is a psychological intervention assisting patients to achieve state of rest (physical relaxation) and inner calm (mental relaxation). Relaxation interventions trigger parasympathetic nervous system, reducing oxygen use, slowing heart rate and breathing, reducing blood pressure, releasing muscle tension, and reducing stress response.

f. Efficacy: Value of relaxation has been generally recognized as a quieting and hypometabolic state achieved during wakefulness. Mind-body strategies, including relaxation, encourage self-efficacy and active participation in healing process.

g. Nurse's role: Relaxation techniques can be used by nurses to guide patient relaxation experience (e.g., jaw relaxation, diaphragmatic breathing, heartbeat or rhythmic breathing, progressive muscle relaxation, meditation, or prayer).

5. Guided imagery

a. Introduction: Guided imagery is a mind-body intervention using creativity, imagination, and sensory recollections to envision and experience images, objects, places, or situations regarded as pleasant. Guided imagery may also be referred to as guided meditation, visualization, or self-guided hypnosis.

b. Description: Guided imagining encourages person to explore an identified environment with triggers to be present in that space by considering whole-body sensory impacts: how it looks, feels, sounds, smells, and even tastes. It is imperative to explore with person what environment they wish to explore through imagery.

c. Theory: Some research supporting guided imagery is based on grounded theory, a systematic methodology largely applied to qualitative research by social scientists. Guided imagery is based on cognitive-behavioral strategies. Focused relaxation engages listener to concentrate on object, sound, or experience to calm mind.

d. Indication: While distracting person from current experience of pain, guided imagery can help to relieve stress and anxiety and promote a feeling of calmness.

e. **Contraindication:** Special considerations should be given to those with cognitive impairment or those suffering from emotional instability, posttraumatic stress disorder, or other mental health disorders. Absolute contraindications include persons experiencing delusions, extreme anger or aggression, or suicidal ideation.

f. Biological effect: Imagining oneself in a scene can provoke a feeling of relaxation and distraction from suffering of pain, stress, anxiety, or other distressing symptoms. Guided imagery has potential to reduce a variety of symptoms in various conditions and contexts. When symptoms interfere with sleep, guided imagery can improve sleep quality by altering how body responds to stress.

g. Efficacy: Research using guided imagery as an intervention for pain and anxiety has generally been small with some conflicting results. Some systematic reviews and meta-analyses have reported a general cost-effective benefit. It has been effectively used to control postoperative, procedural, arthritis, fibromyalgia, and post-trauma pain.

h. Nurse's role: Nurses can prepare themselves to guide patients with visualizations to promote state of relaxation. There are also many commercial audio and audiovisual applications that can lead people through guided imagery sessions.

6. Hypnosis

a. Introduction: Despite being used for centuries, there continue to be numerous explanations of what hypnosis is and how it works.

1) Hypnosis is often considered an altered state of consciousness or altered reality achieved through the use of visualization, relaxation, and suggestion. In 2019, the Hypnosis Definition Committee of the Division 30 of the American Psychological Association (APA) officially defined hypnosis as "a state of consciousness involving focused attention and reduced peripheral awareness characterized by an enhanced capacity for response to suggestion" (*Policy & Procedures Manual of APA Division 30*, p. 5).

2) An important tenet of hypnosis is the person who is hypnotized is always in control,

and thus essentially, the process is always self-hypnosis. Part of the control is understanding that, in order to fully experience hypnosis, the person must allow the hypnotic process to occur.

b. Description: Most simply, hypnosis involves one person guiding or providing suggestions to the person undergoing an altered focus with intention of creating imaging to modify perception, expectation, and memory. This begins with a hypnotic induction involving narrowing focus accompanied by repeated suggestions of relaxation. It is believed the degree to which person can be hypnotized depends upon person's hypnotizability or hypnotic suggestibility (extent to which person positively responds to suggestions made by hypnotist).

c. Theoretical support: As with explanations of hypnosis, diverse theories have been generated. These include:

1) Sociocognitive theories of hypnosis postulate person being hypnotized generates experiences as suggested by hypnotist. Theories in this category are not based upon need for different conscious state to be created.

2) Theory of dissociated experience posits people being hypnotized are able to dissociate by inhibiting cognitions and perceptions to which they normally respond in a particular manner. This then allows them to respond in suggested new way.

3) Relational theory of hypnosis suggests hypnosis results from alterations in boundaries (both intrapersonal and interpersonal), thus enabling person being hypnotized to explore hypnotic suggestions by hypnotist.

d. Indication: Hypnosis has successfully been used with children, teenagers, adults, and geriatric patients in wide variety of situations, including procedures, dental work, burn care, labor, delivery, wound care, and surgical procedures.

1) Hypnosis is used clinically to help patients manage symptoms such as nausea, anxiety, fear, and pain that is acute, persistent, debilitating, and at end of life.

2) Since at least some evidence to date indicates areas of brain involved with relaxation and distraction are different from those involved with hypnosis, these interventions can be used in combination.

3) An important consideration for people using hypnosis to manage pain is the person is in control and thus is empowered with greater self-efficacy.

e. Biological effect: Lateral and medial prefrontal cortices and anterior cingulate areas of brain are involved during hypnosis. A variety of studies involving functional magnetic resonance imaging (fMRI), electroencephalography, positron emission tomography, and somatosensory event–related potentials demonstrated that cortical and subcortical cerebral activity also may be involved in analgesia. Researchers used fMRI to assess cerebral activity during hypnosis and reported increased functional connectivity noted between insula in salience network and dorsolateral prefrontal cortex; decreased connectivity between default mode network and executive control network; and decreased activity in dorsal anterior cingulate cortex.

f. Efficacy: A systematic review reported positive results when hypnosis was used for analgesia, with strength of correlation strongly related to ease of hypnotic suggestibility of participant. The authors suggest analgesic benefit is related to effect of hypnosis on prefrontal cortex and insular and anterior cingulate cortex, which are also involved with pain modulation.

7. Meditation

a. Introduction: Meditation has ancient roots as a contemplative practice emerging from Eastern (particularly Buddhism), Jewish, and Christian spiritual philosophies/traditions. Despite religious origins, today meditation is used both by people with strong spiritual connections and those with no formal religious affiliation. It was and continues to be viewed as a vehicle for gaining awareness and insight, managing pain and suffering, and cultivating focus and compassion. With dedicated practice, benefits of meditation can increase over time. It is often integrated into a self-management program of health and wellness that may include managing pain.

b. Description: Broadly described as a process by which a person turns inward using attentional practices resulting in altered consciousness with expanded awareness, clarity, increased presence, and enhanced insight with self-integration. Person meditating is both alert and relaxed with an effortless, continuous, focused attention. Various meditative methods are classified as either concentration or mindfulness.

1) Concentration methods involve focusing on a single item (e.g., candle flame, flower), word (e.g., peace, love), sound (e.g., om), concept (e.g., love or compassion), or action (e.g., breathing or walking). Focus is often accompanied by a word or phrase mantra.

2) Mindfulness method involves intentionally being present in the moment with attention to what is transpiring, while disengaging from any connection with emotions, concepts, judgments, or opinions. In the 1980s, mindfulness meditation was incorporated into work with patients to gain insights and other tools to ease persistent pain. This work evolved into mindfulness-based stress reduction.

3) Guided meditation is most often used by someone beginning a meditative practice. It involves audio, visual, or interpersonal guidance through relaxation and process. With time, this guidance often is not necessary.

c. Theoretical support: In connection with pain, two theories support meditation:

1) Gate control theory hypothesized within nociceptive process: There is two-way communication with signals transmitted from periphery, then ascending through central nervous system, where modulation occurs to either increase or decrease pain signal. Modulation is influenced by a variety of factors (e.g., psychological, neurohormonal, cognition, interpretation, genetics, and memory). Within this construct, meditation is understood through cerebral and psychological perspectives with cognitive and affective mediators to support people working to manage pain.

2) Brain theory of meditation suggests different areas and functions of brain are employed with different meditative styles (e.g., focus, compassion, loving kindness, and mindfulness), but all share augmented integration of cerebral hemispheres with increased flexibility and facilitation of more efficient cerebral functioning.

d. Indication: Meditation has traditionally been associated with emotional and spiritual health. In recent years, it has been reported to improve physical health and be effective as an intervention for a variety of physical conditions. From pain perspective, it has been effective with helping to manage persistent pain, including fibromyalgia. It is also reported to be beneficial with managing symptoms of diabetes, cardiovascular conditions, cancer, anxiety, depression, eating disorders, obesity, and insomnia, which are all correlated with painful situations. Loving kindness meditation (meditative practice derived from Buddhist tradition with focus on compassion for both self and others) has been used specifically with people living with persistent pain (i.e., persistent low back pain and other nonmalignant pain).

e. Biological effect: Historically, health benefits have been attributed to increased mental clarity and reduction of physical distress. A recent literature review exploring relationship of meditation and yoga with circulating concentrations of brain-derived neurotropic factor (BDNF, a crucial mediator of central nervous system neuroplasticity as well as cognitive function) supports increases in concentrations of circulating BDNF in participants who meditated or pursued other mind-body exercises (e.g., yoga). Another study using a multimodal MRI approach found structural changes in brains of long-term meditators who practiced a type of compassionate meditation (i.e., loving-kindness meditation).

f. Efficacy: A study found meditation was not only independently correlated with less hypercholesterolemia but also less incidence of diabetes, stroke, and coronary artery disease, important findings given that people who develop those specific conditions often have persistent pain. In another study, experienced meditators were compared to sex-matched controls. Meditators were found to have lower stress-induced cortisol and less neurogenic inflammatory response to topical capsaicin application. Meditators also had higher scores on social well-being and resiliency tests.

g. Nursing role: Based upon positive attributes and minimal concerns for use of meditation among people living with many different states of health and illness, it is appropriate for nurses to encourage and support this practice as part of multimodal approach for managing pain. Meditation is a process that requires commitment and practice. Recent technology has expanded availability of meditation instruction and guidance through electronic venues, including telehealth. In addition to benefit for patients with pain, meditation is also an excellent way for nurses to manage stress and enhance their own quality of life.

h. **Caution:** Nurses need to be aware that during meditation, the meditator may become aware of painful past experiences connected with strong emotional responses. It is important to know resources to whom the person can be referred to help process the response.

8. Virtual reality
a. Introduction: Virtual reality (VR) and immersive virtual reality have generated substantial attention, use, excitement, and research during the last two decades. Historically, VR dates to 1929,

when a flight simulator was developed to teach pilots how to fly an aircraft. From a pain management perspective, it evolved from work with mirror therapy and continues to evolve.

b. Description: Active VR involves using interactive technological devices to actively participate in simulated auditory and visual experiences in a computer-generated, multisensory, 3-dimensional artificial environment. Participating person wears a head-mounted display, including headphones and visual input that simulates a virtual environment. There are also devices that enable navigation through the environment (Fig. 15.2). There are a number of manufacturers, and technology varies among them and needs to be considered when reviewing research. Virtual environments vary with potential use, from guided meditations to underwater adventures to pediatric-specific situations.

c. Theoretical support: It is believed the human brain has finite capacity for amount of sensory stimulation it can process, and intense stimulation of VR diverts attention from pain. Similarly, gate control theory has been used to support use of VR because competing pleasant sensations have a modulating effect on pain. It is also theorized VR involves interactions with anterior cingulate cortex of brain involved with nociception.

d. Indication: VR has been used successfully with people experiencing a variety of painful situations, including wound care, burn treatments, venipuncture, various procedures (e.g., episiotomies, biopsies), various sources of pain (e.g., musculoskeletal, neuropathic, persistent, cancer-related), chemotherapy, physical therapy, and rehabilitation, and it has been used as technique when working with patients with fears related to pain.

e. Biological effect: Little is known about physiological effects of VR. Physiological parameters (i.e., blood pressure and heart rate) have been

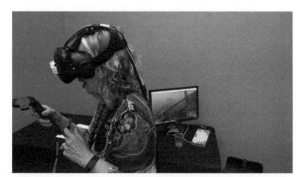

Figure 15.2 Immersive virtual reality. Courtesy ©2008 Ann Quinlan-Colwell.

noted to quiet during VR. A certain number of patients experience what is known as virtual reality sickness, which includes nausea, oculo-motor disturbances, and disorientation. A large systematic review and meta-analysis reported that not only are symptoms affected by technology but also by content. Additional research is needed to identify any correlation with a partici-pant's characteristics, scenarios, and equipment. One concern identified for using VR is whether it is safe to use with children living with epi-lepsy or photosensitive epilepsy; however, to date, there is no evidence this concern is valid.

   f. Efficacy: VR is in its infancy when used for pain management; similarly, so is research involving it. One challenge in confirming effi-cacy is that methodologies used in many stud-ies do not allow for comparison and may be flawed. Also, technology varies with companies and with intended use. Authors of one system-atic review reported VR is promising for use in management of anxiety and pain among patients with cancer. A different systematic review involved randomized control trials using VR with patients in acute inpatient environ-ments. The authors concluded VR has potential use for managing pain and other clinical situa-tions but needs additional research with strong methodology.

   g. Nurse's role:
     1) Nurses are in a position to be actively involved in encouraging use of this new technique in multimodal analgesic plans of care.
     2) Despite the fact VR is generally safe, nurses need to be aware of possible adverse effects and review literature as it becomes available.

D. Energetic therapies
  1. Healing touch
   a. Introduction: Healing touch (HT) is a specific type of hands-on energy healing founded by Janet Mentgen in 1989. It is a noninvasive ther-apy in which practitioners use their hands to reestablish harmony and balance in the energy field of person. It is used to alleviate a variety of symptoms, including pain and stress.
   b. Description: Practitioners use skills they learn through a six-level program in preparation for certification through Healing Touch International, Inc. More than 25 skills are derived from a variety of energy approaches involving both whole-body and focused tech-niques, and they are used with intention of restoring balance in person. After conducting an assessment and scanning the energy field of

person, healing touch practitioner determines which skills are appropriate to use to restore balance within energy field. Additional infor-mation can be obtained through https://www.healingtouchprogram.com/welcome-hti.
   c. Theoretical support: Most recently, two theo-retical bases have been identified.
     1) First is Einstein's theory concept of energy and relativity.
     2) Second theoretical base is Jean Watson's theory of human caring and transpersonal caring.
   d. Indication: HT was designed to assist patients with healing themselves. In addition to often being used to alleviate anxiety, it has been used for a variety of pain-related issues, including postsurgical pain, biopsies, cancer-related pain, and persistent pain in older adults.
   e. Biological effect: Exact mechanism of how HT influences body is not clear. Research to iden-tify mechanism remains needed.
   f. Efficacy: As with many energy-field therapies, it is difficult to directly delineate effectiveness of HT. Generally, efficacy is established through indirect measurement of patient symptoms, including pain and anxiety. Although number of research studies involving HT have markedly increased during last two decades, additional research using strong methodologies is needed.
   g. Nurse's role: Nurses who are interested can undertake education and certification process to become HT practitioners.
  2. Reiki
   a. Introduction: Reiki is believed to have origi-nated over 2,000 years ago in India or Tibet. The term *reiki* is composed of two Japanese words: *rei,* meaning universal, and *ki,* meaning life force; it was discovered by Dr. Mikao Usui from Japan in late 1900s. After learning how to do reiki, Dr. Usui taught his family and then opened a clinic where he could treat the public.
   b. Description: Reiki is a biofield therapy focused on centering and presence. Reiki practitioner uses hand positions over or on a person's chakras to channel energy. It is believed to occur by reiki energy connecting individuals to their own innate spiritual wisdom and highest good. Reiki practitioner is not source of energy or source of healing; instead, practitioner is channel for energy.
   c. Theory: Thought to balance person's biofield and promote body's ability to heal itself. As an emerging area of study, biofield science views energy as part of complex system with capacity to influence the whole system. This science is

based on principle that all living things contain vital life force that creates a biofield (an invisible field of energy around them). Moreover, biofield science suggests complex interactions involving energy-healing therapies may be mediated by processes yet to be discovered.

d. Indication: Reiki has been used to decrease pain, anxiety, fatigue, and stress, along with promoting relaxation and well-being. It has been used with a variety of patient populations including patients with cancer, fibromyalgia, HIV/AIDS, obstetrical procedures, and those recovering from surgery.

e. Biological effect: Most energy therapies in the United States focus on a person's biofield. Although research examining biological effects of energy therapies is still in early stages, many people with pain seek reiki or other energy therapies to find pain relief.

f. Efficacy: Majority of studies have had small sample sizes and did not compare reiki with a control group. Recently, a large-scale effectiveness trial was conducted across the United States. The well-validated 20-item Positive and Negative Affect Schedule was used along with brief self-report measure immediately before (pre) and after (post) each reiki session. Results revealed significant improvement (all p-values were less than 0.001) in pain, fatigue, nausea, appetite, and shortness of breath. Of note, no harmful effects have been reported in any reiki studies.

g. Nurse's role:
   1) Nurses within their clinical setting can provide time and space for patient to receive reiki, typically lasting 15 minutes for a seated session or 45 minutes for full session.
   2) Nurses can also learn reiki to use in their own practice setting or for their own well-being.

3. Therapeutic touch
   a. Introduction: Therapeutic touch (TT) is an evidence-based energy field intervention. It focuses holistic compassionate intention to help person to promote balance and well-being. This is done by TT practitioner using their hands to attune with energy field that surrounds person.
      1) In healthy individuals, energy is balanced and flows without interruption. When there is illness, trauma, or disease, energy becomes disordered.
      2) TT is a process by which practitioner works to rebalance and restore energy field to balanced state. It is currently taught in more than 90 countries.

   b. Description: TT process begins with practitioner centering self, accessing compassion for person, then assessing energy field of person. This is followed by a purposeful and individualized intervention that includes balancing and rebalancing of energy field. Despite the name, one benefit of this therapy is that actual physical touch is not necessary and most frequently does not occur. Generally, practitioner's hands work in an area between 2 to 6 inches above skin of person. Session concludes with reassessment or evaluation and closure. Additional information can be obtained through the Therapeutic Touch International Association website at https://therapeutictouch.org/.

   c. Theoretical support: Several theories support TT.
      1) General underlining theory supporting energy healing, including TT, is quantum theory of physics with concept that vibrating energy fields surround all matter, and when different energy fields are in contact, there is resonance between them.
      2) Science of Unitary Human Beings (Rogers) provided early support.
      3) Recent theoretical support specific to TT is Practice-Based Theory of Healing Through Therapeutic Touch: Advanced Holistic Nursing Practice.

   d. Indication: Initially, most common response to TT is feeling of relaxation, beneficial with both anxiety and pain. TT has been used to help manage many symptoms, including pain, anxiety, agitation, insomnia, vomiting, and fatigue. It has also been used to promote healing in wounds, burns, and fractures, which are painful conditions. Not actually touching the body is an important benefit of TT with patients who have pain and are extremely sensitive to touch, as with neuropathic pain. It can also be a beneficial adjunct during wound care.

   e. Biological effect: Bioeffect of TT was first investigated by Krieger in 1975. Investigators in a more recent study reported that culture fibroblasts, osteoblasts, and tenocytes showed increased proliferation when treated with TT.

   f. Efficacy: Most common initial response to TT is feeling of relaxation. In recent small study with infants, there were significant differences in pain scores and heart rates, with lower respiratory rates in group who received TT.

   g. Nurse's role: If interested, nurses can learn to use TT in their individual practice setting. Since it takes little time to utilize, TT can be an important component of a multimodal analgesic plan of care.

E. Natural Products
  1. Aromatherapy
     a. Introduction: Aromatherapy is use of essential oils for therapeutic purposes when derived from distillate of an aromatic plant (e.g., flowers, leaves, bark, roots, seeds, and skin of many plants). Plants make oils for protection or survival, allowing plant to recover from injury or exposure to pathogens. Plants' oils are stored as microscopic cellular components in cells, glands, ducts, or hairs. Essential oils, which are classified by their family, genus, and species, are complex mixtures of organic molecules. Specific therapeutic properties are effect of chemical composition of particular essential oil.
     b. Description: Aromatherapy involves inhaling or topically applying diluted essential oils derived from flora, including herbs, flowering plants, and trees.
     c. Theory: There are differing theories about biochemical mechanism of action of essential oils. Connection between olfactory system and limbic system is often theorized as causing effect on emotions. Other theories focus on neurobiology and psychological effect of odors on central nervous system and memory.
     d. Indication: Aromatherapy can be part of a complementary treatment plan to promote comfort or well-being in realm of discomfort or stressor (e.g., pain, insomnia, nausea, fatigue, stress, or anxiety). However, to be in accordance with regulatory agencies, the indication for aromatherapy cannot be "diagnosed" and "prescribed" by registered nurses (RNs). In healthcare settings, essential oils are chosen with intention to promote well-being and comfort.
     e. Safety considerations: As with every natural product, there are certain precautions and contraindications regarding use of essential oils:
        1) Only use high-quality pure essential oils.
        2) Follow storage and quality control guidelines (Box 15.1).
        3) During pregnancy, it is important to consult with obstetric providers.
        4) Should not be used on mucous membranes
        5) Some oils cannot be used with patients with seizures, or receiving chemotherapy.
        6) History of adverse reactions or events associated with essential oils
        7) History of profound bronchial hyper-reactivity (e.g., asthma provoked by environmental triggers)
        8) History of migraine and no previous exposure to essential oils
        9) Sensitivity to or dislike of scents
        10) Adverse reactions to botanicals

Box 15.1

Advice for Storing and Controlling Quality of Essential Oils

- Store in cool area (ideally under refrigeration).
- After opening, replace the cap immediately after use.
- Store out of the reach of children.
- Dispose of essential oils that are prone to oxidation within 6 months of purchase or first use.
- Keep out of direct sunlight and away from heat, flames, vaporizers, and candles.

From Tisserand R, Young R. (2013). *Essential Oil Safety-E-book: A Guide for Health Care Professionals*. London: Churchill Livingstone.

---

     f. Biological effect: In general, smell is a chemical reaction perceived by specific receptors in an intact olfactory system to limbic system and hypothalamus, with ensuing release of endorphins.
     g. Efficacy: Recent studies suggest aromatherapy used for promotion of well-being may be a safe adjunctive treatment for a variety of symptoms, including pain, sleep disorders, anxiety, depression, and nausea/vomiting, among others.
     h. Nurse's role: Nurses need to know essential oils are not generally approved by the Food and Drug Administration (FDA). Since most essential oils are concentrated, they need to be diluted before using them. It is recommended RNs complete a professional education course that provides nursing certification.
  2. Herbs and dietary supplements
     a. Introduction: Natural products are biologically based substances found in nature. Examples include herbs (also known as botanicals), vitamins, minerals, probiotics, and essential oils. Use of herbs and dietary supplements is one of oldest forms of medicine, dating back to early Egyptians.
     b. Description: Dietary supplements in the United States include dietary components, metabolites, or extracts used with intent of improving nutritional intake and include herbs, vitamins, minerals, amino acids, foods, and other products. Herbs are plants whose flowers, seeds, or leaves are used to produce flavorings, food, or medicine.
        1) Herbal medicine is considered art and science of using herbs for promoting health and preventing and treating illness.
        2) Western herbology classifies herbs by their therapeutic properties, whereas TCM

categorizes use primarily by imbalance experienced by patient.

   c. Theoretical support: Use of these products varies by philosophical approach. Herbal selection practiced by Western herbology is driven by disease state. TCM considers internal and external threats to individual's life balance and impact herbs may have on adjusting those imbalances.

   d. Indication: Musculoskeletal pain, headache, and dysmenorrhea are common reasons people seek herbal therapies. Some common herbs and supplements used for pain include glucosamine, chondroitin, magnesium, turmeric, Boswellia, and feverfew.

   e. Biological effect: Biological effects of herbs and supplements are particular to properties of each. Some effects include:

     1) Chondroitin is believed to improve cartilage formation through collagen synthesis and chondrocyte metabolism. Glucosamine and chondroitin are often combined.

     2) Magnesium deficiencies are linked to headache pain, particularly hormonally driven migraines.

     3) Turmeric is a spice in powder form believed to have pain-relieving properties, including for postoperative pain.

     4) Feverfew is herb thought to be effective and safe choice to help reduce multiple pain sources, including headaches, migraines, toothaches, and joint pain.

     5) Boswellia has anti-inflammatory effects that have been effective in management of headaches, arthritis, and inflammatory bowel disorders.

   f. Efficacy of herbs is difficult to determine due to variances in plants.

     1) Herbs are not regulated or standardized by the FDA. Differences in plant growth conditions, harvesting, storage, and production can account for variances in herb potency.

     2) Other challenges in determining efficacy lie in failure to define efficacy (e.g., reduced pain, restoration of qi, delay of joint degeneration).

     3) Researchers have conducted rigorous studies with large sample sizes on a variety of natural products, and results show they are *not effective.*

     4) Regardless of definitive supporting research, patients continue to seek pain relief through herbs and supplements.

   g. Nurse's role:

     1) Be knowledgeable about reasons people seek herbal and nutritional supplements,

and be familiar with available options, mechanism of action, and potential adverse effects.

     2) Responsible to assess for product use and educate patients on many medication-to–natural product interactions that can occur

III. Other Systems of Care

A. The National Center for Complementary and Integrative Health recognizes most complementary or integrative therapies can be categorized as mind and body practices or natural products. However, some interventions are classified as "other systems of care," such as Ayurvedic medicine, homeopathy, naturopathy, or TCM.

B. Ayurvedic medicine

   1. Introduction: *Ayurveda* is Sanskrit word for "science of life" and although new in the United States, it has been practiced for over 5,000 years in India, its country of origin.

   2. Description: Focus of Ayurveda is holistic interdependent relationship between person with surrounding world and with their own body, mind, and spirit. These relationships begin with five elements of air, earth, fire, water, and space, which combine to create three doshas: vata (air and space), pitta (fire and water), and kapha (water and earth). Prakriti is balance of person's doshas and describes behavioral, mental, and physical tendencies.

   3. Theoretical support: Person's environment and lifestyle can stimulate imbalance in doshas, called vikriti, resulting in illness. Accumulation of toxins and emotional imbalance can also cause illness.

   4. Indication: Ayurveda may be used to address variety of issues, such as anxiety, stress, or digestive issues; however, there is paucity of research to support its efficacy.

   5. Biological effect: Treatment of imbalances in Ayurveda are based on lifestyle approaches, such as nutrition, herbs, and exercise, with goal of returning right balance.

   6. Efficacy: Research publications in Western healthcare journals are scant; however, there have been reports of Ayurvedic interventions reducing pain and improving function with osteoarthritis.

   7. Nurse's role:

     a. Ayurveda is not a licensed healthcare profession in the United States; most practitioners are licensed in other healthcare professions, such as chiropractic, massage therapy, or nursing.

     b. Although nonherbal interventions (e.g., aromatherapy, diet, yoga) are generally considered safe, one health concern related to Ayurvedic medicine is use of gems, metals, and minerals. Although these metals are intentionally used in preparations to improve equilibrium, some preparations contain mercury, lead, or arsenic and may be toxic in humans.

   c. Ayurvedic medicines are considered dietary supplements as opposed to medications and therefore are not required to meet same safety and efficacy standards.

   d. Ayurveda should not replace conventional medical care, especially when treating serious conditions.

C. Homeopathy
  1. Introduction: Homeopathy was developed as a system of healthcare in Germany more than 200 years ago by a physician, Dr. Samuel Hahnemann, and was introduced to America in the 1820s. The word *homeopathy* is from the Greek *homoios,* meaning similar, and *pathos,* meaning suffering.
  2. Description: Hahnemann considered symptoms and disease as equivalent, which led him to erroneous conclusion that if symptom was relieved, person was cured of disease.
  3. Theoretical support: This system of care is based on several theories, such as "like cures like," that is, an illness can be treated by a substance that produces similar symptoms in people who are healthy, and "the law of minimum dose," suggesting the lower the dose of medication, the more effective it will be.
  4. Indication: Homeopathy may be used to treat a variety of conditions, such as anxiety, stress, or digestive issues; however, there is paucity of research to support its safety and efficacy.
  5. Biological effect: Homeopathic medicines are made from plants, animals, or minerals and then highly diluted. These treatments are assumed to work in accordance with vibrational principle and formulated for unique needs of each person, with goal to promote balance and healing.
  6. Efficacy: While millions of adults use homeopathy, more research is needed because research results have not found homeopathy to be effective for any condition.
  7. Nurse's role: Awareness of state laws in the United States is important, as laws regulating homeopathy vary from state to state. Typically, healthcare professionals who are licensed to practice another health profession are allowed to study and practice homeopathy. A major concern about the use of homeopathy is patients will potentially delay life-saving diagnosis and care.

D. Naturopathy: dietary and lifestyle changes
  1. Introduction: Naturopathic practitioners use variety of interventions, such as dietary and lifestyle changes, herbs and other dietary supplements, stress reduction, and psychotherapy/counseling. Education and licensure depend on practitioner's role.
  2. Description: Naturopathy strives to improve diet and promote healthy lifestyle, which are known to improve pain experience.
  3. Theoretical support: Anti-inflammatory diets and those low in fat (e.g., Mediterranean diet) are believed to reduce C-reactive protein and reduce tumor necrosis factor levels, leading to decreased inflammation. Omega-3 and omega-6 regulate biochemical pain pathways; folate deficiencies are known to cause peripheral neuropathy; and vitamin D deficiencies contribute to musculoskeletal pain.
  4. Indication: Naturopathy can be used for headache management, specifically through diets such as elimination diets (e.g., eliminating all foods with immunoglobulin G antibodies), vegan diets, high-fiber diets, and diets low in sodium and pro-inflammatory fatty acids.
  5. Biological effect: Diet plans are associated with eliminating food triggers, reducing estrogen levels, and including anti-inflammatory increasing antioxidants. Eliminating high fat and tyramines and practicing a high-fiber, high-antioxidant diet has strong support for reducing pain intensity and duration of migraine and headache symptoms. Obesity contributes to inflammation due to increased pro-inflammatory cytokines within adipose tissue. A diet with anti-inflammatory properties was found to reduce pain independent of weight loss.
  6. Efficacy: Although study results are difficult to compare due to diverse research methods often lacking rigor, there is support for pain reduction for individuals with inflammatory and autoimmune conditions (e.g., osteoarthritis, fibromyalgia, and rheumatoid arthritis) who adhere to diet low in saturated fat and unrefined carbohydrates. Nutrients can be helpful in managing pain; however, some are known to interfere with medications used to treat pain. In addition, tyramines enhance adverse effects of monoamine oxidase inhibitors, caffeine interferes with psychotropic medications, and sorbitol slows absorption.
  7. Nurse's role: Implications for nursing practice include awareness of dietary benefits; assessing for dietary factors potentially interfering with pain relief; identifying nutrient-drug interactions; and having awareness that many individuals suffering from pain seek and embrace nutritional advice to reduce pain symptoms and improve quality of life.

Part 4

E. Traditional Chinese Medicine (TCM)
   1. Introduction: Originated in China over 2,500 years ago and is based on Taoist philosophy.
   2. Description: Core beliefs of TCM include:
      a. Importance of harmony between opposing yet complementary forces called *yin* and *yang*; imbalance between yin and yang will result in illness
      b. Five elements of water, fire, earth, wood, and metal, which represent stages of life and explain all bodily functions
      c. Qi is energy that maintains. Qi is considered vital energy behind all physiological processes and flows through animals, plants, people, the earth, and sky. Qi is distributed throughout an organism along a network of meridians, which connect all parts of the organism.
   3. Theoretical support: Although basic beliefs of TCM are of interest, current research efforts are focused on efficacy of specific therapies used in symptom management. More research is welcomed, as holistic perspective of assessment and care characterizing TCM are particularly valuable for patients living with complex conditions such as myofascial pain syndrome.
   4. Indication: TCM uses a variety of therapies, such as acupuncture, auricular acupuncture, tai chi, qi gong, and herbs to prevent and treat disease.
   5. Efficacy: TCM is commonly used throughout Asia; however, there is limited published research regarding its safety and effectiveness.

Bibliography

Ahmad, M., Mohammad, E. B., & Anshasi, H. A. (2020). Virtual reality technology for pain and anxiety management among patients with cancer: a systematic review. *Pain Management Nursing, 21*(3), 601–607.

Aldekhyyel, R. N., Bakker, C. J., Pitt, M. B., & Melton, G. B. (2019). The impact of patient interactive systems on the management of pain in an inpatient hospital setting: a systematic review. *Applied Clinical Informatics, 10*(4), 580–596. doi:10.1055/s-0039-1694002.

Allard, M. E., & Katseres, J. (2018). Using essential oils to enhance nursing practice and for self-care. *The Nurse Practitioner, 43*(5), 39–46. doi:10.1097/01.NPR.0000531915.69268.8f.

Allen, S. (2018). *The Science of Gratitude: a white paper for the John Templeton Foundation.* Greater Good Science Center at UC Berkley.

American Psychological Association (APA). (2019). *Policy & Procedures Manual of APA Division 30: The Society of Psychological Hypnosis.* https://www.apadivisions.org/division-30/leadership/committees/policy-procedures.pdf.

Bagci, H., & Cinar Yucel, S. (2020). A systematic review of the studies about therapeutic touch after the year of 2000. *International Journal of Caring Sciences, 13*(1), 231–241.

Baim, M., Arcari, P., Hoffman, S. D., & Stuart-Shor, E. M. (2020). Cognitive-affective strategies to promote resilience and well-being. In M. A., Blaszko Helming, D. A., Shields, K. M., Avino, & W. E., Rosa (Eds.), *Dossey & Keegan's Holistic Nursing: A handbook for practice* (8th Ed, pp. 551–567). Jones & Bartlett Learning.

Bakir, E., Baglama, S. S., & Gursoy, S. (2018). The effects of reflexology on pain and sleep deprivation in patients with rheumatoid arthritis: A randomized controlled trial. *Complementary Therapies in Clinical Practice, 31,* 315–319.

Bat, N. (2021). The effects of reiki on heart rate, blood pressure, body temperature, and stress levels: A pilot randomized, double-blinded, and placebo–controlled study. *Complementary Therapies in Clinical Practice, 43*(101328), 1–5. doi:10.1016/j.ctcp.2021.101328.

Bauckhage, J., & Sell, C. (2021). When and for whom do psychodynamic therapists use guided imagery? Explicating practitioners' tacit knowledge. *Research in Psychotherapy, 24*(3), 577. doi:10.4081/ripppo.2021.577.

Becker, W. C., Dorflinger, L., Edmond, S. N., Islam, L., Heapy, A. A., & Fraenkel, L. (2017). Barriers and facilitators to use of nonpharmacological treatments in chronic pain. *BMC Family Practice, 18*(1), 41. doi:10.1186/s12875-017-0608-2.

Bertrand, A., Mauger-Vauglin, C. E., Martin, S., Goy, F., Delafosse, C., & Marec-Berard, P. (2019). Evaluation of efficacy and feasibility of foot reflexology in children experiencing chronic or persistent pain. *Bulletin du Cancer, 106*(12), 1073–1079.

Boyce, V. J., & Natschke, M. (2019). Establishing a comprehensive aromatherapy program in patient care settings. *Pain Management Nursing, 20*(6), 532–540. doi:10.1016/j.pmn.2019.06.017.

Boyd, C., Crawford, C., Paat, C. F., Price, A., Xenakis, L., & Zhang, W., et al. Evidence for Massage Therapy (EMT) Working Group. (2016). The impact of massage therapy on function in pain populations—a systematic review and meta-analysis of randomized controlled trials: Part II, cancer pain populations. *Pain Medicine, 17*(8), 1553–1568.

Bruckenthal, P., Marino, M. A., & Snelling, L. (2016). Complementary and integrative therapies for persistent pain management in older adults. *Journal of Gerontological Nursing, 42*(12), 40–48.

Celano, C. M., Beale, E. E., Beach, S. R., Belcher, A. M., Suarez, L., Motiwala, S. R., & Huffman, J. C. (2017). Associations between psychological constructs and cardiac biomarkers following acute coronary syndrome. *Psychosomatic Medicine, 79*(3), 318–326.

Centers for Disease Control and Prevention (CDC). (2016). CDC Guideline for Prescribing Opioids for Chronic Pain. Retrieved from: https://www.cdc.gov/drugoverdose/pdf/prescribing/Guidelines_Factsheet-a.pdf.

Centers for Medicare & Medicaid Services. (2019). Improving drug utilization review controls in Part D. Retrieved from: https://www.cms.gov/Medicare/Prescription-Drug-coverage/PrescriptionDrugCovContra/RxUtilization.

Chen, L., & Michalsen, A. (2017). Management of chronic pain using complementary and integrative medicine. *BMJ, 357,* j1284. doi:10.1136/bmj.j1284.

Cheung, C., Park, J., & Wyman, J. (2016). Effects of yoga on symptoms, physical function, and psychosocial outcomes in adults with osteoarthritis: a focused review. *American Journal of Physical Medicine and Rehabilitation, 95*(2), 139–151.

Cho, E. H., Lee, M., & Hur, M. (2017). The effects of aromatherapy on intensive care unit patients' stress and sleep quality: A non-randomized controlled trial. *Evidence-Based Complementary and Alternative Medicine, 2017,* 2856592-10. doi:10.1155/2017/2856592.

Choudhary, S. (2021). Efficacy of reflexology in prevention of post-operative nausea-vomiting after general surgery.

International Journal of Clinical and Experimental Medicine Research, 5(2), 116–126.

Clark, S. D., Bauer, B. A., Vitek, S., & Cutshall, S. M. (2019). Effect of integrative medicine services on pain for hospitalized patients at an academic health center. *Explore (New York, N.Y.), 15*(1), 61–64. doi:10.1016/j.explore.2018.07.006.

Cooney, M. F., & Quinlan-Colwell, A. (2021). *Assessment and multimodal management of pain.* Elsevier.

Cramer, H., Ward, L., Steel, A., Lauche, R., Dobos, G., & Zhang, Y. (2016). Prevalence, patterns, and predictors of yoga use: results of a US nationally representative survey. *American Journal of Preventative Medicine, 50*(2), 230–235.

Crawford, C., Boyd, C., Paat, C. F., Price, A., Xenakis, L., et al. (2016). Evidence for massage therapy (EMT) working group. The impact of massage therapy on function in pain populations – A systematic review and meta–analysis of randomized controlled trials: Part I, patients experiencing pain in the general population. *Pain Medicine, 17*, 1353–1375.

Croy, I., Luong, A., Triscoli, C., Hofmann, E., Olausson, H., & Sailer, U. (2016). Interpersonal stroking touch is targeted to C tactile afferent activation. *Behavioural Brain Research SreeTestContent1, 297*, 37–40.

Dalhoumi, S., & Bonakdar, R. (2016). Yoga for pain management. In R., Bonakdar, & A., Sukiennik (Eds.), *Integrative Pain Management* (pp. 415–424). Oxford University Press.

Dascal, J., Reid, M., Ishak, W. W., Spiegel, B., Recacho, J., Rosen, B., & Danovitch, I. (2017). Virtual reality and medical inpatients: a systematic review of randomized, controlled trials. *Innovations in Clinical Neuroscience, 14*(1-2), 14–21.

Davodabady, F., Naseri-Salahshour, V., Sajadi, M., Mohtarami, A., & Rafiei, F. (2021). Randomized controlled trial of the foot reflexology on pain and anxiety severity during dressing change in burn patients. *Burns, 47*(1), 215–221.

DeVore, J., Clontz, A., Ren, Dianxu, Cairns, L., & Beach, M. (2017). Improving patient satisfaction with better pain management in hospitalized patients. *Journal for Nurse Practitioners, 13*(1), e23–e27.

Dilek, B., & Necmiye, C. (2020). Usage of aromatherapy in symptom management in cancer patients: a systematic review. *International Journal of Caring Sciences, 13*(1), 537–546.

Drake, G., & De C. Williams, A. C. (2017). Nursing education interventions for managing acute pain in hospital settings: a systematic review of clinical outcomes and teaching methods. *Pain Management Nursing, 18*(1), 3–15. doi:10.1016/j.pmn.2016.11.001.

Dyer, N., Baldwin, A., & Rand, W. (2019). A large-scale effectiveness trial of reiki for physical and psychological health. *The Journal of Alternative and Complementary Medicine, 25*(12), 1156–1162.

Eaton, L. H., Hulett, J. P., Langford, D. J., & Doorenbos, A. Z. (2019). How theory can help facilitate implementing relaxation as a complementary pain management approach. *Pain Management Nursing, 20*(3), 207–213. doi:10.1016/j.pmn.2018.12.008.

Edwards, D. J., Young, H., & Johnson, R. (2018). The immediate effect of Therapeutic Touch and deep touch pressure on range of motion, interoceptive accuracy and heart rate variability: a randomized controlled trial with moderation analysis. *Frontiers in Integrative Neuroscience, 12*, 41. doi:10.3389/fnint.2018.00041.

Engen, H. G., Bernhardt, B. C., Skottnik, L., Ricard, M., & Singer, T. (2018). Structural changes in socio-affective networks: multi-modal MRI findings in long-term meditation practitioners. *Neuropsychologia, 116*, 26–33.

Erich, M., & Quinlan-Colwell, A. (2017). Celebrating 20 years of the Healing Arts Network. *Southern Pain Society Newsletter*, 3–4. Summer.

Erich, M., Quinlan-Colwell, A., & O'Conner-Von, S. (2021). Distraction and relaxation. In M. F., Cooney, & A., Quinlan-Colwell (Eds.), *Assessment and multimodal management of pain* (pp. 586–612). Elsevier.

Esmel-Esmel, N., Tomás-Esmel, E., Tous-Andreu, M., Bové-Ribé, A., & Jiménez-Herrera, M. (2017). Reflexology and polysomnography: changes in cerebral wave activity induced by reflexology promote N1 and N2 sleep stages. *Complementary Therapies in Clinical Practice, 28*, 54–64.

Felix, M. M. D. S., Ferreira, M. B. G., da Cruz, L. F., & Barbosa, M. H. (2019). Relaxation therapy with guided imagery for postoperative pain management: an integrative review. *Pain Management Nursing, 20*(1), 3–9. doi:10.1016/j.pmn.2017.10.014.

Flemons, D. (2020). Toward a Relational Theory of Hypnosis. *American Journal of Clinical Hypnosis, 62*(4), 344–363.

Field, T. (2016). Massage therapy research review. *Complementary Therapies in Clinical Practice, 24*(8), 19–31.

Foley, M. K. H., Anderson, J., Mallea, L., Morrison, K., & Downey, M. (2016). Effects of healing touch on postsurgical adult outpatients. *Journal of Holistic Nursing, 34*(3), 271–279.

Fortney, L. (2018). Recommending meditation. In D., Rakel (Ed.), *Integrative Medicine* (pp. 945–953). Elsevier.

Gardiner, P., D'Amico, S., Luo, M., & Haas, N. (2020). An innovative electronic health toolkit (our whole lives for chronic pain) to reduce chronic pain in patients with health disparities: Open Clinical Trial. *JMIR mHealth and uHealth, 8*(3), e14768.

Goldberg, D. R., Wardell, D. W., Kilgarriff, N., Williams, B., Eichler, D., & Thomlinson, P. (2016). An initial study using healing touch for women undergoing a breast biopsy. *Journal of Holistic Nursing, 34*(2), 123–134.

Groenewald, C. B., Beals-Erickson, S. E., Ralston-Wilson, J., Rabbitts, J. A., & Palermo, T. M. (2017). Complementary and alternative medicine use by children with pain in the United States. *Academic Pediatrics, 17*(7), 785–793. doi:10.1016/j.acap.2017.02.008.

Hall, H., Leach, M., Brosnan, C., & Collins, M. (2017). Nurses' attitudes towards complementary therapies: a systematic review and meta-synthesis. *International Journal of Nursing Studies, 69*, 47–56. doi:10.1016/j.ijnurstu.2017.01.008.

Hanley, M. A., Anderson, M., & Shields, D. A. (2020). Energy healing. In M. A., Blaszko Helming, D. A., Shields, K. M., Avino, & W. E., Rosa (Eds.), *Dossey & Keegan's holistic nursing: A handbook for practice* (8th ed, pp. 311–520). Jones & Bartlett Learning.

Hanley, M. A., Coppa, D., & Shields, D. (2017). A practice-based theory of healing through therapeutic touch: advancing holistic nursing practice. *Journal of Holistic Nursing, 35*(4), 369–381.

Heap, M. (2017). Theories of hypnosis. In G. R., Elkins (Ed.), *Handbook of medical and psychological hypnosis: Foundations, applications, and professional issues* (pp. 9–18). Springer.

Institute for Healthcare Improvement. (2020). Retrieved from http://www.ihi.org/resources/Pages/HowtoImprove/default.aspx.

Jans-Beken, L., Jacobs, N., Janssens, M., Peeters, S., Reijnders, J., Lechner, L., & Lataster, J. (2020). Gratitude and health: an updated review. *The Journal of Positive Psychology, 15*(6), 743–782.

Jeans, Katz, J., & Taenzer, P. (2020). Remembering Ronald Melzack (1929–2019). *Canadian Journal of Pain, 4*(1), 122–124. doi:10.1080/24740527.2020.1757385.

Jensen, M. P., Jamieson, G. A., Lutz, A., Mazzoni, G., McGeown, W. J., Santarcangelo, E. L., et al. (2017). New directions in hypnosis research: strategies for advancing the cognitive and clinical neuroscience of hypnosis. *Neuroscience of Consciousness, 2017*(1), 1–14.

Jiang, H., White, M. P., Greicius, M. D., Waelde, L. C., & Spiegel, D. (2017). Brain activity and functional connectivity associated with hypnosis. *Cerebral Cortex, 27*(8), 4083–4093.

Joint Commission. (2018). New Joint Commission advisory on non-pharmacologic and non-opioid solutions for pain management. Retrieved from: https://www.jointcommission.org/resources/news-and-multimedia/newsletters/newsletters/quick-safety/quick-safety-44-nonpharmacologic-and-non-opioid-solutions-for-pain-management/#.ZAE-qz3MKUk.

Kievisiene, J., Jautakyte, R., Rauckiene-Michaelsson, A., Fatkulina, N., & Agostinis-Sobrinho, C. (2020). The effect of art therapy and music therapy on breast cancer patients: what we know and what we need to find out—A systematic review. *Evidence-Based Complementary and Alternative Medicine, 2020*, 1–14. doi:10.1155/2020/7390321.

Kihlstrom, J. F. (2016). Hypnosis. In *Reference module in neuroscience and biobehavioral psychology: Encyclopedia of mental health* (2nd ed., pp. 361–365). Elsevier.

King, C., Moore, L., & Spence, C. (2016). Exploring self-reported benefits of auricular acupuncture among veterans with posttraumatic stress disorder. *Journal of Holistic Nursing, 34*(3), 291–299.

Kirsch, I. (2017). *Hypnosis: Theory, research and application.* Routledge Taylor & Francis.

Krittanawong, C., Kumar, A., Wang, Z., Narasimhan, B., Jneid, H., Virani, S. S., et al. (2020). Meditation and cardiovascular health in the US. *The American Journal of Cardiology, 131*, 23–26.

Kukimoto, Y., Ooe, N., & Ideguchi, N. (2017). The effects of massage therapy on pain and anxiety after surgery: a systematic review and meta-analysis. *Pain Management Nursing, 18*(6), 378–390.

Labus, N., Wilson, C., & Arena, S. (2019). Mind-body therapies as a therapeutic intervention for pain management. *Home Healthcare Now, 37*(5), 293–294. doi:10.1097/NHH.0000000000000809.

Landry, M., & Raz, A. (2017). Neurophysiology of hypnosis. In G. R., Elkins (Ed.), *Handbook of medical and psychological hypnosis: Foundations, applications, and professional issues* (pp. 19–28). Springer.

Lee, T., Sherman, K., Hawkes, R., Phelan, E., & Turner, J. (2020). The benefits of Tai Chi for older adults with chronic back pain: a qualitative study. *The Journal of Alternative and Complementary Medicine, 26*(6), 456–462.

Mallari, B., Spaeth, E. K., Goh, H., & Boyd, B. S. (2019). Virtual reality as an analgesic for acute and chronic pain in adults: a systematic review and meta-analysis. *Journal of Pain Research, 12*, 2053–2085.

Manworren, R. (2015). Multimodal pain management and the future of a personalized medicine approach to pain. *AORN Journal, 101*(3), 308–314. doi:10.1016/j.aorn.2014.12.009.

Matinella, A., Brugnoli, M. P., Pasin, E., Segatti, A., Concon, E., & Squintani, G. (2017). Laser-evoked potentials (LEPs) in chronic pain conditions during hypnotic analgesia. *Clinical Neurophysiology, 128*(12), e432.

McManus, D. (2020). A phenomenological study of the lived experience of Roman Catholic Sisters and successful aging. *Journal of Holistic Nursing, 38*(4), 350–361.

Meghani, N., Tracy, M., O'Conner-Von, S., Hadidi, N., Mathiason, M., & Lindquist, R. (2020). Generating evidence of critical care nurses' perceptions, knowledge and use of music therapy, aromatherapy and guided imagery. *Dimensions of Critical Care Nursing, 39*(1), 47–57.

Millstein, R. A., Celano, C. M., Beale, E. E., Beach, S. R., Suarez, L., Belcher, A. M., … Huffman, J. C. (2016). The effects of optimism and gratitude on adherence, functioning and mental health following an acute coronary syndrome. *General Hospital Psychiatry, 43*, 17–22. doi:10.1016/j.genhospsych.2016.08.006.

Montgomery, R., & McNamara, S. A. (2016). Multimodal pain management for enhanced recovery: Reinforcing the shift from traditional pathways through nurse-led interventions. *AORN Journal, 104*(6), S9–S16. doi:10.1016/j.aorn.2016.10.012.

Mueller, G., Palli, C., & Schumacher, P. (2018). [Abstract] The effect of Therapeutic Touch on back pain in adults on a neurological unit: an experimental pilot study. *Pain Management Nursing* Online publication 2018 Nov 10. pii: S1524-9042(17)30510-6. doi:10.1016/j.pmn.2018.09.002. PMID: 30425012.

Munkombwe, W. M., Petersson, K., & Elgán, C. (2020). Nurses' experiences of providing nonpharmacological pain management in palliative care: a qualitative study. *Journal of Clinical Nursing, 29*(9-10), 1643–1652. doi:10.1111/jocn.15232.

Nahin, R. L., Boineau, R., Khalsa, P. S., Stussman, B. J., & Weber, W. J. (2016). Evidence-based evaluation of complementary health approaches for pain management in the United States. *Mayo Clinic Proceedings, 91*(9), 1292–1306. doi:10.1016/j.mayocp.2016.06.007.

Naseri-Salahshour, V., Sajadi, M., Abedi, A., Fournier, A., & Saeidi, N. (2019). Reflexology as an adjunctive nursing intervention for management of nausea in hemodialysis patients: a randomized clinical trial. *Complementary Therapies in Clinical Practice, 36*(1), 29–33.

National Center for Complementary and Integrative Health (NCCIH). (2018). Reiki. Retrieved from https://www.nccih.nih.gov/health/reiki.

National Center for Complementary and Integrative Health (NCCIH). (2019). *Pain.* National Institutes of Health website. Retrieved from https://nccih.nih.gov/health/pain.

National Center for Complementary and Integrative Health (NCCIH). (2022). The use and cost of complementary health approaches in the United Stated. Retrieved from https://www.nccih.nih.gov/about/the-use-and-cost-of-complementary-health-approaches-in-the-united-states.

O'Conner-Von, S., & Quinlan-Colwell, A. (2021). Spirituality as a component of multimodal pain management. In M. F., Cooney, & A., Quinlan-Colwell (Eds.), *Assessment and multimodal management of pain* (pp. 673–686). Elsevier.

Oschman, J. L. (2016). Bodywork, energetic, and movement therapies. In J. L., Oschman (Ed.), *Energy Medicine* (pp. 101–112). Elsevier.

Owens, J. E., Menard, M., Plews-Ogan, M., Calhoun, L. G., & Ardelt, M. (2016). Stories of growth and wisdom: a mixed-methods study of people living well with pain. *Global Advances in Health and Medicine, 5*(1), 16–28.

Park, J., Krause-Parello, C., & Barnes, C. (2020). A narrative review of movement-based mind-body interventions: effects of yoga, tai chi, and qigong for back pain patients. *Holistic Nursing Practice, 34*(1), 3–23.

Payrau, B., Quere, N., Breton, E., & Payrau, C. (2017). Fasciatherapy and reflexology compared to hypnosis and music therapy in daily stress management. *International Journal of Therapeutic Massage & Bodywork, 10*(3), 4–13.

Pearlman, A. (2016). Complementary and alternative medicine. In L., Goldman, & A., Schafer (Eds.), *Goldman Cecil Medicine* (25th Ed, pp. 181–184.e1). Elsevier.

Penlington, C. (2019). Exploring a compassion-focused intervention for persistent pain in a group setting. *British Journal of Pain, 13*(1), 59–66.

Phillips, B. C. (2020). Hypnosis in the clinical setting. *Journal of the American Association of Nurse Practitioners, 32*(5), 351–353.

Polomano, R. C., Fillman, M., Giordano, N. A., Vallerand, A. H., Nicely, K. L., & Jungquist, C. R. (2017). Multimodal analgesia for acute postoperative and trauma-related pain. *The American Journal of Nursing, 117*(3 Suppl 1), S12–S26.

Quinlan-Colwell, A. (2021a). Manual therapies for pain management. In M. F., Cooney, & A., Quinlan-Colwell (Eds.), *Assessment and multimodal management of pain* (pp. 652–672). Elsevier.

Quinlan-Colwell, A. (2021b). Additional nonpharmacologic interventions as components of multimodal pain management. In M. F., Cooney, & A., Quinlan-Colwell (Eds.), *Assessment and multimodal management of pain* (pp. 738–769). Elsevier.

Quinlan-Colwell, A. (2021c). Natural products: supplements, botanicals, vitamins, and minerals as a component of multimodal pain management. In M. F., Cooney, & A., Quinlan-Colwell (Eds.), *Assessment and multimodal management of pain* (pp. 687–737). Elsevier.

Quinlan-Colwell, A., & O'Conner-Von, S (2021). Energy healing therapies or biofield therapies as a component of multimodal analgesic pain management. In M. F., Cooney, & A., Quinlan-Colwell (Eds.), *Assessment and multimodal management of pain* (pp. 636–651). Elsevier.

Raffone, A., Marzetti, L., Del Gratta, C., Perrucci, M. G., Romani, G. L., & Pizzella, V. (2019). *Toward a brain theory of meditation Progress in Brain Research* 244, 207–232.

Ringdahl, D. (2023). Reiki. In R., Lindquist, M., Tracy, & M., Snyder (Eds.), *Complementary therapies in nursing: Promoting integrative care* (pp. 447–474). Springer.

Rosenkranz, M. A., Lutz, A., Perlman, D. M., Bachhuber, D. R., Schuyler, B. S., MacCoon, D. G., & Davidson, R. J. (2016). Reduced stress and inflammatory responsiveness in experienced meditators compared to a matched healthy control group. *Psychoneuroendocrinology, 68*, 117–125.

Roth, I., Highfield, L., Cuccaro, P., Wells, R., Misra, S., & Engebretson, J. (2019). Employing evidence in evaluating complementary therapies: Findings from an ethnography of integrative pain management at a large urban pediatric hospital. *Journal of Alternative and Complementary Medicine, 25*(S1), S95–S105.

Rubik, B., Muehsam, D., Hammerschlag, R., & Jain, S. (2015). Biofield science and healing: History, terminology, and concepts. Global Advances in Health and Medicine. *Biofield Special Issue, 4*, 8–14.

Sajadi, S., Kazemi, M., Bakhtar, B., & Ostadebrahimi, H. (2019). Comparing the effects of auricular seed acupressure and foot reflexology on neonatal abstinence syndrome: a modified double blind clinical trial. *Complementary Therapies in Clinical Practice, 36*, 72–76.

Saredakis, D., Szpak, A., Birckhead, B., Keage, H. A., Rizzo, A., & Loetscher, T. (2020). Factors associated with virtual reality sickness in head-mounted displays: a systematic review and meta-analysis. *Frontiers in Human Neuroscience, 14*(6), 1–17.

Sayari, S., Nobahar, M., & Ghorbani, R. (2018). Effect of foot reflexology massage on physiological indices in patients with acute myocardial infarction. *Koomesh, 20*(3), 469–477.

Sundberg, T., Cramer, H., Sibbritt, D., Adams, J., & Lauche, R. (2017). Prevalence, patterns, and predictors of massage practitioner utilization: results of a US nationally representative survey. *Musculoskeletal Science and Practice, 32*, 31–37.

Swain, N., Lennox Thompson, B., Gallagher, S., Paddison, J., & Mercer, S. (2020). Gratitude Enhanced Mindfulness (GEM): a pilot study of an internet-delivered programme for self-management of pain and disability in people with arthritis. *The Journal of Positive Psychology, 15*(3), 420–426.

Tabatabaee, A., Tafreshi, M. Z., Rassouli, M., Aledavood, S. A., AlaviMajd, H., & Farahmand, S. K. (2016). Effect of Therapeutic Touch in patients with cancer: a literature review. *Medical Archives, 70*(2), 142–147. doi:10.5455/medarh.2016.70.142-147.

Thompson, T., Terhune, D. B., Oram, C., Sharangparni, J., Rouf, R., Solmi, M., et al. (2019). The effectiveness of hypnosis for pain relief: a systematic review and meta–analysis of 85 controlled experimental trials. *Neuroscience & Biobehavioral Reviews, 99*, 298–310.

Tick, H., Nielsen, A., Pelletier, K. R., Bonakdar, R., Simmons, S., Glick, R., Ratner, E., Lemmon, R. L., Wayne, P., & Zador, V. Pain Task Force of the Academic Consortium for Integrative Medicine and Health. (2018). Evidence-based nonpharmacologic strategies for comprehensive pain care: the consortium pain task force white paper. *Explore, 14*(3), 177–211.

Tychsen, L., & Thio, L. L. (2020). Concern of photosensitive seizures evoked by 3D video displays or virtual reality headsets in children: current perspective. *Eye and Brain, 12*, 45–48.

Vallerand, A. H., Crawley, J., Pieper, B., & Templin, T. N. (2016). The perceived control over pain construct and functional status. *Pain Medicine, 17*(4), 692–703. doi:10.1111/pme.12924.

Vickers, A., Vertosick, E., Lewith, G., MacPherson, H., Foster, N., Sherman, K., et al. (2018). Acupuncture for chronic pain: update of an individual patient data meta-analysis. *Journal of Pain, 19*(5), 455–474. doi:10.1016/j.jpain.2017.11.005.

Wijaya, R. D., Madjid, T. H., & Alwi, E. H. (2020). The effect of touch and sound therapy to the level of pain and physiological parameters in infants. *IJNP (Indonesian Journal of Nursing Practices), 4*(1), 7–13.

You, T., & Ogawa, E. F. (2020). Effects of meditation and mind-body exercise on brain-derived neurotrophic factor: a literature review of human experimental studies. *Sports Medicine and Health Science, 2*(1), 7–9.

Yu, C. P., Lee, H. Y., & Luo, X. Y. (2018). The effect of virtual reality forest and urban environments on physiological and psychological responses. *Urban Forestry & Urban Greening, 35*, 106–114.

Yu, H., Cai, Q., Shen, B., Gao, X., & Zhou, X. (2017). Neural substrates and social consequences of interpersonal gratitude: intention matters. *Emotion, 17*(4), 589–602. doi:10.1037/emo0000258.

Part 4

CHAPTER 16

Psychosocial Interventions for Pain Management

Chasity Brimeyer, PhD, EdS
Maureen F. Cooney, DNP, FNP-BC, ACHPN,AP-PMN*

Introduction

An individual's pain experience and outcomes can be understood as a dynamic and unique interaction of biological, psychological, and social factors, necessitating an interdisciplinary approach to understanding and treating pain. In addition to pain relief, psychosocial interventions like cognitive behavioral therapy, acceptance and commitment therapy, relaxation training, and biofeedback help to improve emotional well-being, empower individuals to resume daily functioning, and enhance quality of life. Alternative delivery of psychosocial pain interventions, including group formats and digital-based supports, offer solutions to logistical barriers in accessing comprehensive pain management intervention.

I. Biopsychosocial Contributions to Pain

A. Biopsychosocial model
  1. First conceptualized by George Engel in 1977; offers multifactorial approach to pain management
  2. Defines health, disease, and symptoms as products of reciprocal influences of biological, psychological, and social domains, rather than relying on physical or biological factors alone (as in biomedical model) and provides understanding of individual's subjective experience of well-being or illness
  3. Considers complex contributions and interactions of biopsychosocial model factors to understand patient's experience within context of life circumstances comprehensively
    a. Biological factors:
      1) Age, sex, ethnicity
      2) Physical health, neurochemistry, metabolic disorders, hormones, genetic vulnerability, comorbidities
      3) Medication side effects

      4) Lifestyle (e.g., sleep, nutrition)
      5) Stress reactivity
    b. Psychological factors:
      1) Emotions, temperament, self-esteem, attitudes/beliefs
      2) Stress, coping skills, perceptions/perspectives
      3) Trauma
      4) Response to rewards, learning and memory
      5) Health behaviors
    c. Social factors:
      1) Interpersonal relationships, social support dynamics, school or work dynamics, social skills, religion or spiritual belief systems
      2) Gender identity, culture
      3) Family background, family circumstances
      4) Socioeconomics, healthcare access
  4. Provides framework for interprofessional assessment, diagnosis, and treatment; outcomes of a health condition vary greatly based on context with which symptoms, illness, or disease occurs
B. Biopsychosocial model and pain
  1. Pain experience and pain outcomes are multifactorial, not just mechanistic biological process. Pain is dynamic interaction of biological, psychological, and social factors unique to each individual.
    a. Biological factors impacting pain presentation/experience include disease severity, nociception, inflammation, and nervous system function. Certain conditions increase the likelihood of developing pain (e.g., obesity, age, prolonged stress that over-sensitizes nervous system functioning).
    b. Psychological factors impacting pain presentation/experience include stress, coping, pain beliefs, mood/affect, and pain catastrophizing (irrational expectation of the worst).
      1) Anxiety, depression, and/or psychological trauma can increase pain intensity, duration, risk for acute pain to transition to persistent (chronic) pain, and interference with daily functioning.

---

*Section Editor for the chapter.

2) Pain beliefs and prior learning about pain affect whether or not individual engages in behaviors that promote recovery and coping.

c. Social factors impacting pain presentation/ experience: culture, social support, economic factors, family history of pain, health literacy

1) Discord in interpersonal relationships, lack of adequate housing, poverty, lack of access to healthcare and alternative healing modalities, and/or being underinsured influence individual's pain experience and outcomes.

2) Modeling pain coping (accommodating versus avoiding activities and responsibilities, functional disability, pain catastrophizing) influence individual's pain experience and outcomes.

2. Interaction of biological, psychological, and social factors results in different pain experiences and outcomes.

a. Biopsychosocial model led to development of interprofessional pain management to provide more comprehensive, individualized pain treatment that targets all contributing factors.

b. Because individuals with pain differ physically, psychologically, and socially, a one-size-fits-all or medication-only approach to pain treatment is inadequate.

c. Goal of pain management includes learning to identify and modify maladaptive pain-related thoughts, relieve physical discomfort, improve adaptive functioning, and decrease pain interference in daily life; this cannot be accomplished through medical intervention alone (Fig. 16.1).

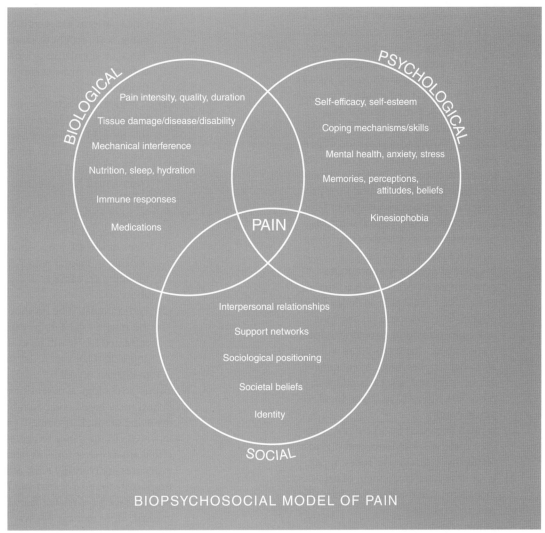

Figure 16.1 **Biopsychosocial model of pain.** *From What causes pain and how does it work?* © Westcoast SCI, Port Coquitlam, BC, Canada. Retrieved from https://westcoastsci.com/blog/ pain-how-it-works-and-management/.

II. Psychosocial Interventions for Pain Management

A. Cognitive and behavioral-based therapies
  1. Cognitive-behavioral therapy (CBT) for pain
     a. Most empirically supported psychosocial intervention for pain management
     b. CBT is based on premise that psychological suffering originates from combination of unhelpful ways of thinking and learned patterns of maladaptive behaviors. Within context of pain, CBT is used to help individuals change negative pain-related beliefs and improve adaptive functioning.
     c. Common elements of cognitive-behavioral therapy include:
        1) Psychoeducation
           a) Provides rationale for how CBT may help to reduce pain and distress
              (1) Lack of sufficient education about pain contributes to poor pain management and lack of effective self-advocacy in pain treatment.
              (2) When used in combination with other treatment strategies, education about biopsychosocial aspects of pain has shown to improve patient self-management and self-efficacy.
           b) Involves providing explanation of persistent pain (pain that does not serve a protective function), how pain signals are transmitted to brain and then processed in central nervous system (e.g., gate control theory, central sensitization), and how psychosocial variables influence pain processing
           c) Is aimed at managing appropriate expectations for procedure for acute or procedural-related pain; includes detailed discussion of all aspects involved in procedure (providing patient with information about where procedure will occur and what supplies, tools, or equipment will be used) and how certain aspects of procedure will feel (e.g., tight, small pinch, numb)
           d) Is often enhanced by take-home reference materials, handouts, and digital platforms (internet references, apps)
           e) Is an important component of pain management and remains understudied and underutilized
        2) Cognitive reframing
           a) Describes process of identifying and then modifying how pain-related thoughts, experiences, beliefs, and/or circumstances are viewed to improve negative emotions.
           b) Involves challenging or disputing unhelpful thoughts with more adaptive evidence or perspective.
           c) Common unhelpful thinking patterns associated with persistent pain include catastrophizing (exaggerated negative focus toward real or anticipated pain and pain events), polarized thinking (inability to see alternatives or solutions regarding pain), filtering (focusing on negative details of situation while ignoring positive or neutral aspects), and external control fallacy (viewing oneself as helpless victim of pain).
           d) Patients are encouraged to first identify and gain awareness of unhelpful thoughts about pain through monitoring their thought patterns.
              (1) Once patterns are identified, patients are taught to examine evidence or alternative perspectives that support or negate unhelpful thoughts.
              (2) If evidence does not support the thought, patient learns to change this thought into more adaptive one (e.g., "Nothing works for my pain" can be reframed to, "There are still treatments I have not tried that may help").
           e) Can be used before, during, or following acute or procedural pain
              (1) Steps of identifying, disputing, and revising unhelpful pain-related thoughts are same as described above.
              (2) For example, "The flu shot will hurt too much! I can't do it" can be reframed to, "It will be over quickly and I can play a game on my phone to distract myself."
        3) Exposure/psychological desensitization
           a) Behaviorally based component of CBT involving gradual, systematic exposure to feared circumstance to decrease associated anxiety over time. Systematic exposures are typically rank-ordered from least- to most-feared and help patients face pain-related fears in gradual, more manageable way.
           b) Premise of exposure therapy is a fear response to pain or pain-related circumstances is conditioned (learned), so fear

response can be deconditioned (unlearned) by experiencing feared circumstance without associated anxiety.

    (1) Fear is anticipatory emotional response to circumstances an individual believes will exacerbate pain.

    (2) Avoidance behaviors are those that prevent or delay encountering feared situation.

    (3) While pain-related fear is not always associated with avoidance behaviors, pain- or fear-avoidance is common among individuals with persistent pain and is typically characterized as avoiding activities of daily living, jobs, school, or even enjoyable activities.

c) Pain is significant, yet modifiable, component that contributes to adaptive functioning (or individual's ability to effectively and independently manage tasks of daily life).

    (1) Anticipating pain exacerbation can negatively influence pain perception.

    (2) In persistent pain, graduated exposure or desensitization is used to decrease fear associated with engaging in activities. This helps individuals resume daily functioning, which can reduce persistent pain.

d) Exposure and desensitization techniques are readily applied to procedural pain.

    (1) If patients demonstrate pain-related anxiety about specific procedures, graduated exposure can be used to decrease fear of the procedure over time.

    (2) For example, successive exposures to needles are paired with relaxation and cognitive reframing skills to reduce anxiety about injections.

4) Distraction

a) Another behaviorally based CBT technique that aims to shift individual's attention away from discomfort or pain toward something more pleasant, relaxing, or engaging. This attentional shift interrupts pain-processing pathways in brain, leaving less perceptual resources to process pain signals.

b) Distraction can be internal to individual, including focusing on adaptive thoughts, or external to individual, including conversation, watching shows, playing games, or using relaxation techniques.

c) Distraction can involve passive engagement (e.g., watching something) or active engagement (e.g., exercising, having a conversation).

d) Patients uniquely respond to distraction efforts; what works for one individual may not be distracting to another. Patients may require assistance with identifying which types of distraction work best for them.

e) Distraction can be done individually or involve others, like caregivers or healthcare providers.

f) Distraction for persistent pain resembles improved daily functioning, such as being engaged in work, school, hobbies, or extracurricular activities.

g) Distraction is commonly used for managing procedural pain, given its efficacy, empirical support, wide range of applicability, and ease of use.

h) Virtual reality programs have been used as a distraction technique to manage acute pain.

    (1) Virtual reality involves using variety of equipment meant to immerse individual in multisensorial, computer-generated environment.

    (2) Individual's attention is diverted from pain while engaging in virtual environment, there by decreasing perceptual resources to process pain signals.

    (3) Virtual reality equipment is increasingly more affordable, portable, and realistic; however, research on efficacy is burgeoning.

d. Evidence base for CBT in pain management

1) Associated with neural changes on functional magnetic resonance imaging

a) Orbitofrontal cortex is associated with cognitive processing of pain perception, decision-making, and pain modulation.

b) Dorsal attention network is associated with goal-directed processing and replacement of attention.

c) Abnormal intrinsic connectivity network (useful for investigating thoughts, behaviors, emotions, and somatic sensations) within orbitofrontal cortex and dorsal attention network are normalized in adult persistent pain patients who completed CBT treatment.

2) Improves general mood and increases positive emotions, motivation, and self-efficacy in

adults, but its effect on pain reduction is more variable. More improvement has been shown in:

   a) Widespread versus focal pain intensity
   b) Certain pain diagnoses (e.g., back pain versus fibromyalgia)
   c) Functional disability versus other components of pain experience

3) Improves quality of life and activities of daily living, persistent headache, myofascial pain, and arthralgia, particularly if effective therapeutic alliance or rapport is established.

4) Improves pain-related behaviors, such as vocalizations of distress, posturing, or withdrawing from activities, in youth with persistent pain.

5) CBT has been shown to be equally or more effective than standard medical care in reducing recurrent abdominal pain in children. It has been associated with positive cognitive coping, more helpful pain appraisal, and reduced expression of pain behaviors in adults.

6) CBT is now considered part of first-line preventive treatment for pediatric headache and migraine, either alone or in combination with medication-based therapies. In adults with persistent musculoskeletal pain, CBT was found to be particularly beneficial for reducing pain-related functional disability.

7) Graduated in vivo (real world) exposure reduces pain, fear-avoidance beliefs and thoughts, and avoidant behaviors.

2. Acceptance and commitment therapy (ACT; pronounced "act")

   a. ACT is a newer treatment approach effectively applied to pain management.

   b. Uses mindfulness, acceptance, identification of valued life directions, and committed action toward goals and values to facilitate "psychological flexibility," or ability to move forward toward one's desired life outcomes despite unwanted thoughts, feelings, or physical symptoms.

   c. With regard to pain management, ACT is employed to increase individual's ability to live full, meaningful life despite discomfort. Patients are encouraged to increase functioning, in accordance with individual values, by shifting focus away from struggling with pain toward pursuing quality of life.

   d. In contrast to CBT, ACT discourages attempts to reframe or challenge unhelpful thoughts, feelings, or physical symptoms and instead teaches patients to accept negative or unhelpful circumstances as inevitable and normal experiences that occur when living a meaningful, values-based life.

   e. ACT relies heavily on use of metaphors and experiential exercises to increase flexible perspectives.

   f. Core ACT processes are:

      1) Mindfulness or "being present"
         a) Involves focusing on present moment rather than ruminating on past events or anticipating future outcomes
         b) Can also assist patient in increasing awareness of all emotional and physical experiences and sensations, not just pain

      2) Acceptance
         a) Involves developing willingness to experience some discomfort in name of pursuing meaningful life, as trying to control pain may result in more distress (e.g., failed treatments, continued pain)
         b) Promotes engagement in values-based action, recognizing it will likely include level of discomfort
         c) Regarding pain, acceptance shifts treatment goals from eliminating pain to living fully despite pain

      3) Cognitive defusion
         a) Refers to skills that change how individuals react to thoughts and feelings
         b) Assists patients in differentiating between having a thought and being negatively influenced or consumed by a thought

      4) Self-as-context
         a) Individual identities can become intertwined with pain. Self-as-context establishes sense of self that is greater than individual's thoughts, feelings, or physical body.
         b) Self-as-context techniques assist individual in discarding labels and self-judgments that inhibit positive behavioral change.

      5) Identifying values
         a) Asks individuals to identify defining characteristics or qualities (e.g., family, hard work, spirituality). Patients then set meaningful goals that improve quality of life, functioning, and meaning-making despite pain.
         b) Assists individuals in refocusing priorities away from pain and toward meaningful engagement

6) Committed action
   a) Involves commitment to valued action despite pain
   b) Individuals are encouraged to live life consistent with their values and goals rather than be inhibited by pain.
g. Evidence base for ACT
   1) Associated with greater reductions in pain, functional disability, pain intensity, and fear of pain compared to standard medical care for youth with general persistent pain
   2) Decreases disability, depressive symptoms, pain-related anxiety, functional disability, analgesic use, and healthcare utilization in adults with general persistent pain
   3) Clinically significant effects have been demonstrated on a range of pain-related outcomes, including improvement in pain acceptance and psychological flexibility. Methodological biases may overestimate treatment effectiveness.
   4) ACT is similar in effectiveness to more traditional cognitive and behavior therapy, like CBT. ACT may be a suitable alternative to CBT, given its focus on valued action rather than controlling the pain experience.
   5) Improvements in pain interference, physical and emotional quality of life, and activity are maintained at follow-up in adults with persistent pain using ACT.

B. Relaxation techniques
   1. Nonpharmacological skills used to decrease individual's pain perception by promoting sense of physical well-being, calm, and comfort
   2. Easy to learn, cost effective, and do not require specialized technology or equipment
   3. Why relaxation is used
      a. When an individual perceives a stressor, stress hormones are released by adrenal glands (e.g., adrenaline, norepinephrine, cortisol) and trigger a series of physical responses (e.g., increased heart rate, vasoconstriction, sweating, increased muscle tension), commonly called the "fight or flight" response, to assist person in addressing stressor.
         1) Body can overreact to non–life-threatening circumstances, resulting in chronic stress.
         2) Chronic stress keeps hypothalamic-pituitary-adrenal (HPA) axis, and thereby the sympathetic nervous system, activated.
         3) Chronic stress alone worsens pain, in addition to exacerbating other physical and psychological conditions that can indirectly worsen pain (e.g., obesity, poor sleep, anxiety, depression).

b. Relaxation techniques counter stress response and decrease chronic stress by inducing "relaxation response," which engages parasympathetic nervous system to restore physiological functioning to normal. Relaxation response interrupts pain processing.
   4. Common relaxation techniques include:
      a. Diaphragmatic breathing
         1) Involves slow, rhythmic breathing from diaphragm muscle rather than thoracic or chest area
         2) Decreases work or effort of breathing, encourages full oxygen/carbon dioxide exchange (which has positive benefits for heart rate and vasodilation), and engages vagus nerve (which triggers relaxation response from parasympathetic nervous system)
         3) Has positive impact on respiratory, cardiovascular, cardiorespiratory, and autonomic nervous systems
         4) Is most commonly used relaxation technique
         5) Continues to have uncertain long-term benefit for persistent pain
         6) Has been associated with acute pain reduction, but results have been inconsistent
         7) Diaphragmatic breathing may be effective in obtaining subjective relaxation response and diverting individual's focus from painful stimuli to exercise of breathing, serving as distraction.
      b. Guided imagery
         1) Sometimes referred to as guided meditation or visualization
         2) Involves focused attentional process where individual uses soothing words and/or music to evoke imaginary sensory images that bring about positive physical and emotional changes
         3) May alter cortical processing associated with centrally mediated pain
         4) Videos, audio, or scripts are used to describe objects, places, or events that evoke calmness.
            a) Common scenes include sunsets, beaches, and floating on water.
            b) Some imagery is more pain-focused, encouraging individual to modify shape, color, or intensity of pain to promote relief.
         5) Frequently paired with other relaxation tools, such as diaphragmatic breathing
         6) Shown to decrease pain intensity for variety of pain types, including spontaneous pain,

evoked pain, paresthesias, and acute/postoperative pain

7) Less effective for paroxysmal pains

8) Underutilized pain management tool, in part due to lack of quality training programs for non-behavioral health providers

c. Progressive muscle relaxation

1) Muscle tension is thought to be one aspect of body's stress response.

2) Used to gradually loosen or relieve tension in muscles; involves successively contracting and releasing muscle groups while focusing on different sensations of tension versus relaxation that result

3) Commonly paired with other relaxation techniques, such as diaphragmatic breathing and guided imagery

4) Greater awareness of muscle tension can intercept pain before it increases.

5) Evidence base for progressive muscle relaxation:

a) May reduce negative mood states and improve sleep quality, which can indirectly improve pain perception for both acute and persistent pain

b) Associated with improvement in health-related quality of life, fatigue, and treatment-related pain

c) Offers feasible intervention that decreases headache frequency and stress

C. Biofeedback/biofeedback-assisted relaxation therapy

1. Provides auditory, visual, or tactile feedback about physiological processes regulated by autonomic nervous system (e.g., heart rate, muscle tension, respiratory rate) to increase individual's voluntary control over these processes. These physiological processes are implicated in body's stress response and thus contribute to pain.

2. Instruction on relaxation techniques, combined with information or feedback about body's response, can be used to make positive physical changes in body (e.g., slower pace and better quality of breath, reduction in muscle tension, and increased blood flow)

3. Helps to decrease sympathetic arousal, promote specific and overall relaxation, and enhance individual's sense of self-control

4. Visual feedback is often displayed using numbers, graphs, or interactive displays (games where actions are correlated with positive physical changes).

5. Biofeedback modalities have different pain management benefits. Common sensors or modalities include:

a. Pace and quality of breath

b. Skin conductance for emotional/stress reactivity

c. Photoplethysmography for heart rate and blood-volume changes (used to assess heart rate and respiration coherence for overall well-being)

d. Surface electromyography (sEMG) for muscle tension

e. Thermistor/thermal warming for general relaxation and headache treatment

f. sEMG and thermal biofeedback for tension-type headaches and migraines offer most empirical treatment support.

6. Barriers to implementation include need for expensive equipment, specialized training, and lack of insurance coverage.

7. Evidence base for biofeedback therapy:

a. Correlated with reduction in noradrenaline (neurotransmitter involved in intrinsic pain modulation)

b. Associated with improvement in overall well-being, depression, and pain-related disability in patients with persistent low back pain

c. Associated with long-term benefits in reducing pain intensity and pain-related outcomes (affect, cognitive, and behavior)

d. Meta-analytic review demonstrated:

1) Biofeedback therapy can lead to immediate and long-term improvements in pain intensity, muscle tension, and other pain-related outcomes (depression, coping, and functional disability).

2) Research remains sparse and with methodological flaws (variability in sample size, characteristics, modality, and lack of control groups). Nevertheless, biofeedback may be promising individual or adjunctive pain therapy.

D. Other formats for pain intervention

1. Group therapy

a. Cost-effective, efficient means of providing traditional psychosocial intervention for pain while also promoting social support and parent or family training

b. Acceptable, feasible, non-stigmatizing resources that may address barriers to accessing interprofessional pain care, including time, cost, and logistical concerns

c. Can be run on weekends or condensed into time-limited interventions (e.g., one day) to reduce school or work absences

d. Small but positive effects have been found in daily functioning, depression symptoms, and pain catastrophizing for adolescents with persistent pain.

e. Small but positive effects have been found in reducing pain intensity for adults with persistent pain.

2. Virtual/online/digital-based programs

   a. Digital pain intervention programs are interactive psychosocial treatments for pain and provide alternative to in-person interventions.

      1) Programs are delivered online, via texting, or apps.

      2) Programs vary considerably in content but typically involve adapting psychoeducation, CBT, ACT, parent training, and relaxation training programs for internet or smartphone formats.

      3) Programs can be synchronous (live) or self-paced.

   b. Internet-based and smartphone app interventions may help to reduce waiting lists and stigma; however, self-guided programs may lack therapeutic feedback or guidance.

      1) Automated text-based programs for smartphones have been used to deliver coping strategies, pain psychoeducation, and treatment adherence support with positive benefit for both adults and children.

      2) Apps for pain management, including symptom monitoring, medication usage, relaxation instruction, and pain education (e.g., activity pacing) are well-accepted and easily accessible means of basic pain-related support. While promising, more empirical support is needed. (Search "relaxation for pain relief," "relaxation for pain management," "pain management," and "pain diary" in app stores.)

      3) Improvements in function, mood, confidence in managing pain, anxiety, and pain interference have been demonstrated, in addition to reduced healthcare costs. Duration of pain may moderate program engagement.

      4) While digital-based pain interventions address barriers of access to services, high attrition rates, low motivation, lack of therapeutic support, and technology-related issues negatively impact treatment fidelity.

III. Implications for Nurses

A. Be knowledgeable about how social, emotional, family, and cultural factors; health literacy; and learning styles impact individuals' pain presentation and engagement in pain treatment. Use this knowledge to advocate within treatment team for biopsychosocial approach to pain care (versus emphasis on physiological management alone).

B. Provide education about how pain processing/nervous system functioning, psychological factors, and social factors influence one another and affect symptoms to foster a good working alliance with patients.

C. Implement basic psychosocial supports in nursing care, including encouraging healthy patient expectations (e.g., treatment course), being fully present with patients, strengthening verbal and nonverbal communication skills to convey empathy, teaching relaxation skills to patients, providing patients opportunities to discuss their concerns and barriers to care, and monitoring patient distress, coping, and pain interference.

D. Model provision of basic psychosocial supports for patient's medical treatment team.

E. Triage patients to specialized behavioral healthcare with observation of increased distress and pain interference. Be familiar with referral sources for cognitive therapies (CBT, ACT) and relaxation training (biofeedback). Build resource bank for digital relaxation training (apps, handouts, videos) to provide to patients.

F. Some strategies can be used by nurses to prevent compassion fatigue, such as practicing mindfulness and personal application of relaxation techniques.

Bibliography

Boersma, K., Södermark, M., Hesser, H., Flink, I. K., Gerdle, B., & Linton, S. L. (2019). Efficacy of a transdiagnostic emotion-focused exposure treatment for chronic pain patients with comorbid anxiety and depression: a randomized controlled trial. *Pain, 160,* 1708–1718. http://dx.doi.org/10.1097/j.pain.0000000000001575.

Buck, C., Keweloh, C., Bouras, A., & Simoes, E. J. (2021). Efficacy of short message service text messaging interventions for postoperative pain management: systematic review. *Journal of Medical Internet Research, 9*(6). doi:10.2196/20199.

Coakley, R., Wihak, T., Kossowsky, J., Iversen, C., & Donado, C. (2018). The comfort ability pain management workshop: a preliminary, nonrandomized investigation of a brief, cognitive, biobehavioral, and parent training intervention for pediatric chronic pain. *Journal of Pediatric Psychology, 43*(3), 252–265. doi:10.1093/jpepsy/jsx112.

Gōmez-de-Regil, L., & Estrella-Castillo, D. F. (2020). Psychotherapy for physical pain in patients with fibromyalgia: a systematic review. *Pain Research and Management.* https://doi.org/10.1155/2020/3408052.

Herbert, M. S., Afari, N., Liu, L., Heppner, P., Rutledge, T., Williams, K., et al. (2017). Telehealth versus in-person acceptance and commitment therapy for chronic pain: a randomized noninferiority trial. *The Journal of Pain, 18*(2), 200–211. https://dx.doi.org/10.1016/j.jpain.2016.10.014.

Huestis, S. E., Kao, G., Dunn, A., Hilliard, A. T., Yoon, I. A., Golianu, B., et al. (2017). Multi-family pediatric pain group therapy: capturing acceptance and cultivating change. *Children, 4,* 106–121.

Hughes, L. S., Clark, J., Colclough, J. A., Dale, E., & McMillan, D. (2017). Acceptance and Commitment Therapy (ACT) for chronic pain: a systematic review and meta-analyses. *Clinical Journal of Pain, 33*(6), 552–568. doi: 10.1097/AJP.0000000000000425.

Joypaul, S., Kelly, F., McMillan, S. S., & King, M. A. (2019). Multidisciplinary interventions for chronic pain involving education: a systematic review. *PLoS ONE, 14*(10). https://doi.org/10.1371/journal.pone.0223306.

Kaur, J., Ghosh, S., Sahani, A. K., & Sinha, J. K. (2020). Mental imagery as a rehabilitative therapy for neuropathic pain in people with spinal cord injury: a randomized controlled trial. *Neurorehabilitation and Neural Repair, 34*(11), 1038–1049. doi:10.1177/1545968320962498.

Kent, P., O'Sullivan, P., Smith, A., Haines, T., Campbell, A., McGregor, A. H., et al. (2019). RESTORE-Cognitive functional therapy with or without movement sensor biofeedback versus usual care for chronic, disabling low back pain: study protocol for a randomized controlled trial. *BMJ Open, 9*(8). doi:10.1136/bmjopen-2019-031133.

Kisaarslan, M., & Aksoy, N. (2020). Effect of progressive muscle relaxation exercise on postoperative pain level in patients undergoing open renal surgery: a nonrandomized evaluation. *Journal of PeriAnesthesia Nursing, 35*(4), 389–396. https://doi.org/10.1016/j.jopan.2019.12.003.

Meints, S. M., & Edwards, R. R. (2018). Evaluating psychosocial contributions to chronic pain outcomes. *Program of Neuropsychopharmacological and Biological Psychiatry, 20*(87), 168–182. doi:10.1016/j.pnpbp.2018.01.017.

Palermo, T. M., Murray, C., Aalfs, H., Abu-El-Haija, M., Barth, B., Bellin, M. D., et al. (2020). Web-based cognitive-behavioral intervention for pain in pediatric acute recurrent and chronic pancreatitis: protocol of a multicenter randomized controlled trial from the study of chronic pancreatitis, diabetes and pancreatic cancer (CPDPC). *Contemporary Clinical Trials, 88.* https://doi.org/10.1016/j.cct.2019.105898.

Pielech, M., Vowles, K. E., & Wicksell, R. (2017). Acceptance and commitment therapy for pediatric chronic pain: theory and application. *Children, 4*(10). doi:10.3390/children4020010.

Pim, T. J., Williams, L. J., Reay, M., Pickering, S., Lota, R., Coote, L., et al. (2020). An evaluation of a digital pain management programme: clinical effectiveness and cost savings. *British Journal of Pain, 14*(4), 238–249. doi:10.1177/2049463719865286.

Pourmand, A., Davis, S., Marchak, A., Whiteside, T., & Sikka, N. (2018). Virtual reality as a clinical tool for pain management. *Current Pain and Headache Reports, 22*, 53–59. https://doi.org/10.1007/s11916-018-0708-2.

Semerci, R., & Kostak Akgün, M. (2020). The efficacy of distraction cards and kaleidoscope for reducing pain during phlebotomy: a randomized control trial. *Journal of PeriAnesthesia Nursing, 35*, 397–402. https://doi.org/10.1016/j.jopan.2020.02.003.

Sielski, R., Rief, W., & Glombiewski, J. A. (2017). Efficacy of biofeedback in chronic back pain: a meta-analysis. *International Journal of Behavioral Medicine, 24*, 25–41. doi:10.1007/s12529-016-9572-9.

Thurnheer, S. E., Gravestock, I., Pichierri, G., Steurer, J., & Burgstaller, J. M. (2018). Benefits of mobile apps in pain management: systematic review. *JMIR Mhealth Uhealth, 6*(10). doi:10.2196/11231.

Wren, A. A., Ross, A. C., D'Souza, G., Almgren, C., Feinstein, A., Marshall, A., et al. (2019). Multidisciplinary pain management for pediatric patients with acute and chronic pain: a foundational treatment approach when prescribing opioids. *Children, 6*, 33–55.

Yoshino, A., Okamoto, Y., Okada, G., Takamura, M., Ichikawa, N., et al. (2018). Changes in resting-state brain networks after cognitive-behavioral therapy for chronic pain. *Psychological Medicine, 48*, 1148–1156. https://doi.org/10.1017/S0033291717002598.

Part 4

CHAPTER 17
Pharmacological Pain Management Strategies

Linda Mary Vanni, MSN, PMGT-BC, ACNS-BC, NP, AP-PMN
Theresa J. Di Maggio, MSN, CRNP, PPCNP-BC
Maureen F. Cooney, DNP, FNP-BC, ACHPN, AP-PMN*

Introduction

This chapter provides an overview of medication therapies commonly used in multimodal pain management, with a focus on their pharmacological properties and monitoring parameters. It identifies pharmacological pain management therapy for medications with the U.S. Food and Drug Administration (FDA) approval for pain management and other FDA approved medications used off-label. Inclusion of medications used off-label is due to a multitude of practitioners prescribing the products for pain treatment. Schedule I controlled substances are not discussed in this chapter. *The following material is considered general foundational concepts. Content on the specific management of children and older adults are located at the end of the chapter. All dosing information should be considered as a general guide for adults and not a specific dosing prescription for any individual; clinical judgment is always required. Additionally, content presented in tables and boxes does not imply recommended order of use.*

I. Pharmacokinetics

A. Pharmacokinetics is the study of a medication's movement throughout the body—the interaction of a medication and the body in terms of absorption, distribution, metabolism, and excretion (ADME). Knowledge of pharmacokinetics is essential for nurses. Mastery of ADME facilitates appropriate assessment, administration, and intervention when delivering patient care.
1. Absorption: movement of a medication into systemic circulation. The rate and extent of absorption determines when a medication becomes available to exert its action, influencing duration and intensity of medication action.
2. Solubility: Water-soluble medications are absorbed more rapidly than lipid-soluble medications.
3. Concentration: High medication concentrations are absorbed more rapidly at site of administration compared to lower concentrations.
4. pH: pH affects solubility and compartmentalization of medications within the human body.

Gastrointestinal tract pH varies depending on location within intestinal tract.
5. Gastric emptying rate: rate at which stomach empties into duodenum. An increase or decrease of gastric emptying rate affects exposure time to both higher and lower pH environments.
6. Blood flow: Heat or massage at site of administration increases blood flow and rate of absorption. Vasoconstrictors and shock conditions decrease blood flow and rate of absorption.
7. Surface area: Rapid absorption occurs from the surface of the cell membrane, such as pulmonary alveolar epithelium, intestinal mucosa, or layers of the skin. The larger the surface area, the more absorption may occur.
8. Bioavailability: Percentage of active medication absorbed and available to tissues after administration. Absorption varies with different routes of administration.

B. Absorption
1. Gastric absorption primarily occurs in stomach and small intestine. Medications are impacted by decomposition via gastric secretion and dilution prior to reaching the intestine. Various dosage forms are impacted differently.
2. An increase in absorption rate can be facilitated by:
   a. Upright position
   b. Empty stomach
   c. Drinking water
3. Small intestine absorption:
   a. Highly vascular area
   b. Numerous villi
   c. Larger absorption area than stomach
   d. Increased intestinal motility decreases absorption.
4. Medication bioavailability is affected by extent of first-pass metabolism and physical characteristics of medication.
   a. Solid form: Tablets need to disintegrate before being absorbed into the small intestine. Enteric-coated tablets and controlled- or sustained-release tablets delay medication dissolution and are

*Section Editor for the chapter.

241

absorbed more slowly. Capsule and powder forms are absorbed more quickly.

    b. Liquid form: Liquids are absorbed more rapidly than solid form.

5. Capacity to absorb medications:

    a. Emesis reduces bioavailability.

    b. Surgeries, such as gastric bypass, can cause a reduction in absorption and bioavailability of extended release (ER) preparations due to decreased surface area absorption and pH changes.

C. Potential routes: (alphabetical order)

1. Cutaneous: Absorption includes topical application to mucous membranes (e.g., conjunctiva, nasopharynx, oropharynx, vagina, colon, urethra, and urinary bladder) for localized effects.

2. Enteral:

    a. Used in individuals unable to consume orally but having an intact gastrointestinal (GI) tract (e.g., nasally or surgically placed gastrostomy or jejunal tube)

    b. Location of tube determines differences in absorption and onset of action.

    c. Standardization of medication administration procedure can minimize potential complications.

3. Epidural: refers to medication injected in space outside the dura mater

    a. Diffusion through dura mater must take place for this route to be effective.

    b. There is some vascular uptake with initial administration.

4. Intra-arterial: Medication injected directly into an artery and dependent on blood flow; metabolism is circumvented.

5. Intramuscular (IM):

    a. IM route is not recommended for pain management because it is painful.

      1) Absorption is variable, unpredictable, and delivers a large bolus in an intermittent and infrequent schedule, creating peaks and troughs in blood levels. Absorption rate depends on blood flow.

      2) Absorption is generally more rapid with administration in deltoid or vastus lateralis muscles.

      3) Absorption in gluteus maximus is slower in obese or emaciated patients, and especially in women because of increased subcutaneous (SC) fat.

      4) Absorption can also be affected by repeated injections causing scar tissue or lipodystrophy.

    b. First-pass metabolism is circumvented.

6. Intraperitoneal: Medications are injected into peritoneal cavity. Absorption occurs through large surface area of abdomen, from which medication then enters into portal vein circulation. First-pass metabolism can occur.

7. Intrathecal: refers to medication injected directly into spinal subarachnoid space, bypassing blood-brain barrier (BBB)

    a. Large dose reductions are required compared to other delivery routes. Some medications must be reduced by a factor of more than 100.

    b. No literature to support using standard equal analgesic conversion table when determining initial dosing. Use caution with dosing due to risks of severe adverse events, including mortality.

8. Oral:

    a. Preferred method of delivery

    b. Onset of action significantly slower than parenteral

    c. First-pass effect/metabolism (hepatic):

      1) Oral medications pass through portal vein into liver before entering general circulation.

      2) Only a small fraction of medication is available for distribution to produce effect.

9. Parenteral: (intravenous [IV])

    a. Dependent on blood flow

    b. Administered directly into systemic circulation

    c. Administration should be slow to prevent adverse effects.

    d. Circumvents first-pass metabolism

    e. Quick onset

10. Pulmonary: Inhalation/intranasal absorption uses large surface area of pulmonary epithelium and mucous membranes.

    a. Entry into systemic circulation is virtually instantaneous.

    b. First-pass metabolism is circumvented.

    c. Rapid absorption related to high vascularity and permeability of nasal tissues

    d. Nebulized opioids are commonly used to treat dyspnea in palliative care.

    e. Metered-dose spray, atomizer, or nasal dropper can be used for intranasal route.

11. Rectal:

    a. Absorption delivers medication into superior, middle, and inferior rectal vein.

      1) Medications absorbed into middle and inferior rectal veins directly reach systemic circulation without first-pass effect, resulting in higher absorption.

      2) Superior rectal vein drains into portal system and exposes medication to first-pass metabolism.

    b. Dissolution of medications occurs slowly with irregular, unpredictable, and incomplete absorption.

      1) High degree of variability in medication absorption between different individuals.

2) Extent of absorption depends on rectal content, localized irritation, and medication retention.

c. Use of rectal route is generally considered safe in oncology patients unless patient is thrombocytopenic, neutropenic, or immunosuppressed secondary to risk of perirectal abscess.

d. Rectal administration is contraindicated for patients with rectal lesions, lower gastrointestinal bleeding, diarrhea, fissures, inflammation, or previous colorectal surgery.

12. Subcutaneous:
   a. Medication administered beneath skin into connective tissue or fat under dermis
   b. Medication solubility and vasoconstriction of blood vessels cause delays in absorption. Absorption is generally slow.
   c. With continuous medication administration, rate of delivery into systemic circulation is comparable to IV infusion.
   d. First-pass metabolism is circumvented.
   e. General consensus recommends a maximum volume for bolus SC infusion to be 1.5 to 3 mL to avoid pain at site or issues with absorption.

13. Sublingual and Buccal:
   a. Absorption from oral mucosa of mouth delivers medication directly into venous blood flow going to superior vena cava with minimal first-pass effect, resulting in higher absorption.
   b. Sublingual: under tongue; most permeable region in oral cavity.
   c. Buccal: between teeth and mucous membrane of cheek. When applied properly, there is minimal systemic absorption.

14. Topical (skin):
   a. Absorption produces localized effect with minimal systemic effect.
   b. Can be obtained from medications (normally lipid soluble) formulated in ointments or transdermal patches
   c. Creams and ointments are semisolid forms intended for topical use only. The difference between ointments and creams is percentage of base used.
      1) *Creams* have >20% water and normally <50% hydrocarbons and polyols as vehicle for medication substance.
      2) *Ointments* have <20% water and >50% polyols, giving them an oil-based semisolid consistency.
      3) If a large surface area coverage is needed, a cream preparation should be used. Ointments are more suitable for smaller skin surface areas.
   d. Gel preparations are clear, transparent, and semisolid and contain solubilized active substance. Gel preparations have fastest onset of action, followed in order by creams and then ointments.
   e. Skin must be intact to prevent an increase in systemic absorption of potentially toxic chemicals. Massaging skin enhances absorption.
   f. Transdermal (passive) cutaneous permeation of medications is primarily mediated by diffusion. Diffusion into systemic circulation varies depending on thickness of lipophilic, keratinous stratum corneum, allowing formation of depot in subcutaneous fat tissue.
   g. Transdermal (iontophoresis) iontophoretic delivery requires creation of an external electrical current from positive and negative terminals. Through this mechanism, positively charged, ionizable medication is actively transported into systemic circulation in a non-saturable manner. No need for formation of subcutaneous fat depot.

15. Compounded medications:
   a. Formulation involving one or more medication products not commercially available (e.g., ketamine, amitriptyline, clonidine, gabapentin, baclofen, and opioids). Compounding pharmacies produce analgesics in vehicles that can be applied topically to target various pain sites specific to individuals.
   b. Compounded medications are not FDA-approved (FDA does not verify safety or effectiveness of compounded medications).
   c. Compounding pharmacies are registered, licensed, and have oversight from state licensing boards.

D. Distribution
   1. Transport of medication in body fluids from bloodstream to various bodily tissues and sites of action. Volume of distribution defines medication concentration in the body.
   2. Factors affecting medication distribution:
      a. Cardiac output alterations affect volume of fluid distribution.
      b. Regional permeability of capillaries in muscle, skin, and organs varies. First distribution is to organs with largest circulatory supply and then redistributes to areas with less blood flow.
      c. Medication accumulation occurs in tissues, especially with lipid-soluble medications.
      d. Protein binding occurs, especially albumin and alpha-1-acid glycoprotein for basic medications.
      e. Distribution varies with age, gender, and disease state.

Part 4

f.   Obesity increases volume of distribution if medication is distributed in both lean and fat tissues.

g.   BBB allows for distribution of lipid-soluble medications into brain and cerebrospinal fluid.

3.   Barriers to distribution:

a.   Lipid-insoluble medications require other mechanisms to pass through BBB.

b.   Placental barrier has membranous layers separating the blood vessels of mother and fetus.

1)   Barrier is nonselective.

2)   Allows passage of lipid-soluble and lipid-insoluble medications, providing fetus with little protection.

3)   Steroid, opioid, and anesthetic agents easily cross placental barrier.

4.   Body fluid distribution:

a.   Cerebrospinal fluid distribution is restricted by BBB.

1)   Blood flow in central nervous system (CNS) is permeable to nonpolar, lipid-soluble medications.

2)   Strongly ionized medications normally are not permitted to enter CNS from systemic circulation.

b.   Plasma protein binding results in decreased medication availability for tissue distribution (e.g., only unbound medication can cross tissue membranes).

1)   Competitive binding for plasma protein sites can displace other protein-bound medications.

a)   Displaced protein-bound medications continue to circulate in bloodstream.

(1)   Remaining inactive

(2)   Creating a medication reservoir or storage depot

(3)   Toxicity may result

b)   Caution needs to be taken with combining medications. For example: When warfarin is at a stable dose and phenytoin is added to medication regimen, it displaces warfarin. Competing for binding sites takes place, releasing more free medication of warfarin and increasing risk of toxicity (hemorrhage).

2)   Binding site availability.

a)   Available protein levels: When there is a low albumin level in blood, there is less albumin to bind with and more free medication available to travel to point of action. Toxicity could result if normal dosage is given.

3)   Adipose tissue binding is more likely to occur with lipid-soluble medications, as adipose tissue has low blood flow and is a stable reservoir.

E.   Metabolism

1.   Chemical reaction involved in biotransformation to a more water-soluble compound(s) or metabolite(s), which is ionized at a physiological pH (i.e., 7.0 to 7.4)

2.   Occurs in plasma, kidneys, small intestine, brain, and liver. Liver is primary organ for medication metabolism:

a.   Liver has dual blood supply: 25% from hepatic artery, 75% from portal vein.

b.   Hepatic blood flow affected by:

1)   Severe cardiovascular dysfunction

2)   Starvation

3)   Renal insufficiency

4)   Genetic polymorphism

5)   Chronic liver disease

6)   Age

c.   Gaps (i.e., fenestrae) between endothelial cell lining of hepatic sinusoids allow plasma to make contact with microvilli of hepatocytes. Cytochrome P450 (CYP450) enzymes are located in smooth endoplasmic reticulum cell structure inside hepatocyte. These enzymes create chemical alterations of medication.

3.   Process

a.   Phase I: CYP450 monooxygenase system:

1)   First-pass hepatic effect:

a)   Oral medications pass through portal vein into liver, entering general circulation.

b)   When certain medications are metabolized by hepatic microsomal enzyme system, only a small fraction of medication is available for distribution to produce effect.

c)   First-pass hepatic effect can result in complete elimination of medication, resulting in no pharmacological effect.

2)   CYP450 oxidation:

a)   Phase I metabolism consists of three types of chemical reactions:

(1)   Oxidation: About 90% of medication oxidation involves the following enzymes: CYP1A2, CYP3A4, CYP2C9, CYP2C19, CYP2D6, and CYP2E1.

(2)   Reduction

(3)   Hydrolysis

b)   CYP3A4 and CYP2D6 isoenzymes

(1)   Most prevalent CYP isoenzymes

(2)   Exist predominantly in liver but also in extrahepatic tissues, including brain, lungs, intestine, and kidneys

c)   Substrate: any medication metabolized by these enzymes (Table 17.1)

Table 17.1

Select Examples of Cytochrome P450 (CYP 450) Substrates, Inhibitors, and Inducers

Substrate Definition: Medication that is metabolized by the CYP450 enzyme		Inhibitor Definition: Medication that prevents the binding of the substrate to the CYP450 enzyme		Inducer Definition: Medication that increases the CYP450 enzyme metabolism of the substrate	
Isozyme: CYP1A2					
Acetaminophen	Imipramine	Amiodarone	Grapefruit juice	Insulin	Smoking
Amitriptyline	Naproxen	Cimetidine	Isoniazid	Omeprazole	Cruciferous
Caffeine	Ondansetron	Ciprofloxacin	Ketoconazole	Phenobarbital	vegetables
Cyclobenzaprine	Propranolol	Clarithromycin	Levofloxacin	Phenytoin	Char-grilled meats
Desipramine	Ropivacaine	Erythromycin	Norfloxacin	Rifampin	
Diazepam	Verapamil	Fluvoxamine	Paroxetine	Ritonavir	
Haloperidol	R-warfarin				
Isozyme: CYP3A4					
Alfentanil	Dronabinol	Cannabinoids	Indinavir	Carbamazepine	—
Alprazolam	Fentanyl	Ciprofloxacin	Itraconazole	Dexamethasone	
Amitriptyline	Imipramine	Clarithromycin	Ketoconazole	Ethosuximide	
Bupivacaine	Lidocaine	Erythromycin	Propofol	Phenobarbital	
Cannabinoids	Midazolam	Fluconazole	Ritonavir	Phenytoin	
Carbamazepine	Prednisone	Fluoxetine	Verapamil	Primidone	
Cocaine	Ropivacaine	Fluvoxamine	Oliceridine	Rifampin	
Codeine	Sertraline	Grapefruit juice		St. John's wort	
Cyclobenzaprine	Temazepam				
Dexamethasone	Trazodone				
Dextromethorphan	Triazolam				
Diazepam					
CYP2C9					
Amitriptyline	Ibuprofen	Amiodarone	Ketoconazole	Phenobarbital	—
Diclofenac	Imipramine	Fluconazole	Paroxetine	Rifampin	
Fluoxetine	Phenytoin	Fluvoxamine	Ritonavir		
Glipizide	S-warfarin	Itraconazole	Sertraline		
		Isoniazid	Trimethoprim		
CYP2C19					
Citalopram	Pantoprazole	Cimetidine	Omeprazole	Phenobarbital	—
Diazepam	Phenytoin	Fluoxetine	Paroxetine	Rifampin	
Indomethacin	Propranolol	Fluvoxamine	Ritonavir		
Omeprazole	Topiramate	Ketoconazole	Sertraline		
CYP2D6					
Amitriptyline	Meperidine	Amiodarone	Fluoxetine	Dexamethasone	—
Amphetamine	Metoclopramide	Celecoxib	Methadone	Carbamazepine	
Codeine	Mexiletine	Cimetidine	Oliceridine	Phenobarbital	
Cyclobenzaprine	Morphine	Citalopram	Paroxetine	Phenytoin	
Desipramine	Nortriptyline	Cocaine	Ritonavir	Rifampin	
Dextromethorphan	Ondansetron	Desipramine	Sertraline	Tramadol	
Doxepin	Oxycodone				
Fluoxetine	Paroxetine				
Haloperidol	Tramadol				
Hydrocodone	Trazodone				
Imipramine	Venlafaxine				
CYP2E1					
Acetaminophen	Methoxyflurane	Disulfiram		Acetone	Isoniazid
Alcohol	Ropivacaine			Alcohol	Obesity
Halothane	Sevoflurane			Fasting	
Isoflurane	Theophylline				

Note: Table information is a guideline only and is not inclusive of all medications or brand names in class. Information listed in the tables is attributed to published literature and manufacturer's package insert. Some dose adjustments are based on clinical practice experience. Caution is needed for those with severe hepatic/renal dysfunction due to limited studies. UpToDate information can be found in common tertiary references. Tables refer to adult dosing and routes of administration only.

Note: The listing of medications in the following tables and boxes relates to adult dosing and does not imply recommended order of use.

d) Enzyme inhibition: Most common type of inhibition reaction is reversible at CYP450 active site.
  (1) Competitive inhibition occurs when inhibitor prevents binding of substrate to active site on the enzyme. This type of inhibition can be reversed by giving more substrate.
  (2) Noncompetitive inhibition occurs when inhibitor binds to another site on enzyme to form an inactive complex. This type of inhibition cannot be overcome by adding more substrate.
e) Enzyme induction: This adaptive response protects cells by increasing detoxification activity of liver enzymes, thereby decreasing length of medication effect.
  (1) CYP2E1 is alcohol-inducible enzyme with significant role in metabolism of acetaminophen.
  (2) CYP2E1 catalyzes oxidation of acetaminophen to produce hepatotoxic metabolite N-acetyl-p-benzoquinone imine. Long-term ethanol use induces CYP2E1 production and increases production of acetaminophen toxic metabolite.
f) Genetic polymorphism: Distribution within a population for inheriting liver enzymatic activity is controlled at a single genetic locus.
  (1) Medications metabolized by CYP2D6 have lower interaction potential than those metabolized by CYP3A4.
  (2) Genetic variation of CYP2D6 can lead to significant variability in metabolism of opioid medications, such as hydrocodone, codeine, and to a lesser extent, oxycodone.
  (3) CYP2D6 rapid metabolizers can experience reduced efficacy with medications, such as hydrocodone, or can experience increased risk of toxicity with codeine (a prodrug).
  (4) Prevalence of CYP2D6 allelic variants is 5% to 10% in Caucasians (non-Hispanic). An estimated 1% to 7% Caucasian (non-Hispanic) are rapid metabolizers.
  (5) Among persons of Asian descent, <1% are poor metabolizers, and there are no reports of rapid metabolizers in this population.
  (6) Poor metabolism is highly variable in persons of African descent, ranging from 0% to 34%, and rapid metabolizers are also highly variable from 9% to 30%.
b. Phase II
  1) Conjugation reactions are biosynthetic.
  2) Metabolic process combines medications, or phase I metabolites, to small endogenous substances. Medications and metabolites combine with glucuronic acid, sulfate, glycine, or glutathione; this allows medications and metabolites to be detoxified.
  3) Glucuronosyltransferases:
    a) Uridine diphosphate-glucuronosyltransferases (UGTs) are enzymes that produce glucuronidation reactions. With morphine administration, morphine undergoes CYP450 enzyme metabolism, which produces three metabolites, two of which undergo phase II conjugation with glucuronic acid to form morphine-3-glucuronide (M3G) and morphine-6-glucuronide (M6G).
    b) The glucuronidation of morphine, buprenorphine, and nalorphine involves UGT1A1. UGT1A3/1A4 is involved in glucuronidation of lamotrigine and tricyclic antidepressants (TCAs), including amitriptyline, doxepin, imipramine, desipramine, and nortriptyline. UGT2B7 is involved in glucuronidation of benzodiazepines.
F. Excretion
  1. Process whereby medications and active and inactive metabolites are eliminated primarily through kidneys. Excretion may also occur through liver, bile, feces, lungs, sweat, and salivary and mammary glands.
  2. Clearance: volume of blood completely cleared of medication in a unit of time
  3. Elimination half-life ($t_{1/2}$): Measure of time for half the medication to be cleared by kidneys. Half-life depends on volume of distribution and clearance of medication.
  4. Types of excretion
    a. Renal excretion
      1) Affected by adequate blood supply to kidneys, maturity of kidneys, presence or absence of kidney disease, and urinary pH. Some medications (e.g., nonsteroidal anti-inflammatory drugs [NSAIDs]) decrease renal blood flow and glomerular filtration rate (GFR).
      2) Occurs through passive glomerular filtration, active tubular secretion, and partial reabsorption.

a) Free medications and water-soluble metabolites are filtered by glomeruli.
b) Protein-bound medications do not pass through glomerular filtration system.
c) After filtration, lipid-soluble medications are not excreted but reabsorbed by tubular nephron and reenter systemic circulation.
d) Non-ionized, water-soluble medications bypass the glomerular filtration system and go through hepatic metabolism before returning to kidneys for excretion.

b. Hemodialysis
1) Substances normally excreted by kidney, either completely or partially, can be dialyzed out.
2) If medication is dialyzable, supplemental dosing will be needed after completion of dialysis run (cycle) to keep medication level therapeutic (Table 17.2).
c. Mammary glands
1) Weak acids, such as barbiturates, are less concentrated in breast milk.
2) There may be a cumulative effect in infant because of infant's immature metabolism.

Table 17.2

Opioid Use During Renal Failure and Dialysis

Opioid	Comments About Use During Renal Failure	Comments About Use During Dialysis
Morphine	Avoid use. Metabolites can accumulate, and adverse effects can be prolonged.	Choose another opioid if possible. Parent drug and metabolites are removed by dialysis, but "rebound" accumulation can occur between dialysis sessions as drug and metabolites re-equilibrate between CNS and plasma.
Codeine	Do not use. Metabolites can accumulate and cause serious adverse effects.	Do not use. Parent drug and metabolites can accumulate and cause serious adverse effects.
FentaNYL[a,b]	Use cautiously. Appears safe, particularly for short-term use. Metabolites are inactive, but accumulation of parent drug may occur. Cautious use and careful monitoring of adverse effects are advised with long-term use and continuous intravenous or intraspinal infusion.	Not removed by dialysis. Appears safe, particularly for short-term use. Metabolites are inactive, and no adverse effects have been reported during dialysis. In most cases, no dose adjustments are necessary, but use caution during and after titration. FentaNYL may absorb onto one type of filter, in which case changing the filter is recommended.
HYDROcodone	Use cautiously, monitor adverse effects closely, and adjust dose as needed. Metabolite can accumulate, causing neuroexcitation.	Parent drug can be removed, but metabolite can accumulate and may pose risk.
HYDROmorphone	Use cautiously, carefully monitor for adverse effects, and adjust dose as needed. Metabolite can accumulate, causing neuroexcitation, but the drug has been used safely in patients with renal failure. May be an option in patients with ESRD who are unable to tolerate other opioids.	Parent drug can be removed, but metabolite can accumulate and may pose a risk. Use cautiously and monitor patient closely during dialysis.
Meperidine	Do not use. Metabolite accumulation increases adverse effects.	Do not use. No data on drug or metabolites during dialysis, but risk of adverse effects is plausible.
Methadone[a]	Use with caution, as methadone is associated with increased risks in all patient populations. No clear increased risk in ESRD, as it is eliminated primarily by hepatic metabolism, but more research regarding its excretion is needed. Parent drug and metabolites are excreted into the gut, and renal excretion varies widely.	Metabolites are inactive, but use with caution because parent drug is not removed by dialysis.
OxyCODONE	Further research is needed to make conclusive recommendations. Parent drug and metabolite (oxyMORphone) can accumulate. If used, administer with great caution and carefully monitor adverse effects.	Monitor closely for adverse effects, as there is insufficient research to provide conclusive evidence of safety. In a small study (n = 20), a limited amount of oxycodone and noroxycodone were dialyzed (Samolsky Dekel et al., 2017).

CNS, central nervous system; *ESRD,* end-stage renal disease.
[a]Not dialyzed; considered "safe," but cautious titration and close monitoring for a protracted period are recommended in patients with renal failure or undergoing dialysis (Dean, 2004).
[b]The other fentaNYLs (i.e., remifentanil, SUFentanil, and alfentanil) have been designated as safe for use in patients with renal impairment (Wellington & Chia, 2009), but further research and clinical experience with their use in these patients is warranted.

From Pasero, C., & McCaffery, M. (2011). *Pain assessment and pharmacologic management* (p. 364). St. Louis, MO: Mosby. Data from Dean, M. (2004). Opioids in renal failure and dialysis patients. *Journal of Pain Symptom Management,* 28(5), 497–504; Johnson, S. J. (2007). Opioid safety in patients with renal or hepatic dysfunction. *Pain Treatment Topics.* Retrieved February 2 2009 from http://www.pain-topics.org; Kurella, M., Bennett, W. M., & Chertow, G. M. (2003). Analgesia in patients with ESRD: A review of available evidence. *American Journal of Kidney Disease,* 42(2), 217–225; Wellington, J., & Chia Y. Y. (2009). Patient variables influencing acute pain management. In R. S. Sinatra, O.A. de Leon-Casasola, B. Ginsberg, E. R. Viscusi (Eds.), *Acute Pain Management,* Cambridge, New York Cambridge University Press. © 2011, Pasero, C., & McCaffery, M. May be duplicated for use in clinical practice.

5. Therapeutic medication monitoring:
   a. Medication levels
      1) C_{max}: Peak medication level (i.e., maximum concentration)
      2) C_{min}: Trough medication level (i.e., minimal concentration)
      3) T_{max}: Time to achieve maximum concentration
      4) T_{min}: Time to achieve minimum concentration
      5) Steady state: Achieved when plasma medication level remains constant and does not peak or trough significantly
      6) Concentration at steady state (Css) depends on medication elimination and frequency of administration. It takes approximately four medication half-lives to reach a 95% steady-state plasma concentration.
   b. Laboratory monitoring is important to help determine appropriate pharmacotherapy selection, dose modification, and monitoring of medication safety profile.
      1) Renal monitoring:
         a) Serum creatinine (SCr) is a measurement of waste product from muscle metabolism. Normally, SCr is produced at a consistent rate. Because it is filtered and excreted by kidneys, SCr has become a standard way to measure kidney function at a given point in time.
         b) Creatinine clearance (CrCl) is commonly used to measure the estimated GFR and adjust medication doses. For adults within a hospital or outpatient clinic, equations such as Cockcroft-Gault, or Modification of Diet in Renal Disease (MDRD), are used to estimate CrCl. These equations take into account patient characteristics, such as age, sex, and body size.
      2) Hepatic monitoring:
         a) Aspartate aminotransferase (AST) is an enzyme commonly used to monitor for hepatic damage. It may also indicate other medical conditions (e.g., certain cardiac issues or trauma).
         b) Alanine aminotransferase (ALT) is an enzyme often used as a marker for hepatic damage. Elevated levels are more often related to hepatic injury versus other organ damage in comparison to AST levels.
         c) Hepatic monitoring maybe helpful in determining appropriate acetaminophen administration.

      3) Hematologic monitoring: Platelet counts can help determine risk of bleeding. Some medications (e.g., NSAIDS) or medication delivery routes may increase risk of bleeding.
      4) Cardiac monitoring:
         a) Rate-corrected QT interval (QTc) is measured with electrocardiography. Prolongation and development of torsades de pointes have been associated with methadone and has resulted in an FDA black box warning.
         b) Health history, concurrent medications, and continued monitoring of QTc are necessary to reduce adverse effects, including death.

II. Pharmacodynamics

A. Pharmacodynamics
   1. Effect of a medication at its site of action, including drug/receptor interactions, dose/response relationship, medication interactions, and physiological variation (e.g., age, sex, and genetics)
   2. Involves response or effect of tissues to specific chemical agents at various sites in body. Effects of medication on body may be in form of increasing, decreasing, or replacing enzymes, hormones, or body metabolic functions.
B. Medication/receptor interaction
   1. Receptor: A reactive cellular site that binds with medication to produce effect. This lock-and-key effect creates a complementary relationship between a certain portion of the medication molecule and the cell receptor site. Example: Methadone-specific receptor awaits dose of methadone for binding to occur.
   2. Affinity: ability of medication to bind at receptor site
   3. Efficacy: ability of medication to initiate biological activity in medication/receptor interaction
   4. Agonist: produces the effect
   5. Antagonist: reverses, or produces no effect, by competing with (blocking) agonist at the receptor
      a. Competitive antagonism: Involves an agent with same affinity for the receptor as the agonist. This competition reduces effect of agonist at receptor site.
      b. Example: A patient received epidural morphine and develops pruritus. A lower dose of antagonist (e.g., naloxone 0.05 mg IV) reverses the pruritus, whereas a higher dose of antagonist (e.g., naloxone 0.4 mg IV) reverses side effect *and* analgesic effect of morphine.

C. Nonreceptor interactions
   1. Some medications require no receptor site affinity to create action. These enter a cell or accumulate along a membrane, where they influence chemical or physical function along the cell membrane.
   2. Example: Amide local anesthetics inhibit Na ion channels, stabilizing neuronal cell membranes and inhibiting nerve impulse initiation and conduction.
D. Medication/enzyme interaction
   1. Medication can produce its effect by interacting with a cellular enzyme.
   2. Enzyme produces a catalyst, and medications can inhibit action of specific enzyme, producing an altered response.
   3. Example: Steroidal medications are manufactured by enzyme action on plant steroids.
E. Nonspecific medication interaction
   1. Cell membranes are lipoproteins that regulate flow of ions and metabolites and maintain electrochemical propensity between interior and exterior surfaces of cell.
   2. Example: General anesthetics are lipid soluble and therefore able to cross cell membranes.

III. Adverse medication reactions

A. Reactions can vary from minor to severe and include:
   1. Exaggerated medication response (e.g., prolonged morning sedation following nighttime diphenhydramine)
   2. Unwanted effect on an organ system different from that being treated (e.g., impact of NSAIDs on platelet function)
   3. Allergic or hypersensitivity reaction: Anaphylactic reactions involve an immune response created by antigen binding to immunoglobulin E antibodies. Symptoms may include hives, swelling, or anaphylaxis.
   4. Idiosyncratic reaction: Medication interaction causing either increased or decreased response (e.g., torsades de pointes [QTc prolongation] results from inhibition

of haloperidol metabolism by CYP2D6 when methadone is started) (Box 17.1).
   5. Side effect: a dose-related, expected reaction based on pharmacological activity of agent frequently observed in the general population (e.g., constipation or pruritis from opioids)
   6. Overdose or toxic effects result from excessive medication levels (e.g., high opioid dose results in respiratory depression).
   7. Pseudoallergic (nonimmunologic) reaction. Example: Administration of morphine by IV or oral routes can cause nonimmunologic degranulation of mast cells to release histamine in a dose-dependent fashion. Patients who are sensitive to changes in histamine levels may experience an itching or burning sensation, most commonly on face, chest, and trunk.
B. Variables affecting adverse medication reactions:
   1. Patient variables:
      a. Age (when considering medication implications, age ranges are often referred to as neonate, pediatric, adult and elderly)
      b. Genetic factors (e.g., CYP450 enzyme deficiencies)
      c. Comorbidities
   2. Medication variables:
      a. Route of administration
      b. Product formulation
      c. Duration of therapy
   3. Medication-induced diseases. Example: NSAIDs causing aplastic anemia
C. Medication interaction: Change in magnitude or duration of a response to one medication in the presence of another medication. This change results in increase or decrease in concentration of medication at site of action.
   1. Addictive effect: Two medications with similar pharmacological action are taken and produce a summed effect. Example: aspirin and ibuprofen effect on platelets
   2. Synergistic effect: Two medications with a combined effect greater than the sum of each medication acting alone produce an increased effect.

Box 17.1

Examples of High-Risk Medications for QTc Prolongation

Amiodarone	Chlorpromazine	Clarithromycin	Disopyramide
Droperidol	Erythromycin	Haloperidol	Loperamide
Methadone	Oliceridine	Pentamidine	Pimozide
Procainamide	Quetiapine	Quinidine	Sotalol
Thioridazine	—	—	—

Example: intravenous opioids combined with oral NSAIDs, COX-2 inhibitors, or acetaminophen versus intravenous opioids alone

3. Potentiation: One medication increases effect of a second medication. Example: Diazepam may potentiate the effect of alcohol.

IV. Multimodal analgesia

A. Multimodal analgesia: rational combination of optimal doses of individual analgesics with differing mechanisms of actions
1. Incorporates pharmacological, nonpharmacological, and integrative and complementary interventions
2. Multimodal regimens must be individualized to the patient, keeping in mind patient's preexisting medical conditions, reason for each medication's use, and possible side effects of each medication.
3. Theoretically, different analgesics with different mechanisms of action
B. Rationale for using multimodal analgesic techniques:
1. May have synergistic effects when used in combination
2. May prevent or treat acute pain and postoperative pain; further studies are needed to correlate use of multimodal analgesia in reducing persistent pain syndromes.
3. More effective than using single medications in high doses
4. Reduces complications and side effects experienced when using higher doses of a single analgesic (e.g., reduced opioid-related adverse effects)
5. Nonopioid medications are increasingly being used as co-analgesia before, during, and after surgery.
C. Possible components of multimodal analgesia
1. Acetaminophen
2. NSAIDs
3. Opioid analgesic medications
4. Alpha-2-delta ligands (e.g., gabapentin and pregabalin)
5. Ketamine
6. Alpha-2 adrenergic receptor agonists (e.g., clonidine, tizanidine, dexmedotomidine)
7. Local anesthetics via neuraxial analgesia, peripheral nerve blocks, systemic infusion, topical administration, subcutaneous or intra-articular infiltration

V. Preemptive Aanalgesia

A. Preemptive analgesia: Interventions are given prior to nociception (typically preoperatively) because analgesic intervention started before nociception is more effective than same intervention after nociception. Preemptive analgesia has had conflicting evidence.
B. Preventive analgesia: All-encompassing term including all multimodal perioperative efforts to decrease postoperative pain. Preventive analgesia in perioperative period reduces postoperative pain scores, reduces analgesic consumption, and may prevent central sensitization and persistent pain syndromes.
C. Recommended components of preoperative interventions to improve postoperative pain control include:
1. Preoperative education and evaluation:
a. Develop comprehensive, individualized pain management plan and educate patient (and family).
b. Establish realistic goals.
c. Patients on opioid therapy prior to surgery should have their prescribed opioids continued unless there is a plan to taper or stop them safely.
2. Preemptive oral and IV medications (off-label use)
a. Acetaminophen
b. Celecoxib
c. Gabapentinoids
d. Ketamine
e. Lidocaine
f. Opioids: Preemptive opioids have conflicting evidence and are *not* recommended as an intervention to decrease postoperative pain.
3. Local, regional, and neuraxial therapies
a. SC infiltrations, intra-articular infiltrations, and regional anesthetic techniques may be used for specific procedures if studies have demonstrated benefit.
b. Neuraxial analgesics, including epidurals or intrathecal therapies, are often considered for major thoracic and abdominal procedures.

VI. Pharmacology/pharmaceutics

Note: Medication doses listed in this section are those recommended for use in adults. Pediatric doses are described in a later section.
A. Alpha-2 agonists:
1. Alpha-2 agonists (Table 17.2) are used for treatment in neuropathic pain, spasticity, opioid withdrawal, and opioid-induced hyperalgesia.
2. Multiple activities occur via G protein linked–mechanisms, including inhibition of cyclic adenosine monophosphate formation and the opening of potassium ion (K^+) channels.
3. Work at peripheral, spinal, and brainstem sites
4. Mechanisms of analgesia are unknown.
5. Shown to potentiate action of opioids and local anesthetics

B. Anticonvulsants
   1. Sodium ion (Na⁺) channel–blocking anticonvulsants (Table 17.3)
      a. Inhibit sustained high-frequency neuronal firing by blocking voltage-dependent Na⁺ channels after an action potential
      b. Reduce excitability in sensitized C-nociceptors
   2. Other anticonvulsants have multiple mechanisms of action (Table 17.4)

      a. Blocking Na⁺ channels
      b. Increasing synthesis and activity of gamma-aminobutyric acid A (GABAA), which is an inhibitory neurotransmitter in brain
   3. Anticonvulsants binding to alpha-2-delta subunit of calcium channel (Table 17.5)
      a. Reduce neurotransmitter release
      b. Inhibit neuronal excitability

Table 17.3

Alpha-2 Agonists

Generic Name	Route(s)	Half-life	Known Active Metabolites (Half-life)	Renal Dose Adjustment Recommended	Hepatic Dose Adjustment Recommended
Clonidine	TP, OT, Neuraxial	12.7 to 13.7 hours, 12.5 to 16 hours (epidural)	No	Yes	No
Dexmedetomidine	IV	2 to 2.67 hours	No	Noᵃ	Yes
Tizanidine	OC, OT	2.5 hours	No	Yes	Yes

IV, intravenous; *OC*, oral capsule immediate release; *OT*, oral tablet immediate release; *TP*, transdermal patch.

ᵃUse caution, and individualize dosing based on other comorbidities.

Table 17.4

Commonly Used Anticonvulsants: Sodium Ion Channel Blocking

Generic Name	Route(s)	Half-life	Known Active Metabolites (Half-life)	Renal Dose Adjustment Recommended	Hepatic Dose Adjustment Recommended
Carbamazepine	OC, OS, OT, OER, OCT	25 to 65 hours initially, then 12 to 17 hours after 3 to 5 weeks due to auto-induction	Carbamazepine-10,11-epoxide (6.1 hours)	No	Yes
Lamotrigine	OCT, OER, OT, ODT	25.4 to 70.3 hours	No	Yes	Yes
Oxcarbazepine	OS, OT OER	2 hours, 7 to 11 hours for OER	10-monohydroxy metabolite (9 to 11 hours)	Yes	Yes
Phenytoin	OS, OT, OCT, IV, OER	7 to 42 hours	No	Noᵃ	Yes

IV, intravenous; *OC*, oral capsule immediate release; *OCT*, oral chewable tablet; *ODT*, oral dissolvable tablet; *OER*, oral tablet/capsule extended release; *OS*, oral liquid solution; *OT*, oral tablet immediate release.

ᵃUse caution, and individualize dosing based on other comorbidities.

Table 17.5

Anticonvulsants: Multiple Mechanisms of Action

Generic Name	Route(s)	Half-life	Known Active Metabolites (Half-life)	Renal Dose Adjustment Recommended	Hepatic Dose Adjustment Recommended
Topiramate	OC, OER, OT	21 hours (OT, OC), 31 to 56 hours (OER)	No	Yes	Noᵃ
Valproic acid, Divalproex sodium	OC, OS, OER, IV	9 to 16 hours	No	Noᵃ	Yes

IV, intravenous; *OC*, oral capsule immediate release; *OER*, oral tablet/capsule extended release; *OS*, oral liquid solution; *OT*, oral tablet immediate release.

ᵃUse caution, and individualize dosing based on other comorbidities.

Part 4

Part 4

c. Perioperative use of gabapentin and pregabalin can provide significant opioid-sparing analgesic efficacy and reduced opioid-related side effects.

  1) Gabapentin 600 mg to 1200 mg or pregabalin 150 mg to 300 mg administered orally 1 to 2 hours prior to surgery have been studied. These medications can also be continued postoperatively.

  2) Higher doses of gabapentin (>300 mg) used in a recent study were associated with respiratory depression.

  3) Systematic reviews and meta-analysis support use as an adjuvant analgesic.

  4) May be associated with side effects, particularly sedation and dizziness

  5) Pregabalin is a schedule V controlled substance.

  6) Gabapentin is not a federally controlled substance, but individual states may classify as schedule V in their prescription monitoring systems.

C. Antidepressants

  1. TCAs (Table 17.6) inhibit presynaptic neuronal reuptake of norepinephrine and serotonin (5-hydroxytryptamine [5-HT]) at the descending tract.

  2. Selective serotonin reuptake inhibitors (SSRIs) (Table 17.7) inhibit presynaptic neuronal reuptake of serotonin.

  3. Serotonin norepinepherine (also referred to as noradrenaline) reuptake inhibitors (SNRIs) (Table 17.8) inhibit reuptake of serotonin and norepinephrine.

  4. Atypical antidepressants (Table 17.9)

    a. Bupropion

      1) Second-generation non-TCA

      2) Inhibits reuptake of norepinephrine and dopamine

    b. Mirtazapine

      1) Tricyclic structural analogue with nonselective receptor activities

      2) Main mechanism involves antagonist activity at central presynaptic alpha-2 adrenergic

---

Table 17.6

Anticonvulsants: Alpha-2-Delta Subunit Calcium Channel Binding (FDA-Approved Pain Indications for Anticonvulsants)

Generic Name	Route(s)	Half-life	Known Active Metabolites (Half-life)	Renal Dose Adjustment Recommended	Hepatic Dose Adjustment Recommended
Gabapentin	OC, OT, OS, OER	5 to 7 hours	No	Yes	No[a]
Pregabalin	OC, OS	6.3 hours	No	Yes	No[a]

OC, oral capsule immediate release; *OER,* oral tablet/capsule extended release; *OS,* oral liquid solution; *OT,* oral tablet immediate release.

[a]Use caution, and individualize dosing based on other comorbidities.

Table 17.7

Tricyclic Antidepressants

Generic Name	Route(s)	Half-life	Known Active Metabolites (Half-life)	Renal Dose Adjustment Recommended	Hepatic Dose Adjustment Recommended
Amitriptyline	OT	9 to 25 hours	Nortriptyline (15 to 39 hours), 10-hydroxyamitriptyline, amitriptyline-*N*-oxide, 10-hydroxynortriptyline	No	Yes
Desipramine	OT	14.3 to 24.7 hours	2-Hydroxydesipramine (21.8 hours)	No[a]	No[a]
Doxepin	OC, OS, topical cream, OT	15.3 hours	*N*-desmethyldoxepin (31 hours)	No[a]	Yes
Imipramine	OT, OC	6 to 18 hours	Desipramine (12 to 36 hours), 2-hydroxyimipramine (6 to 18 hours), 2-hydroxydesipramine (12 to 36 hours)	No	No
Nortriptyline	OC, OS, OER	15 to 39 hours	10-hydroxynortriptyline	No	No[a]

OC, oral capsule immediate release; *OER,* oral tablet/capsule extended release; *OS,* oral liquid solution; *OT,* oral tablet immediate release.

[a]Use caution, and individualize dosing based on other comorbidities.

Table 17.8

Selective Serotonin Reuptake Inhibitors

Generic Name	Route(s)	Half-life	Known Active Metabolites (Half-life)	Renal Dose Adjustment Recommended	Hepatic Dose Adjustment Recommended
Citalopram	OT, OS	35 hours	Didesmethylcitalopram, citalopram-N-oxide	No[a]	Yes
Escitalopram	OS, OT	27 to 32 hours	S-desmethylcitalopram (59 hours), S-didesmethylcitalopram	No[a]	Yes
Fluoxetine	OC, OER, OS, OT	4 to 6 days	Norfluoxetine (9.3 days)	No[a]	Yes
Fluvoxamine	OT, OER	15.6 hours (OT), 16.3 hours (OER)	Fluvoxamine acid	Yes	Yes
Paroxetine	OT, OER, OS	15 to 21 hours	No	Yes	Yes
Sertraline	OS, OT, OER	27.2 hours	Desmethylsertraline (62 to 104 hours)	No	Yes

OC, oral capsule immediate release; OER, oral tablet/capsule extended release; OS, oral liquid solution; OT, oral tablet immediate release.

[a]Use caution, and individualize dosing based on other comorbidities.

Table 17.9

Serotonin Norepinephrine Reuptake Inhibitors

Generic Name	Route(s)	Half-life	Known Active Metabolites (Half-life)	Renal Dose Adjustment Recommended	Hepatic Dose Adjustment Recommended
Desven-lafaxine	OER	10 to 11.1 hours	No	Yes	Yes
Duloxetine	OER	8 to 17 hours	No	Yes	Yes
Milnacipran	OT / OER	6 to 8 hours	No	Yes	No
Venlafaxine	OT, OER	5 hours	O-desmethylvenlafaxine (11 hours)	Yes	Yes

OER, oral tablet/capsule extended release; OT, oral tablet immediate release.

receptors, which enhances activity of norepinephrine and serotonin (5-HT$_2$ and 5-HT$_3$).

   3) Is potent antagonist of histamine H$_1$-receptors

  c. Nefazodone

   1) Chemically related to trazodone

   2) Serotonin 5-HT$_2$ blockade

   3) Less alpha-1 blockade

  d. Trazodone

   1) Inhibits serotonin reuptake

   2) Blocks serotonin 5-HT$_2$

   3) An antagonist at alpha-1 adrenergic receptors

  e. For FDA-approved pain indications for antidepressants, see Table 17.10.

  f. Herbals: There are many herbal medications and supplements used to treat depression and pain. The focus for this chapter is on FDA-approved antidepressants; see Integrative

and Complementary Therapy chapter for more information on herbals.

D. Antihistamines:

  1. H$_1$ antihistamines: (first generation) (Table 17.11) bind to histamine, muscarinic, alpha-adrenergic, and serotonin receptors to reduce transmission of itch and pain from afferent C-type nerve fibers in periphery.

  a. Diphenhydramine and promethazine are commonly used for allergic rhinitis, treatment of opioid-induced itching, general pruritus, nausea, and vomiting.

  b. Hydroxyzine is commonly used for allergic rhinitis, anxiety, acute pain (off-label use), opioid-induced itching, general pruritus, nausea, and vomiting.

  c. Other first-generation antihistamines are primarily used for allergic rhinitis.

Table 17.10

Atypical Antidepressants

Generic Name	Route(s)	Half-life	Known Active Metabolites (Half-life)	Renal Dose Adjustment Recommended	Hepatic Dose Adjustment Recommended
Bupropion	OT, OER	14 to 21 hours	Hydroxybupropion, erythrohydrobupropion, and threohydrobupropion	Yes	Yes
Mirtazapine	OT, ODT	26 hours (males), 37 hours (females)	Desmethyl mirtazapine	Yes	Yes
Nefazodone	OT	2 to 4 hours	Hydroxynefazodone, desethyl hydroxyne-fazodone, and m-chlorophenylpiperazine	No[a]	Yes
Trazodone	OT, OER	7 hours (OT), 10 hours (OER)	m-chlorophenylpiperazine	No	No[a]

ODT, oral dissolvable tablet; *OER,* oral tablet/capsule extended release; *OT,* oral tablet immediate release.

[a]Use caution, and individualize dosing based on other comorbidities

Table 17.11

FDA-Approved Pain Indications for Anticonvulsants and Antidepressants

Medication	FDA-Approved Indications
Carbamazepine	Trigeminal neuralgia and glossopharyngeal neuralgia
Duloxetine	Diabetic peripheral neuropathic pain, fibro-myalgia, persistent musculoskeletal pain
Gabapentin	Postherpetic neuralgia
Milnacipran	Fibromyalgia
Pregabalin	Fibromyalgia, diabetic peripheral neuro-pathic pain, neuropathic pain associated with spinal cord injury-related, postherpetic neuralgia
Topiramate	Migraine prophylaxis (immediate release only)

FDA, U.S. Food and Drug Administration.

Hudson, OH: Wolters Kluwer, Inc. Updated periodically.

2. H_2 antihistamines (second generation) (Table 17.12) have a slower dissociation rate from histamine receptor, less CNS penetration, and minimal activity with non-histamine receptors.
E. Anxiolytics
  1. Benzodiazepines:
    a. Bind directly to GABAA receptor/chloride (Cl^-) ion channel complex to modulate binding of gamma-aminobutyric acid (GABA) (inhibitory neurotransmitter)
    b. Primary use is for anxiolytic (Table 17.13), anticonvulsant, and antispasmodic activity.
    c. Schedule IV controlled substance
    d. Highly synergistic with opioids
  2. Benzodiazepine receptor antagonist:
    a. Flumazenil is a benzodiazepine receptor antagonist used for complete or partial reversal of sedation induced by benzodiazepines.
    b. Does not have anxiolytic effects

    c. Should be administered intravenously over 15 seconds when used for reversal of moderate to deep sedation and general anesthesia
    d. Should be administered intravenously over 30 seconds when used for suspected benzodiazepine overdose
    e. Onset of action is 1 to 2 minutes, with 80% response within 3 minutes.
    f. Withdrawal symptoms may occur in patients using benzodiazepines for a prolonged period and in whom dependence or tolerance or both may have developed.
    g. May result in seizures related to benzodiazepine withdrawal. Seizure occurrence may be more likely to occur in patients on benzodiazepines long-term or following TCA overdose.
    h. Re-sedation may occur if a large single dose or cumulative dose of benzodiazepine has been administered along with neuromuscular-blocking agent and multiple anesthetic agents.
  3. Non-benzodiazepine anxiolytic: buspirone (Table 17.14)
    a. Presynaptic serotonin 5-HT1A agonist of azapirone chemical class that decreases neuronal firing and reduces synthesis and release of serotonin
    b. No interaction occurs with GABA receptors.
    c. Primarily used for anxiety disorders
    d. Does not cause as much sedation as benzodiazepines
F. Hypnotics
  1. Benzodiazepine hypnotics (Table 17.15)
    a. Pharmacologic effects by directly binding to GABAA receptor/Cl^- ion channel complex to modulate binding of GABA
    b. Schedule IV controlled substance

Table 17.12

First-Generation (H$_1$) Antihistamines

Generic Name	Route(s)	Half-life	Known Active Metabolites (Half-life)	Renal Dose Adjustment Recommended	Hepatic Dose Adjustment Recommended
Chlorpheniramine	OT, OER, OS	20 hours	—	No	Yes
Cyproheptadine	OS, OT	16 hours	—	No[a]	Yes
Diphenhydramine	OT, OC, OS, topical cream, IV, IM, ODT	4 to 8 hours	—	Yes	Yes
Hydroxyzine	IM, OS, OT, OC	3 to 20 hours	Cetirizine (25 hours)	No[a]	Yes

IM, intramuscular; *IV,* intravenous; *OC,* oral capsule immediate release; *ODT,* oral dissolvable tablet; *OER,* oral tablet/capsule extended release; *OS,* oral liquid solution; *OT,* oral tablet immediate release.

[a]Use caution, and individualize dosing based on other comorbidities.

Table 17.13

Second-Generation (H$_2$) Antihistamines

Generic Name	Route(s)	Half-life	Known Active Metabolites (Half-life)	Renal Dose Adjustment Recommended	Hepatic Dose Adjustment Recommended
Cetirizine	OS, OT OCT, ODT, OC	8.3 hours	No	Yes	Yes
Desloratadine	OT, ODT, OS	19–40 hours	3-OH-desloratadine	Yes	Yes
Fexofenadine	OT, OS	14.4 hours	No	Yes	No
Levocetirizine	OS, OT	7–9 hours	No	Yes	No
Loratadine	OS, OCT, OT, OC, ODT	8.4 hours	Descarboethoxyloratadine (17.5 hours)	Yes	Yes

OC, oral capsule immediate release; *OCT,* oral chewable tablet; *ODT,* oral dissolvable tablet; *OS,* oral liquid solution; *OT,* oral tablet immediate release.

Table 17.14

Anxiolytics: Benzodiazepines

Generic Name	Route(s)	Half-life	Known Active Metabolites (Half-life)	Renal Dose Adjustment Recommended	Hepatic Dose Adjustment Recommended
Alprazolam	OT, ODT, OER, OS	11.2 hours (OT), 12.5 hours (ODT), 10.7 to 15.8 hours (OER)	4-Hydroxy-alprazolam, alpha-hydroxy-alprazolam	No[a]	Yes
Chlordiazepoxide	OC, IV, IM	24 to 48 hours	Desmethylchlor-diazepoxide, demox-epam (14 to 95 hours)	Yes	Yes
Clonazepam	OT, ODT	30 to 40 hours	No	No[a]	No[a]
Clorazepate	OT	2.29 hours	Nordazepam (2 days)	No	Yes
Diazepam	IV, IM, OS, OT, Rectal	20 to 48 hours	*N*-desmethyl-diazepam (100 hours), nordaze-pam (194 hours)	No[a]	Yes
Lorazepam	OT, IV, OS, IM	12 to 14 hours	No	No[a] (IV form not recommended)	Yes
Midazolam	IV, OS, IM, intranasal (not approved)	1.8 to 6.4 hours	Alpha-hydroxy-midazolam (1 hour)	Yes	Yes
Oxazepam	OC	8.2 hours	No	No	No[a]
Benzodiazepine Receptor Antagonist					
Flumazenil	IV	41 to 79 minutes	No	No	Yes

IM, intramuscular; *IV,* intravenous; *OC,* oral capsule immediate release; *ODT,* oral dissolvable tablet; *OER,* oral tablet/capsule extended release; *OS,* oral liquid solution; *OT,* oral tablet immediate release.

[a]Use caution, and individualize dosing based on other comorbidities.

Part 4

2. Non-benzodiazepine hypnotics (Table 17.16)
   a. Structurally unrelated to benzodiazepines but interact in a more targeted manner at one GABAA receptor
   b. Used for short-term management of insomnia
   c. Less anxiolytic and anticonvulsant activity
   d. Schedule IV controlled substance
3. Other hypnotics: ramelteon (Table 17.17)
   a. Full agonist of melatonin receptors MT_1 and MT_2 within suprachiasmatic nucleus of hypothalamus, area responsible for circadian rhythms and synchronization of sleep/wake cycle
   b. Melatonin decreases sleep latency and increases sleep time without causing hangover, addiction, or withdrawal effects.

G. Induction anesthetics (Table 17.18)
   1. Ketamine:
      a. Analgesic agent and general anesthetic agent
      b. Binds to phencyclidine receptor on *N*-methyl-D-aspartate (NMDA) channel NMDA receptor antagonist
      c. NMDA receptor is a ligand-gated ion channel activated by glutamate. NMDA receptors have been linked to nociceptive signal transmission and opioid tolerance.
      d. Channel is highly permeable to calcium.
      e. Noncompetitively inhibits glutamate activation
      f. Best understood as an adjuvant analgesic
      g. Used off-label in low IV and oral (PO) doses to produce analgesia
      h. May decrease hyperalgesia and central sensitization

Table 17.15

Non-Benzodiazepine Anxiolytics

Generic Name	Route(s)	Half-life	Known Active Metabolites (Half-life)	Renal Dose Adjustment Recommended	Hepatic Dose Adjustment Recommended
Buspirone	OT	2.4 to 2.7 hours	1-Pyrimidinyl piperazine (4.8 to 6.1 hours)	Yes	Yes

OT, oral tablet immediate release.

Table 17.16

Benzodiazepine Hypnotics

Generic Name	Route(s)	Half-life	Known Active Metabolites (Half-life)	Renal Dose Adjustment Recommended	Hepatic Dose Adjustment Recommended
Flurazepam	OC	2.3 hours	*N*-1-Desalkyl-flurazepam (47 to 100 hours), *N*-1-hydroxyethyl-flurazepam (16 hours)	No[a]	Yes
Temazepam	OC	3.5 to 18.4 hours	No	No[a]	No
Triazolam	OT	2.3 hours	Alpha-hydroxytri-azolam (4 hours)	No	Yes

OC, oral capsule immediate release; *OT*, oral tablet immediate release.

[a]Use caution, and individualize dosing based on other comorbidities.

Table 17.17

Non-Benzodiazepine Hypnotics

Generic Name	Route(s)	Half-life	Known Active Metabolites (Half-life)	Renal Dose Adjustment Recommended	Hepatic Dose Adjustment Recommended
Eszopiclone	OT	5 to 6 hours	No	No	Yes
Zaleplon	OC	1 hour	No	No[a]	Yes
Zolpidem	OT, OER, SL, Oral spray	2.5 to 2.6 hours (OT), 2.8 hours (OER), 2.5 to 2.85 hours (SL), 2.7 to 3 hours (oral spray)	No	No[a]	Yes

OC, oral capsule immediate release; *OER*, oral tablet/capsule extended release; *OT*, oral tablet immediate release; *SL*, sublingual tablet.

[a]Use caution, and individualize dosing based on other comorbidities.

Table 17.18

Other Hypnotics

Generic Name	Route(s)	Half-life	Known Active Metabolites (Half-life)	Renal Dose Adjustment Recommended	Hepatic Dose Adjustment Recommended
Ramelteon	OT	1 to 2.6 hours	M-II (2 to 5 hours)	No	Yes

OT, oral tablet immediate release.

Table 17.19

Induction Anesthetics

Generic Name	Route(s)	Half-life	Known Active Metabolites (Half-life)	Renal Dose Adjustment Recommended	Hepatic Dose Adjustment Recommended
Dexmedetomidine	IV	2 to 3 hours	No	No[a]	Yes
Ketamine	IV, IM	2 to 2.67 hours	Norketamine, dehydronorketamine	No	Yes
Propofol	IV	1.5 to 2.4 hours	No	No[a]	No[a]

IM, intramuscular; *IV,* intravenous.

[a]Use caution, and individualize dosing based on other comorbidities.

i. Evidence-based consensus guidelines on infusions for acute pain management by American Society for Regional Anesthesia (ASRA)/American Academy of Pain Management (AAPM) developed in 2018.
1) A review of 39 clinical trials, examining efficacy of low-dose IV bolus or continuous infusion of ketamine for postoperative pain, using reduction of pain scores or reduction of opioid consumption as primary endpoint. Findings support the premise the use of ketamine results from reduced opioid consumption more than from reduction in pain score. There were no major complications when given up to 48 hours after surgery.
2) Ketamine IV given preoperatively as bolus dose and intraoperatively as IV infusion may decrease postoperative pain medication use. Ketamine can be continued as continuous IV infusion at lower dose postoperatively if desired.
3) Schedule III controlled substance
2. Propofol:
   a. Ultrashort-acting general anesthetic
   b. Unrelated to benzodiazepines and barbiturates
   c. Mechanism of action is uncertain.
3. Dexmedetomidine:
   a. Selective alpha-2 adrenoreceptor agonist
   b. Decreases norepinephrine release
   c. Has analgesic and sedative properties
   d. Does not produce reliable amnesia
   e. FDA approved as a sedative

H. Local anesthetics (Table 17.19) and regional analgesia
1. Block conduction of nerve impulses by decreasing or preventing an increase in permeability of excitable membranes to Na^+, producing anesthesia to reduce pain
2. Classified by their structure as either amino ester or aminoamide. Generic name can be used to determine if it is an amino ester or an aminoamide. If there is more than one "i" in the name, it is an aminoamide.
3. Used in treating patients undergoing procedures, as well as patients with acute, persistent, and cancer pain
4. IV lidocaine infusions may be prescribed for some types of pain, such as renal colic and postoperative pain, and may be administered by unit nursing staff according to organizational policies and protocols and with appropriate nursing education.
5. New formulations allow prolonged delivery through various routes and catheters (i.e., IV, SC, IM, intra-articular, perineural, intrapleural, epidural, intrathecal, and topical) as either a single bolus injection or a continuous infusion.
6. IV and oral preparations of local anesthetics have been used to treat neuropathic pain syndromes, but the evidence is conflicting.
   a. Systematic review of 16 randomized control trials during perioperative period with total of 395 patients receiving IV lidocaine compared to 369 controls suggests:
   1) Lidocaine IV in perioperative period is safe and has advantages of significant reduction in postoperative pain intensity and opioid consumption for patients undergoing laparoscopic and open abdominal surgery, as well as in ambulatory surgery patients.

2) Mechanisms of action responsible for analgesic benefit include lidocaine's selective depression of pain transmission in spinal cord and reduction in neural discharge of active A-delta and C peripheral nerve fibers, which are uniquely sensitive to effects of lidocaine without creating hemodynamic disturbance or local anesthetic systemic toxicity (LAST).

3) Lidocaine IV infusion is typically given as an IV bolus followed by a continuous infusion through the end of surgery.

7. Local, regional, and neuraxial therapies (see Interventional chapter)

a. SC infiltrations, intra-articular infiltrations, and regional anesthetic peripheral nerve block techniques may be used for specific procedures if studies have demonstrated benefits.

1) Studies of peripheral nerve blocks involving surgeries of upper extremities show effectiveness of nerve blocks in axillary, supraclavicular, and interscalene regions.

2) Literature also supports use of peripheral nerve blocks in other locations, such as intercostal, ilioinguinal, penile, interpleural, or plexus.

b. Local anesthetic agents can be administered via a single injection or through placement of a catheter in or around a surgical or trauma site for continuous infusion.

c. A multi-organizational panel with input from the American Society of Anesthesiologists and subsequent approval by the ASRA recommends use of site-specific regional anesthetic techniques as a component of multimodal analgesia for management of postoperative pain when they can be applied and maintained safely.

d. Advantages include:
1) Provide superior analgesia
2) Opioid sparing, and in some cases may eliminate need for opioids
3) May improve patient satisfaction

e. Liposomal bupivacaine
1) FDA approved in 2011
2) Slow-release local anesthetic
3) Given via a single injection infiltration into transversus abdominis plane. Use in bunionectomy and hemorrhoidectomy.
4) Approved indications: In patients aged 6 years and older for single-dose infiltration to produce postsurgical local analgesia. In adults as an interscalene, brachial plexus nerve block to produce postsurgical regional analgesia. Limitations of use, safety, and efficacy have not been established in other nerve blocks.

f. Bupivacaine with meloxicam
1) Extended-release solution
2) Indications (updated 12/2021): in adults for soft-tissue or periarticular instillation to produce postsurgical analgesia for up to 72 hours after foot and ankle, small-to-medium open abdominal, and lower extremity total joint arthroplasty surgical procedures

8. Oral local anesthetic: conflicting data on efficacy of mexiletine for painful diabetic neuropathy and central post-stroke pain

9. Topical local analgesics (Table 17.20)
a. Limited to mucous membranes and skin
b. Not suitable for injection because of irritating or ineffective properties
c. Mechanism of action same as with injectable local anesthetics

10. Local anesthetic potential adverse effects
a. Allergic-type reactions
1) Reactions are rare, with biggest concern being anaphylaxis.
a) Prompt detection and treatment are essential.
b) Important to differentiate reactions related to allergy from those due to systemic toxicity.
2) Amino ester group is most likely to cause allergic reaction compared to aminoamides.
3) If history of allergy, ask patient which local anesthetic was used and what type of reaction occurred.

Table 17.20

Commonly Used Local Anesthetics: Classification, Onset, and Duration

Local Anesthetic	Onset	Duration
Bupivacaine	Slow	Long
Bupivacaine/meloxicam	Slow	Long
Chloroprocaine	Very quick	Short
Etidocaine	Quick	Long
Lidocaine	Quick	Medium
Liposomal bupivacaine	Slow	Long
Mepivacaine	Quick	Medium
Prilocaine	Quick	Medium
Procaine	Slow	Short
Ropivacaine	Slow	Long
Tetracaine	Slow	Long

Retrieved from http://www.nysora.com/mobile/regional-anesthesia/foundations-of-ra/3492-local-anesthetics-clinical-pharmacology-and-rational-selection.html.

4) Can be localized or systemic
   a) Local reaction: Contact dermatitis presents with localized rash and pruritus; delayed swelling at site.
   b) Systemic reaction: Immediate urticaria and anaphylaxis may result in cardiovascular or CNS reactions or methemoglobinemia.
b. Local anesthetic systemic toxicity (Box 17.2)
   1) Local anesthetic agents have a vasodilatory effect; when plasma concentration is high, toxicity can occur.
   2) Cardiovascular reactions can result in myocardial suppression, bradycardia, hypotension, and cardiovascular collapse.
   3) CNS reactions
      a) Minor (e.g., lightheadedness and dizziness)
      b) Moderate (e.g., difficulty focusing, tinnitus, or circumoral numbness)
      c) Severe (e.g., muscle twitching, convulsions, loss of consciousness, or even death); may also involve transient neurological symptoms, such as prolonged anesthesia and paresthesia

I. Skeletal muscle relaxants (Table 17.21)
   1. Baclofen
      a. Activates $GABA_B$ receptors reducing release of neurotransmitters and amino acids
      b. Acts specifically at spinal end of upper motor neurons to cause muscle relaxation
   2. Benzodiazepines (Table 17.13)
      a. Diazepam has been widely studied.
      b. Not likely first-line medication because of abuse potential and likelihood of multiple interactions
   3. Botulinum toxin
      a. Types A, B are neurotoxins produced by *Clostridium botulinum*.
      b. Works at presynaptic membrane of neuromuscular junction
      c. Prevents calcium-dependent release of acetylcholine
      d. Creates state of temporary denervation
   4. Carisoprodol
      a. Centrally acting skeletal muscle relaxant
      b. Precise mechanism of action is unknown.
      c. Benefits are most likely from sedative side effects.
      d. Additive effects occur with other CNS depressants.
      e. Generally avoided
      f. Psychological dependence reported with long-term use.
      g. Metabolized to meprobamate, which has anxiolytic and sedative effects
      h. Schedule IV controlled substance
   5. Chlorzoxazone
      a. Centrally acting skeletal muscle relaxant
      b. Acts on spinal cord and subcortical levels by depressing polysynaptic reflexes
   6. Cyclobenzaprine
      a. Centrally acting skeletal muscle relaxant pharmacologically related to TCAs
      b. Primarily acts as antispasmodic at brainstem rather than at spinal cord level
   7. Dantrolene
      a. Interferes with calcium ion (Ca2+) release from sarcoplasmic reticulum in skeletal muscles
      b. Reduces excitation/contraction coupling
   8. Metaxalone
      a. Centrally acting muscle relaxant
      b. Mechanism of action unknown
   9. Methocarbamol
      a. Centrally acting skeletal muscle relaxant
      b. Suppresses spinal polysynaptic reflexes

Box 17.2

Local Anesthetic Systemic Toxicity

Precautions
- The first consideration is prevention. To assure optimal patient care, healthcare providers, including nurses, should screen the patient for a past history of reaction to local anesthetics, renal or hepatic dysfunction, preexisting heart block or heart conditions, and history of respiratory acidosis.
- Toxicity may occur more often in pregnancy, in the very old or very young, and in those with hypoxia.
- Toxicity usually occurs from inadvertent intravascular injection, excessive dose or rate of injection, or delayed clearance of the medication.
- Close assessment and monitoring can detect side effects before they cause patient harm.

Management of Local Anesthetic Systemic Toxicity
- At first signs of change, get help, administer oxygen.
- If underventilation or apnea, immediate attention to establishment and maintenance of patent airway.
- If necessary, use benzodiazepines to control seizures and basic and advanced cardiac life support (ACLS) for management of cardiac arrhythmias.
- Use lipid emulsion 20% therapy according to American Society for Regional Anesthesia (ASRA) checklist for treatment of local anesthetic systemic toxicity (LAST) pharmacologic treatment protocol.
- American Society of Regional Anesthesia and Pain Medicine (2018). Checklist for treatment of local anesthetic systemic toxicity. Retrieved from https://www.asra.com/advisory-guidelines/article/3/checklist-for-treatment-of-local-anesthetic-systemic-toxicity.

Part 4

Table 17.21

Topical Compounds for Pain Management (Prescription Required)

U.S. Food and Drug Administration Approved, Commercially Available	Off-Label Use, Pharmacy Compounded	U.S. Food and Drug Administration Approved, Commercially Available	Off-Label Use, Pharmacy Compounded
Anticonvulsants		**Topical Preparations of Opioids**	
• None	• Carbamazepine 2% • Gabapentin 8%		• Hydromorphone, various percentages • Morphine, various percentages • Methadone, various percentages
Antidepressants			
• Doxepin 5% cream (FDA approved for pruritus, use for pain is off-label)	• amitriptyline 2% • nortriptyline, various percentages	**Other**	
Local Anesthetics		• 8% Capsaicin: dermal patch. Must be performed by a healthcare provider.	• Baclofen 5% • Orphenadrine, various percentages • Cyclobenzaprine 0.5%, 1%, 2% • Clonidine 0.2% • Guanethidine 1%, 2%

• Lidocaine
  • 2% viscous solution for oral use
  • 2% cream, gel
  • 3% cream, lotion
  • 4% patch, cream, solution
  • 5% patch, cream, ointment
  • Intradermal powder 0.5 mg
• Lidocaine 2.5% and Prilocaine 2.5%
• Cetacaine
• Benzocaine
  • 7.5% gel
  • 10% gel, ointment, liquid
  • 20% gel, liquid, ointment, solution, swab, otic solution
	• Lidocaine
	  • 2%, 4%, 5% compounded in various products
	  • FDA warning on the risk of potentially fatal arrhythmias with compounded lidocaine products
	• Prilocaine, various products
	• Bupivacaine, various products
	• Tetracaine, various products
	• Dyclonine
	• Pramoxine
		Examples of Over-the-Counter Topical Compounds	

		Local Anesthetics	
		• Lidocaine 0.5% spray, gel, cream, ointment	
		• Lidocaine 2.5% spray	
		• Lidocaine 4% gel, cream	
		• Lidocaine 5% cream	
		• Benzocaine 6.3% liquid, gel	
		• Benzocaine 20% cream, spray	
		• Pramoxine 1% cream, ointment, aerosol, pads	
		• Pramoxine 1% cream, ointment, aerosol, pads	
Topical Preparations of Nonsteroidal Anti-inflammatory Drugs		**Salicylates***	
• Diclofenac 1.3% transdermal patch • Diclofenac 1% gel • Diclofenac 3% gel • Diclofenac solution 1.5%, 2%	• Diclofenac, various percentages • Ketoprofen 4%, 5%, 10% • Flurbiprofen 5% • Ibuprofen 2% • Indomethacin, various percentages • Piroxicam 0.5%, 2%	• Methyl salicylate 30% cream	
		• Trolamine salicylate 10% cream	
		Counterirritants	
		• Menthol 16% ointment	
		• Menthol 5% transdermal	
Topical Preparations of *N*-methyl-D-aspartate Receptor Antagonists		• Menthol 1.3% and camphor 1.3% ointment	

• No approved, commercially available products	• Ketamine 5%, 10%, 15%, 20%
	• Dextromethorphan, various percentages
	• Amantadine, various percentages
		• Capsaicin
		  • 0.025% cream, 0.075% lotion, 0.1% gel, 0.15% patch
		  • 0.015% roll-on	

FDA, U.S. Food and Drug Administration.

*All aspirin and salicylate products are contraindicated in children.

10. Orphenadrine
    a. Muscarinic H₁ receptor antagonist
    b. Inhibits norepinephrine transporter
    c. NMDA receptor ion channel blocker
11. Tizanidine
    a. Centrally acting alpha-2 agonist
    b. Acts as antispasmodic medication

    c. Causes presynaptic inhibition of motor neuron activity

J. Nonopioid analgesics
    1. Acetaminophen (Table 17.22)
        a. Nonopioid analgesic with mechanism of action for pain relief not entirely clear

Table 17.22

Skeletal Muscle Relaxants

Generic Name	Route(s)	Half-life	Known Active Metabolites (Half-life)	Renal Dose Adjustment Recommended	Hepatic Dose Adjustment Recommended
Baclofen	OT, IT	3 to 6.8 hours (systemic), 1.5 hours (IT)	No	Yes	No
Carisoprodol	OT	8 hours	Meprobamate (10 hours)	No[a]	Yes
Chlorzoxazone	OT	1.1 hours	No	No[a]	Yes
Cyclobenzaprine	OER, OT	18 hours, 32 hours (OER)	No	No[a]	Yes
Dantrolene	OC, IV	10.8 hours (IV), 8.7 hours (oral)	5-hydroxydan-trolene	No[a]	Yes
Metaxalone	OT	8 to 9 hours	No	Yes	Yes
Methocarbamol	IV, IM, OT	0.9 to 2 hours	No	No[a] (IV form not recommended)	No[a]
Orphenadrine	IV, OT, OER	13.2 to 20.1 hours	No	No[a]	No[a]
Tizanidine	OC, OT	2 hours	No	Yes	Yes

IM, intramuscular; *IT,* intrathecal; *IV,* intravenous; *OC,* oral capsule immediate release; *OER,* oral tablet/capsule extended release; *OT,* oral tablet immediate release.

[a]Use caution, and individualize dosing based on other comorbidities.

b. Inhibits prostaglandin synthetase in CNS to produce pain relief and fever
c. Reinforces descending inhibitory serotonergic pain pathways
d. Has some interactions with endocannabinoid system that may contribute to analgesia
e. Has an opioid-sparing effect and may reduce opioid consumption by 30%–40%
f. Administered as a single dose (typically 1000 mg one hour prior to procedure)
g. Ideally administered around-the-clock postoperatively unless contraindicated
h. Adjustment recommended for both renal and hepatic concerns.
i. Adult dose 325–1000 mg every 4–6 hours. Max: not to exceed 4000 mg from all sources
2. NSAIDs (Table 17.23)
   a. Inhibit production of prostaglandins at spinal cord and periphery
   b. Have an opioid-sparing effect and can reduce opioid consumption by 30% to 40%
   c. Ideally administered around-the-clock postoperatively unless contraindicated
   d. Nonselective cyclooxygenase (COX) inhibitors
      1) COX-1 is expressed in most cells and is the primary enzyme isoform that converts arachidonic acid to prostaglandins.
      2) Nonselective NSAIDs inhibit COX-1 and prevent formation of prostaglandin mediators that trigger inflammation. They have antipyretic, analgesic, and anti-inflammatory effects.
         a) Normally, prostaglandins regulate gastrointestinal cytoprotection, renal

vasodilation, renal Na^+ and Cl^- reabsorption, platelet aggregation, fever, and uterine contraction.
   b) Inhibition of prostaglandin synthesis via COX-1 by NSAIDs may produce gastrointestinal irritation, renal ischemia, electrolyte imbalances (Na^+ retention), and increased bleeding.
e. Selective NSAIDs
   1) The COX-2 enzyme isoform is produced in tissues after injury or in proliferative diseases (e.g., cancer) and is induced by inflammatory stimuli and cytokines (i.e., bacterial lipopolysaccharide, interleukins, and tumor necrosis factor).
   2) Selective NSAIDs (i.e., "COX-2 inhibitors") (Table 17.24)
      a) Inhibit COX-2 and reduce inflammation at the tissue site but exert no effect on COX-1
      b) COX-2 inhibitors retain analgesic and anti-inflammatory properties but have lower rates of gastrointestinal toxicity.
      c) Celecoxib 200 to 400 mg orally should be considered 30 to 60 minutes before major surgery.
      d) Celecoxib is contraindicated in coronary artery bypass graft surgery.
K. Opioids
   1. Receptor agonists (Table 17.25)
      a. Exogenous opioids selective for either mu receptors, kappa receptors, or delta receptors that mimic endogenous endorphins, enkephalins, or dynorphin A to produce supraspinal or spinal analgesia

Part 4

Table 17.23

Miscellaneous Analgesics

Generic Name	Route(s)	Half-life	Known Active Metabolites (Half-life)	Renal Dose Adjustment Recommended	Hepatic Dose Adjustment Recommended
Acetaminophen	OC, OS, OT, OCT, ODT, OER, rectal, IV	2 to 3 hours	No	Yes	Yes
Dihydroergotamine	IV, IM, intranasal	9–10 hours	8-hydroxy-dihydroergotamine	Yes	Yes
Dronabinol	OC	19 to 36 hours	11-Hydroxy-Δ^9-tetrahydrocannabinol (TCH)	No[a]	No[a]
Ergoloid mesylates	OT	3.5 hours	No	No[a]	No[a]
Ergotamine tartrate	SL, OT, rectal	1.5 to 2 hours	No	No[a]	No[a]
Nabilone	OC	2 hours	Isomeric carbinols (35 hours), diol (35 hours)	No[a]	No[a]
Tapentadol	OT, OER	4 to 5 hours	No	Yes	Yes
Tramadol	Nasal spray, OER, OT	5.6 to 6.7 hours (OT), 6.5 to 10 hours (OER)	O-Desmethyl-tramadol (6.7 to 7 hours)	Yes	Yes

IM, intramuscular; *IV,* intravenous; *OC,* oral capsule immediate release; *OCT,* oral chewable tablet; *ODT,* oral dissolvable tablet; *OER,* oral tablet/capsule extended release; *OS,* oral liquid solution; *OT,* oral tablet immediate release; *SC,* subcutaneous; *SL,* sublingual.

[a]Use caution, and individualize dosing based on other comorbidities.

Table 17.24

Nonselective Nonsteroidal Anti-inflammatory Drugs

Generic Name	Route(s)	Half-life	Known Active Metabolites (Half-life)	Renal Dose Adjustment Recommended	Hepatic Dose Adjustment Recommended
Aspirin[a]	OT, OER, OCT, RS, Oral gum	20 to 60 minutes	Salicylic acid half-life of 6 hours	Yes	Yes
Choline magnesium trisalicylate	OT	9 to 17 hours	—	Yes	No
Diclofenac	OC, OT, OER, oral powder for solution, ophthalmic solution, topical gel	OC, OT, OS: 1 to 2 hours	—	Yes	Yes
	OC	2 hours		—	
	TP	12 hours		—	
	IV	2.29 hours		—	
	Topical solution	79 hours		—	
	Topical cream	—		—	
Diflunisal	OT	8 to 12 hours	—	Yes	Yes
Etodolac	OC, OT, OER	3.3 to 11.3 hours (OC), 7.6 to 8.4 hours (OER)	—	Yes	Yes
Fenoprofen	OC, OT	3 hours	—	No	No
Flurbiprofen	OT, ophthalmic solution	4.7 to 5.7 hours	—	Yes	Yes
Ibuprofen	OC, OT, OS	1.8 to 2.44 hours	—	Yes	No
	IV			—	
	Topical cream				
Indomethacin	OC, OER	4.5 to 7.6 hours	—	Yes	No[a]
	OS, RS			—	
Ketoprofen	OC	0.9 to 3.3 hours (OC)	—	Yes	Yes
	OER	3.4 to 7.4 hours		—	

Table 17.24

Nonselective Nonsteroidal Anti-inflammatory Drugs—cont'd

Generic Name	Route(s)	Half-life	Known Active Metabolites (Half-life)	Renal Dose Adjustment Recommended	Hepatic Dose Adjustment Recommended
Ketorolac	OT, IM, IV, ophthalmic solution	6.1 to 7 hours	—	Yes	Yes
	Nasal spray	—		—	
Meclofenamate	OC	1.3 hours	—	Yes	No
Mefenamic acid	OC	2 hours	—	Yes	No[a]
Meloxicam	OT, OS, OC	15 to 20 hours	—	Yes	Yes
Nabumetone	OT	24 hours	—	Yes	Yes
Naproxen	OT, OER, OS	12 to 17 hours	—	Yes	Yes
Piroxicam	OC	50 hours	—	Yes	Yes
Salsalate	OT	1 hour	—	Yes	No
Sulindac	OT	7.8 hours	sulfide: 16.4 hours	Yes	Yes
Tolmetin	OC, OT	5 hours		Yes	No

IM, intramuscular; *IV,* intravenous; *OC,* oral capsule immediate release; *OCT,* oral chewable tablet; *OER,* oral tablet/capsule extended release; *OS,* oral liquid solution; *OT,* oral tablet immediate release; *TP,* transdermal patch.

[a]Use caution, and individualize dosing based on other comorbidities.

Table 17.25

Cyclooxygenase-2 Selective Nonsteroidal Anti-inflammatory Drugs

Generic Name	Route(s)	Half-life	Known Active Metabolites (Half-life)	Renal Dose Adjustment Recommended	Hepatic Dose Adjustment Recommended
Celecoxib	OC, powder	11 hours	—	Yes	Yes

OC, oral capsule immediate release.

b. Play an important role in analgesic treatment of acute moderate to severe pain during and after surgery

c. Pure mu-agonists (Table 17.26) typically require only a small percentage (10% to 20%) of available receptors to be occupied to produce maximum pharmacological response.

d. Most are schedule II controlled substances.

2. Equianalgesic: approximately "equal" analgesia when referring to opioids. Equianalgesic charts list routes and rough estimates of opioid potency (Table 17.27).

3. Incomplete cross tolerance

   a. Prolonged opioid use can result in tolerance evidenced by shorter duration of action and requiring increased doses to accomplish the same level of analgesia.

   b. Cross tolerance may develop with opioids acting on the same receptor site.

   c. When using equianalgesic dosing, clinicians must expect that patient has incomplete cross tolerance to new opioid. A dose reduction of at least 50% of new opioid equianalgesic dose

should be made to prevent overdosing because patient is not as tolerant to new opioid.

   d. Assessment of response to new medication is necessary, as additional medication maybe required.

   e. Incomplete cross tolerance is influenced by genetic polymorphism.

4. Common opioid side effects

   a. Nausea and vomiting

      1) Difficult to differentiate whether cause is from opioid or other sources

      2) Mechanism of action may involve stimulation of vestibular system providing direct input via histamine and cholinergic pathways into vomiting center.

      3) Chemoreceptor trigger zone may be exposed.

      4) Interventions:

         a) Decrease dose or change opioids.

         b) Administer antiemetics and/or antihistamines (may potentiate sedation).

   b. Urinary retention

      1) May be caused by relaxation of detrusor muscle at floor of bladder

Table 17.26

Opioid Receptor Agonists

Opioid Receptor	Endogenous Opioid	Exogenous Opioid	Antagonist
Delta	Enkephalin	Levorphanol Methadone	Naloxone Naltrexone Buprenorphine
Kappa	Dynorphin A	Butorphanol (partial) Levorphanol Nalbuphine Pentazocine (partial)	Buprenorphine Naloxone Naltrexone
Mu	Enkephalin Beta-endorphin	Alfentanil Buprenorphine (partial) Butorphanol (partial) Codeine Fentanyl Hydrocodone Hydromorphone Levorphanol Meperidine Morphine Methadone Oliceridine Oxycodone Oxymorphone Pentazocine (partial) Remifentanil Sufentanil Tramadol	Nalbuphine (partial) Naloxone Naltrexone Pentazocine

2) Seen with increasing age and more often in males
3) Interventions:
  a) Monitor urine output.
  b) Straight catheterization for urinary retention
  c) Reduce or change opioid.
  d) Low-dose naloxone infusion
c. Itching
1) Common side effect
2) Mechanism unknown
3) True anaphylactic allergic reactions to opioids are extremely rare.
4) Reaction at injection site is due to histamine release.
5) Interventions:
  a) Decrease dose.
  b) Switch opioids.
  c) Consider low-dose antihistamine (may potentiate sedation).
  d) Low-dose naloxone infusion
  e) Nalbuphine
d. Constipation:
1) Common side effect

2) Pain and opioids slow peristalsis.
3) Immobility, poor diet, and dehydration slow peristalsis.
4) Interventions:
  a) Monitor bowel sounds and elimination patterns.
  b) Educate patient and family.
  c) Other options include hydration, ambulation, high-fiber diet, stool softener, peristaltic agent, hyperosmotic laxative, and methylnaltrexone.
e. Confusion:
1) Inadequate pain management
2) Seen with opioid administration and impaired renal function
3) Interventions:
  a) Determine baseline mental status.
  b) Assess for mental status changes and etiology.
f. Opioid-induced sedation and respiratory depression (see chapter 12)
5. Patient-controlled analgesia (PCA)
a. PCA is a method of analgesic administration in which patient self-administers predetermined amounts of analgesia (usually opioids) through a specialized delivery administration system.
b. PCA infusion devices (pumps) are specifically designed to deliver intermittent patient-activated dosing, with or without a continuous (basal) infusion.
c. PCA dose is amount administered each time patient activates pump once lockout period has passed
d. Lockout interval is predetermined period during which patient cannot receive doses.
e. Continuous (basal) rate is amount that infuses continuously, regardless of activation of PCA or patient assessment and may avoid peaks and valleys of pain, analgesia, and sedation.
f. For postoperative patients, post-anesthesia care unit (PACU) is the place to initiate PCAs to avoid delays following transfer to general care units. Titration to effect (rapid acceleration) is a common method of administering fast-acting opioids to elevate serum opioid level and provide patient with proper analgesia prior to starting PCA.
g. Benefits and expected outcomes:
1) Improved pain relief with activity
2) Patient has some control over pain relief.
h. Routes of PCA administration include enteral, IV, subcutaneous, epidural, and regional.
1) Considerations for enteral PCA administration:
  a) Management of acute pain
  b) May be considered for patients who are capable of understanding the

Table 17.27A

Opioid Agonists

Generic Name *Origin* [chemical class]	Route(s)	Half-life	Known Active Metabolites (Half-life)	Renal Dose Adjustment Recommended	Hepatic Dose Adjustment Recommended
Alfentanil *Synthetic* [phenylpiperidine]	IV	90 to 111 minutes	—	Yes	Yes
Codeine *Natural opioid* [phenanthrenes]	OT, OS	3 hours	Morphine (3 hours)	Yes	Yes
Fentanyl *Synthetic* [phenylpiperidine]	TP, IV, mucous membrane lozenge/ troche	Varies	—	Yes	Yes
	IV PCA	2 to 12 hours			
	TP	20 to 27 hours			
	Iontophoretic transdermal system	3 to 12 hours			
	Buccal film, TIRF	14 hours			
	Sublingual spray, TIRF	5.25 to 11 to 99 hours			
	Mucous membrane lozenge, TIRF	7 hours			
	Intranasal, TIRF	15 to 24.9 hours			
	Buccal tablet, TIRF	11 hours			
	Sublingual tablet, TIRF	100 to 200 mcg is 5.02 to 6.67 hours; 400 to 800 mcg is 10.1 to 13.5 hours			
Hydrocodone *Semi-synthetic* [phenanthrenes]	OER	8 hours	—	Yes	Yes
	OER	7 to 9 hours			
Hydromorphone *Semi-synthetic* [phenanthrenes]	OT, OER, OS, RS	—	—	Yes	Yes
	IV	2.3 hours			
	OER PCA	11 hours			
Levorphanol *Semi-synthetic* [phenanthrenes]	OT IV PCA	11 to 16 hours	—	No	Yes
Meperidine *Synthetic* [phenylpiperidines]	OT, OS, IV	Meperidine (3.2 to 3.7 hours)	Normeperidine (24 to 48 hours)	Yes	Yes
Methadone *Synthetic* [diphehnylheptanes]	OT, OS, IV	8 to 59 hours	—	Yes	Yes
Morphine *Natural opioid* [phenanthrenes] Oliceridine *Synthetic – organic* No chemical class identified	OC, OT, OER, OS, IV, IT	2 to 4 hours	Morphine-6-glucuronide (M6G; 18.2 plus or minus 13.6 hours)	Yes No	Yes Yes
	IV	1.5 to 4.5 hours	None currently known		
	—	—			
	IV, PCA	1.3 to 3 hours			
Oxycodone *Semi-synthetic* [phenanthrenes]	OC, OT, OER, OS	— 3.5 to 4 hours 4.5 to 8 hours	—	Yes	Yes

(Continued)

Table 17.27A						
Opioid Agonists—cont'd						
Generic Name ***Origin*** **[chemical class]**	**Route(s)**	**Half-life**	**Known Active Metabolites (Half-life)**	**Renal Dose Adjustment Recommended**	**Hepatic Dose Adjustment Recommended**	
Oxymorphone *Semi-synthetic* [phenanthrenes]	OT, OER, IV	7.25 to 9.43 hours	—	Yes	Yes	
Remifentanil *Synthetic* [phenylpiperidines]	IV	3 to 10 minutes	—	No	No	
Sufentanil *Synthetic* [phenylpiperidines]	IV	164 min	—	No[a]	No[a]	
Pentazocine *Synthetic* [benzomorphans]	IV	2 to 3 hours	—	No	Yes	

IT, intrathecal; *IV*, intravenous; *mcg*, microgram; *OC*, oral capsule immediate release; *OER*, oral tablet/capsule extended release; *OS*, oral liquid solution; *OT*, oral tablet immediate release; *PCA*, patient-controlled analgesia; *RS*, rectal suppository; *TIRF*, transmucosal immediate release fentanyl; *TP*, transdermal patch.

[a]Use caution, and individualize dosing based on other comorbidities.

relationship between pain, taking an oral dose, and pain relief and can physically self-administer medication

  i. PCA administration and monitoring

    1) Avoid continuous infusions in high-risk patients. Assess risk/benefit ratio for individual patients. The Institute for Safe Medication Practices recommends continuous infusions be used *only* with opioid-tolerant patients.

    2) Use additional respiratory monitoring (e.g., capnography) in high-risk patients. Avoid depending on pulse oximetry if patient is receiving supplemental oxygen.

    3) Continue to assess sedation and respiratory status, decreasing or stopping PCA if sedation is detected.

  j. SC analgesia (continuous, PCA, or both)

    1) SC and IV opioid infusions produce similar levels and provide comparable analgesia and side effects.

    2) Less invasive, less expensive, and provides easy access when IV or oral routes are not possible

    3) Infusions and boluses are limited to absorption of opioid at SC site; thus, reduced infusate volume or more frequent site rotation may be needed.

    4) Local toxicity or chemical irritation from opioid is uncommon. More likely to occur with higher concentrations and/or higher doses.

    5) Problems at site include scarring, variation of absorption, and possible unpredictable analgesia.

    6) Morphine and hydromorphone are most commonly used. Fentanyl is generally not used due to inability to concentrate, and larger volumes may be painful.

    7) Common sites are subclavicular area, anterior chest wall, and abdomen.

6. Dependence, tolerance, and use disorders (see chapter 22)

  a. Physical dependence: manifested by physical need to continue administration of a medication to prevent withdrawal symptoms; an expected physiological response to continuous use of opioids and does not imply substance use disorder (SUD)

  b. Opioid tolerance: need to take more of a medication to achieve same effect; it too is a normal process and does not imply SUD

  c. Opioid use disorder (OUD): problematic pattern of opioid use leading to clinically significant impairment or distress, as manifested by at least two *Diagnostic and Statistical Manual of Mental Disorders*, fifth edition (*DSM-5*) criteria occurring within a 12-month period

  d. SUD: cluster of cognitive behavioral and physiological symptoms indicating the individual continues using substance despite significant substance-related problems

7. Tapering (weaning) in the context of long-term opioid use

  a. Preoperative

    1) Current literature supports an association between preoperative opioid use, worsened postoperative pain, surgical outcomes, length of stay, and financial costs.

    2) Preoperative opioid reduction may result in substantial improvement in outcomes, but conclusive evidence is lacking. Three-month period is optimal for preoperative weaning to occur.

Table 17.27B

Frequently Published Equianalgesic Dose Chart With Opioid Pharmacokinetic Information

A Guide to Using Equianalgesic Dose Charts[a]

- *Equianalgesic* means approximately the same pain relief.
- The equianalgesic chart is a guideline for selecting doses for opioid-naïve patients. Doses and intervals between doses are titrated according to individuals' responses.
- The equianalgesic chart is helpful when switching from one drug to another or switching from one route of administration to another[b].
- Doses in this equianalgesic chart suggest a ratio for comparing the analgesic effects of one drug to those of another.
- The longer a patient has been receiving an opioid, the more conservative the starting dose of a new opioid should be.

Opioid	Oral (PO) (Over ~4 h) Traditional	Parenteral (IV/subq/IM[c]), (Over ~4 h)	Onset (min)	Peak (min)	Duration (h)[d]	Half-Life (h)
Mu agonists	—	—	—	—	—	—
Morphine	30 mg	10 mg	30 to 60 (PO)	60 to 90 (PO)	3 to 6 (PO)	2 to 4
	—	—	30 to 60 (MR)[e]	90 to 180 (MR)[e]	8 to 24 (MR)[e]	—
	—	—	30 to 60 (R)	60 to 90 (R)	4 to 5 (R)	—
	—	—	5 to 10 (IV)	15 to 30 (IV)	3 to 4 (IV)[d,f]	—
	—	—	10 to 20 (subq)	30 to 60 (subq)	3 to 4 (subq)	—
Codeine	200 mg NR	130 mg	30 to 60 (PO)	60 to 90 (PO)	3 to 4 (PO)	2 to 4
	—	—	10 to 20 (subq)	ND (subq)	3 to 4 (subq)	—
FentaNYL	—	100 mcg IV1 mcg/h of TD fentaNYL is approximately equal–2 mg/24 h of oral morphine[i]	5 (OT)[g] 5 (B)[g] 3 to 5 (IV) 12 to 16 h (TD)	15 (OT)[g] 15 (B)[g] 15–30 (IV) 24 h (TD)	2 to 5 (OT)[g] 2 to 5 (B)[g] 2 (IV)[d,f] 48 to 72 (TD)	3 to 4[h] >24 (TD)
HYDROcodone	30 mg[j] NR	—	30 to 60 (PO)	60 to 90 (PO)	4 to 6 (PO)	4
HYDROmorphone	7.5 mg	1.5 mg[k]	15 to 30 (PO) 15 to 30 (R)	30 to 90 (PO) 30 to 90 (R)	3 to 4 (PO) 3 to 4 (R)	2 to 3
	—	—	5 (IV)	10 to 20 (IV)	3 to 4 (IV)[d,f]	—
	—	—	10–20 (subq)	30–90 (subq)	3–4 (subq)	—
Levorphanol	4 mg	2 mg	30 to 60 (PO) 10 (IV) 10 to 20 (subq)	60 to 90 (PO) 15 to 30 (IV) 4 to 6 (IV)[b,e] 4 to 6 (IV) 60 to 90 (subq) 4 to 6 (IV) 4 to 6 (IV)	4–6 (PO) 4–6 (subq)	12 to 15
Meperidine Not recommended for analgesic purposes: information provided to rotate off meperidine to another opioid	300 mg NR	75 mg	30 to 60 (PO) 5 to 10 (IV)	60–90 (PO) 10 to 15 (IV)	2 to 4 (PO) 2 to 4 (IV)[d,f]	2 to 3
	—	—	10 to 20 (subq)	15 to 30 (subq)	2 to 4 (subq)	—
Methadone	(See Boxes 11.17–11.19 and Table 11.11)	—	—	—	—	—
OxyCODONE	20 mg	—	30 to 60 (PO) 30 to 60 (MR)[l]	60 to 90 (PO) 90 to 180 (MR)[l]	3 to 4 (PO) 8 to 12 (MR)[l]	2 to 3 (short acting) 4.5 (MR)[l]
	—	—	30 to 60 (R)	30 to 60 (R)	3 to 6 (R)	—

(Continued)

Table 17.27B

Frequently Published Equianalgesic Dose Chart With Opioid Pharmacokinetic Information—cont'd

Opioid	Oral (PO) (Over ~4 h) Traditional	Parenteral (IV/ subq/IM[c]), (Over ~4 h)	Onset (min)	Peak (min)	Duration (h)[d]	Half-Life (h)
OxyMORphone	10 mg (10 mg R)	1 mg	30 to 45 (PO)	30 to 90 (PO) 60 (MR)[m]	4 to 6 (PO) 12 (MR)[m]	7 to 11 (PO 2 (parenteral)
	—	—	15 to 30 (R)	120 (R)	3 to 6 (R)	
	—	—	5 to 10 (IV)	15 to 30 (IV)	3 to 4 (IV)[d,f]	
	—	—	10 to 20 (subq)	ND (subq)	3–6 (subq)	

B, buccal; *IM*, intramuscular; *IV*, intravenous; *MR*, oral modified-release; *ND*, no data; *NR*, not recommended; *OT*, oral transmucosal; *PO*, oral; *R*, rectal; *subq*, subcutaneous; *TD*, transdermal.

[a]This table provides equianalgesic doses and pharmacokinetic information about selected opioid drugs. Characteristics and comments about selected mu opioid agonist drugs can be found in Table 11.7.

[b]An expert panel was convened for the purpose of establishing a new guideline for opioid rotation and recently proposed a two-step approach (Fine, P. G., & Portenoy, R. K. [2009]. Ad Hoc Expert Panel on Evidence Review and Guidelines for Opioid Rotation. Establishing "best practices" for opioid rotation: conclusions of an expert panel. *Journal of Pain & Symptom Management*, 38[3], 418–425.). The approach presented in the text for calculating the dose of a new opioid can be conceptualized as the panel's Step One, which directs clinicians to calculate the equianalgesic dose of the new opioid based on the equianalgesic table. Step Two suggests that clinicians perform a second assessment of patients to evaluate the current pain severity (perhaps suggesting that the calculated dose be increased or decreased) and to develop strategies for assessing and titrating the dose and to determine the need for breakthrough doses and calculate those doses.

[c]The intramuscular route for opioid administration should be avoided and information is therefore omitted.

[d]Duration of analgesia is dose dependent; the higher the dose, usually the longer the duration.

[e]As in, for example morphine modified-release products. Some products have duration of 8 hours, and others are 12 to 24 hours. Refer to the product information for specific medications.

[f]The intravenous route produces the highest peak concentration of the drug, and the peak concentration is associated with the highest level of toxicity (e.g., sedation). To decrease the peak effect and lower the level of toxicity, intravenous boluses may be administered more slowly (e.g., morphine 5 mg over a 15-min period), or smaller doses may be administered more often (e.g., morphine 2 mg every 1 to 1.5 hours).

[g]The delivery system for transmucosal fentaNYL influences potency (e.g., buccal fentaNYL is approximately twice as potent as oral transmucosal fentaNYL).

[h] At steady state, slow release of fentaNYL from storage in tissues can result in a prolonged half-life (e.g., 4 to 5 times longer).

[i]This is the ratio that is used clinically.

[j]Equianalgesic data are not available.

[k]The recommendation that 1.5 mg of parenteral HYDROmorphone is approximately equal to 10 mg of parenteral morphine is based on single-dose studies. With repeated dosing of HYDROmorphone (as during patient-controlled analgesia), it is more likely that 2 to 3 mg of parenteral HYDROmorphone is equal to 10 mg of parenteral morphine.

[l]As in, for example, modified-release oxyCODONE.

[m]As in modified-release oxyMORphone.

[n]Used in combination with mu agonist opioids, this drug may reverse analgesia and precipitate withdrawal in opioid-dependent patients.

[o]In opioid-naive patients who are taking occasional mu agonist opioids, such as HYDROcodone or oxyCODONE, the addition of butorphanol nasal spray may provide additive analgesia. However, in opioid-tolerant patients, such as those receiving around-the-clock morphine, the addition of butorphanol nasal spray should be avoided because it may reverse analgesia and precipitate withdrawal.

Data from Pasero, C., & McCaffery, M. *Pain assessment and pharmacologic management* (pp. 444–446). St. Louis, MO: Mosby. Data from American Pain Society. (2003). *Principles of analgesic use in the treatment of acute pain and chronic cancer pain*. Glenview, IL, Author; Breitbart, W., Chandler, S., Eagel, B., Ellison, N., Enck, R. E., Lefkowitz, M., & Payne, R. (2000). An alternative algorithm for dosing transdermal fentanyl for cancer-related pain. *Oncology*, 14(5), 695–705 (see discussion in same issue, pp. 705,709–710,712,17; Coda, B. A., Tanaka, A, Jacobson, R. C., Donaldson, G., & Chapman, C. R. (1997). Hydromorphone analgesia after intravenous bolus administration. *Pain*, 71(1), 41–48; Dormer, B., Zenz, M., Trvba, M., & Stnunpf, M. (1996). Direct conversion from oral morphine to transdermal fentanyl: A multicenter study in patients with cancer pain. *Pain*, 64(3), 527–534; Dunbar, P. J., Chapman, C. R., Buckley, F. P., & Gavin, J. R. (1996). Clinical analgesic equivalence for morphine and hydromorphone with prolonged PCA. *Pain*, 68,226–270; Fine, P. G., Portenoy, R. K., & Ad Hoc Expert Panel on Evidence Review and Guidelines for Opioid Rotation. (2009). Establishing best practices for opioid rotation: Conclusions of an expert panel. *Journal of Pain Symptom Management*, 38(3), 418–425; Gutstein, H. B., & Akil, H. (2006). Opioid analgesics. In L. L. Brunton, J. S. Lazo, & K. L. Parker (Eds.), *Goodman & Gilman's The pharmacological basis of therapeutics* (11th ed.). New York: McGraw-Hill; Hanks, G., Cherny, N. I., & Fallon, M. (2004). Opioid analgesic therapy. In D. Doyle, G. Hanks, N. I. Cherny, & K. Calman, (Eds.), *Oxford textbook of palliative medicine* (3rd ed.)., New York: Oxford Press; Johnson, R. E., Fudala, P. J., & Payne, R. (2005). Buprenorphine: Considerations for pain management. *Journal of Pain Symptom Management*, 29(3), 297–326; Kaiko, R. F., Lacouture, R, Hopf, K., Brown, J., & Goldenheim, P. (1996). Analgesic onset and potency of oral controlled release (CR) oxycodone CR and morphine. *Clinical Pharmacology & Therapeutics*, 59(2), 130–133; Knotkova, H., Fine, P. G., & Portenoy, R. K. (2009). Opioid rotation: The science and limitations of the equianalgesic dose table. *Journal of Pan Symptom Management*, 38(3), 426–439; Lawlor, P., Turner, K., Hanson, J., & Bruera, E. (1997). Dose ratio between morphine and hydromorphone in patients with cancer pain: A retrospective study. *Pain*, 72(1, 2), 79–85; Manfredi, P. L, Borsook, D., Chandler, S. W., & Payne, R. (1997). Intravenous methadone for cancer pain unrelieved by morphine and hydromorphone: Clinical observations. *Pain*, 70, 99–101; Portenoy, R. K. (1996). Opioid analgesics. In R. K. Portenoy, & R. M. Kanner (Eds.), *Pain management: Theory and practice*. Philadelphia, FA Davis; Sittl, R., Likar, R., & Nautrup, B. P. (2005). Equipotent doses of transdermal fentanyl and transdermal buprenorphine in patients with cancer and noncancer pain: Results of a retrospective cohort study. *Clinical Therapeutics*, 27(2), 225–237; Skaer, T. L (2004). Practice guidelines for transdermal opioids in malignant pain. *Drugs*, 64(23), 2629–2638; Skaer, T. L. (2006). Transdermal opioids for cancer pain. *Health and Quality of Lift Outcomes*, 4, 24; Vogelsang, J., & Hayes, S. R. (1991). Butorphanol tartrate (Stadol): A review. *Journal of Post Anesthesia Nursing*, 6(2),129–135; Weinberg, D. S., Inturrisi, C E., Reidenberg, B., Moulin, D. E., Nip, T. J., Wallenstein, S., … Foley, K. M. (1988). Sublingual absorption of selected opioid analgesics. *Clinical Pharmacology & Therapeutics*, 44, 335–342; Wilson, J. M., Cohen, R. I., Kezer, E. A., Schange, S. J., & Smith, E. R. (1995). Single and multiple-dose pharmacokinetics of dezocine in patients with acute and chronic pain. *Journal of Clinical Pharmacology*, 35, 395–403. ©2011, Pasero, C., & McCaffery, M. May be duplicated for use in clinical practice.

Part 4

3) Additional aspects of preoperative opioid weaning should include:
   a) Nurturing a commitment to overall biopsychosocial-spiritual health
   b) Strong focus on reducing pain catastrophizing
   c) Bolstering self-efficacy and resilience
b. Postoperative
   1) If taken on regular schedule, physical tolerance can develop in previously opioid-naïve postoperative patients in as few as 5 days in some cases.
   2) All patients placed on opioids should be educated on physical withdrawal symptoms.
   3) All postoperative patients should be instructed to call healthcare providers before taking more or less of prescribed pain medication.
   4) Literature advises tapering opioids by 6 weeks after most major surgeries to preoperative dose or lower in the absence of clinically meaningful improvements in function and pain, using 20% weekly dose reductions.
c. Health and Human Services "HHS Guide for Clinicians on the Appropriate Dosage Reduction or Discontinuation of Long-Term Opioid Analgesics" for tapering chronic opioid use
   1) Individualize
   2) Longer duration of opioid therapy make take longer to taper.
   3) Common tapers involve dose reduction of 5% to 20% every 4 weeks.
   4) Slower tapers: 10% per month or slower
   5) Faster tapers: 10% of original dose each week until 30% of original dose is reached, followed by weekly decrease of 10% of remaining dose
      a) Faster tapers may trigger withdrawal.
      b) Once smallest dose is reached, interval can be extended.
   6) Multimodal base should be continued to help alleviate emotional and physical stress.
   7) Pauses can be built into the taper plan to allow the patient extra time for physical and psychological adjustment to new dose.
   8) Ultrarapid detoxification under anesthesia is associated with substantial risks and should not be used.
   9) Taper is considered successful as long as patient is making progress.
8. Tapering (weaning) in the context of iatrogenic exposure
a. Iatrogenic exposure: drug dependence that develops as result of medical treatment (e.g., prolonged opioid use during a hospital stay)

b. Withdrawal syndrome: multisystem symptoms occurring with an abrupt decrease or complete cessation of licit or illicit drug (e.g., nicotine, cannabinoids opioids, benzodiazepines, alcohol or alpha 2-agnosts) to which the body has become dependent
c. Taper/weaning: slow and systematic decrease in medications to which patient has become dependent to avoid withdrawal syndrome
   1) Use of standardized weaning protocol has been associated with shorter wean duration, decreased medication consumption, shorter intensive care unit (ICU) stays, and shorter length of stays.
   2) Several tapering or weaning methods are available in literature.
   3) Generally speaking:
      a) Length of exposure should guide length of wean (e.g., a patient exposed for 7 days should not require a 14 day wean).
      b) <5-day exposure: often does not require a dedicated wean and can be managed with intermittent medications as needed
      c) 6- to 10-day exposure: Consider weaning 20% of the initial dose (5-day wean).
      d) 11- to 20-day exposure: Consider weaning 10% of initial dose daily (10-day wean).
      e) >21 day exposure: Consider weaning 10% of initial dose every 2 days (20-day wean).
d. Withdrawal assessment is discussed in chapter 12.
9. Risk evaluation and mitigation strategy
a. "Food and Drug Administration Amendments Act of 2007" gave FDA authority to require manufacturers to develop risk evaluation and mitigation strategy (REMS) programs for safe prescribing of specifically identified high-risk products.
b. REMS is a strategy designed to manage known or potential risks associated with a biologic product or medication to ensure the benefits outweigh risks.
c. In 2012, FDA approved REMS for ER and long-acting (LA) opioid medications used to treat moderate to severe pain. In the setting of a growing problem of prescription medication use and abuse, REMS were designed to introduce safety measures to improve prescribing and safer use of ER and LA opioid analgesics, while continuing to provide access to these medications for patients in pain.
d. As part of REMS, all ER, LA, and immediate-release (IR) opioid-manufacturing companies must provide education for healthcare professionals.

1) Content is directed at prescribers and other healthcare professionals, including pharmacists and nurses.
2) Continuing education opportunity for the course is provided.
e. Focuses on responsibilities for appropriate prescribing of ER/LA/IR opioids
f. Learning outcomes from education include but are not limited to:
   1) Understanding how to assess patients for treatment with ER/LA/IR opioid analgesics
   2) How to initiate, adjust, manage ongoing, and discontinue ER/LA/IR analgesic therapy
   3) Knowing product-specific information
   4) Providing education to patients and caregivers about the medication, including instruction on safe storage and disposal
   5) Content is not intended to be exhaustive and not intended to be a substitute for a more comprehensive pain management course.
10. Partial agonists (Table 17.27)
    a. Exogenous opioids with mixed delta-, mu-, and kappa-receptor activity to produce spinal analgesia; require 75% to 100% receptor occupancy to produce maximum response.
    b. Buprenorphine
       1) Partial mu-agonist and weak kappa-antagonist

2) Schedule III controlled substance
3) Conflicting opinions whether buprenorphine should be stopped preoperatively and for what duration
4) FDA issues Drug Safety Communication (1/12/22) concerning dental problems with buprenorphine medicines dissolved in the mouth.
   a) Dental problems may include tooth decay, cavities, oral infections, and loss of teeth.
   b) May be serious and have been reported even in patients with no history of dental issues
c. Butorphanol
   1) Partial mu-agonist and partial kappa-agonist
   2) Schedule IV controlled substance
d. Nalbuphine: partial mu-antagonist and kappa-agonist
e. Pentazocine: partial mu-agonist and partial kappa-agonist; schedule IV controlled substance
11. Opioid antagonists (Table 17.28)
    a. Nonselective for a receptor, central acting
    b. Competitively interact at opioid receptors to displace opiate
    c. Capable of producing relief of opioid-induced constipation or pruritus at low doses and reversal of analgesia and recovery from respiratory depression at higher doses

Table 17.28

Opioid Partial Agonists

Generic Name	Route(s)	Half-life	Known Active Metabolites (Half-life)	Renal Dose Adjustment Recommended	Hepatic Dose Adjustment Recommended
Buprenorphine	IV, sublingual tablet	31 to 35 hours (sublingual formulation)	—	No	Yes
	Buccal film	27.6 hours	—		
	TP	26 hours	—		
	IV	1.2 to 7.2 hours	—		
Buprenorphine/ Naloxone	Buccal film	16.4 to 27.5 hours (bupren-orphine), 1.9 to 2.4 hours (naloxone)	—	No	Yes
	Sublingual film	24 to 42 hours (bupren-orphine), 2 to 12 hours (naloxone)	—	No	Yes
	Sublingual tablet	24 to 42 hours (bupren-orphine), 2 to 12 hours (naloxone)	—	No	Yes
Butorphanol	IV, nasal spray	2.89 to 9.17 hours (nasal spray)	Hydroxy-butorphanol; half-life 18 hours	Yes	Yes
	IV	2.06 to 8.79 hours	—	—	—
Nalbuphine	IV	2.2 to 2.6 hours	—	No	Yes

IV, intravenous; *TP*, transdermal patch.

d. May induce acute withdrawal in a patient with opioid tolerance, dependence, or both
e. Naloxone is an opioid antagonist.
   1) Injectable solution IV/IM/SC, intranasal spray, and auto-injector (IM/SC) are available in community for opioid overdose.
      a) Rapid onset of action: IV within 2 minutes; IM/SC within 2 to 5 minutes; intranasal approximately 8 to 13 minutes
      b) Duration of action: approximately 30 to 120 minutes, depending on route of administration; IV shorter than IM/SC.
   2) Treatment of respiratory depression or arrest
      a) Duration of naloxone reversal is shorter than most opioids; repeated doses are usually needed, as patients are at risk for repeated respiratory depression.
      b) Individuals require ongoing monitoring for an additional 90 to 120 minutes to ensure no recurrence of respiratory depression. Continued monitoring may be necessary, depending on factors such as opioid, dose, route, and concurrent medications.
      c) Naloxone administration should be in conjunction with other rescue measures.
f. Naltrexone is an opioid antagonist
   1) Comes in two forms:
      a) Oral tablets for opiate or alcohol dependence treatment
      b) IM, ER, suspension for alcohol or opioid dependence treatment
   2) Low-dose naltrexone (LDN), off-label use as treatment of autoimmune disease pain and other chronic pain syndromes
   3) Modes of purposed action include reducing inflammatory response and increased levels of endogenous opioids.
g. Selective for mu-receptor, peripheral acting agents
   1) Alvimopan oral tablet for postoperative ileus
   2) Methylnaltrexone SC injection for opioid-induced constipation
   3) Naloxegol oral tablets for opioid-induced constipation
L. Steroids
   1. Glucocorticoids (Table 17.29).
      a. Bind to glucocorticoid receptor in cellular cytoplasm
      b. Exogenous steroid binding activates the receptor by changing the transcription of target genes.
         1) Results in multiple anti-inflammatory actions, including blocking production and release of cytokines (e.g., interleukins and tumor necrosis factor) and inhibiting immunoglobulin E–dependent histamine release from basophils
         2) Cortisol, the endogenous glucocorticoid, is suppressed with the administration of exogenous glucocorticoid steroids.

Table 17.29

Opioid Antagonists

Generic Name	Route(s)	Half-life	Known Active Metabolites (Half-life)	Renal Dose Adjustment Recommended	Hepatic Dose Adjustment Recommended
Alvimopan	OC	10 to 17 hours	Amide hydrolysis metabolite (10 to 18 hours)	Yes	Yes
Methylnaltrexone	SC	8 hours	—	Yes	No
Naloxegol	OT	6 to 11 hours	—	Yes	Yes
Naloxone	IV	30 to 81 minutes	—	No	No
	IM or SC	—			
	Nasal spray	2.08 to 2.1 hours			
Naltrexone	OT	Biphasic: 3.9 to 10.3 hours for the first 24 hours, followed by 96 hours with continued therapy	—	Not studied in severe impairment	Not studied in severe impairment
	IV	5 to 10 days	6β-Naltrexol (5 to 10 days)		

IM, Intramuscular; *IV,* intravenous; *OC,* oral capsule immediate release; *OT,* oral tablet immediate release; *SC,* subcutaneous.

272**PART 4** • Management

2. Mineralocorticoids (Table 17.30)
   a. Bind to the mineralocorticoid receptors in the kidney, colon, salivary glands, sweat glands, and hippocampus
   b. The endogenous analogue, aldosterone, is converted to cortisone, which interacts with mineralocorticoid receptors, resulting in multiple physiological functions, predominantly effecting electrolyte and water homeostasis.
M. Serotonin agonists (Table 17.31)
   1. Agonists bind to serotonin 5-HT$_{1B}$ and 5-HT$_{1D}$ receptors located on the trigeminal nerve.
      a. Lead to inhibition of firing of serotoninergic neurons and reduction in the synthesis and release of serotonin
      b. Results in vasoconstriction of dural blood vessels

2. Serotonin syndrome, or serotonin toxicity
   a. Increased serotonergic activity within the CNS, which is often observed in the setting of therapeutic medication use, drug/drug interactions, or medication overuse
   b. Diagnosis is based on clinical symptoms, which can include mental status changes, neuromuscular abnormalities, or autonomic hyperactivity.
   c. Serotonin syndrome may result in mild symptoms or may lead to death.
   d. When developing a pain management plan for a patient, evaluation of current medications should occur to minimize risk.
   e. Medications that may precipitate serotonin syndrome are those that:
      1) Increase release of serotonin (e.g., amphetamines)

Table 17.30

Glucocorticoid Steroids

Generic Name	Route(s)	Half-life	Known Active Metabolites (Half-life)	Renal Dose Adjustment Recommended	Hepatic Dose Adjustment Recommended
Betamethasone	Topical cream, topical lotion, topical ointment, topical foam, topical spray, OS	5.6 hours		No	No[a]
Dexamethasone	OT, OS, IV, ophthalmic solution	1.88 to 2.23 hours		No	No[a]
Methylprednisolone	OT, IV	2 to 3 hours		No	No[a]
Prednisone	OT, OS, OER	2 to 3 hours	Prednisolone (2 to 4 hours)	No	No[a]
Triamcinolone	OT, IV, mucous membrane paste, nasal spray, topical cream, topical lotion, topical ointment, topical spray			No	Yes
	IV	88 minutes			
	Nasal spray	3.1 hours			

IV, Intravenous; *OER,* oral tablet/capsule extended release; *OS,* oral liquid solution; *OT,* oral tablet immediate release.

[a]Use caution, and individualize dosing based on other comorbidities.

Table 17.31

Mineralocorticoid Steroids

Generic Name	Route(s)	Half-life	Known Active Metabolites (Half-life)	Renal Dose Adjustment Recommended	Hepatic Dose Adjustment Recommended
Cortisone	OT	1 to 2 hours	Hydrocortisone	—	—
Fludrocortisone	OT	3.5 hours	—	No	No[a]
Hydrocortisone	OT, RS, IV, rectal cream and enema, topical cream, lotion, and ointment, otic solution	1 to 2 hours		No	Yes

IV, intravenous; *OT,* oral tablet immediate release; *RS,* rectal suppository.

[a]Use caution, and individualize dosing based on other comorbidities.

Table 17.32

Serotonin Agonists

Generic Name	Route(s)	Half-life	Known Active Metabolites (Half-life)	Renal Dose Adjustment Recommended	Hepatic Dose Adjustment Recommended
Almotriptan	OT	3 to 4 hours		Yes	Yes
Eletriptan	OT	4 to 5 hours		No[a]	Yes
Frovatriptan	OT	26 hours		No[a]	Yes
Naratriptan	OT	6 hours		Yes	Yes
Rizatriptan	ODT, OT	2 to 3 hours	*N*-monodesmethyl Rizatriptan	No[a]	No[a]

[a]Behm, L.B., & Leinum, C.J. (2018). *Overview of pain management pharmacology.* (Czarnecki & Turner, eds). Elsevier.

   2) Inhibit reuptake of serotonin (e.g., SSRIs, TCAs, tramadol, cyclobenzaprine)
   3) Inhibit serotonin metabolism (e.g., monoamine oxidase inhibitors [MAOIs])
  f. Patients should be provided education about potential side effects of prescribed medications and the importance of not starting other medications (such as, St. John's wort) without discussing it with their provider first.
N. Miscellaneous (Table 17.32)
  1. Tramadol
    a. Weakly binds to mu-opioid receptors
    b. Inhibits reuptake of norepinephrine and serotonin
    c. Monitor for serotonin syndrome.
    d. May increase risk of seizure activity
    e. Schedule IV controlled substance
  2. Tapentadol
    a. Binds mu-opioid receptors in CNS
    b. Causes inhibition of norepinephrine reuptake, modulating ascending pain pathway
    c. Schedule II controlled substance
  3. Ergot alkaloids
    a. Ergoloid mesylates, dihydroergotamine, and ergotamine tartrate
    b. Interacts with adrenergic, dopaminergic, and serotonin receptors. These serotonergic effects result in reversal of vasodilation and decrease in neurogenic inflammation.
    c. At therapeutic doses, they also produce peripheral vasoconstriction by stimulating alpha-adrenergic receptors.
    d. Commonly used as analgesic for management of vascular headaches
  4. Ziconotide
    a. An N-type calcium channel blocker, nonopioid
    b. Binds to N-type calcium channels on primary nociceptive afferent nerves in dorsal horn of spinal cord

    c. Derived from the venom of a marine snail (genus *Conus*)
    d. Available for intrathecal administration only
    e. FDA approved for treatment of persistent pain
    f. Prior authorization required and may be cost prohibitive.

VII. Pain Management Pharmacology in Special Populations

A. Older adults
  1. Physiological age-related impairments in older adults
    a. Absorption
      1) Increased gastric activity contributes to slower absorption in older adults.
      2) Decreased absorption
        a) Decreased intestinal blood flow
        b) Increased gastric emptying
        c) Decreased motility of gastrointestinal tract
    b. Distribution
      1) Medication remains in tissue longer and acts for longer duration due to:
        a) Decreased lean body mass
        b) Increased body fat (which increases volume of distribution of lipid-soluble medications)
        c) Decreased total body water volume (decreased volume of distribution for water-soluble medications leads to higher peak plasma concentrations)
        d) Decreased muscle and soft-tissue mass
      2) Protein-binding capacity of medications is influenced by nutritional status of older adults.
    c. Metabolism
      1) Decreased liver mass
      2) Decreased hepatic blood flow
      3) Decreased microsomal enzyme activity

Table 17.33

Medications to Avoid or Use Cautiously in Older Adults

Medication	Considerations
Opioids	
Meperidine	Oral meperidine has decreased analgesic efficacy due to first-pass metabolism. It may cause delirium and agitation postoperatively in older adults. The neurotoxic metabolite, normeperidine, can cause tremors, myoclonus, generalized seizures, confusion, and mood alterations in older adults, especially when renal impairment is present or patient has heart failure. Naloxone should not be given to treat normeperidine toxicity.
Pentazocine	Pentazocine causes hallucinations, dysphoria, delirium, and agitation in older adults.
Codeine	The dose of codeine needed for pain relief has increased incidence of side effects, such as nausea and constipation. Also, due to genetics, codeine is ineffective in many people.
Butorphanol	—
Nonsteroidal Anti-Inflammatory Drugs (Oral)	
Aspirin >325 mg/day Diclofenac Diflunisal Etodolac Fenoprofen Ibuprofen Indomethacin Ketoprofen Ketorolac (oral and parenteral) Meclofenamate Mefenamic acid Meloxicam Nabumetone Naproxen Oxaprozin Piroxicam Sulindac Tolmetin Tramadol	Gastrointestinal symptoms: Dyspepsia, nausea, vomiting, diarrhea, constipation, reflux, and ulcerations. Signs and symptoms in older adults may be insidious: light-headed, dizzy, fatigue, falls, delirium, low red blood cell count, and black tarry stools. Renal symptoms: A person may have subclinical symptoms. Signs of renal dysfunction range from an increase in creatinine clearance (CrCl) to acute renal failure. Sodium and water retention may occur, leading to bilateral lower extremity edema. When lower extremity edema occurs in older adults, renal and cardiac function should be evaluated. Hematological symptoms: Decreased platelet aggregation, which increases bleeding time. Aspirin binds with the platelet for the life of the platelet and can increase bleeding time for 2 to 3 weeks. Bone marrow depression from NSAIDs may occur, but it is rare. Central nervous system symptoms: Sedation, drowsiness, confusion, headache, depression, or psychosis. Aspirin may produce tinnitus. Hepatic symptoms: Elevated hepatic laboratory values. It is uncommon for NSAIDs to produce hepatitis or hepatic failure. Reduce dose in renal-impaired Immediate release: Reduce dose Extended release: Avoid
Antidepressants (Alone or in Combination)	
Amitriptyline Amoxapine Clomipramine Desipramine Doxepin >6 mg/day Imipramine Nortriptyline Paroxetine Protriptyline Trimipramine	May cause potent anticholinergic side effects, such as dry mouth (creating discomfort and risk of choking), constipation (creating discomfort and obstruction from fecal impaction), urinary retention, delirium, sedation, and orthostatic hypotension
Skeletal Muscle Relaxants	
Carisoprodol Chlorzoxazone Cyclobenzaprine Metaxalone Methocarbamol Orphenadrine	Have anticholinergic adverse effects, sedation, increased risk of falls, and fractures
Benzodiazepines	
Alprazolam Chlordiazepoxide Clonazepam Clorazepate Diazepam Estazolam Flurazepam Lorazepam Oxazepam Quazepam Temazepam Triazolam	Sedatives and hypnotics have a long duration of action. They increase potential for falls, fractures, cognitive impairment, and delirium in older adults.

NSAID, nonsteroidal anti-inflammatory drug.

4) Decreased medication clearance or elimination because of reduced hepatic blood flow and function of medication-metabolizing enzymes

5) Increased elimination half-life as a result of reduction of metabolic clearance

6) Decline in capacity of liver to break down and convert medications and their metabolites

d. Excretion and elimination is decreased because of:

1) Decreased glomerular filtration and tubular reabsorption rates, which may result in prolonged analgesic effects

2) Decreased creatinine clearance

3) Decreased renal mass and blood flow

4) Decreased clearance of medications can lead to longer elimination half-life (time it takes plasma concentration in bloodstream to be reduced by 50%).

5) Creatinine clearance (CrCl) may decrease in older adults, even though serum creatinine may not change.

   a) After 40 years of age, CrCl decreases 10% every 10 years.

   b) If CrCl decreases to <30 m/L min, excretion of medication decreases significantly. For renally eliminated medications, dose adjustment may be necessary when CrCl is <60 mL/min.

2. Pharmacological interventions

a. Acetaminophen is the preferred nonopioid for mild to moderate pain in older adults and may reduce need for opioids for acute pain.

1) Maximum daily doses are significantly lower in the elderly and frail older adults. The dose should be reduced 50% to 75% in older adults with reduced liver functions and a history of alcohol abuse.

2) Acetaminophen may mask the fever of infection.

3) Obtain information on over-the-counter and prescription medications to calculate total acetaminophen dose to avoid accidental overdose.

b. Topical anesthetics and analgesics may manage pain with fewer systemic adverse effects.

1) Lidocaine patch 5% may be used as adjuvant to relieve neuropathic pain.

2) Lidocaine 2.5%/prilocaine 2.5% can be used as a local anesthetic for venipuncture or accessing ports or arteriovenous fistulas.

3) Capsaicin cream effectiveness depends on pain type, distribution, and individual responses.

4) Topical NSAIDs (e.g., voltaten gel or cream) have fewer side effects compared to oral NSAIDs.

5) Topical corticosteroids: Long-term use may cause localized thinning of skin, which may further decrease integrity of an older adult's skin.

c. NSAIDs: Most oral NSAIDs should be avoided in older adults because of high risk of systemic adverse effects.

1) Celecoxib and ibuprofen can be used short term with gastroprotective agents and careful monitoring in those with no cardiovascular risk.

2) Misoprostol lessens risk of gastrointestinal bleeding but creates other issues related to its adverse effects and polypharmacy concerns (e.g., *C. difficile* infection, fractures).

3) Use topical NSAIDs for localized pain.

d. Adjuvants

1) Antidepressants are not recommended for older adults.

2) Anticonvulsants for neuropathic pain should be used with caution. Side effects include dizziness, drowsiness, and sedation. Should not be used if history of falls.

3) Corticosteroids

   a) Long-term use should be avoided.

   b) Use lowest dose for shortest effective time.

   c) Inhaled and topical forms are more localized and less systemic.

   d) Side effects may include hyperglycemia, weight gain, neuropsychiatric symptoms, osteoporosis, and increased risk of peptic ulcer disease or gastrointestinal issues.

e. Opioids

1) May be used for acute, cancer, and persistent pain severe enough to impact function and quality of life and not relieved with nonpharmacological interventions and other medications. Conduct risk/benefit analysis and discussion with patient and family regarding pain-relief goals.

2) Start low and go slow. Assess functional status.

3) Avoid in patients with history of falls or fractures.

4) Choose medications with short half-lives and fewer side effects, especially for opioid-naïve older adults. Start at 25% to 50% lower than standard adult dose and adjust doses slowly.

5) Use around-the-clock dosing instead of as needed for continuous pain, particularly in those with cognitive impairments or who are nonverbal.

6) Initiate or increase bowel regimen and continue to assess bowel function.

7) Assess for medication interactions. Minimize number of CNS-acting medications due to increased risk of falls.

8) Assess for any renal and hepatic impairment.

9) Consider long-acting analgesics only in those who are not opioid naïve with moderate to severe pain impacting function and/or quality of life.

10) Assess for opioid abuse, misuse, and diversion. Provide education to patient and family about physical dependence, tolerance, and substance use disorders.

3. Beer's criteria
   a. Evidence-based, graded tool developed by Mark H. Beers in 1991
   b. Continually used over the years by American Geriatrics Society
   c. Goals:
      1) Improve medication selection for older adults (at least 65 years old).
      2) Educate prescribers to avoid medication adverse effects.
      3) Help evaluate care quality.
      4) Determine medication use trends for older adults.
   d. Criteria:
      1) Include medications that should be typically avoided in older adults.
      2) Medications that should be avoided in older patients with certain conditions
      3) Medications that should be used with caution because of benefits that may offset risks, medication interactions, and changes in dosing based on kidney function
      4) Decisions on medication should take into account a variety of factors, including stopping medications when no longer beneficial.
   e. Key points for pain management pharmacology in older adults:
      1) Avoid tramadol use: risk of hyponatremia from syndrome of inappropriate antidiuretic hormone secretion.
      2) Avoid prescribing opioids with benzodiazepines or gabapentinoids due to increased risk of severe respiratory depression.
      3) NSAIDs and COX-2 inhibitors:
         a) Should not be used in older patients with heart failure; may be considered with caution in those with well-controlled heart failure
         b) NSAIDs: high rate of GI bleed in patient use for 3 to 6 months

B. Infants and children
   1. Safety and efficacy of medications are impacted by:
      a. Age and growth
         1) Neonate
            a) Birth to 1 month of age
            b) Principle that age and growth affect medication response is particularly important in neonatal period.
            c) In immediate postnatal period, medications given to mother may have been received by neonate via placenta.
            d) Medications may be transmitted from mother to baby via breast milk.
         2) Infant: 1 month to 1 year
         3) Child: 1 year to onset of puberty
         4) Adolescent: onset of puberty to adulthood
   b. Pharmacokinetics
      1) Absorption
         a) Gastrointestinal
            (1) Gastric emptying, which affects drug absorption, historically was thought to be prolonged in newborns and premature babies, reaching older child rates at 6 months. A recent meta-analysis on almost 1,500 patients between 29 weeks gestation and adulthood found the type of water, milk, and solid food to account for differences in gastric emptying rates more so than age.
            (2) Gastric acidity reaches adult levels by 12 years of age.
            (3) Breastfeeding (or feeding of expressed milk to) infants is contraindicated if mother is using illicit drugs (see exceptions for methadone use in supervised methadone program, below). Detailed information on specific medications and their safety in breast milk is available at Drugs and Lactation Database (LactMed) from the U.S. National Library of Medicine (NLM) at National Institutes of Health (NIH).
         b) Rectal: unpredictable
         c) Skin: Thickness of keratinized stratum corneum affects extent and rapidity of absorption. Newborns and infants have thinner keratinized stratum corneum, which may impact topical medication absorption.
      2) Distribution
         a) Water and fat composition
            (1) High body water and low plasma protein results in increased volume of distribution of water-soluble drugs in neonates and young infants. This results in need for higher doses of water-soluble drugs to attain desired affect.

(2) Low body fat may result in lower doses of lipid-soluble drugs in newborns.
b) Low plasma protein levels result in lower drug-binding capacity.
  (1) This is of particular significance for drugs that are highly protein-bound and also have narrow therapeutic index.
  (2) Concentrations of albumin and globulin are lower in newborns. By end of first year of life, they reach adult levels. Alpha-1-acid lipoprotein concentration is lower in newborns.
  (3) Fetal albumin has a lower affinity for drugs; therefore, dosing in premature infants is much lower because free or unbound drug is increased, resulting in higher total plasma concentration of active drug.
  (4) Protein binding is affected by presence of bilirubin, which can displace medications from binding to albumin, resulting in increase in "free" (active form) of drug. This can cause drug toxicity in neonates. Examples of drugs highly protein-bound include NSAIDS and diphenhydramine.
  (5) Lower protein binding in addition to larger body water in neonate results in increased volume of distribution of drugs in babies. The BBB in newborns is considered to be more permeable.
c) Distribution is generally decreased in neonates, particularly those that are premature. Distribution increases to adult values during first few months of life.
3) Metabolism/biotransformation
a) Cytochrome P450 enzyme system in term babies is about 50% of adult levels. Each activity (sulfation/oxidation, glycation/reduction and glucuronidation/conjugation) matures at different rates, so some drugs are effectively metabolized and others are poorly metabolized.
b) For most drugs, biotransformation is decreased in neonates, increases from 1 to 5 years of age, and then decreases after puberty to adult levels.
4) Renal excretion
a) GFR in the full-term newborn is approximately 10 to 20 mL at birth. At this age, kidneys are inefficient at drug

elimination, which leads to prolonged elimination half-lives of many drugs. Drugs with low therapeutic indices may exhibit toxic effects in neonates. GFR increases rapidly during first weeks of life and reaches adult levels at approximately 3 to 5 months.
b) Tubular secretion is low at birth, but capacity reaches adult values in 2 to 3 months.
c) Clearance of some drugs may be greater in infants compared to older children or adults due to disproportionate development of renal filtration and secretion in relation to reabsorption.
2. Pediatric pharmacologic interventions
a. Many medications used to treat pain in adults may be considered for use in children if dosed appropriately.
  1) Many analgesics used in adults are not approved for use in the pediatric population by the FDA.
  2) Children may require cardiac and respiratory monitoring not typically used for adults receiving the same analgesics, but this in no way replaces skilled assessments and observation by nursing staff in an inpatient setting.
b. Not all medications used in an inpatient setting are considered safe for home use, particularly for infants.
c. Pediatric patients are at increased risk (compared to adults) of experiencing harm from medications due to their weight (including incorrect weight estimates), body surface area, immature renal and hepatic function, difficulty in communicating adverse symptoms and pain severity, or associated symptoms.
d. Children with obesity present additional considerations for appropriate medication dosing, particularly those medications with narrow therapeutic windows.
  1) Recommended to dose many medications (e.g., dexmedetomidine, ketamine, lorazepam, midazolam, morphine) based on ideal body weight and titrate if needed
  2) Prescriber must always consider that per kg dose calculations should not exceed safe maximum doses for specific drug.
e. Use simplest and ideally least painful route to administer medications.
  1) Route selection
    a) Enteral
      (1) Always ask child or parent about child's preference for oral medications. Many children are not able to swallow pills and may require chewable tablets or liquid medication.

(2) When using liquid medication, the smallest volume possible is preferred. Caution should be used when placing liquid medications in formula; an infant or toddler may or may not consume in a timely fashion.

(3) If a tablet is safe to be crushed (e.g., not time-released or enteric-coated preparation), place it in a small volume of liquid (e.g., syrup) or soft food (e.g., pudding) immediately prior to administration.

b) IM injection: Should be avoided whenever possible. Most children will deny pain and suffer in silence rather than receive an IM injection. Alternate routes should be considered.

c) Intranasal: Many medications are irritating to nasal mucosa and have a bitter or unpleasant taste. This is not a common administration route for most medications, and care should be exercised when using with undesirable tastes or burning sensation, as next time the route is attempted, the child may vigorously protest.

d) Parenteral/IV

(1) Caution must be exercised with infants due to their prolonged elimination half-lives and potential for medication to accumulate and result in respiratory depression.

(2) PCA for opioid administration

(a) PCA has proven to be safe and effective in children when dosed correctly and with appropriate monitoring in place.

(b) Children with typical cognitive development tend to understand the concept of pushing a button to receive pain relief between 7 and 8 years of age.

(c) Children may require more instruction and reinforcement than adults to understand how to use a PCA pump. Younger children should be evaluated frequently for their understanding of correct use of PCA button, as they are at risk to receive either too much or too little pain medication if they do not understand the lag time between pushing PCA button and receiving pain relief.

(d) Advantages of PCA are the same in children as in adults (e.g.,

timely administration, lower doses, ability to titrate to effect).

(e) Basal (or continuous) infusions may be advantageous in younger children, who may not always remember to push PCA button when experiencing pain. However, continuous infusions place child at increased risk of opioid-induced sedation and respiratory depression. The Institute for Safe Medication Practices (ISMP) recommends continuous rates be used only with opioid-tolerant patients.

(f) Pulse oximetry is commonly used for monitoring pediatric patients.

(g) Although use of capnography is ideal, children may or may not tolerate the required nasal cannula.

(3) Authorized agent-controlled analgesia or parent/nurse-controlled analgesia

(a) This delivery technique is referred to as authorized agent-controlled analgesia (AACA) by the American Society of Pain Management Nursing (ASPMN).

(b) This delivery technique is beneficial for infants and children who are unable to understand the concept of PCA due to their age and/or developmental level. Nurses and parents must be formally educated and authorized to safely act as infant's or child's agent to deliver analgesic medication.

(c) Advantage of AACA is an infant or child who is not developmentally able to utilize PCA is not subjected to delays that occur when a parent has to call a nurse to bedside to medicate a child in pain. This avoids lag time of nurse obtaining opioids from a locked medication cabinet, finding another nurse for double-check process, and then returning with medication to bedside.

(d) Having anyone other than the patient push PCA button removes the inherent safety feature of PCA (e.g., if patients get sleepy from opioid, they stop pushing PCA button). When others, even if authorized, push PCA button for patient who is unable to do so, there is a risk sedation may not be noticed and opioids could continue to be administered, placing patients at increased risk for respiratory depression. This continues to be a topic of controversy in pediatrics; education and monitoring are key to safety.

(e) Some institutions continue to ban use of AACA by both nurses and parents, and some institutions allow only nurses and not parents to push PCA button. Many institutions have found AACA by nurses and parents to be safe and effective with appropriate education and monitoring.

(f) Not all parents opt to participate with AACA. For some parents, this responsibility is too stressful for them to assume, and for other parents, it offers a sense of control and satisfaction that they are able to help their child. Nurses and prescribers must assess parent(s)' comfort level before assigning this responsibility to parent.

(g) In one study of AACA, parents were not more satisfied with AACA than nurse-administered intermittent as-needed opioids.

(h) Refer to ASPMN position statement for additional information.

e) Rectal

(1) Similar to its use in adults, the rectal route provides variable absorption but can be useful when oral and IV routes are not available.

(2) Many children dislike use of suppositories. Use of rectal route is not appropriate in children who are victims of known or suspected sexual abuse.

(3) When using suppositories, dosing options are limited. Cutting a suppository in a quarter or half does not guarantee a quarter or half a dose because active drug may not be distributed evenly throughout suppository.

(4) Consult with pharmacy about options for using liquid

formulations rectally when no other route is available.

f) Sublingual

(1) Limited sublingual medications are available for children.

(2) Children are not likely to leave a bitter-tasting medication in their mouths long enough for sublingual absorption.

g) Transdermal

(1) Few medications are available in dosing low enough for children.

(2) Children must be observed to assure they are not placing hot or cold packs over a transdermal patch.

(3) A child who may pick or place patch in their mouth is not a candidate for transdermal patch unless access to patch can be restricted or child is in a closely observed setting.

f. Medications

1) This section is intended to augment previous content by discussing concepts specific to children as opposed to providing a comprehensive review of previous content.

2) See Dose Adjustment of Recommended Analgesics in Chronic Kidney Disease (Table 17.34).

3) Prescribers and clinicians must always weigh risks and benefits of individual medications.

4) Use of multimodal analgesia with or without regional techniques may lower dose, frequency, and duration of opioid requirements to manage children's pain.

5) Select medication classes.

a) Antidepressants

(1) The FDA joint advisory committee recommended a U.S. Black Box warning for all antidepressant drugs, indicating increased risk of suicidal thinking and behavior (suicidality) in pediatric patients and young adults (18 to 24 years of age) with major depressive disorder and other psychiatric disorders. Following this warning, antidepressant use sharply declined not just among children.

(2) Most antidepressant use in pediatrics is off-label for any indication.

(3) Children treated with antidepressants for any indication require close monitoring and observation for clinical worsening of depression, suicidality, and unusual behavior, especially for first 1 to 2 months of treatment or during periods of dose adjustment.

Table 17.34

Dose Adjustment of Recommended Analgesics in Chronic Kidney Disease (CKD)[a]

Drug (Applicable Population)	Kidney Function by GFR, mL/min/1.73 m²[b]	RECOMMENDED DOSING				DIALYZABILITY		
		Dose/Interval Adjustment	Initial (Maximum Dose)	Interval	Protein Binding (Molecular Weight)	Conventional HD	High-Permeability HD	PD
Methadone (C)[c]	>50	None	PO: 0.1 mg/kg (NA)	3 to 4 doses q 4 to 6 hr, then q 8 to 12 hr	85% to 90% (309.453 Da)	Not dialyzable	Unlikely, limited data	Not dialyzable
	30 to 50	Yes		No load, begin q 6 to 8 hr				
	29	No load, decrease frequency		No load, begin q 8 to 12 hr				
	<10 or HD or PD	No load, decrease frequency		No load, begin q 12 to 24 hr				
Oxycodone (I, C, A)[c]	≥50	None	PO: 0.05 to 0.1 mg/kg (<50 kg: 5 to 10 mg; ≥50 kg: 20 mg)	q 4 to 6 hr	38% to 45% (315.369 Da)	Give 50% of usual dose after dialysis	≥30%; give 50% of usual dose after dialysis	Give 50% of usual dose
	10 to 50	75% of usual dose	0.0375 to 0.75 mg/kg					
	<10	50% of usual dose	0.025 to 0.5 mg/kg					
Tramadol (≥17yr)[c,d]	>30	None	PO: 50 to 100 mg (400 mg/day)	q 4 to 6 hr	20% (263.381 Da)	Not dialyzable	≥30%: decrease frequency to q 12 hr, dose after dialysis	No data available
	<30	Decreased frequency	PO: 50 to 100 mg (200 mg/day)	q 12 hr				

A, adolescents; C, children; CRRT, continuous renal replacement therapy; eGFR, estimated glomerular filtration rate; GFR, glomerular filtration rate; HD, hemodialysis; I, infants; IM, intramuscular; IV, intravenous; NA, no accepted maximum dose; PD, peritoneal dialysis; PO, oral.

[a]Given the dynamic nature of pharmacology, consult pharmacology resources before prescribing medications. (All dosing from Lexicomp online and Aronoff's *Drug Prescribing in Renal Failure: Guidelines for Adults and Children.*)

[b]Use estimated eGFR to determine dosing of medications based on renal function. The eGFR is calculated by bedside Schwartz equation, where eGFR = (0.413 × height in cm)/(serum creatinine in mg/dL).

[c]Increase as tolerated to optimize pain relief; monitor vital signs.

[d]Immediate release.

From Reis A, Luecke C, Davis TK, Kakajiwala A. *J Pediatr Pharmacol Ther.* 2018 May/Jun; 23(3): 192–202.

Part 4

(4) Patient's family must be educated to closely observe patient and discuss any concerns with prescriber immediately.

(5) Tricyclic antidepressants are used off-label in pediatrics. Neither amitriptyline nor nortriptyline are approved for use in pediatric patients, however, nortriptyline is available as solution, which can be useful; for children who are not able to take tablets.

(6) SSRIs–associated behavioral activation, such as restlessness, hyperkinesis, hyperactivity, and agitation, is 2 to 3 times more likely in children compared to adolescents, and it is more common in adolescents than in adults. Vomiting is also more common in children and adolescents.

b) Select anticonvulsants
(1) Neuropsychiatric adverse events (e.g., behavioral problems), thought disorders (e.g., problems with concentration), and hyperkinesis (e.g., hyperactivity and restlessness) have been reported in clinical trials in children 3 to 12 years of age. Children with cognitive delays may be at increased risk for these adverse effects.

(2) Gabapentin remains first-line treatment for neuropathic pain given its overall safety profile.

(3) Topiramate is FDA-approved for preventive treatment of headaches in children 12 years of age and up.

(4) Pregabalin has been used in adolescents with fibromyalgia.

(5) Anticonvulsants can help reduce opioid use in postoperative pain in children.

c) Select benzodiazepines
(1) Benzodiazepines may have detrimental effects on brain development in children ≤3 years of age with repeated or lengthy exposure. This has been demonstrated in animal studies, and based on human clinical data, it is thought short exposures are not likely to have same negative consequences.

(2) Diazepam is commonly used to treat muscle spasms. Some dosage forms may contain benzyl alcohol or sodium benzoate/benzoic acid. Large amounts of benzyl alcohol

have been associated with potentially fatal toxicity in neonates.

(3) Lorazepam is often used to treat acute anxiety or insomnia in pediatric patients for a brief period, although its safety and efficacy have not been established for patients younger than 12 years of age.

(4) Midazolam is often used with procedural sedation given its quick onset and short duration of action.

d) Select general anesthetics
(1) Patients ≤3 years of age may be at risk with repeated or lengthy exposure to sedatives for detrimental effects on brain development. Multiple animal studies have shown detrimental effects on the developing brain. Studies in humans have shown cognitive and behavioral problems. Additional study and exploration are needed to ensure these findings are not due to patient's underlying conditions.

(2) Ketamine should not be used in infants ≤3 months of age or in any child with hydrocephalus due to concerns of apoptosis.

(3) Post-recovery agitation does not appear to be lessened by premedication with benzodiazepines as previously thought, and co-administration of ketamine and benzodiazepine increases airway events, including oxygen desaturation.

e) Acetaminophen/NSAIDs
(1) Oral formulations are available in multiple concentrations, and care must be taken to prevent dosing errors.

(2) Acetaminophen
(a) Acetaminophen is commonly administered in pediatric population. Parents must be cautioned that many over-the-counter preparations contain acetaminophen, which can lead to overdoses in home environment.

(b) Acetaminophen is eliminated more slowly in newborns due to slower GFR and tubular secretion compared to children and adults. It is necessary to lengthen interval between doses for preterm and term neonates ≤10 days of age.

(c) Safe maximum enteral doses:
1. Preterm 28 to 32 weeks: 40 mg/kg/day
2. 33 to 37 weeks or term neonates <10 days of life: 60 mg/kg/day
3. Term neonates ≥10 days of life: 75 mg/kg/day
4. Children and adolescent: 75 mg/kg/day or 4,000 mg/day

(d) IV acetaminophen
1. Should not be used for patients on a ketogenic diet, as premixed formulation from manufacturer contains 38.50 mg of carbohydrate per mL.
2. Experts do not recommend use of IV acetaminophen in infants <32 weeks post-menstrual age (PMA) until pharmacokinetic and pharmacodynamic studies are conducted in this age group.
3. Acetylsalicylic acid (ASA): Not recommended for children since a link was found between use of aspirin in children with respiratory or viral illness and development of Reyes syndrome.
4. Ibuprofen
(a) Commonly used in children. Product labeling is for infants 6 months of age and older.
(b) Studies comparing ibuprofen to oral morphine for children's home pain management demonstrated little difference in efficacy.
5. Ketorolac: There is no good evidence to support or reject the supposition that ketorolac is superior to other NSAIDs or that it is associated with serious side effects in treating pediatric pain following surgery.

f) Select opioids
(1) An infant's chronological age or days post-birth, not gestational age or number of weeks in utero, determines infant metabolism of opioids. Due to reduced albumin and alpha-1 glycoprotein concentrations, infants have an increased sensitivity to opioid CNS depressant effects.

(2) Codeine
(a) Codeine is not recommended in pediatric population due to life-threatening respiratory depression and death.
(b) In reported cases of respiratory depression and death following tonsillectomy and/or adenoidectomy, many children were found to be ultrarapid metabolizers of codeine due to CYP-450 2D6 polymorphisms.
(c) U.S. Black Box warning states codeine is contraindicated in pediatric patients <12 years of age and in any pediatric patient <18 years of age following tonsillectomy and adenoidectomy.
(d) A case report discusses death of a breast-fed neonate whose mother took codeine for episiotomy pain; mother was found to be an ultrarapid metabolizer.

(3) Fentanyl
(a) Transdermal administration is limited by child's weight, as patch cannot be trimmed to obtain dosing for small children. Approved by the FDA for use in children ≥2 years of age who have moderate to severe pain, are opioid tolerant, and are currently receiving opioids.
(b) No data are reported for infants whose dermal differences (skin thickness) may affect dosing.

(4) Methadone
(a) Single doses of methadone are frequently administered in operating room at start of procedures as part of multimodal analgesia protocols.
(b) If child is comfortable after initial dose or two of methadone, dose must be lowered or interval extended to avoid potential overdose.
1. If over-sedation occurs with initial dosing, methadone should be discontinued.
2. Half-life in children is 14 hours, with a range between 3.8 and 62 hours.

(c) Infants of mothers who are actively participating in a supervised methadone program (i.e., medication-assisted treatment for opioid use disorder) and negative for HIV and other illicit drugs may breastfeed according to Centers for Disease Control and Prevention (CDC) and American Academy of Pediatrics (AAP).

(5) Morphine
(a) Widely used in infants and children, and one of few opioids extensively studied in pediatric population
(b) Careful titration is required for infants <6 months of age. Starting doses for infants <6 months of age are often 25% of usual pediatric dose (0.05 to 0.1 mg/kg/dose).
(c) Morphine elimination half-life is significantly prolonged in preterm (and term) infants compared to children.
1. Infants <2 months of age have decreased rate of elimination due to decreased renal clearance and immature CYP450 system in liver.
2. Glucuronidation reaches adult levels between 2 and 6 months of age. Morphine-6-glucuronide has a very different ADME profile than does morphine and can put infants at increased risk for respiratory depression. Morphine and its metabolites present additional challenges in children receiving dialysis and are generally avoided.

(6) Oxycodone
(a) Pharmacokinetics of oxycodone have been found to be highly variable in patients <6 months of age, and risk of side effects may be greater in infants <2 months of age.
(b) Dosing for infants ≤6 months of age is typically 0.025 to 0.05 mg/kg enterally every 4 to 6 hours as needed. For infants >6 months and children, dosing recommendations increase to 0.1 to 0.2 mg/kg

(until adult dosing recommendations are reached) every 4 to 6 hours as needed.

g) Local anesthetics
(1) Bupivacaine and ropivacaine
(a) Bupivacaine and ropivacaine are both amides and metabolized by CYP450 enzymes in the liver, which accounts for some differences found between infants and older children and adults.
(b) Amide local anesthetics have diminished clearance in infants <3 months of age; clearance reaches adult levels at approximately 8 months of age.
(c) Pharmacokinetic studies in infants <6 months of age receiving bupivacaine infusions epidurally for >48 to 72 hours showed bupivacaine levels continued to increase at 48 to 72 hours, suggesting appropriately dosed infusion rates can result in toxicity if continued past 48 to 72 hours.
(d) Infants <30 days of age had slower clearance of ropivacaine and higher unbound drug than did those ≥30 days of age.
(2) Chloroprocaine
(a) Hydrolyzed primarily by plasma cholinesterases, which accounts for some differences between infants, children, and adults
(b) Chloroprocaine may be considered safer due to low risk of medication accumulation compared to amide local anesthetics such as bupivacaine and ropivacaine.
(c) Infusion rates studied in children 1 to 9 years of age demonstrated levels of unbound ropivacaine were stable and below toxic level.
(3) See Procedural Sedation chapter for information on topical local anesthetics and methemoglobinema.

Bibliography

Aarons, L., Sadler, B., Pitsiu, M., Sjovall, J., Henriksson, J., & Molnar, V. (2011). Population pharmacokinetic analysis of ropivacaine 2′6-pipecoloxylidide from pooled data in neonates, infants, and children. *British Journal of Anesthesia, 107*(3), 409–424.

Agins, A. (2003). Drug Interactions. *Orlando National Advanced Practice Conference*, p. 450, Orlando, Fl, USA.

American Geriatric Society. (2020). Beers criteria for inappropriate medication use in older patients: an update from the AGS. *Am Fam Physician, 101*(1), 56–57.

American Medical Association. (2018). AMA Opioid Task Force Helping Guide. https://www.end-opioid-epidemic.org.

American Pharmacists Association. (2020). *Pediatric and Neonatal Dosage Handbook*. Hudson, OH: Lexi-Comp.

American Society of Pain Management Nursing. (2018). Position paper on ethical pain management of the patient suffering from addictive disease. https://www.aspmn.org.

Anghelescu, D. L., Burgoyne, L. L., Oakes, L. L., & Wallace, D. A. (2005). The safety of patient-controlled analgesia by proxy in pediatric oncology patients. *Anesthesia and Analgesia, 101*(6), 1623–1627.

Atkinson, T. J., & Fudin, J. (2014). Interactions between pain medications and illicit street drugs. *Practical Pain Management, 14*(7).

Baxter, K. J., Hafling, J., Sterner, J., Patel, A. U., Giannopoulos, H., Heiss, K. F., & Raval, M. V. (2018). Effectiveness of gabapentin as a postoperative analgesic in children undergoing appendectomy. *Pediatric Surgery International, 34*(7), 769–774.

Beckman, E. J. (2017). Analgesia and sedation in hospitalized children in Sedation and Analgesia. *PedSAP 2017 Book, 3*, 7–30.

Behm, L.B., & Leinum, C.J. (2018). *Overview of pain management pharmacology*. (Czarnecki & Turner, eds). Elsevier.

Berde, C. B., Beyer, J. E., Bournaki, M. C., Levin, C. R., & Sethna, N. F. (1991). Comparison of morphine and methadone for prevention of postoperative pain in 3-to-7-year-old children. *The Journal of Pediatrics, 119*(1 pt 1), 136–141.

Berde, C. B., Sethna, N. F., Holzman, R. S., Reigy, P., & Gondek, E. J. (1987). Pharmacokinetics of methadone in children and adolescents in the perioperative period. *Anesthesiology, 67*, A519.

Bhatnagar, M., & Pruskowski, J. (2021). Opioid Equivalency. In *StatPearls [Internet]*. Treasure Island (FL): StatPearls Publishing. https://www.ncbi.nlm.nih.gov/books/NBK535402/.

Bland, C. M., Quidley, A. M., Love, B. L., Yeager, C., McMichael, B., & Bookstaver, P. B. (2016). Long-term pharmacotherapy considerations in the bariatric surgery patient. *American Journal of Health-System Pharmacy, 73*(16), 1230–1242.

Bosenberg, A. (2004). Pediatric regional anesthesia update. *Paediatric Anaesthesia, 14*, 398–402.

Bril, V., England, J., Franklin, G. M., Backonja, M., Cohen, J., Del Toro, D., & Zochodne, D. (2011). Evidence-based guideline: Treatment of painful diabetic neuropathy: Report of the American Academy of Neurology, the American Association of Neuromuscular and Electrodiagnostic Medicine, and the American Academy of Physical Medicine and Rehabilitation. *Neurology, 76*(20), 1758–1765.

Brubaker, L., Kendall, L., & Reina, E. (2016). Multi-modal Analgesia: a systematic review *of* local NSAIDs for non-ophthalmologic post-operative pain management. *International Journal of Surgery, 32*, 155–166.

Centers for Disease Control and Prevention. (2020). *Breastfeeding: contraindications*. Author. From www.cdc.gov.

Centers for Disease Control (2018). *CDC Guideline for Prescribing Opioids for Chronic Pain*. From www.cdc.gov/drugoverdose/prescribing/guideline.

Chin, M.L. (2019). Multimodal analgesia: Role of non-opioid analgesics. from https://www.asra.com/guidelines-articles/original-articles/article-item/legacy-b-blog-posts/2019/08.

Chou, R., Gordon, D. B., de Leon-Casasola, O. A., Rosenberg, J. M., Bickler, S., Brennan, T., … Wu, C. L. (2016). Management of postoperative pain: a clinical practice guideline from the American Pain Society, the American Society of Regional Anesthesia and Pain Medicine, and the American Society of Anesthesiologists' Committee on Regional Anesthesia, Executive Committee, and Administrative Council. *Journal of Pain, 17*(2), 131–157.

Claus, C. F., Lytle, E., Tong, D., Sigler, D., Lago, D., Bahoura, M., … Soo, T. E. (2019). The effect of ketorolac on posterior thoracolumbar spinal fusions: a prospective double-blinded randomised placebo-controlled trial protocol. *BMJ Open, 9*, e025855. doi:10.1136/bmjopen-2018-025855.

Cockcroft, D. W., & Gault, M. H. (1976). Prediction of creatinine clearance from serum creatinine. *Nephron, 16*(1), 31–41.

Cohen, M. R., Weber, R. J., & Moss, J. (2009). Patient-controlled analgesia: making it safer for patients. A continuing education program for pharmacists and nurses. *Institute for Safe Medication Practices*. https://www.ismp.org/prfdevelopment//PCAMonograph.pdf.

Cooney, M. F., Czarnecki, M. L., Dunwoody, C., Eksterowicz, N., Merkel, S., Oakes, L., & Whurman, E. (2013). Authorized agent controlled analgesia: ASPMN Position Statement Revision. *Pain Management Nursing, 14*(3), 176–181.

Cooney, M. F., & Quinlan-Colwell, A. (2021). *Assessment and multimodal management of pain. An integrative approach*. St. Louis, Missouri: Elsevier.

Cote, C. J., Lerman, J., & Anderson, B. J. (2013). *A practice of anesthesia for infants and children*. Philadelphia: Elsevier.

Culp, W. C., Jr., & Culp, W. C. (2011). Practical application of local anesthetics. *Journal of Vascular and Interventional Radiology, 22*(2), 111–118.

Czarnecki, M. L., Hainsworth, K., Simpson, P. M., & Weisman, S. J. (2015). Opioid administration for postoperative pain in children with developmental delay: parent and nurse satisfaction. *Journal of Pediatric Surgical Nursing, 4*(1), 15–27.

Dalal, P. G. (2015). The need to treat maternal pain in the breastfeeding mother: Are opioids safe? *Pain Medicine, 16*(4), 630–631.

Difference between ointment cream paste gel lotion Jelly. PharmaEducation. (2023, September 26). https://pharmaeducation.net/difference-between-ointment-cream-paste-gel/.

Deer, T. R., Smith, H. S., Cousins, M., Doleys, D. M., Levy, R. M., Rathmell, J. P., … Webster, L. R. (2010). Consensus guidelines for the selection and implantation of patients with noncancer pain for intrathecal drug delivery. *Pain Physician, 13*(3), E175–E213.

Eidelman, A. I., & Schanler, R. J. (2012). Section on breastfeeding. American Academy of Pediatrics policy statement: breastfeeding and the use of human milk. *Pediatrics, 129*(3), e827–e841.

Food and Drug Administration (2022). Buprenorphine: Drug Safety Communication - FDA warns about dental problems with buprenorphine medicines dissolved in the mouth to treat opioid use disorder and pain. From www.fda.gov/safety.

Food and Drug Administration (2018). FDA Safety Communication: FDA review results in new warnings about using general anesthetics and sedation drugs in young children and pregnant women. From www.fda.gov.

Green, C. J., & Tay, Y. C. (2016). Techniques in opioid administration. *Anesthesia & Intensive Care, 17*(9), 454–459.

Gudin, J. (2012). Opioid therapies and cytochrome P450 interactions. *Journal of Pain and Symptom Management, 44*(6S), S4–S14. http://dx.doi.org/10.1016/j.jpainsymman.2012.08.013.

Gudin, J., & Fudin, J. (2020). A narrative pharmacological review of buprenorphine: a unique opioid for the treatment of chronic pain. *Pain and Therapy, 9,* 41–54. https://doi.org/10.1007/s40122-019-00143-6.

Gudin, J., & Fudin, J. (2020). Peripheral opioid receptor antagonists for opioid-induced constipation: a primer on pharmacokinetic variabilities with a focus on drug interactions. *Journal of Pain Research, 13,* 447–456. https://doi.org/10.2147/JPR.S220859.

Hah, J. M., Bateman, B. T., Ratliff, J., Curtin, C., & Sun, E. (2017). Chronic opioid use after surgery: implications for perioperative panagement in the face of the opioid epidemic. *Anesthesia and analgesia, 125*(5), 1733–1740. https://doi.org/10.1213/ANE.0000000000002458.

Hale, T. W., & Rowe, H. E. (2017). *Medications & mother's milk: a manual of lactational pharmacology.* Springer Publishing Company.

Hunter, O. O., Wong, A., Leng, J., & Mariano, E. R. (2021). Educating nurses on intravenous lidocaine for postoperative pain management. *Pain Management Nursing, 22*(1), 94–99.

Ivani, G., & Mossetti, V. (2008). Regional anesthesia for postoperative pain control in children: focus on continuous central and perineural infusions. *Paediatric drugs, 10*(2), 107–114. https://doi.org/10.2165/00148581-200810020-00005.

Institute for Safe Medication Practices. (2009). *ISMP medication safety alert: beware of basal opioid infusions with PCA therapy.* Institute for Safe Medication Practices (ISMP). https://www.ismp.org/newsletters/acutecaare/articles/20090312.asp.

Jouguelet-Lacoste, J., La Colla, L., Schilling, D., & Chelly, J. E. (2015). The use of intravenous infusion or single dose of low-dose ketamine for postoperative analgesia: a review of the current literature. *Pain Medicine, 16*(2), 383–403.

Jungquist, C. R. (2018). Preventing opioid-induced respiratory depression in the hospitalized patient with obstructive sleep apnea. *Journal of PeriAnesthesia Nursing, 33*(5), 601–607.

Koren, G., Cairns, J., Chitayat, D., Gaedigk, A., & Leeder, S. J. (2006). Pharmacogenetics of morphine poisoning in a breastfed neonate of a codeine-prescribed mother. *The Lancet, 368*(9536), 704.

Knezevic, N. N., Tverdohleb, T., Knezevic, I., & Candido, K. D. (2018). The role of genetic polymorphisms in chronic pain patients. *International Journal of Molecular Sciences, 19*(6), 1707. doi:10.3390/ijms19061707.

Lancaster, R. J., Wren, K., Hudson, A., Leavitt, K., Albala, M., & Tischaefer, D. (2019). Intravenous lidocaine for chronic neuropathic pain: a systematic review addressing nursing care. *Pain Management Nursing, 21*(2), 194–200. https://doi.org/10.1016/j.pmn.2019.06.008.

Lee, C. S., Merchant, S., & Chidambaran, V. (2020). Postoperative pain management in pediatric spinal fusion surgery for idiopathic scoliosis. *Pediatric Drugs, 22*(6), 575–601.

Lembke, A., Ottestad, E., & Schmiesing, C. (2019). Patients maintained on buprenorphine for opioid use disorder should continue buprenorphine through the perioperative period. *Pain Medicine, 20*(3), 425–428. doi:10.1093/pm/pny019.

Lexicomp. (2016). *[Website].* Hudson, OH: Wolters Kluwer, Inc. Updated periodically.

Lundeberg, S. (2015). Pain in children—are we accomplishing the optimal pain treatment? *Pediatric Anesthesia, 25*(1), 83–92.

Mallinckrodt Pharmaceuticals. Acetaminophen prescribing information. Hazelwood, MO: Author.

Mattia, C., & Coluzzi, F. (2015). A look inside the association codeine-paracetamol: clinical pharmacology supports analgesic efficacy. *European Review for Medical and Pharmacological Sciences, 19*(3), 507–516.

McAnally, H. (2017). Rationale for and approach to preoperative opioid weaning: a preoperativeoptimization protocol. *Perioperative Medicine, 6*(19). https://doi.org/10.1186/s13741-017-0079-y.

McCarthy, G. C., Megalla, S. A., & Habib, A. S. (2010). Impact of intravenous lidocaine on postoperative analgesia and recovery from surgery: a systematic review of randomized control trials. *Drugs, 70*(9), 1149–1163.

McNichol, E. D., Rowe, E., & Cooper, T. E. (2018). Ketorolac for postoperative pain in children (Review). *Cochrane Database of Systematic Reviews, 7.* doi:10.1002/14651858.CD012294.pub2.

McPherson, M. L. (2019). *Demystifying opioid conversion calculations: a guide for effective dosing.* Bethesda, MD: American Society of Health-System Pharmacists.

Micromedex Healthcare Series. (2016). *[Internet database].* Greenwood Village, CO: Thomson Micromedex. Updated periodically. Retrieved from http://www.micromedexsolutions.com.

Mikhaeil, J., Ayoo, K., Clarke, H., Wąsowicz, M., & Huang, A. (2020). Review of the Transitional Pain Service as a method of postoperative opioid weaning and a service aimed at minimizing the risk of chronic post-surgical pain. *Anaesthesiology Intensive Therapy, 52*(2). doi: https://doi.org/10.5114/ait.2020.96018.

Muhly, W. T., Sankar, W. N., Ryan, K., Norton, A., Maxwell, L. G., DiMaggio, T., … Flynn, J. M. (2016). Rapid recovery pathway after spinal fusion for idiopathic scoliosis. *Pediatrics, 137*(4), e201515.

National Institute of Child Health and Human Development. (Internet). Drugs and Lactation Database (LactMed). Bethesda, MD. Retrieved December 29, 2022.

Neal, J. M., Woodward, C. M., & Harrison, T. K. (2017). The American Society of Regional Anesthesia and Pain Medicine Checklist for Managing Local Anesthetic Systemic Toxicity: 2017 Version. *Regional Anesthesia and Pain Medicine, 43*(2), 150–153.

Neal, J. M., Barrington, M. J., Fettiplace, M. R., Gitman, M., Memtsoudis, S. G., Mörwald, E. E., et al. (2018). The Third American Society of Regional Anesthesia and Pain Medicine Practice Advisory on Local Anesthetic Systemic Toxicity. *Regional Anesthesia and Pain Medicine, 43*(2), 113–123.

Obaid, M., Kaye, A. D., Kaye, A., Belani, K., & Urman, R. D. (2017). Emerging roles of liposomal bupivacaine in anesthesia practice. *Journal of Anaesthesiology: Clinical Pharmacology, 33*(2), 151–156.

Pokela, M. L., Seppala, T. S., & Olkkola, K. T. (2005). Marked variation in oxycodone pharmacokinetics in infants. *Pediatric Anesthesia, 15,* 560–565.

Poonai, N., Datoo, N., Cashin, M., Drendel, A., Shu, R., Lepore, N., … Bartley, D. (2017). Oral morphine versus ibuprofen at home for postoperative orthopedic pain in children: a randomized controlled trial. *Canadian Medical Association Journal, 189,* E1252–E1258. doi:10.1503/CMAJ.170017.

Quinlan, J., Rann, S., Bastable, R., & Levy, N. (2019). Perioperative opioid use and misuse. *Clinical medicine (London, England), 19*(6), 441–445. https://doi.org/10.7861/clinmed.2019.0227.

Reis, A, Luecke, C., David, T. K., & Kakajiwala, A. (2018). Pain management in pediatric chronic kidney disease. *Journal of Pediatric Pharmacology and Therapeutics, 23*(3), 194–195.

Ross, E. L., Mixon, M. A., Valdez, & Reiter, P. D (2015). Development of recommendations for dosing of commonly prescribed medications in critically ill obese children. *American Journal Health System Pharmacy, 72*(7), 542–556.

Rowbotham, D. J., & McIntrye, P. E. (2003). *Clinical pain management: acute pain*. London: Arnold.

Schecter, N. L., Berde, C. B., & Yaster, M. (2003). *Pain in infants, children, and adolescents*. Baltimore: Lippincott Williams & Wilkins.

Schwenk, E. S., Viscusi, E. R., Buvanendran, A., Hurley, R. W., Wasan, A. D., Narouze, S., … Cohen, S. P. (2018). Consensus guidelines on the use of intravenous ketamine infusions for acute pain management from the American Society of Regional Anesthesia and Pain Medicine, the American Academy of Pain Medicine, and the American Society of Anesthesiologists. *Regional Anesthesia and Pain Medicine, 43*(5), 456–466. doi:10.1097/AAP.0000000000000806.

Seth, P. L. (1993). Percutaneous absorption of ibuprofen from different formulations. Comparative study with gel, hydrophilic ointment and emulsion cream. *Arzneimittelforschung, 43*(8), 919–921. PMID: 8216453.

Stewart, C. F., & Hampton, E. M. (1987). Therapy Review: effect of maturation on drug disposition in pediatric patients. *Clinical Pharmacy, 6*, 548–564.

The Joint Commission on Accreditation of Healthcare Organizations. (2004). Patient controlled analgesia by proxy. Sentinel Event Alert, Issue 33. https://www.jointcommission.org/sentinel_event_alert_issue_.33_patient_controlled_analgesia_by_proxy/.

Trevena, Inc. (2020). Olinvyk package insert. https://olinvyk.com/docs/OLINVYK_Final_Label_Ver%20002_Nov2020_1103.pdf.

Trofimovitch, D., & Baumrucker, S. J. (2019). Pharmacology update: Low-dose naltrexone as possible nonopioid modality for some chronic, nonmalignant pain syndromes. *American Journal of Hospice & Palliative Care, 36*(10), 907–912. doi:10.1177/1049909119838974.

Urits, I., Viswanath, O., Orhurhu, V., Gress, K., Charipova, K., Kaye, A. D., & Ngo, A. (2019). The utilization of mu-opioid receptor biased agonists: Oliceridine, an opioid analgesic with reduced adverse effects. *Current Pain and Headache Reports, 23*(5), 31. doi:10.1007/s11916-019-0773-1.

UpToDate. (2016). *[Website]*. Hudson, OH: Wolters Kluwer Inc. from. http://www.uptodate.com/.

Usach, I., Martinez, R., Festini, T., & Peris, J. E. (2019). Subcutaneous injection of drugs: Literature review of factors influencing pain sensation at the injection site. *Advance Therapuetics, 36*(11), 2986–2996. doi:10.1007/s12325-019-01101-6. Epub 2019 Oct 5. PMID: 31587143; PMCID: PMC6822791.

U.S. Food and Drug Administration. (2016). FDA blueprint for prescriber education for extended-release and long-acting opioid analgesics. From http://www.accessdata.fda.gov/drugsatfda_docs/rems/ERLA_opioids_2016-04-26_FDA_Blueprint.pdf.

U.S. Department of Justice. (2016). Controlled substance schedules. from http://www.deadiversion.usdoj.gov/schedules/.

U.S. Department of Health and Human Services. (2019). *Pain Management Best Practices Inter-Agency Task Force Report: Updates, Gaps, Inconsistencies, and Recommendations*. U.S. Department of Health and Human Services from website: https://www.hhs.gov/ash/advisory-committees/pain/reports/index.html.

Vadivelu, N., Mitra, S., Schermer, E., Kodumudi, V., Kaye, A. D., & Urman, R. D. (2014). Preventive analgesia for postoperative pain control: a broader concept. *Local and Regional Anesthesia, 7*, 17–22.

Van den Anker, J., Reed, M., Allegaert, K., & Kearns, G. (2018). Developmental changes in pharmacokinetics and pharmacodynamics. *The Journal of Clinical Pharmacology, 58*((Suppl) 10), S10–S25. doi:10.10021/jcph.1284.

Vyas, D., Quinones Cardona, V., Carroll, A., Markel, C., Young, M., & Fleishman, R. (2022). Standardized Scoring Tool and Weaning Guideline to Reduce Opioids in Critically Ill Neonates. *Pediatric quality & safety, 7*(3), e562. https://doi.org/10.1097/pq9.0000000000000562.

Voepel-Lewis, T., Marinkovic, A., Kostrezewa, A., Tait, A.R., & Malviya, S. (2008). The presence of and risk factors for adverse events in children receiving patient-controlled analgesia by proxy or patient-controlled analgesia after surgery. *Anesthesia and Analgesia, 107*(1), 70–75.

Walker, S. M. (2015). Pain after surgery in children: clinical recommendations. *Current Opinion in Anesthesiology, 28*(5), 570–576.

Weingarten, T. N., Jacob, A. K., Njathi, C. W., Wilson, G. A., & Sprung, J. (2015). Multimodal analgesic protocol and postanesthesia respiratory depression during phase 1 recovery after total joint arthroplasty. *Regional Anesthesia and Pain Medicine, 40*(4), 330–336.

Wolkerstorfer, A., Handler, N., & Buschmann, H. (2016). New approaches to treating pain. *Bioorganic & Medicinal Chemistry Letters, 26*(4), 1103–1119.

CHAPTER 18
Cannabinoids for Pain Management

Marian Wilson, PhD, MPH, RN, PMGT-RN
Tracy Klein, PhD, ARNP, FAAN, FAANP
Maureen F. Cooney, DNP, FNP-BC, ACHPN, AP-PMN*

This chapter provides information necessary to understand cannabis use within the context of pain management. Persistent pain is a common condition reported by patients for the medical use of cannabis. The state of science to date on cannabis for pain, its pharmacokinetics and pharmacodynamics, aspects of law, policy, and nursing education are covered. Principles of assessment, screening, and treatment are outlined, including recommendations for shared decision-making regarding cannabis for pain management and screening for cannabis use disorder, cannabis withdrawal, and adverse effects. Content is based on nursing's ethical principles, guidelines from expert authorities, and available research evidence.

I. Cannabis Overview

A. Cannabis sativa (cannabis)
 1. Cannabis sativa is a plant with a complicated molecular profile used medicinally for thousands of years.
 2. Other commonly used terms are marijuana or hemp, the latter of which is a variety grown for industrial use.
B. More than 700 varieties of cannabis exist and are made up of numerous compounds, including 100 different cannabinoids, which are responsible for medical effects.
 1. Cannabinoids are fatty compounds found in cannabis, other plants, and humans.
  a. Endogenous cannabinoids ("endocannabinoids") are present naturally within human body and likely have natural role in pain modulation.
  b. Exogenous cannabinoids are those that are administered in either synthetic or plant-based products.
  c. Both types of cannabinoids interact with cannabinoid receptors present in what is known as the body's endocannabinoid system.

2. Cannabidiol (CBD) and Δ^9-tetrahydrocannabinol (THC) are best-known cannabinoids and are also identified in highest concentrations in cannabis.
 a. CBD is typically described as "nonpsychoactive" endocannabinoid, although its true effects in the body are widespread and poorly defined.
 b. CBD was originally identified in the 1940s.
 c. CBD may be protective against some of psychoactive and cognitive negative effects of THC when used concurrently.
3. THC produces main psychoactive effects of cannabis, which may include paranoia, perceptual and cognitive alterations, and anxiety.
 a. Its structure was identified in the 1960s, leading to development of synthetic THC for medicinal use. In 1985, pharmaceutical companies received approval to begin developing THC preparations (e.g., dronabinol and nabilone) for therapeutic use, and as a result, cannabinoids were reintroduced into the armamentarium of willing healthcare providers.
 b. Products such as dronabinol were approved for treating chemotherapy-induced nausea and vomiting and weight loss.
 c. Hemp products contain low to no THC.
C. To date, there is total of over 550 compounds in addition to 100 cannabinoids isolated from cannabis.
 1. Science is still emerging regarding how CBD and THC interact with other substances present in cannabis, particularly if used for medical purposes.
 2. The entourage effect recognizes synergy among various cannabis components.
  a. Terpenes are aromatic compounds that create characteristic scent of many plants.
  b. More than 150 terpenes have been identified in cannabis plants.
   1) Positive contribution of terpenes to other cannabis plant ingredients has been called the entourage effect.
   2) Terpenes contribute to flavor and smell of cannabis; they vary considerably from plant to plant.

---

*Section Editor for the chapter.

3) Myrcene, α-pinene, limonene, and linalool are some identified terpenes.
4) Terpenes may have anti-inflammatory properties.

c. Synergy between terpenes and cannabinoids may have medical benefits; this needs additional research.

II. Cannabis Pharmacology

A. Endocannabinoid system

1. Endocannabinoid system is widespread neuromodulatory network.

   a. Consists of endogenous cannabinoids (endocannabinoids), cannabinoid receptors, and enzymes responsible for synthesis and degradation of endocannabinoids
   b. Cannabinoids, whether endogenous or exogenous, act on cannabinoid receptors to regulate physiologic, behavioral, immunologic, and metabolic functions.
   c. Recognized as an endogenous pain control pathway
   d. Key role is resolving pain through mechanisms including sensory, emotional, and cognitive aspects of pain.

2. Cannabinoid receptors are located on cell plasma membranes and in intracellular compartments in endoplasmic reticulum.

   a. CB_1 and CB_2 are distinct G protein–coupled receptors with unique locations and functions.
   b. While CB1 and CB2 are best-known types of cannabinoid receptors, many subcategories exist.
   c. Receptors are located throughout body, including brain, skin, and peripheral tissues.
   d. This complexity accounts for potential medical effects still being discovered and confirmed.

B. Pharmacokinetics (movement of drug through body)

1. Vary based on formulation, route of administration, and patient-specific factors
2. Lack of standardization in retail market makes it challenging to predict patient effects.
3. Choice of product and administration method depends on patient preference and treatment goals.

   a. Individuals report using cannabis for sleep disturbance, depressive symptoms, anxiety, and posttraumatic stress disorder.
   b. Majority of adults think cannabis provides pain relief.

4. Cannabis can be classified as THC dominant, CBD dominant, or THC/CBD intermediate.

   a. THC dominant is defined as 5:1 ratio of THC to CBD.
   b. CBD dominant is 1:5 ratio of CBD to THC.
   c. Intermediate is 0.2:1 THC/CBD.

5. Absorption is much slower with oral cannabis.

   a. Mean concentration levels are reached in 1 to 3 hours but are variable depending on delivery agent and patient-specific variation.
   b. Oral formulations may be preferred when symptom relief is required over longer time.

6. Bioavailability varies depending on administration routes.

   a. Absorption can vary as much as 20% to 30% with oral products and 10% to 60% with inhaled products.
   1) Smoking cannabis produces a rapid high with short duration of effect.
   2) Oral route has resulted in many emergency room admissions.
      a) Edible products have delayed onset, much greater long-term potency, and longer duration.
      b) Because it takes longer to feel the impairing effects of oral products, overconsumption of THC occurs; this scenario creates serious risk for impairment.

   b. Smoking is most common route of cannabis administration.
   1) Smoking onset of effects is rapid (within 3 to 10 minutes).
   2) Bioavailability when smoking can range from 10% to 35%.
   3) Using vaporizer to administer cannabis avoids respiratory risks associated with smoking yet has comparable pharmacokinetics.

   c. Both THC and CBD are highly lipophilic, and bioavailability can be increased by administration in an oil preparation; cannabinoids may accumulate in adipose tissue.

7. Miscellaneous factors affecting cannabis metabolism, absorption, and response include:

   a. Organ tissue and liver function differences
   b. Recent meals ingested
   c. Depth of inhalation and breath holding with smoking
   d. Comorbid conditions
   e. Cannabis use history
   1) Cannabis-naïve people may experience stronger initial effects.
   2) Tolerance is likely and anticipated with long-term cannabis use; reduced response over time may require higher doses for same effect.
   3) Periodic drug holidays of 48 hours will reduce tolerance and allow for lowering of therapeutic dose needed to extend effects of THC-containing products.

8. Drug interactions can lead to variations in pharmacokinetics.
   a. Due to THC and CBD being metabolized in liver, potential exists for drug-drug interactions related to interference with hepatic enzymes.
   b. CBD potentially interacts with various cytochrome P450 (CYP450) enzymes involved in drug metabolism, which raises concerns about possible drug-drug interactions.
      1) Immunosuppressants, chemotherapy drugs, antiepileptics, antidepressants, opioids, and antipsychotics are examples of medications having metabolic drug-drug interactions with cannabis.
      2) Numerous potential interactions are listed for FDA-approved synthetic cannabis products (Table 18.1).
C. Pharmacodynamics (what drug does to body)
   1. Pharmacodynamics of cannabis products are varied and remain under study.
   2. Relative to pain symptom management, cannabis products may influence a number of pain and pain-related symptoms.
   3. Cannabinoid receptors are present at all levels of pain processing, including regions involved with pain transduction, transmission, perception, and modulation.
   4. Activation of CB_1 and CB_2 receptors results in inhibition of pain transmission and blocking detection of pain signals.
   5. Cannabinoids are thought to influence pain pathway by acting simultaneously on multiple pain targets within both peripheral and central nervous systems.
      a. In periphery:
         1) CB_1 receptors are found in peripheral sensory nerve endings, and both CB_1 and CB_2 are in dorsal root ganglion.

   2) CB_2 receptors are predominantly located in immune cells and in periphery and much less present in central nervous system compared to CB_1 receptors.
   3) CB_2 receptors regulate immune responses and inflammatory pathways throughout body.
   b. In spinal cord:
      1) CB_1 receptors are found in dorsolateral funiculus, in surroundings of central canal, and in superficial dorsal horn.
      2) CB_2 is expressed on glial cells restricted to lumbar spinal cord, on some neurons within brainstem, and on glial cells in cerebellum and cortex.
      3) When cannabinoids activate CB receptors in spinal cord, pain signals are unable to be transmitted, and behavioral responses to noxious stimuli (i.e., pain) are suppressed.
      4) In supraspinal sites, CB_1 receptors are found in areas of brain involved in pain processing, perception, and modulation (e.g., thalamus, amygdala, periaqueductal gray matter, hypothalamus, and cerebellum).
   c. Persistent neuropathic pain can be treated, in part, with inhibition of descending supraspinal pain pathways via the endocannabinoid system.
   d. Expression of CB_1 receptors in brainstem cardiorespiratory control center is very low compared to opioids, resulting in little risk of respiratory depression and no known overdose deaths with overuse or misuse.
D. Impact of cannabinoids on pain
   1. Because pain is a multidimensional experience, it is thought cannabinoids assist pain relief by acting on correlated symptoms. Analyses of prescription data from Medicare Part D enrollees in states with medical access to cannabis suggest significant reduction in prescriptions of conventional pain medications.

Table 18.1

U.S. FDA-Approved Cannabis-Derived Products

Generic	Brand Name	Active Ingredient	Approved Indications	Severe Adverse Effects
Nabilone	Cesamet	Synthetic THC	Refractory chemotherapy-induced emesis in adults	Seizures, angioedema[a]
Dronabinol	Marinol	Synthetic THC	Refractory chemotherapy-induced nausea and vomiting; anorexia associated with weight loss in AIDS	Bradycardia, seizures[a]
Cannabidiol	Epidiolex	Purified CBD	Two rare and severe forms of epilepsy in children	Liver injury, suicide attempt[b]

[a]Prescribers' Digital Reference (PDR), 2021.

[b]U.S. Food and Drug Administration, 2018.

AIDS, acquired immune deficiency syndrome; *CBD*, cannabidiol; *THC*, Δ⁹-tetrahydrocannabinol.

2. Analgesic effects from cannabinoids result from inhibition of release of neurotransmitters and neuropeptides from presynaptic nerve endings, modulation of postsynaptic neuron excitability, and reduction of neural inflammation.

3. CB_2 receptors may contribute to pain relief by modulating dopamine release as well as by acting on opioid and serotonin receptors that can assist with mood and opioid withdrawal symptoms.

4. Some evidence supports cannabinoids target affective aspects of pain, inducing anti-anxiety effects and reducing negative affect. Therefore, its use may improve perception of pain and coping.

5. Moderate evidence suggests that cannabinoids are effective in improving short-term sleep outcomes in patients with persistent pain.

6. THC has well-known effects on thoughts and on emotions mediated through endocannabinoid system that can indirectly influence pain.

E. Adverse effects associated with cannabis

1. Cannabis side effects can be dose limiting (e.g., patient may need to try different ratios of THC/CBD).

2. Adverse effects can be attributed mainly to THC that can cause psychoactive adverse events depending on dose and person's previous tolerance.

a. Acute marijuana intoxication can result in neuropsychiatric symptoms, including agitation, psychosis, and anxiety.

b. Other psychological side effects reported include mania, euphoria, dysphoria, suicidal ideation, schizophrenia, mood disorders, depression, panic attacks, paranoia, and cognitive alterations. Neuropsychiatric symptoms such as agitation, psychosis, and anxiety may be managed with benzodiazepines.

c. Other mental health conditions can worsen with cannabis use.

3. Most common adverse effects attributed to CBD-only products include elevated liver enzymes, somnolence, sedation, fatigue, dizziness, sleep disturbance, diarrhea, decreased appetite, and infections.

4. Cannabis hyperemesis syndrome has been identified as a gut-brain axis disorder characterized by episodic nausea and vomiting worsened by cannabis intake.

a. Strict criteria for diagnosis is lacking, although it is associated with long-term or increased cannabis use and is generally found among adults.

b. Presentation includes severe, cyclic nausea; intractable vomiting; and compulsively taking hot showers or baths for relief.

c. While general gastrointestinal symptoms respond to antiemetics, antiemetics may be ineffective for hyperemesis syndrome.

d. Volume depletion with acute kidney injury has been reported.

e. Cessation of cannabis use is most effective.

5. Cannabis use has been associated with alterations in cognition, including learning, memory, and attention. Reaction time, information processing, and motor coordination can be depressed or impaired depending on dose and type of cannabis used.

6. Substantial evidence shows long-term cannabis smoking worsens respiratory symptoms and results in more frequent chronic bronchitis episodes.

7. Cannabis use disorder (CUD) is a diagnosable mental health disorder recognized by *Diagnostic and Statistical Manual of Mental Disorders, Fifth Edition* (*DSM-5*) and defined as a problematic pattern of cannabis use.

a. Specific criteria must be met, such as social and behavioral impairments, cravings, and physiological adaptation.

b. Adults with pain are more vulnerable to adverse cannabis use outcomes such as CUD.

c. In 2019, CUD was most common substance use disorder, affecting approximately 4.4 million people aged 12 or older in the United States, or 1.6% of U.S. adult population.

1) About 9.3% of those using cannabis meet diagnostic criteria for CUD.

2) Younger age is associated with greater risk of CUD.

3) Pain is risk factor for developing CUD.

d. Currently, no FDA-approved medications exist to treat CUD, and scant evidence supports use of any specific medications.

1) Moderate evidence suggests antidepressants do not reduce cannabis use or improve abstinence.

2) Cognitive behavioral therapy and motivational enhancement therapy with abstinence-based incentives provide the most effective improvements to date for CUD.

3) Research is needed to explore interventions for CUD in context of pain conditions.

8. Cannabis withdrawal syndrome is diagnostic indicator of CUD.

a. Cannabis withdrawal, although not life threatening, can be unpleasant.

b. Occurs among nearly half of all adults who use cannabis regularly, including those using cannabis for pain.

c. Regular intake of cannabis is thought to down-regulate CB_1 receptors, resulting in mood and behavioral symptoms.

d. Commonly reported withdrawal symptoms are sleep difficulties, irritability, depressed mood, and anxiety.

e. More severe withdrawal symptoms have been associated with increased severity of CUD, younger adults with mental health problems, smoking cannabis, female sex, longer history of use, and greater frequency of use.

f. Withdrawal symptoms start to decrease within 48 hours for most patients, and CB_1 receptors return to normal function within 4 weeks of abstinence.

F. Specific population considerations
   1. Adolescents
      a. Thirty-three percent (33%) of all eighth-, tenth-, and twelfth-graders report lifetime cannabis use.
      b. Initiation of cannabis use in adolescence has been associated with later CUD.
      c. Use of high THC content, such as concentrates for nonmedical use, has been linked to higher risk of substance use problems in adolescents.
      d. Insufficient research is available to evaluate medical use of cannabis for approved conditions by adolescents. Concerns exist regarding use initiated in adolescence while brain development is still occurring.
   2. Pregnancy considerations
      a. Insufficient human subject research exists regarding fertility and neonatal effects.
      b. While harms of THC fetal exposure have been reported in observational studies, there is absence of published literature regarding CBD use and long-term use of THC during pregnancy.
      c. THC can cross placenta and is excreted in human breast milk, risking toxicity to the developing brain.
      d. Exposure to cannabis in utero is associated with an increased risk of decreased birth weight.
      e. Prenatal exposure is linked to higher odds of newborn being placed in neonatal intensive care unit.
   3. Older adults
      a. Have increased risks of adverse effects with cannabis use
      b. Polypharmacy increases risk due to known interactions with cannabis and pharmaceuticals, including when cannabis is used concurrently with other central nervous system–depressant drugs.
      c. Drugs with known cardiac toxicity (e.g., amphetamine, cocaine, and atropine) taken with cannabis provide additive hypertension and tachycardic effects.

d. Increased cognitive vulnerability in older adults can lead to increased risk of sedation and subsequent falls.

e. Individuals with renal or hepatic conditions have additional adverse risks related to pharmacokinetic changes that can occur as renal and liver function declines. This risk is more common in older adults.

   4. Alternatives to cannabis should be considered, particularly in medically complex patients.
   5. Inhaled cannabis is not recommended when preexisting conditions of asthma, bronchitis, emphysema, or any pulmonary disease are known.

III. Current Evidence Surrounding Cannabis and Pain

A. Evidence may exist for using cannabis to treat the following conditions (limited to certain populations, symptoms, formulations, routes, and dosages):
   1. Cachexia
   2. Chemotherapy-induced nausea and vomiting
   3. Pain (from cancer or rheumatoid arthritis)
   4. Persistent pain (fibromyalgia): only modest reduction found
   5. Neuropathies
   6. Spasticity
   7. Reduction of posttraumatic stress disorder nightmares

B. Evidence for pain efficacy
   1. Most common reasons adults report medical cannabis use are pain, anxiety, and depression/mood.
   2. Strongest evidence to date is for neuropathic pain where blinded and controlled studies are available, yet high-quality evidence remains lacking.
      a. A review of 16 studies involving 1,750 adults with persistent neuropathic pain, pain intensity, sleep disturbance, and psychological distress showed improvement with use of THC-containing cannabis products.
      b. Potential benefits may still be outweighed by potential harms.
   3. Canadian Pain Society revised their statement in 2014 to recommend cannabinoids as third-level therapy for persistent neuropathic pain, while acknowledging sufficient quality research is lacking.
   4. In majority of animal studies, CBD is shown to act as analgesic; however, human studies show conflicting results.

C. Cannabis and mental health comorbidities
   1. Mental health conditions are among more commonly studied pain comorbidities in available cannabis research.

2. Cannabis use is associated with lack of improvement in mental health symptoms.
3. Major depressive disorder is risk factor for problematic cannabis use, and frequency of cannabis use is linked to developing CUD.
4. Mood disorders are common in people with persistent pain. Research has demonstrated for some people with persistent pain, opioid and cannabis co-use is associated with elevated anxiety and depression symptoms.
5. Cannabis use may be higher among people with higher levels of anxiety, depression, and suicidal ideation.
6. Addictive disorders:
   a. Insufficient evidence exists to support cannabinoids as an effective treatment for achieving abstinence from addictive substances.
   b. With opioid overdose deaths increasing, cannabis has been suggested as potential harm-reduction strategy (by being used as substitute for opioids).

IV. Issues Surrounding Cannabis Research

A. Limitations of available data need to be addressed to build confidence in evidence regarding cannabis for pain.
   1. High-quality research has been limited by regulations and policies restricting access to cannabis products for research purposes.
   2. Inability to conduct robust randomized controlled trials with available cannabis varieties limits ability to evaluate both potential usefulness and harms.
      a. Lack of standardization in cannabis dosing, products, and administration complicates ability to formulate conclusions with recommendations for clinical practice.
      b. One obstacle to cannabis research is inability to easily blind study participants to effects of THC.
      c. Added challenge specific to pain research is multiple pain types and pain pathways along with comorbid symptoms, such as depression, anxiety, and sleep disturbances.
   3. Much of available cannabis research is lower-level evidence, such as cohort, observational studies.
      a. Problems with low-quality studies include confounding variables, heterogeneity of cannabis products, and variety in type and severity of pain conditions.
      b. Small samples and studies of short duration are also noted as limitations to high-quality evidence regarding cannabis use for pain, along with modest reported effects.

   c. Variability in research methodology limits available knowledge regarding safety and efficacy of cannabis in medical conditions.
   4. According to National Academies of Sciences, Engineering, and Medicine (NASEM) (2017), funding bias has been noted whereby more funding has gone toward finding harms of cannabis versus therapeutic effects.
   5. Long-term safety on cannabis for pain is poorly studied; questions about hyperalgesia and tolerance are unanswered.
   6. Conflicting evidence often will both support and not support improvements in persistent pain symptoms when using cannabis. Assessing resources for reliance, quality, and bias is essential. For example:
      a. Conclusion of one European expert panel review is that only neuropathic pain has sufficient evidence to recommend cannabis-based medicines; therefore, in cancer and non-neuropathic, non-cancer pain, use of cannabis-based medicines should be regarded as individual therapeutic trial.
      b. NASEM 2017 report on cannabis and health effects found substantial evidence that some cannabis products are effective for treatment of persistent pain in adults. Report relied on single meta-analysis of 28 studies with large confidence intervals, which could raise questions about the reliability of the results.
      c. Systematic review of 104 studies concluded cannabis is unlikely to benefit most people with chronic noncancer pain and may cause harms, such as disorientation, dizziness, and cognitive disturbances.
   7. Deficits of research and contrasts in literature highlight need for personalized decision-making until greater confidence in existing research can be reached.

V. Law and Policy Impacting Cannabis Use

A. Federal legislation and policy regarding cannabis use through 2021
   1. Before 1936, cannabis was available over the counter and used for variety of ailments.
   2. By 1936, every state passed law to restrict cannabis use, thereby limiting access.
   3. In 1970, drug laws and policies were consolidated into Controlled Substances Act, and cannabis was placed into Schedule 1 category. Rescheduling under federal law can occur through legislative or administration process only.

4. In 2016, *United States Pharmacopeia*, a comprehensive source for medicine standards, developed standards for quality attributes of cannabis for medical use under direction of its Botanical Dietary Supplements and Herbal Medicines Expert Committee.

5. In 2018, U.S. farm bill removed hemp classified with less than 0.3% THC by dry weight from designation as controlled substance, allowing majority of CBD products meeting this definition to be sold over the counter.

6. As of 2021, cannabis remains a Schedule I substance under federal law, meaning it is determined to have high potential for abuse, has no currently accepted medical use in the United States, and lacks accepted safety for use under medical supervision.

B. State legislation and policy regarding cannabis use through 2021

1. In 1996, California legalized "medical marijuana" under Proposition 215, and many states have followed suit, specifying certain qualifying conditions for marijuana "authorizations."

2. In 2012, Colorado was first state to allow purchase of cannabis for adult use (also called "recreational" use), which has increased access for adults to purchase cannabis to self-manage symptoms if they choose.

3. As of November 2020, 36 states and 4 territories had authorized cannabis for medical use.
   a. While cannabis has remained illegal at federal level, 15 states and 3 territories permit use for adults without medical authorization.
   b. Each state's law indicates qualifying diagnoses for medical marijuana authorizations from providers. In general, conditions need to be "serious" and "debilitating" in order to qualify.
      1) Persistent pain is most common qualifying condition reported by people with medical cannabis use authorizations, representing 64.9% of all qualifying conditions in 2016.
      2) While most qualifying conditions are supported by evidence, in some cases evidence is minimal. For example, cannabis as an opioid replacement therapy for opioid use disorder has been added by some states as a qualifying condition, despite limited evidence.
      3) Laws should be checked for updates frequently, using reliable sites where qualifying conditions and marijuana registry protocols are outlined by state. An example of one such site is National Conference of State Legislatures: https://www.ncsl.org/research/health/state-medical-marijuana-laws.aspx.

4. Number of medical cannabis patients has risen as more states legalize medical cannabis. As cannabis becomes more accessible with "adult use" laws, declines have occurred in medical cannabis authorizations.

C. Nursing practice regulations

1. National Council of State Boards of Nursing (NCSBN) provides guidelines (*The NCSBN National Nursing Guidelines for Medical Marijuana*) listing principles of essential knowledge for safe and knowledgeable nursing care of patients using medical or recreational cannabis:
   a. "The nurse shall have a working knowledge of the current state of legalization of medical and recreational cannabis use and of principles of a medical marijuana program (MMP).
   b. The nurse shall have a general understanding of the endocannabinoid system, cannabinoid receptors, cannabinoids, and the interactions between them.
   c. The nurse shall have an understanding of cannabis pharmacology and the research associated with the medical use of cannabis.
   d. The nurse shall be aware of the facility or agency policies regarding administration of medical marijuana" (NCSBN *Guidelines*, 2018, pp. S24–S25). Clinical care guidelines are detailed and include:
      1) "As part of the clinical encounter for a patient using cannabis for medical use, the nurse shall conduct an assessment related to the following: Signs and symptoms of cannabis adverse effects.
      2) The nurse shall communicate the findings of the clinical encounter to other healthcare providers and note such communication in documentation.
      3) The nurse shall be able to identify the safety considerations for patient use of cannabis" (NCSBN *Guidelines*, 2018, pp. S25–S26).

2. NCSBN maintains nurses shall follow ethical principles requiring approaching patients without judgment regarding choice of treatment or preferences in managing pain or other distressing symptoms.

3. Advanced practice registered nurses (APRNs) who plan to or do "authorize" cannabis must be acutely aware of differences in state laws and requirements to minimize legal sanction.
   a. Cannabis is a Schedule I controlled substance and therefore cannot be prescribed nor can it be dispensed by pharmacies.
   b. Some MMPs specify APRNs can certify/authorize qualifying condition.
      1) MMP is official jurisdictional resource for cannabis use for medical purposes.
      2) MMPs vary greatly by state and can be found on state Department of Health or National Conference of State Legislatures websites.

Part 4

c. According to NCSBN, "To authorize" has been defined as "any act of certification, attestation, or other method for a practitioner to affirm that a patient may benefit from medical cannabis" (NCSBN *Guidelines,* 2018, p. S6). This is differentiated from and is "explicitly not" a prescription.

　1) NCSBN does not explicitly track which states permit nurses (by policy or law) to "authorize" or discuss cannabis with their patients.

　2) Nurses must consult individual licensing boards regarding current law and policy regarding medical and adult use of cannabis.

　3) MMPs may require specific course or training in order for provider to participate in certifying MMP qualifying condition.

d. APRNs are advised to consult their facility policies and state law prior to any cannabis authorization.

e. APRNs can inform only patients with qualifying conditions of right to try and possibly benefit from cannabis (APRNs cannot prescribe).

f. Patients can then register for medical marijuana card and go to dispensary of their choosing. Dispensary then provides recommendations for use.

4. Personal use of cannabis by nurses

a. Boards of Nursing regard personal use of cannabis by nurses the same as any other controlled substance, so nurses must remain aware of legality and impacts on their nursing license.

b. Working while impaired, even if marijuana has been recommended for medical reasons, can be grounds for nursing license discipline or denial.

c. Nurses must remain aware cannabis is federally illegal, so its possession on premises receiving federal funds may need to be addressed.

d. Employers may have policies restricting use of cannabis under any condition.

VI. Nursing Care of Patient Using Cannabis

A. Therapeutic communication is priority in conversations regarding cannabis use. Nurses should talk to patients about their cannabis use as law and their license allows.

1. Shared decision-making framework can be useful and begin with patient or clinician bringing up topic of cannabis use.

2. Historically, some clinics required pain agreements for opioid prescribing and disallowed concurrent use of cannabis with opioids.

a. As a result, some patients may not feel comfortable discussing cannabis use with health professionals and fear it will interfere with their care (e.g., ability to access opioids for pain).

b. Nurses can alleviate patient stress by establishing trust before asking about cannabis use.

B. Nursing assessment should include physical, mental health, and substance use assessment.

1. Review of pain and related symptoms should include inquiries regarding pharmacological (including both prescribed and illicit) and all non-pharmacological pain management strategies.

2. Specific questions about cannabis can be asked as appropriate; consider the following:

a. Past and current use

b. Reason(s) for use

c. Perceived benefits and risks

d. Cannabis source, route, dose, frequency, and duration

e. Usual positive and negative effects (e.g., side effects, signs of withdrawal, impairment, signs of overuse)

　1) Harm reduction approaches attempt to reduce adverse consequences of substance use and emphasize practical goals.

　2) Cannabis side effects can be dose limiting (e.g., patient may need to try different ratios of THC/CBD).

3. Assessment should include evaluation of mental illness and substance use disorders, including CUD.

a. National Institute on Drug Abuse has published *Brief Screener for Tobacco, Alcohol, and Other Drugs* and *Screening to Brief Intervention (S2BI),* tools that can assist in identifying problematic cannabis use.

b. These tools are freely available at https://www.drugabuse.gov/nidamed-medical-health-professionals/screening-tools-resources/chart-screening-tools. Results of substance use screening tools should be reviewed and brief interventions applied when indicated for problematic use.

C. Plan

1. After assessment, nurses, together with patients, can create priority list and make recommendations based on legal options.

2. Include discussion on alternatives for symptom management, legal and clinic practice policies, and how cannabis use may affect patient responsibilities (e.g., employment, family, driving).

3. Patient options can be discussed as law and nursing licensure allows (e.g., availability of cannabis for medical or adult [recreational] use).

a. Ethical considerations should include patient's quality of life priorities and their subjective viewpoints.

b. Nurses' and other health professionals' personal opinions or judgments about cannabis use should not impede patient access to legal options for care.

4. Discuss source(s) of products including cannabis (e.g., medical cannabis products need to be purchased at dispensaries).

   a. Healthcare practitioners often defer specifics on dosage or administration plans to dispensary staff.
   b. Costs may be a consideration for patients in their decision to use medically authorized cannabis versus private or retail sources.
   c. Although several cannabinoid products are FDA approved in the United States, they remain off label for pain conditions (see Table 18.1).

5. *NCSBN National Nursing Guidelines for Medical Marijuana* can be used as resource focusing on:

   a. Nursing care for patient using medical cannabis
   b. Standards for APRN authorization of cannabis
   c. Curriculum considerations for nursing education programs

D. Intervention: patient education

1. Patient preferences and health beliefs should be considered and education tailored accordingly.
2. Teach patients to track cannabis products (e.g., source, route, dose) and report response using daily log or symptom management smartphone app.
3. Patient safety priorities

   a. Most common side effects should be reviewed; side effects may be dose limiting or intolerable.
   b. Slow upward titration is particularly important for any THC-containing product due to psychoactive effects.
   c. Patients should be educated about possibility of tolerance, CUD, and learning to recognize withdrawal signs.
   d. Patients who drive should be aware cannabis use is associated with an increased risk of being involved in motor vehicle crashes.
   e. Safe storage of cannabis products includes avoiding access by minors or pets (particularly edibles).

      1) Cannabis products are constantly evolving with market changes, and packaging can be appealing to children.
      2) Homegrown or mass-marketed products lack standardization in quality control.
      3) Advertisements and consumer sites serve as another source of information patients need to consider for accuracy.

   f. Immunocompromised patients should be aware cannabis and cannabinoid preparations (e.g., gels, tinctures, drops, sprays) can pose serious risk if not prepared in sterile environment.

E. Special considerations

1. Childhood exposure

   a. Acute intoxication of cannabis may occur more commonly with edibles having variable THC content, synthetic "street drug" cannabis products, and accidental poisoning in young children.
   b. Unintentional cannabis exposure in children has been shown to increase in states after legalization of adult use cannabis.
   c. Children generally present with central nervous system depression. Treatment consists primarily of supportive care.

2. Postoperative care: Currently, there are no agreed-upon standards regarding co-use of opioids and cannabis. Patients using both should be monitored for adverse effects.
3. Preoperative planning should include assessment of cannabis use. Patients may require more opioids post-op or may experience cannabis withdrawal symptoms.
4. Nursing leaders:

   a. Nursing leaders should proactively address organizational issues and institutional policies so that patients entering hospitals, assisted living, or other facilities will receive clear guidance on expectations regarding cannabis use when they enter facilities.
   b. Nursing education on cannabis is needed for RNs and APRNs in academic and clinical settings, recognizing nurses in practice have not likely received much preparation.

Bibliography

Aviram, J., & Samuelly-Leichtag, G. (2017). Efficacy of cannabis-based medicines for pain management: a systematic review and meta-analysis of randomized controlled trials. *Pain Physician, 20*(6), E755–E796.

Azcarate, P. M., Zhang, A. J., Keyhani, S., Steigerwald, S., Ishida, J. H., & Cohen, B. E. (2020). Medical reasons for marijuana use, forms of use, and patient perception of physician attitudes among the US population. *Journal of General Internal Medicine, 35*(7), 1979–1986.

Bahji, A., Stephenson, C., Tyo, R., Hawken, E. R., & Seitz, D. P. (2020). Prevalence of cannabis withdrawal symptoms among people with regular or dependent use of cannabinoids: a systematic review and meta-analysis. *JAMA Network Open, 3*(4), e202370.

Bahorik, A. L., Sterling, S. A., Campbell, C. I., Weisner, C., Ramo, D., & Satre, D. D. (2018). Medical and non-medical marijuana use in depression: longitudinal associations with suicidal ideation, everyday functioning, and psychiatry service utilization. *Journal of Affective Disorders, 241*, 8–14.

Baraniecki, R., Panchal, P., Malhotra, D. D., Aliferis, A., & Zia, Z. (2021). Acute cannabis intoxication in the emergency department: the effect of legalization. *BMC Emergency Medicine, 21*(1), 32.

Part 4

Baron, E. P. (2018). Medicinal properties of cannabinoids, terpenes, and flavonoids in cannabis, and benefits in migraine, headache, and pain: an update on current evidence and cannabis science. *Headache, 58*(7), 1139–1186.

Boehnke, K. F., Gangopadhyay, S., Clauw, D. J., & Haffajee, R. L. (2019). Qualifying conditions of medical cannabis license holders in the United States. *Health Affairs (Millwood), 38*(2), 295–302.

Boggs, D. L., Nguyen, J. D., Morgenson, D., Taffe, M. A., & Ranganathan, M. (2018). Clinical and preclinical evidence for functional interactions of cannabidiol and Δ^9-tetrahydrocannabinol. *Neuropsychopharmacology, 43*(1), 142–154.

Booth, J. K., & Bohlmann, J. (2019). Terpenes in *Cannabis sativa* – from plant genome to humans. *Plant Science, 284*, 67–72.

Bonnet, U., & Preuss, U. W. (2017). The cannabis withdrawal syndrome: current insights. *Substance Abuse and Rehabilitation, 8*, 9–37.

Bradford, A. C., & Bradford, W. D. (2016). Medical marijuana laws reduce prescription medication use in Medicare part D. *Health Affairs, 35*(7), 1230–1236.

Brown, J. D., & Winterstein, A. G. (2019). Potential adverse drug events and drug-drug interactions with medical and consumer cannabidiol (CBD) use. *Journal of Clinical Medicine, 8*(7), 989.

Buppert, C., & Klein, T. A. (January 2021). Certifying medical cannabis: what APRNs need to know. In *Medscape Nurses.* https://www.medscape.com/viewarticle/943249.

Cohen, K., Weizman, A., & Weinstein, A. (2019). Positive and negative effects of cannabis and cannabinoids on health. *Clinical Pharmacology and Therapeutics, 105*(5), 1139–1147.

Connective Rx. *PDR Drug Information.* (2021). https://www.pdr.net.

Coughlin, L. N., Ilgen, M. A., Jannausch, M., Walton, M. A., & Bohnert, K. M. (2020). Progression of cannabis withdrawal symptoms in people using medical cannabis for chronic pain. *Addiction.* https://doi.org/10.1111/add.15370.

Cuttler, C., Spradlin, A., & McLaughlin, R. J. (2018). A naturalistic examination of the perceived effects of cannabis on negative affect. *Journal of Affective Disorders, 235*, 198–205.

Drug Enforcement Administration (DEA). (2021). *Drug Scheduling.* https://www.dea.gov/drug-scheduling.

Dharmapuri, S., Miller, K., & Klein, J. D. (2020). Marijuana and the pediatric population. *Pediatrics, 146*(2), e20192629.

Ferber, S. G., Namdar, D., Hen-Shoval, D., Eger, G., Koltai, H., Shoval, G., et al. (2020). The "Entourage Effect": terpenes coupled with cannabinoids for the treatment of mood disorders and anxiety disorders. *Current Neuropharmacology, 18*(2), 87–96.

Gates, P. J., Sabioni, P., Copeland, J., Le Foll, B., & Gowing, L. (2016). Psychosocial interventions for cannabis use disorder. *Cochrane Database of Systematic Reviews, 2016*(5), CD005336.

Hasin, D. S., Shmulewitz, D., Cerdá, M., Keyes, K. M., Olfson, M., Sarvet, A. L., et al. (2020). U.S. adults with pain, a group increasingly vulnerable to nonmedical cannabis use and cannabis use disorder: 2001–2002 and 2012–2013. *The American Journal of Psychiatry, 177*(7), 611–618.

Häuser, W., Finn, D. P., Kalso, E., Krcevski-Skvarc, N., Kress, H. G., Morlion, B., et al. (2018). European Pain Federation (EFIC) position paper on appropriate use of cannabis-based medicines and medical cannabis for chronic pain management. *European Journal of Pain, 22*(9), 1547–1564.

Hill, K. P. (2019). Medical use of cannabis in 2019. *JAMA, 322*(10), 974–975.

Ibsen, M. S., Connor, M., & Glass, M. (2017). Cannabinoid CB_1 and CB_2 receptor signaling and bias. *Cannabis and Cannabinoid Research, 2*(1), 48–60.

Joshi, N., & Onaivi, E. S. (2019). Endocannabinoid system components: overview and tissue distribution. *Advances in Experimental Medicine and Biology, 1162*, 1–12.

Keyhani, S., Steigerwald, S., Ishida, J., Vali, M., Cerdá, M., Hasin, D., et al. (2018). Risks and benefits of marijuana use: a national survey of U.S. adults. *Annals of Internal Medicine, 169*(5), 282–290.

Klumpers, L. E., & Thacker, D. L. (2019). A brief background on cannabis: from plant to medical indications. *Journal of AOAC INTERNATIONAL, 102*(2), 412–420.

Kondo, K., Morasco, B. J., Nugent, S., Ayers, C., O'Neil, M. E., Freeman, M., et al. (2020). Pharmacotherapy for the treatment of cannabis use disorder: a systematic review. *Annals of Internal Medicine, 172*(6), 398–412.

Kosiba, J. D., Maisto, S. A., & Ditre, J. W. (2019). Patient-reported use of medical cannabis for pain, anxiety, and depression symptoms: systematic review and meta-analysis. *Social Science & Medicine, 233*, 181–192.

LaFrance, E. M., Glodosky, N. C., Bonn-Miller, M., & Cuttler, C. (2020). Short and long-term effects of cannabis on symptoms of post-traumatic stress disorder. *Journal of Affective Disorders, 274*, 298–304.

Leung, J., Chan, G. C., Hides, L., & Hall, W. D. (2020). What is the prevalence and risk of cannabis use disorders among people who use cannabis? A systematic review and meta-analysis. *Addictive Behaviors*, 106479. doi:10.1016/j.addbeh.2020.106479.

Lu, H. C., & Mackie, K. (2016). An introduction to the endogenous cannabinoid system. *Biological Psychiatry, 79*(7), 516–525.

Lucas, C. J., Galettis, P., & Schneider, J. (2018). The pharmacokinetics and the pharmacodynamics of cannabinoids. *British Journal of Clinical Pharmacology, 84*(11), 2477–2482.

MacCallum, C. A, & Russo, E. B. (2018). Practical considerations in medical cannabis administration and dosing. *European Journal of Internal Medicine, 49*, 12–19.

Mead, A. (2019). Legal and regulatory issues governing cannabis and cannabis-derived products in the United States. *Frontiers in Plant Science, 10*, 697.

Meier, M. H., Docherty, M., Leischow, S. J., Grimm, K. J., & Pardini, D. (2019). Cannabis concentrate use in adolescents. *Pediatrics, 144*(3).

Millar, S. A., Stone, N. L., Yates, A. S., & O'Sullivan, S. E. (2018). A systematic review on the pharmacokinetics of cannabidiol in humans. *Frontiers in Pharmacology, 9*(1365).

Missouri Division of Professional Registration (n.d.). Amendment 2 Medical Marijuana. https://health.mo.gov/safety/cannabis/about-us.php#:~:text=Amendment%202%20became%20Article%20XIV,safe%20access%20to%20medical%20marijuana.

Mlost, J., Bryk, M., & Starowicz, K. (2020). Cannabidiol for pain treatment: focus on pharmacology and mechanism of action. *International Journal of Molecular Sciences, 21*(22), 8870.

Mu, A., Weinberg, E., Moulin, D. E., & Clarke, H. (2017). Pharmacologic management of chronic neuropathic pain:

review of the Canadian Pain Society consensus statement. *Canadian Family Physician, 63*(11), 844–852.

Mücke, M., Phillips, T., Radbruch, L., Petzke, F., & Häuser, W. (2018). Cannabis-based medicines for chronic neuropathic pain in adults. *Cochrane Database of Systematic Reviews, 3*(3), CD012182.

Nashed, M. G., Hardy, D. B., & Laviolette, S. R. (2021). Prenatal cannabinoid exposure: emerging evidence of physiological and neuropsychiatric abnormalities. *Frontiers in Psychiatry, 11*, 624275.

National Academies of Sciences, Engineering, and Medicine (NASEM). (2017). *The Health Effects of Cannabis and Cannabinoids: the Current State of Evidence and Recommendations for Research*. Washington, DC: National Academies Press.

National Conference of State Legislatures (NCSL). (2023). *State Medical Cannabis Laws*. https://www.ncsl.org/research/health/state-medical-marijuana-laws.aspx.

National Council of State Boards of Nursing (NCSBN). (2018). The NCSBN National Nursing Guidelines for Medical Marijuana. *Journal of Nursing Regulation July 2018, Supplement, 9*(2), S3–S59. https://ncsbn.org/public-files/The_NCSBN_National_Nursing_Guidelines_for_Medical_Marijuana_JNR_July_2018.pdf.

National Institute on Drug Abuse. (2021). *Screening and Assessment Tools Chart*. https://www.drugabuse.gov/nidamed-medical-health-professionals/screening-tools-resources/chart-screening-tools.

National Institute on Drug Abuse. (n.d.). *Screening for Drug Use in General Medical Settings: Quick Reference Guide.* Version 2. https://nida.nih.gov/sites/default/files/pdf/screening_qr.pdf.

Patel, J., & Marwaha, R. (2022). *Cannabis Use Disorder*. In *StatPearls [Internet]*. Treasure Island, FL: StatPearls Publishing.

Perisetti, A., Gajendran, M., Dasari, C. S., Bansal, P., Aziz, M., Inamdar, S., et al. (2020). Cannabis hyperemesis syndrome: an update on the pathophysiology and management. *Annals of Gastroenterology, 33*(6), 571–578.

Rogers, A. H., Bakhshaie, J., Buckner, J. D., Orr, M. F., Paulus, D. J., Ditre, J. W., et al. (2019). Opioid and cannabis co-use among adults with chronic pain: relations to substance misuse, mental health, and pain experience. *Journal of Addictive Medicine, 13*(4), 287–294.

Substance Abuse and Mental Health Services Administration (SAMHSA). (2019). *Key Substance Use and Mental Health Indicators in the United States: Results from the 2018 National Survey on Drug Use and Health* (HHS Publication No. PEP195068, NSDUH Series H54). Rockville, MD: Center for Behavioral Health Statistics and Quality, Substance Abuse and Mental Health Services Administration. https://www.samhsa.gov/data/sites/default/files/cbhsq-reports/NSDUHNationalFindingsReport2018/NSDUHNationalFindingsReport2018.htm.

Sarma, N. D., Waye, A., ElSohly, M. A., Brown, P. N., Elzinga, S., Johnson, H. E., et al. (2020). Cannabis inflorescence for medical purposes: USP considerations for quality attributes. *Journal of Natural Products, 83*(4), 1334–1351.

Starowicz, K., & Finn, D. P. (2017). Cannabinoids and pain: sites and mechanisms of action. *Advanced Pharmacology, 80*, 437–475.

Stockings, E., Campbell, G., Hall, W. D., Nielsen, S., Zagic, D., Rahman, R., et al. (2018). Cannabis and cannabinoids for the treatment of people with chronic noncancer pain conditions: a systematic review and meta-analysis of controlled and observational studies. *Pain, 159*(10), 1932–1954.

Urits, I., Gress, K., Charipova, K., Habib, K., Lee, D., Lee, C., et al. (2020). Use of cannabidiol (CBD) for the treatment of chronic pain. *Best Practice & Research Clinical Anaesthesiology, 34*(3), 463–477.

U.S. Food and Drug Administration. (2018). Press announcements. https://www.fda.gov/news-events/press-announcements/fda-approves-first-drug-comprised-active-ingredient-derived-marijuana-treat-rare-severe-forms.

Vučković, S., Srebro, D., Vujović, K. S., Vučetić, Č., & Prostran, M. (2018). Cannabinoids and pain: new insights from old molecules. *Frontiers in Pharmacology, 9*, 1259.

Werneck, M. A., Kortas, G. T., de Andrade, A. G., & Castaldelli-Maia, J. M. (2018). A systematic review of the efficacy of cannabinoid agonist replacement therapy for cannabis withdrawal symptoms. *CNS Drugs, 32*(12), 1113–1129.

Wilson, M., Klein, T., Bindler, R. J., & Kaplan, L. (2021). Shared decision-making for patients using cannabis for pain symptom management in the United States. *Pain Management Nursing, 22*(1), 15–20.

Woodhams, S. G., Chapman, V., Finn, D. P., Hohmann, A. G., & Neugebauer, V. (2017). The cannabinoid system and pain. *Neuropharmacology, 124*, 105–120.

Part 4

CHAPTER 19

Interventional Pain Management

Jason Sawyer, RN-EC, BScN, MN, NP, BC
Mary Milano Carter, MS, NP-BC, AP-PMN, PMGT-BC
Maureen F. Cooney, DNP, FNP-BC, ACHPN, AP-PMN*

INTRODUCTION

This chapter provides an overview of commonly used peripheral nerve blocks, epidurals, and trigger point injections and nurses' role in caring for patients undergoing interventional pain management techniques. Interventional techniques may be provided by qualified pain management specialists from different specialties, including anesthesiology, physical medicine and rehabilitation, or medicine; for simplification, the term *anesthesiologist* or *anesthesia provider* is used to identify the interventional pain management specialist. Content provided in this chapter is foundational and often applied to adult patients, but acute pain interventions such as epidurals and nerve blocks are also provided for children.

I. Overview

A. Interventional pain management involves procedures such as nerve blocks, epidurals, and trigger point injections to diagnose and treat pain independently or with other modalities. Interventions may involve use of medications in targeted areas or ablation of targeted nerves.

B. American Society of Perianesthesia Nurses and Association of periOperative Registered Nurses are additional resources for nurses involved in interventional pain management.

C. Purpose

1. Often used in conjunction with other multimodal analgesia interventions to provide effective analgesia while limiting opioid use and associated adverse effects and risks; may be used for acute, persistent, and end-of-life pain conditions

2. Use in acute pain management:
   a. May be used with surgery, trauma, or other acute processes
   b. Often provided perioperatively by anesthesiologists, including those specializing in regional anesthesia or persistent pain

c. Peripheral or truncal techniques (e.g., nerve blocks) use local anesthetic (LA) to temporarily block nerve impulses to targeted area, thus blocking sensation and reducing pain. LA administered close to specific nerves involved in surgical (or traumatic) site inhibit neural conduction from pain site to spinal cord and decrease spinal cord sensitization.

d. Neuraxial analgesic techniques (e.g., epidural injection or infusion) are used in management of acute pain to provide segmental analgesia. These techniques can be effective for thoracic, abdominal, obstetric, gynecologic (GYN), urologic, and lower extremity orthopedic conditions by reducing afferent transmission of nociceptive signaling and reducing risks of central sensitization.

3. Use in persistent pain management:
   a. Interventional pain management may be indicated for those unable to attain adequate pain relief and functional improvement despite medical management and use of nonpharmacological interventions.
   b. Persistent pain is often associated with a neuropathic pain component not easily treated by pharmacological interventions but may be amenable to interventional pain management approaches, including use of advanced implantable therapies.

D. Mechanism of pain relief (See Chapter 1 for more information on physiology.)

1. Key nerve fiber types in nociception are A, B, and C fibers.
   a. Nerve fibers have different diameters, conduction speeds, myelination, and sensitivity to LAs.
      1) A and B fibers are myelinated, which allows for more rapid conduction.
      2) C fibers are unmyelinated and conduct more slowly.
2. A fibers include A-alpha ($A\alpha$), A-beta ($A\beta$), A-delta ($A\delta$), and A-gamma ($A\gamma$).

---

a. Aα are myelinated fibers of motor and proprioception.
b. Aβ are myelinated fibers of touch, pressure, and proprioception.
c. Aδ and Aγ are less myelinated fibers of pain, temperature, and touch/motor.
3. B fibers are least myelinated, impacting preganglionic sympathetic autonomic fibers.
4. C fibers are unmyelinated fibers of pain, temperature, and touch.
5. Nerve fibers and LAs
   a. LAs are thought to impact nerve conduction on gradient of small to larger fibers and myelinated to unmyelinated, but there are clinical exceptions.
   b. LAs act at cell membrane to prevent generation and conduction of nerve impulses. LAs block conduction by decreasing or preventing the large transient increase in permeability of excitable membranes to Na$^+$ that normally is produced by slight depolarization of membrane. This action is due to direct interaction with voltage-gated Na$^+$ channels.
   c. As anesthetic action progressively develops in nerve, threshold for electrical excitability gradually increases, rate of rise of action potential declines, and impulse conduction slows.
   d. These factors decrease the probability of propagation of action potential, and nerve conduction eventually fails.
E. Local anesthetics (LAs)
   1. LA agents are classified under two categories: esters and amides. Use this handy mnemonic tip for remembering: LAs (generic name) with one "i" are esters and LAs with two "i"s are amides (Box 19.1).
   2. Amides
      a. Metabolized in liver and more stable than esters
      b. Considered one of safest drug classes with respect to allergies

---

Box 19.1

Classifications of LOCAL ANESTHETICS

Generic Name	Structural Classification
Cocaine	Ester
Chloroprocaine	Ester
Prilocaine	Ester
Lidocaine	Amide
Mepivacaine	Amide
Bupivacaine	Amide
Ropivacaine	Amide
Levolbupivacaine	Amide

---

3. Esters are less stable in solutions and are hydrolyzed in plasma by pseudocholinesterase.
4. LA mechanism of action
   a. Primarily target voltage-gated sodium (Na$^+$) channels in sympathetic and somatic (sensory and motor) nerve membranes and prevent propagation of neural impulses
   b. Must cross nerve membrane through its lipid bilayer to access its binding site
   c. Less than 5% of LA reaches nerve membrane.
5. Factors impacting onset of action
   a. Route of administration, volume, concentration, type of nerve fibers, and patient factors all impact effect of LAs.
   b. Generally, enough volume of LA must be infused to block impulse conduction in at least three nodes of Ranvier on nerve axon to provide an effective block.
6. Local anesthetic systemic toxicity (LAST)
   a. Incidence estimated at 0.18% and has been decreasing over time. True incidence likely underreported.
   b. Occurs most likely in context of unintentional vascular injection or excessive systemic absorption.
   c. Presentation usually occurs within 60 seconds of LA injection, but case reports have documented LAST 15 minutes and even 1 hour after injection, which is extremely rare.
   d. LAST may occur on continuum with CNS excitability such as oral metallic taste and ringing in ears, followed by seizure activity, then evolving to CNS, respiratory, and cardiac depression.
      1) CNS symptoms occur exclusively in approximately 40% of LAST episodes, while 30% may experience combined CNS and CV symptoms, and 25% experience CV symptoms only.
      2) Clinicians should have high index of suspicion of LAST when a patient presentation suddenly changes within proximity of high-dose LA injection.
      3) Approximately 20% of LAST episodes happen outside hospital setting.
   e. Risk factors for LAST include being very young and very old; low muscle mass; female sex; and comorbidities of heart and blood, metabolic, and liver disease. Risk for LAST also differs between block type.
   f. Treatment
      1) Preparation (e.g., IV access; oxygen availability; standard monitoring before, during, and for 30 minutes after injection). Having standardized protocol can be helpful.
      2) Immediate treatment (e.g., stop infusion, airway management, advanced cardiac life support [ACLS] algorithm—may be altered for LAST)

3) IV 20% lipid emulsion therapy immediately after airway management. Lipid infusion may act as a shuttle to take LAs from organs of high LA affinity (brain and heart) and distribute LA to muscles and liver for removal from system.
4) Seizure management (if needed), as seizure activity can increase metabolic acidosis. Benzodiazepines are considered the first line.
5) Cardiovascular support (if needed)—follow ACLS algorithm.
g. American Society of Regional Analgesia (www.asra.com) and New York School of Regional Analgesia (www.nysora.com) are two of many resources practitioners can access for most up-to-date information on LAST care.

II. Nursing's Role With Interventional Procedures

A. General considerations
1. Advocate for appropriate use of interventional modalities to improve quality of pain management. Assure patient understanding of expected side effects and precautions of each interventional technique.
2. Be familiar with institutional polices and governing body standards.
3. Advocate for evidence-based monitoring practices (some published recommendations are based on consensus of a few experts).
B. Procedural considerations
1. Preprocedure nursing care
a. Provide education before and after procedure as appropriate.
b. Verify informed consent is obtained.
c. Assess:
1) Pertinent medical and anesthetic history (e.g., malignant hyperthermia)
2) NPO status (depending on type of procedure and anesthesia)
3) Baseline vital signs
4) Weight
5) Medications (especially anticoagulants; any current implanted devices)
6) Allergies (including latex)
7) Mental status—consider psychological screening
8) History of tobacco, alcohol, and substance use
9) Preprocedural labs
10) Ensure immediate availability of oxygen and oxygen delivery devices, resuscitative and intubation equipment, reversal agents, suction apparatus, and appropriate monitoring devices.

2. Periprocedure
a. Determine IV access on case-by-case basis per organizational policy.
b. Monitoring based on preprocedure assessment, procedure performed, sedation used, and organizational guidelines
1) At minimum, vital signs at baseline and after procedure
2) Consider:
a) Cardiac monitor
b) Pulse oximeter and/or capnography
c) More frequent blood pressure and pulse monitoring (e.g., every five minutes)
3) Monitor rate and quality of respirations.
4) Monitor level of consciousness.
5) Assess skin condition.
c. Assure sterile technique is maintained during procedure.
d. Attend to risk of radiation exposure with use of fluoroscopy.
3. Postprocedure
a. Monitor vital signs per organizational policy.
b. Assess for bleeding.
c. Assess level of consciousness, reflexes, and respiratory function as appropriate to procedure.
d. Monitor pain.
e. Note and address allergic reactions to medications given.
f. Determine sensation and motor strength of targeted extremity if LA was injected near nerve root or epidural space.
g. Provide patient education.
1) Explain what to expect from procedure.
2) Describe potential side effects or complications and how to contact clinicians if concerns arise.
C. Special considerations
1. Local anesthetics
a. Be familiar with treatment of LAST (see above); assure lipids and emergency equipment are readily available. Long-acting amide anesthetics (e.g., bupivacaine, ropivacaine) have higher rate of toxicity and fatality.
b. Monitor for symptoms listed above (e.g., drowsiness, headache, confusion, seizures, and cardiac arrest).
c. Anticipate need for safety measures when LAs are used in peripheral nerve or epidural blocks, as they may decrease sensation and cause motor blockade leading to increased risk for injuries and falls.
2. Epidural analgesia
a. IV access should be maintained throughout epidural infusion. IV fluid bolus may be needed if hypotension noted.

b. Assess blood pressure and heart rate frequently following initial administration of epidural LA due to potential hypotension and bradycardia.

c. Assess sensory (dermatomal) levels of neuraxial blockade by evaluating ability to sense input (i.e., perceive temperature differences, differentiation of sharp/dull sensation, numbness, and/or motor weakness) when LAs are used.

1) Decreased sensation and pain indicate a functioning catheter with adequate medication dose and rate.

2) Recognize impact of LAs and location of epidural catheter tip on numbness or weakness in context of expected sensory and motor deficits related to injury or surgical intervention.

3) Complete loss of sensation or motor weakness, or back pain warrants notification of anesthesia provider, decrease (or discontinuation) of LA infusion, and further assessment of potential complications, such as epidural hematoma or abscess.

d. Assess patient's lower extremity strength while receiving LA, especially prior to ambulating. If weakness is present, notify appropriate care provider as outlined in organizational policy.

e. Implement fall awareness and prevention methods for patients who have received LA or who are receiving LA via epidural catheters. LA at L2-L3 level and lower increases fall risks due to changes in proprioception and decreased anterior thigh muscle strength.

f. Be familiar with organizational policy, guidelines, and protocols enabling nurses to address and manage complications or emergency situations.

g. Recognize benefits and risks of LAs within context of each patient's comorbidities.

h. Consider role of LAs in any side effects the patient experiences.

i. Recognize risk factors for LA adverse effects and signs and symptoms of uncommon but serious adverse effects associated with interventional pain catheters such as LAST, compartment syndrome, and falls.

3. Catheters in place

a. Assess and take appropriate action upon identification of side effects/adverse effects of interventional catheter infusions. (See above for epidural administration.)

b. Understand common complications related to interventional procedures are associated with catheter (leakage/dislodgement) or block failure.

1) Verify catheter placement with anesthesia provider before beginning infusion to prevent complications.

2) If catheter migrates in or out, contact anesthesia provider for direction.

3) If catheter becomes completely dislodged (pulled out), it is necessary to check to assure tip of catheter is present and document.

c. If MRI is required, consult anesthesia provider to determine need for catheter removal.

d. Consult organizational policy and anesthesia provider to determine whether medications likely to increase bleeding risks should be held while interventional catheters are in place and at insertion, manipulation, or removal.

e. Regularly assess catheter insertion site for presence of intact dressing, and notify anesthesia provider if there is drainage at site or any signs of infection.

f. Change catheter solution, tubing, and dressing; adjust infusion rates; and remove catheters according to organizational policies and state board of nursing requirements.

g. Avoid unnecessary interruption in closed system for catheter infusion systems to reduce infection risks.

III. Interventional Procedures for Acute Pain Management

A. Peripheral nerve block (PNB) overview

1. Deposit medications in vicinity of peripheral nerve or between tissue planes to provide pain control; it can be single injection or continuous infusion of medications via catheter.

2. Most commonly used medications are LAs, specifically ropivicaine or bupivacaine.

3. Benefits

a. Safety: Most nerve block catheters are safe enough to use in community, with patient or family member removing catheter at home.

b. May be used for inpatient or outpatient depending upon patient's overall health, type of surgery, and ability to manage at home

c. Evidence supports PNBs as opioid sparing, and opioids may not be needed in some situations.

4. Methods of delivering LAs in PNBs

a. A single injection of LA is sufficient for pain expected to last a few hours.

b. Manual intermittent bolus, continuous infusion, and automated programmable bolus through peripheral nerve catheter are three strategies available for pain expected to linger for longer than a few hours.

c. Heterogeneity of operator technique, choice of LA, concentration, volume, and bolus interval are factors that influence effectiveness of PNB.

d. Technological and human availability impact use of intermittent bolus dosing.

e. Ideally, combination of infusion and intermittent bolus is available, and choice can be customized for each patient as response to therapy is evaluated.

5. Adjuvants to optimize LA effects
   a. Dexamethasone
      1) Mechanism of action is most likely stimulation of glucocorticoid receptors on neural membrane, decreasing excitability of C-fibers. Exact mechanism of action is unknown.
      2) Increases duration of block by 233–488 minutes depending on whether short-acting (e.g., ropivacaine) or long-acting (e.g., bupivacaine) LA is used
      3) May reduce opioid consumption and postoperative nausea and vomiting (PONV)
      4) Unclear if benefit is from systemic effect or direct impact at nerve block site
   b. Epinephrine
      1) Alpha-1-adrenoreceptor vasoconstrictor
      2) Often administered to evaluate if LA has inadvertently been injected intravascularly
      3) When used with bupivacaine (not ropivacaine), may extend duration of block by approximately 60 minutes
      4) Primary value is in delaying systemic absorption of LA, possibly reducing risk of systemic toxicity.
   c. Dexmedetomidine
      1) Currently off-label use in PNBs
      2) Alpha-2-antagonist with 8 times higher selectivity compared to clonidine. When used in PNBs, mechanism of action relies on blocking hyperpolarization, leading to vasoconstriction.
      3) Main side effects include bradycardia and hypotension.
      4) Studies suggest use may provide slightly faster onset of sensory and motor blockade and may extend duration of analgesia.
   d. Liposomal LA delivery
      1) Liposomes consist of hydrophilic head and two hydrophobic tails, which create vesicle to hold LA.
      2) LA (bupivacaine) is gradually released as vesicles break down over time.
      3) Approved initially for wound infiltration but has been expanded to include certain nerve blocks
      4) Should not be mixed with other LAs due to concerns of premature release of bupivacaine. A 20-minute delay is recommended if another LA has been previously injected.

e. Other medications studied as adjuncts and requiring further study include buprenorphine, magnesium, clonidine, and opioids.

6. Risks associated with PNB
   a. Neurological complications
      1) Incidence of long-term nerve injury has remained constant at approximately 2–4/10,000, even with widespread use of ultrasound-guided techniques, and is highly variable among different PNBs.
      2) Incidence of neurological adverse events is similar in general anesthetic and nerve block populations undergoing joint arthroplasties.
      3) Several large databases indicate PNBs are not an independent risk factor for peripheral nerve injury.
      4) Transient postoperative neurological symptoms in patients receiving PNBs are common but increasingly rare over time.
         a) Depending upon the study, reported frequency ranges from 0% to 2% at 3 months, 0% to 0.8% at 3 months, and 0% to 0.2% at 1 year.
         b) It is important to note the mere presence of PNB does not imply it is sole contributor to deficit or even a contributor at all.
      5) Key factors contributing to peripheral nerve injury
         a) Location: Interscalene, brachial plexus, femoral, and sciatic blocks may be at increased risk. Retrospective reviews indicate these blocks are not independent risk factors for peripheral nerve injury.
         b) Surgeries that involve significant trauma, prolonged tourniquet time, excessive nerve stretching, inflammation, and ischemia
         c) Preexisting neuropathies either local or distal to site of nerve blockade
         d) Needle trauma
         e) Local anesthetic toxicity
         f) Excessive localized pressure
   b. Falls
      1) Extremity weakness, especially of lower extremities, may pose increased fall risk if weight bearing occurs before effect of LA has resolved.
      2) Large retrospective analysis of inpatient falls after total knee arthroplasty in patients with continuous femoral nerve block (FNBs) showed most falls occurred more than 12 hours after FNBs were removed.
      3) To reduce fall risk, practice has shifted toward blockade of sensory nerves rather than nerves with both sensory and motor components.

c. Compartment syndrome (CS)
  1) Consensus on CS diagnosis is not clear.
    a) Classically, "6 Ps" have been used to diagnose CS.
      (1) Pain
      (2) Paresthesia
      (3) Pallor
      (4) Paralysis
      (5) Poikilothermia (inability to maintain constant core temperature)
      (6) Pulselessness
    b) More recently, pain out of proportion to injury and pain with passive stretch have been suggested.
  2) Caused by elevated pressure in osteofascial compartments, which can lead to ischemic tissue damage. Irreversible changes in functional outcomes can occur after 6 hours.
  3) Incidence of CS ranges from 0.7/100,000 in females to 7.3/100,000 in males.
    a) Commonly occurs in diaphyseal long bone fractures of distal extremities
    b) Tibial shaft fractures: 3% to 15%; forearm diaphyseal: 3%; distal radius fractures: 0.25%
  4) Role of nerve blocks in CS is controversial. One hypothesis is pain relief of nerve block masks increased pain considered to be hallmark of CS.
B. Types of PNBs
  1. Fascial plane blocks (FPBs) overview
    a. Best used as component of multimodal analgesia and unlikely to be sole analgesic
    b. Becoming increasingly common, in large part due to improved ultrasound technology, access to this technology, and critical mass of operators with skills to perform blocks
    c. Truncal nerve blocks (nonspinal) placed in two main body areas (abdominal wall and thoracic wall).
    d. FPBs involve deposit of LA between two fascia layers, targeting cutaneous sensory nerve blockade, with goal of nociceptive sensory afferent inhibition.
    e. Many systematic reviews attest to efficacy and safety. Results of studies should be interpreted with caution due to significant heterogeneity in terms of LA medication, dose, volume, use (e.g., single shot, infusion, intermittent bolus), operator experience, block location, and type of surgery.
    f. Mechanism of action: bulk flow and diffusion
      1) High volume of LA is placed between fascial planes. This can be done as a single injection, continuous infusion, or intermittent bolus. Tissue distention from injectate,

known as hydrodissection, creates pressure manipulated in part by the natural movement of fascial layers that occur with patient motion.
      2) Fluids also diffuse out of fascia due to concentration gradient. LA leaves fascial layer through permeable collagen fibers of fascia and blood vessels.
    g. Factors impacting efficacy of FPBs
      1) Individual differences lead to heterogeneity in results across populations.
      2) Cutaneous innervation is complex, with significant overlap of nerve branches from multiple segments often innervating an area of skin.
      3) Contralateral innervation is well described, particularly in anterior torso.
      4) Pain from visceral or deep somatic structures is generally minimally relieved by FPBs.
  2. Types of FPB:
    a. Transversus abdominus plane (TAP) blocks
      1) Commonly used for abdominal surgeries and includes three approaches depending on site of pain and dermatome involved:
        a) Subcostal TAPS cover dermatomes T6–9.
        b) Posterior TAPS cover dermatomes T9–12.
        c) Lateral TAPS cover dermatomes T10–12.
      2) Oblique-subcostal approach, covering dermatomes T6-L1
        a) Provides coverage of sensory nerves to anterolateral abdominal wall, which is primarily innervated by anterior rami of TL spine
        b) May reduce pain intensity and opioid consumption
        c) May reduce incidence of PONV and time to first analgesic request
    b. Rectus sheath (RS) plane block
      1) Used for midline abdominal surgeries. Depending on method of use, coverage can extend from xyphoid to symphysis pubis.
      2) For laparotomies, RSB may significantly reduce opioid use and pain scores compared to placebo; however, pain intensity difference is not likely clinically relevant.
      3) PONV, sedation, and constipation may be reduced, and patient satisfaction increased.
      4) Rare but unique complications of RS block include LAST and injury of superior and inferior epigastric arteries.
    c. Thoracic wall blocks (TWB): posterolateral chest wall

1) Erector spinae (ES) plane block
   a) Injection of LA into fascial plane between tips of transverse process and erector spinae muscle
   b) LA spreads approximately 3–6 dermatomes in epidural space, and 6–11 dermatomes in intercostal (IC) area are possible.
   c) Spread is craniocaudal more than medial-lateral.
   d) Epidural spread, if it occurs, tends to be unilateral, limiting impact on sympathetic system (i.e., hypotension).
   e) Proximity to spinal nerves results in somatic and visceral analgesia to area affected by LA, and sympathetic blockade may be observed.
   f) Action may be due to effect of LA on nerves passing within erector spinae plane or muscle (branches of dorsal rami) and compartmentalized nerves contiguous with ES plane block (spinal nerve roots, ventral rami, brachial plexus).
2) Paravertebral block (PVB)
   a) Unilateral block impacting dorsal and ventral rami and sympathetic chain as they exit spinal canal
   b) Operationally more challenging than newer FPBs
   c) Provides benefit for several procedures, including breast surgery, and thoracotomy; some evidence for cholecystectomy, renal, and hepatic surgery

3. Thoracic wall blocks: anterolateral chest wall
   a. Serratus anterior plane blocks (SAPs)
      1) Injection of LA superficial or deep in serratus anterior muscle
      2) Target lateral cutaneous branches of intercostal nerves.
      3) Efficacy in breast surgery, thoracotomy, and anterior rib fractures and being studied in cardiac and thoracic surgeries
      4) Potential for T2–T9 dermatomal distribution

4. Pectoralis (PEC) I and II
   a. Injection of LA into fascial plane between pectoralis major and minor muscles (PECS I)
   b. PEC II is separate injection, usually during same needle pass and injects superficially to serratus plane muscle. Very similar to SAP block.
   c. Used predominantly in breast cancer or reconstructive surgery; some evidence for use as adjunctive pain relief in upper arm fistula creation and insertion of implantable cardiovascular devices

5. Brachial plexus blocks (upper arm)
   a. Indicated for surgery involving shoulder through fingertips
   b. Anterior rami of spinal nerves of C5–C8 and T1 form roots of brachial plexus
   c. Brachial plexus innervates shoulder and upper arm, branching into network of nerves derived from anterior rami of lower four cervical and first thoracic spinal nerves.
   d. Anterior rami give rise to three trunks (superior, middle, and inferior) that emerge between scalenus medius and scalenus anterior on posterior triangle of neck.
   e. These trunks are covered by axillary sheath, a lateral extension of prevertebral fascia; each trunk divides into anterior and posterior division behind clavicle, at apex of axilla.
   f. Brachial plexus can be blocked by various methods, depending on area affected and length of time block is needed.
   g. Brachial plexus can be accessed at various locations depending on targeted site. Interscalene, infraclavicular, supraclavicular, and axillary blocks are brachial plexus blocks.
      1) Interscalene block
         a) Indications: shoulder, arm, or elbow trauma, disease, or surgery
         b) LA infused into interscalene groove
         c) May not consistently block entire posterior aspect of shoulder
      2) Infraclavicular block
         a) Indications: hand, wrist, elbow, or distal wrist trauma, disease, or surgery
         b) LA infused into deeper location
         c) Infraclavicular technique decreases risk of accidental catheter dislodgement.
         d) Technique should be avoided in patients with coagulation risks secondary to closeness of subclavian and axillary artery and vein.
      3) Supraclavicular block
         a) Indicated for rapid onset, predictable dense block that covers majority of upper extremity except shoulder
         b) Indications: elbow or hand surgery
         c) LA infused above clavicle, where three main nerve structures (sensory, motor, and sympathetic) are confined to small area
         d) Not used for continuous infusions unless catheter is tunneled due to proximity to neck and risk of dislodgement; few studies currently available regarding use of continuous block

4) Axillary block
   a) Indications: forearm and hand trauma, disease, or surgery
   b) LA infused along axillary brachial plexus sheath, which is highly vascular area with potential for inadvertent intravascular administration of LAs
6. Lower extremity nerve blocks
   a. Lumbar plexus block (technically truncal but used to treat lower extremities)
      1) Indications: hip, anterior thigh, and knee trauma, disease, or surgery
      2) LA infused into deep muscle bed to provide analgesia along entire plexus, including thigh, knee, and below knee
      3) May be combined with sciatic nerve block to obtain pain relief for entire leg
   b. Femoral nerve block
      1) Indications: trauma or surgery to anterior thigh and knee
      2) LA infused into femoral nerve sheath
   c. Fascia iliaca (femoral and lateral femoral cutaneous)
      1) Indications: trauma or surgery of knee, anterior or lateral thigh
      2) LA infused along fascia iliaca
   d. Sciatic nerve block
      1) Indications: surgery or trauma of knee, tibia, ankle, or foot
      2) LA infused along sciatic nerve
      3) May result in analgesia of entire leg below knee, except for medial aspect of lower leg
C. Epidural analgesia
   1. General concepts
      a. Definition: injection of analgesic medication(s), most commonly LA with or without opioids, opioids alone, or other less commonly used medications (e.g., clonidine) into area around nerve roots within epidural "space"
      b. The epidural space lies between walls of vertebral canal and dura mater and is composed of layers of fat, connective tissue, an extensive venous plexus, and is traversed by spinal nerve roots (Fig. 19.1).
      c. *Neuraxial analgesia* is a general term describing delivery of analgesic medications to epidural and/or subarachnoid or intrathecal space.
      d. Mechanism of action is through reduction of afferent transmission of nociceptive signaling.
      e. Medication may be injected into epidural space during preoperative, intraoperative, postoperative, or peripartum periods to provide postoperative, trauma, or disease-related pain relief.
      f. Analgesic medication is administered into epidural space corresponding to dermatomes of painful area.

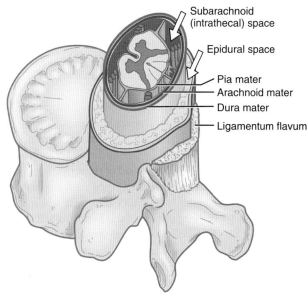

Figure 19.1 Spinal anatomy. The spinal cord extends from the foramen magnum to the first or second lumbar vertebral space. The subarachnoid space (intrathecal space) is filled with cerebrospinal fluid that continuously circulates and bathes the spinal cord. The epidural space is a potential space filled with blood vessels, fat, and a network of nerve extensions. (From Harding, M. M., et al. [2017] Medical-Surgical Nursing: Assessment and Management of Clinical Problems, 10th ed. St Louis: Elsevier.)

   g. Medication into epidural space may be injected as single injection, as continuous infusion, or as continuous infusion with provider or patient-delivered bolus doses (patient-controlled epidural analgesia [PCEA]).
   2. Benefits of epidural analgesia
      a. Medications can be delivered to epidural space, thus reducing systemic effects.
      b. May provide effective analgesia for labor and delivery, orthopedic surgery, open abdominal surgeries, thoracotomies, and rib fractures, as well as other conditions
      c. Aids in prevention of central sensitization
   3. Epidural opioids
      a. Bind at respective opioid receptor sites in substantia gelatinosa of dorsal horn
      b. Neuraxial medications have affinity for spreading rostrally (towards brain) or caudally (towards base of spinal column).
      c. Lipophilic opioids (fat soluble)—fentanyl
         1) Diffuse rapidly through dura, then exit aqueous CSF and quickly penetrate lipid-rich spinal tissue as well as surrounding vasculature
         2) Rapid diffusion accounts for rapid onset of action (5 minutes) and rapid clearance as medication is diffused into vasculature for systemic distribution or stored in epidural fat.

3) Significant systemic action; therefore, epidural opioid dosing is similar to IV dosing

4) Less risk of delayed respiratory depression than hydrophilic opioids

d. Hydrophilic (water-soluble) opioids
1) Morphine
a) Slower distribution to and clearance from epidural space and spinal cord
b) Due to its water solubility, morphine will remain in CSF and may spread rostrally over a period of time.
c) Can cause delayed respiratory depression up to 24 hours after dose administration; unclear if this is due to active metabolite or rostral spread in CSF
d) Pharmacokinetics differ based on injection site (thoracic vs lumbar). Site impacts rostral spread, and there are more systemic side effects if given thoracically.
2) Hydromorphone
a) Similar to morphine but more potent
b) Delayed respiratory depression after 4–6 hours instead of up to 24 hours

e. Side effects and complications of neuraxial opioids:
1) Side effects of epidural opioids are same as those experienced when opioids are delivered by other routes.
2) Advancing sedation and respiratory depression require discontinuation of opioid and administration of naloxone for opioid reversal.
3) Nausea, vomiting, sedation, and respiratory depression tend to happen less frequently when administered epidurally versus systemically.
4) Urinary retention, pruritus, and hemodynamic depression tend to occur more frequently, but this is dependent on dose of opioid/LA administered.

4. Epidural LAs
a. LAs exhibit rostral spread at speed of CSF circulation and may take 10–20 minutes to move from injection site to head.
b. LAs attenuate sensations of touch, temperature, pinprick, and pain.
c. More effective at inhibiting pain from short duration stimuli than longer duration
d. Presence of sensory blockade does not reliably predict effective pain control.
e. Blockade of cutaneous stimuli does not mean visceral or deep structures will have pain control.
f. Sympathetic blockade closely mimics sensory blockade.

g. Factors impacting LA epidural analgesia
1) Extremes of height
2) BMI
3) Age: 40% less dose required for older patients (e.g., 60–70 years old) compared to younger patients (20–30 years old)
4) Individual anatomical variances
5) Total dose of LA is more significant than either rate or concentration.
6) Catheter tip placement
a) Low thoracic mostly cephalad
b) High thoracic mostly caudal

h. Side effects and complications of epidural LA
1) LAST (described above) is possible with epidural administration.
2) Decreased systemic vascular resistance, vasodilation, and hypotension may result from LA block of sympathetic nerve fibers and may lead to bradycardia from blockade of sympathetic cardiac accelerator fibers located at T1–T4 spinal levels.
3) LA neurotoxicity due to direct effects of LA on neural tissue.
4) Cauda equina syndrome, possibly permanent, may result from damage to spinal nerve roots and lead to acute loss of neurologic function below termination (conus) of spinal cord.
5) Transient neurologic symptoms characterized by acute radicular pain without motor deficit that resolves within 24 hours
6) Urinary retention from lumbar LA administration due to S2–S4 nerve root blockade; resolves with discontinuation of LA
7) Motor weakness of lower extremities, especially with lumbar epidural, is usually temporary and increases fall risk.

i. Potential complications of epidural puncture and catheter placement
1) Dural puncture
a) Inadvertent puncture through dura may occur at time of catheter insertion.
b) Symptoms of postdural puncture headache (PDPH) include dull, aching, or throbbing headache. It may be frontal, occipital, or diffuse in location.
c) Headache is usually of moderate to severe intensity.
d) May be accompanied by stiff neck, photophobia, visual disturbances, and nausea and vomiting
e) Headache may worsen with movement, sitting, or standing; patient will feel better when lying down.
f) Treatment includes:
(1) Conservative measures may resolve headache within a week: supine

positioning, hydration, cold or heat, nonopioid analgesics.

(2) Some evidence to support use of caffeine benzoate 300 mg by mouth daily or caffeine sodium benzoate 500 mg IV once or twice daily (adult dosing, for reference only).

(3) Epidural blood patch: aseptic withdrawal and then prompt injection of 15–20 mL of the patient's venous blood into epidural space, at or one level below, initial puncture site

2) Epidural hematoma

   a) Results from accumulation of blood causing pressure on spinal cord; may lead to permanent spinal cord damage and loss of function and is considered a medical emergency

   b) Patients are at greatest risks for hematoma formation during time of epidural puncture, catheter placement, and removal.

   c) Risks

      (1) Advanced age, female sex, obesity

      (2) Difficult or traumatic epidural needle or catheter placement

      (3) Coagulopathy, liver disease, cancer, major surgery, or pelvic or long bone fractures

      (4) Prolonged bedrest

      (5) Thrombocytopenia, administration of anticoagulants, antithrombotics, and thrombolytics. American Society of Regional Anesthesia (ASRA) has published evidence-based guidelines to reduce bleeding risks associated with medication administration, especially with use of anticoagulation.

   d) Symptoms

      (1) May appear within 48 hours of epidural placement

      (2) New or progressive neurological symptoms such as increasing numbness and motor block

      (3) Onset of acute, axial back pain often at level of hematoma

      (4) Urinary or fecal incontinence

      (5) Increased pain with coughing, sneezing, or straining

   e) Early detection of symptoms (within first 6–8 hours of presentation) is important to minimize severe neurological outcomes.

   f) Epidural hematoma is diagnosed by MRI following removal of epidural catheter or, in some cases, by CT scan.

   g) Treatment involves neurosurgical consultation and immediate laminectomy and hematoma evacuation. In some cases, when symptoms improve quickly and when hematoma is small, surgery may be deferred.

   h) Prognosis depends on level of hematoma formation and timing of intervention.

3) Epidural catheter migration or displacement

   a) Catheter may migrate into subarachnoid space, blood vessel, or tissue.

      (1) Migration to subarachnoid space increases risk for respiratory depression; LAs increase numbness and motor block.

      (2) Migration to blood vessel increases risk for LA toxicity and increased pain control.

   b) Catheter may stay in epidural space but migrate higher or lower than intended, resulting in analgesia/anesthesia above or below intended site.

   c) Signs of migration or displacement include leaking at insertion site and/or loss or reduction in analgesia. Having nurses document catheter depth during site assessment can be helpful in identifying migration.

   d) Catheter may be inadvertently dislodged (pulled out) completely.

4) Epidural infection or abscess

   a) Epidural injections and catheters are placed and cares (e.g., dressing changes) performed under aseptic conditions. It is recommended to maintain a closed system, when possible, to reduce infection risks.

   b) Risk factors for infection include preexisting infections, pancreatitis, gastrointestinal (GI) bleeding, and drug or alcohol abuse.

   c) There is no consensus about recommendations for hang time of epidural solutions, tubing, or dressing changes. Usually epidural catheters are not continued for more than 5 days, and many organizations recommend not changing tubing during this time to maintain system integrity.

   d) Signs and symptoms

      (1) Infection should be considered if there are changes in sensory and motor function.

      (2) Early stages: may be difficult to identify but may include fever, increasing backache, headache, or redness and tenderness at injection site

(3) Signs of *serious* infection:
  (a) Neck stiffness, photophobia, fatigue, confusion, altered mental status, nausea, vomiting
  (b) Kernig sign may indicate meningitis. Increased radicular pain, advancing motor deficit, and other neurological signs.
(4) Bowel and bladder dysfunction may indicate epidural abscess and possible cauda equina.
(5) Increased white blood count, ESR, and C-reactive protein in CSF may indicate neuraxial infections.
e) Anesthesia provider should be notified of any signs of infection. Imaging and systemic antibiotics may be required.

IV. Interventional Therapies for Persistent Pain

A. Some interventions and medications listed above for acute pain are also used for persistent pain.
B. LAs, steroids, or NSAIDs are used for various interventional techniques.
  1. LAs provide localized numbness of injected area. Lidocaine has fast onset (minutes) and short duration (two hours); bupivacaine has 30-minute onset but duration of up to 8 hours.
  2. Corticosteroids or NSAIDs will reduce inflammation. Low-solubility corticosteroid agents, such as triamcinolone, should *not* be used for soft tissue injection due to increased risk of surrounding tissue atrophy.
C. Trigger point injections
  1. Musculoskeletal trigger points are palpable bands of tense muscle fibers causing local and referred pain, usually caused by underlying pathology, and can occur all over body.
  2. Indication: painful trigger points
  3. Areas of spasm (trigger points) are identified with manual palpation for treatment.
  4. Procedure: Trigger points can be dry needled, or medication can be injected. Skin is prepared with alcohol or chlorhexidine; aspirate to ensure needle is in muscle and not vessel; use fanning technique, and needle is removed.
D. Joint and bursa injections
  1. Intraarticular (joint) injection
    a. Used for diagnostic or therapeutic reasons
    b. LAs and corticosteroids injected into joint space. Low-solubility corticosteroid agents (e.g., triamcinolone or methylprednisolone) should be used as they remain at site longer.
    c. Hyaluronates are injected for viscosupplementation. Injection of gel-like substances

(hyaluronates) into joint supplements the viscous properties of synovial fluid.
    d. Platelet-rich plasma (PRP) and stem cell therapy are regenerative medical treatments for a variety of joint issues. Platelets are retrieved from patient's blood and stem cells from patient's bone marrow; both trigger healing response.
    e. Procedure: joint space identified, skin prepared with povidone/iodine or chlorhexidine, needle inserted into joint space, medication instilled, and needle removed
  2. Extraarticular injections into bursa (outside joint)
    a. Injection of steroid and/or LA to outside of joint cavity
    b. Indications: pain with palpation over bursa or soft tissue conditions, including bursitis, tendonitis or tendinosis, ganglion cysts, neuromas, entrapment syndromes, or fasciitis
    c. Procedure: Painful bursa site is palpated; skin is prepared with povidone/iodine or chlorhexidine; needle is inserted into bursa area only, not into joint; and medication is instilled into area (amount depends on bursae location).
E. Spinal procedures
  1. Epidural injections
    a. Controversy exists regarding efficacy; however, efficacy in managing a multitude of chronic spinal conditions was found in one systematic review.
    b. Indications: See below for indications specific to method.
    c. Procedure: medication(s) (e.g., steroid, LA, opioid, or some combination of these) injected into epidural space
      1) Fluoroscopy with contrast dye may be used to confirm needle placement.
      2) All medications injected into epidural space must be preservative free.
      3) All contrast material injected into epidural or intrathecal space must be nonionic.
    d. Epidural methods: Cervical, thoracic, or lumbar injection can be accomplished by one of three approaches:
      1) Translaminar: preferred for generalized spinal pain, spinal stenosis, multiple-level disc herniations and bulges, multiple-level disc degeneration, and posterior disc herniations
      2) Transforaminal: preferred for pain (usually unilateral) generating from one or two specific nerve roots verified on CT scan, myelography, or MRI and through physical assessment. Note: transforaminal approach with steroids for cervical injection is often avoided due to the proximity of vascular

structures and risks for cerebral vascular events.

   3) Caudal: indicated when there is extensive scar tissue from prior surgery, as alternative to other approaches, and as assurance of steroid placement close to sacral nerves

  2. Facet (apophyseal joint) blocks (Fig. 19.2)

    a. Steroid, with or without LA, is injected into facet joints (true synovial joints connecting adjacent vertebrae posteriorly) or median branch block of posterior primary ramus. Can be cervical, thoracic or lumbar. These injections may be diagnostic or therapeutic.

    b. Indications: facet syndrome related to inflammation, arthritis, or segmental instability; focal tenderness over facet joint; persistent low back pain with or without radiation; back pain with evidence of disc disease; facet arthritis; postlaminectomy syndrome; recurrent disc disease

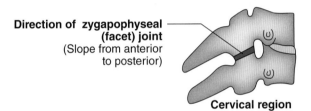

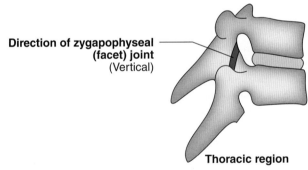

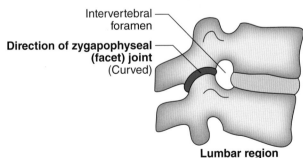

Figure 19.2 The direction of zygapophyseal (facet) joints in cervical, thoracic, and lumbar regions of the vertebral column shown in the lateral view. Note the orientation of facet joints in three different regions. (From Singh, V. [2023] General Anatomy with Systemic Anatomy Radiological Anatomy Medical Genetics, 4th ed. Philadelphia: Elsevier.)

    c. Procedure: injection of LA and steroid into area surrounding posterior ramus nerve, innervating joint, which decreases inflammation and eliminates pain; performed using fluoroscopy

  3. Minimally invasive lumbar decompression (MILD)

    a. Indications: spinal stenosis confirmed on imaging to be due to ligamentum flavum hypertrophy of greater than 2.5 mm; severe symptomatic lumbar spinal stenosis with neurogenic claudication

    b. Procedure: Hypertrophied ligamentum flavum is debulked by percutaneously removing small portions of ligament.

  4. Vertebral body augmentation

    a. Percutaneous vertebroplasty

     1) Therapeutic radiologically guided procedure consists of percutaneous injection of surgical cement into fractured or neoplastic site at vertebral body.

     2) Indications: compression fracture due to osteoporosis, compression fractures from either malignant or nonmalignant cause, symptomatic vertebral hemangiomas

     3) Procedure: Requires procedural (moderate) sedation. Deep sedation or general anesthesia is used if patient cannot tolerate prone position. Vertebral body is injected with polymethyl methacrylate (PMMA) bone cement. Fluoroscopy and contrast are used to monitor flow of cement into undesirable locations, such as epidural space or inferior vena cava. Patient is asked to lie flat for approximately 2 hours for cement to cure.

    b. Kyphoplasty

     1) Similar to vertebroplasty, kyphoplasty is a therapeutic, radiologically guided procedure consisting of percutaneous injection of surgical cement into fractured or neoplastic site at vertebral body, developed to overcome limitations of vertebroplasty.

     2) Indications: osteoporotic vertebral fractures, compression fractures related to neoplasms, prevention of sequelae of immobility

     3) Procedure: In addition to procedure for vertebroplasty, balloon is introduced into vertebra through cannula, which is then inflated to reduce fracture. After balloon is deflated, it leaves space that may then be filled with viscous PMMA.

  F. Sympathetic blocks

    1. LA injected to block pain transmission at sympathetic chain ganglion. In cancer pain, may involve use of neurolytic medication (e.g., 98% alcohol) to destroy ganglion.

Part 4

2. Indications: visceral, ischemic, neuropathic, and sympathetically mediated pain
3. Specific sympathetic ganglion selected depends on type and location of pain.
   a. Stellate ganglion block
      1) Indications: painful conditions of upper extremities such as complex regional pain syndrome (CRPS) I and II, phantom limb pain, ischemic extremity pain, and visceral pain conditions such as pancreatitis
      2) Block expected to cause vasodilation and increased temperature of affected extremity
      3) Sympathetic block to head and affected arm causes myosis, ptosis, and enophthalmos on side of block, and may lead to throat numbness. Swallowing may be impacted.
      4) Arm on injected side may be weak, and there may be venous engorgement on hand and forearm.
   b. Lumbar sympathetic block
      1) Indications: CRPS of lower extremities (to increase perfusion), vascular pain of lower limbs, phantom limb pain
      2) Block expected to cause vasodilatation and increased temperature of affected extremity
      3) Lower extremity on injected side may be weak, and there may be venous engorgement on hands and forearms.
   c. Celiac plexus block
      1) Indications: Afferent nociceptive fibers targeted to block intractable benign or malignant upper abdominal pain unresponsive to less aggressive therapies.
      2) Blocks liver, gallbladder, pancreas, mesentery, and GI tract from stomach to transverse colon.
      3) Common side effects include orthostatic hypotension and diarrhea, which are usually transient.
   d. Pudendal block
      1) Pudendal nerve arises from sacral plexus, and pain is usually unilateral.
      2) Indications: pudendal neuralgia or entrapment (pelvic pain), GYN procedures, anorectal procedures, prostate biopsy, and indwelling catheter pain
   e. Superior hypogastric/ganglion of impar
      1) Indications: visceral pain of lower abdomen in conditions such as pelvic pain, scar tissue formation, perineal pain from coccydynia, rectal pain, and pelvic malignancies
      2) Ganglion of impar block usually requires bowel prep prior to block to reduce risks in case of inadvertent bowel perforation.
4. Side effects/risks of sympathetic blocks
   a. Hypotension due to vasodilation of blood vessels associated with specific blocked ganglion.
   b. Sympathetic block involving extremities (e.g., stellate ganglion or lumbar sympathetic blocks) causes vasodilation of affected extremity.
   c. Fluoroscopy with contrast is used to reduce risk to nerves, blood vessels, and nearby structures during needle placement.
   d. Fluoroscopy is used to reduce risk of intravascular injection of LA, which could lead to LAST.
   e. Blocks of ganglia near spine increase risk of spinal headache, infection, bleeding, segmental nerve injury, transient backache and stiffness, complete spinal block causing temporary paralysis after LA injection, respiratory arrest, and post block neuralgia.
5. Nursing considerations for sympathetic blocks (specifics will be based on organizational policies):
   a. Ensure IV catheter patency.
   b. Continuous oxygen saturation monitoring during procedure
   c. Cardiac monitoring and verbal monitoring
   d. Monitoring of blood pressure, pulse, and respirations every 5 minutes
   e. If stellate or lumbar plexus block, monitoring of extremity temperature before block, at conclusion of block, and during immediate postprocedure period
   f. Continue monitoring until stable, usually 30–60 minutes after completion of procedure.
G. Somatic nerve blocks
   1. Various nerves may be blocked to diagnose or treat painful conditions associated with somatic nerve distributions.
   2. LA with or without steroid injected to temporarily block pain transmission. In serious pain conditions such as cancer pain, block may involve use of neurolytic medication such as highly concentrated alcohol or phenol to destroy nerve.
      a. Intercostal (IC) nerve block
         1) LA injection into one or more IC spaces with duration of 10–12 hours or, if neurolysis with alcohol or phenol, 6–12 months.
         2) Indications: postherpetic neuralgia along thoracic dermatome; surgical incisions; fractured ribs; rib metastasis; chest tubes; dislocation of costochondral joints at sternum; chest pain associated with pleurisy; pain associated with herpes zoster or intercostal nerve entrapment in abdominis rectus sheath; and postoperative pain from thoracotomy, sternotomy, and after renal surgery through flank incisions
         3) Poses risk for pneumothorax. Assess for dyspnea, shortness of breath, and unusual chest pain, and report to provider.

b. Occipital nerve block
   1) LA injected near unilateral or bilateral occipital nerves
   2) Indications: diagnostic or therapeutic for headaches, occipital neuralgia, or painful occiput conditions
   3) Poses risk for glossopharyngeal nerve involvement. Assess and report difficulty swallowing and hoarseness.
c. Genicular nerve block
   1) Injection near superior lateral, superior medial, inferior lateral, or inferior medial genicular nerves that innervate knee
   2) Indications: persistent pain after knee surgeries, persistent knee pain from OA in nonoperative patient
   3) Poses risk for unintended common peroneal nerve block. Assess for foot drop.
d. Ilioinguinal nerve block
   1) Injection near ilioinguinal and iliohypogastric nerves of abdomen that innervate groin and suprapubic pain
   2) Indications: post inguinal hernia repair pain or other inguinal surgery pain, mons pubis pain, anterior scrotum pain, and suprapubic pain
e. Sacroiliac (SI) joint injection
   1) Injection near sacroiliac joint on affected side
   2) Indications: sacroiliitis, SI joint dysfunction
   3) Risk for spinal block. Assess motor strength and sensation
f. Sciatic block
   1) Injection near sciatic nerve for pain in affected lower extremity, posterior thigh, knee, and below
   2) Indications: sciatica from spinal nerve compression or any pain of lower extremity
   3) May cause motor and sensory block of extremity. Assess fall risk.
g. Suprascapular nerve block
   1) Injection near suprascapular nerve, which branches off brachial plexus and is primary sensory nerve for shoulder joint
   2) Indications: adhesive capsulitis, bursitis, arthritis, ineffective or contraindicated intraarticular injections
   3) Advise patients of need for immediate follow-up with physical therapy after block.
h. Lateral femoral cutaneous nerve block
   1) Injection of lateral femoral cutaneous nerve, which innervates anteriolateral thigh
   2) Indications: meralgia parasthetica, postoperative hip or spine surgery pain

H. Botulinum toxin type A injections
   1. Botox purified neurotoxin blocks neuromuscular conduction by binding to receptor sites on motor nerve terminals, entering nerve terminals, and inhibiting release of acetylcholine.
   2. When injected intramuscularly in therapeutic doses, localized chemical denervation and muscle paralysis is produced.
   3. Surface anatomy, electromyography (EMG), or electrical stimulation used to guide nerve site selection
   4. Indications: migraine headaches; strabismus and blepharospasm associated with dystonia; intractable dystonias, spasms, and tremors; spasticity; rigidity resulting from extrapyramidal disorders; muscle tension; chronic cervical pain; migraine headache; Temporomandibular Joint (TMJ) Disorders; whiplash injury; hemifacial pain; low back pain; myofascial pain; piriformis syndrome; postlaminectomy syndrome
   5. Patient teaching:
      a. Treat site tenderness with over-the-counter (OTC) analgesics and ice packs.
      b. Avoid physical exertion for 24 hours.
      c. Inform patient: clinical benefit is seen in one to three days and peaks in four to six weeks, lasting about three to five months; injection site tenderness may worsen with rubbing or pressing injection sites in first 12 hours.
I. Neuroablative techniques
   1. Involve destruction of selected nerve(s) for purpose of pain relief
   2. Indications: cancer-related pain in those with limited life expectancy and for pain refractory to other interventions
   3. Generally, not recommended for benign pain due to high failure rates and risks for neurological complications
   4. Some blocks and procedures described in earlier sections may be performed as neuroablative if nerve destruction is needed.
   5. Neurolysis or neurectomy is neuroablative technique accomplished by injecting nerve destroying substances such as ethyl alcohol 50%–100% or phenol 6.6%–10% in glycerin into selected nerve(s).
      a. Late causalgia (burning sensation) is common after procedure.
      b. Usual targets are sensory nerves, but motor deficits may occur if mixed nerves are ablated.
      c. Risk for unintentional damage to other structures
      d. Nursing implications:
         1) Alcohol neurolysis
            a) Painful if LA is not used prior to injection
            b) Anticipate need for analgesics.
            c) Inform patient neurolysis occurs rapidly.

        d) Position with affected nerve root *up*, as alcohol is *hypobaric* and medication will *rise*.

    2) Phenol neurolysis

        a) No pain on injection

        b) At least 15 minutes until effective

        c) Position with affected nerve *down*, as phenol is *hyperbaric* and medication will *follow gravity*.

6. Radiofrequency electrocoagulation involves ablation of nerve by heat using radiofrequency current applied by an electrode.

    a. Tissue is heated by ionic movement, and cell death occurs by thermal coagulation necrosis.

    b. Indications: facet joint syndromes, pain related to sympathetic ganglion conditions

    c. May be performed in an outpatient setting

    d. Procedure may be repeated if necessary.

    e. Rare complications include numbness, motor paralysis, longer-term increased pain.

7. Intradiscal electrothermal therapy (IDET) and intradiscal electrothermal annuloplasty involve use of cannula to apply heat to seal crack(s) in disc wall (annular tears).

    a. High temperature may destroy small nerve fibers growing into cracks and invaded degenerated disc, causing back pain.

    b. Indications: internally ruptured discs or limited disc herniations nonresponsive to other interventions

    c. Complications include discitis, infection, bleeding, nerve damage, pain, retention of foreign body if catheter shearing occurs, and paralysis.

J. Intraspinal infusions

  1. Implantable epidural port system

    a. Indication: painful conditions requiring *long-term* infusion of medications into epidural space for analgesia

    b. Description:

      1) Epidural catheter is threaded percutaneously around flank to front of body.

      2) Catheter is connected to epidural port, which is implanted over lower ribs for stability.

      3) Port allows easy access to epidural space so external infusions can be connected to port via nonboring needle or medication can be directly injected into port through nonboring needle.

  2. External percutaneous long-term (tunneled) epidural catheter

    a. Indication: painful conditions requiring *short-term* (several weeks) infusion of medications into epidural space for analgesia

    b. Description:

      1) Epidural catheter is threaded percutaneously around flank to front of body, where it exits and is connected to ambulatory infusion pump. It is secured by percutaneous adhering cuff.

      2) Requires regular dressing changes over exit site

      3) Povidone-iodine may be used to prepare site to access catheter. Alcohol is contraindicated because of potential for migration into epidural space, causing nerve destruction.

      4) Filter (0.22 micron) without surfactant is used for medication administration.

  3. Implanted infusion pumps

    a. Indications: spasms related to SCI, cancer pain, or persistent low back pain. Allows for minimal amounts of opioid to be delivered into CNS to provide substantial relief without significant systemic side effects.

    b. Description:

      1) Implanted device continually infuses concentrated analgesic medication into intrathecal or epidural space.

      2) Small pump placed in abdomen or buttock area delivers medication by way of internalized catheter to intrathecal or epidural space.

      3) Pumps are manufactured with varied flow rates, sizes, and volume capacities and can be programmed externally using telemetry.

    c. Criteria for patient selection:

      1) Pain refractory to conventional therapy

      2) Intolerable side effects from other routes of administration

      3) Physiologically stable and able to tolerate insertion and implantation

      4) Pain is responsive to trial of epidural or intrathecal medication administration.

      5) Psychological evaluation indicates emotional stability.

      6) Adequate social support system in place to facilitate care

      7) Life expectancy of months to years to warrant cost of device insertion

      8) Insertion and care are financially feasible (insurance or self-payment), including cost of delivery system, medications, needles, supplies, and visits for refills.

    d. Contraindications:

      1) Anticoagulant therapy immediately before, during, and immediately after implantation

      2) Coagulation disorders

      3) Intraspinal infection

      4) Active or untreated systemic bacterial infection

      5) Patient is averse to implant

      6) Lack of appropriately trained and experienced personnel to support device management after implantation

    e. Nursing implications:

      1) Acute pain following pump implantation may occur at pump pocket site or back incision site and may require analgesic administration.

2) Educate patient to:
   a) Avoid wearing constrictive clothing or belt over site of pump placement.
   b) Notify provider of impending air travel plans, as pumps are altitude sensitive.
   c) If using hot tub or heating pad, do so with caution.
   d) Alert provider of any fever, as elevated body temperature may increase intrathecal pump infusion rate.
   e) Carry identification card and Medi-alert information at all times.
   f. Pumps are MRI compatible, but settings must be verified following MRI exposure.
4. Intraspinal medication management
   a. All intraspinal solutions must be preservative free to reduce risk for neurotoxicity.
   b. Preservative-free morphine and ziconotide for pain and baclofen for spasticity are only U.S. Food and Drug Administration (FDA)-approved medications, but other opioids, LAs, gamma aminobutyric acid (GABA) agonist, and other adjuvants are used off-label.
   c. Pump is refilled by trained healthcare provider accessing internalized port.
   d. Frequency of refill depends on size of reservoir and rate of infusion.
   e. Intraspinal infusions are often used in combination with systemic adjuvant analgesics.
   f. Opioid infusions:
      1) Equianalgesic conversion ratio for oral to intravenous to epidural to intrathecal opioids becomes smaller as route proceeds from oral, to intravenous, to epidural, to intrathecal administration; depends on meningeal permeability of specific opioid.
      2) Meningeal permeability is affected by lipophilicity of opioid, its molecular weight, and possibly structure.
      3) Hydrophilic opioids such as morphine have direct spinal effect, so when administered into intrathecal space, they will bind to mu opioid receptors in dorsal horn and have effect.
         a) Intrathecal concentration of hydrophilic opioids will remain elevated for longer periods of time than lipophilic opioids and will have greater risk of respiratory depression due to rostral spread (higher toward respiratory center).
         b) Lipophilic opioids (e.g., fentanyl) work primarily through supraspinal effect, which occurs secondary to systemic absorption. When administered epidurally, fentanyl is rapidly absorbed systemically and, with

prolonged infusion, will achieve plasma levels similar to IV infusion.
   g. N-type (neuronal specific) calcium channel blocker (ziconotide) infusion:
      1) Derived from venom of fish-eating marine snail, *Conus magus*
      2) Only administered through intrathecal route; generally used as monotherapy
      3) Indicated for pain refractory to intrathecal morphine
      4) Acts through selective blockade of pre-synaptic neuronal N-type calcium channels in spinal cord
      5) Initiated at low doses (e.g., 2.4 mcg/day) via intrathecal pump and titrated up slowly (e.g., by 2.4 mcg/day, two or three times per week or less to maximum of 19.2 mcg/day) to minimize risk of adverse effects
      6) Serious adverse effects: neuropsychiatric/cognitive effects (confusion, depression, hallucinations, somnolence), presyncopal and syncopal episodes, gait disturbances, elevated creatinine kinase
      7) Contraindicated in patients with history of major psychiatric illness/psychosis
   h. Baclofen infusion
      1) GABA agonist-modulated hypertonia secondary to upper motor neuron pathology
      2) Indications: chronic spinal spasticity of cerebral or spinal origin for those unresponsive to oral therapy or who experience intolerable CNS adverse effects at effective doses
      3) Not recommended for epidural, IC, or IM administration
      4) Serious adverse effects: hypotonia, somnolence, headache, convulsion. Massive overdose may lead to coma and death.
      5) Abrupt discontinuation of intrathecal baclofen may be life threatening and result in high-fever altered mental status, severe rebound spasticity, muscle rigidity, rhabdomyolysis, multiorgan system failure, and death.
      6) Patient selection must consider ability of patient to follow-up at scheduled pump refill dates to avoid risk of withdrawal.
   i. Off-label medications and adjuvants are sometimes used when FDA-approved medications are ineffective or poorly tolerated.
      1) Opioids: hydromorphone, fentanyl, methadone
      2) Alpha-2-agonists: clonidine, dexmedetomidine, tizanidine
      3) NMDA receptor antagonist: ketamine

Part 4

Bibliography

Abdelsalam, K., & Mohamdin, O. (2016). Ultrasound-guided rectus sheath and transversus abdominis plane blocks for perioperative analgesia in upper abdominal surgery: A randomized controlled study. *Saudi Journal of Anaesthesia, 10*(1), 25. https://www.saudija.org/article.asp?issn=1658-354X;year=2016;volume=10;issue=1;spage=25;epage=28;aulast=Abdelsalam.

Ahmed, S., Subramaniam, S., Sidhu, K., Khattab, S., Singh, D., Babineau, J., & Kumbhare, D. A. (2019). Effect of local anesthetic versus botulinum toxin-A injections for myofascial pain disorders. *Clinical Journal of Pain, 35*(4), 353–367.

Albrecht, E., Kern, C., & Kirkham, K. (2015). A systematic review and meta-analysis of perineural dexamethasone for peripheral nerve blocks. *Anaesthesia, 70*(1), 71–83.

Baeriswyl, M., Kirkham, K. R., Kern, C., & Albrecht, E. (2015). The analgesic efficacy of ultrasound-guided transversus abdominis plane block in adult patients: a meta-analysis. *Anesthesia & Analgesia, 121*(6), 1640–1654.

Bakshi, S. G., Mapari, A., & Shylasree, T. (2016). REctus Sheath block for postoperative analgesia in gynecological ONcology Surgery (RESONS): a randomized-controlled trial. *Canadian Journal of Anesthesia/Journal Canadien d'Anesthésie, 63*(12), 1335–1344. https://link.springer.com/content/pdf/10.1007/s12630-016-0732-9.pdf.

Barksdale, P., & Yager, M. (2014). *Clinical practice guideline peripheral nerve blocks in upper and lower extremity*. Chicago: National Association of Orthopaedic Nurses, SmithBucklin.

Bashandy, G. M. N., & Elkholy, A. H. H. (2014). Reducing postoperative opioid consumption by adding an ultrasound-guided rectus sheath block to multimodal analgesia for abdominal cancer surgery with midline incision. *Anesthesiology and Pain Medicine, 4*(3).

Bicket, M. C., Gupta, A., Brown, C. H. IV & Cohen, S. P. (2013). Epidural injections for spinal pain: A systematic review and meta-analysis evaluating the "control" injections in randomized controlled trials. *Anesthesiology, 119*(4), 907–931.

Bicket, M. C., Horowitz, J. M., Benzon, H. T., & Cohen, S. P. (2015). Epidural injections in prevention of surgery for spinal pain: systematic review and meta-analysis of randomized controlled trials. *Spine Journal, 15*(2), 348–362.

Bos, E. M., Hollmann, M. W., & Lirk, P. (2017). Safety and efficacy of epidural analgesia. *Current Opinion in Anaesthesiology, 30*(6), 736–742.

Bourne, E., Wright, C., & Royse, C. (2010). A review of local anesthetic cardiotoxicity and treatment with lipid emulsion. *Local and Regional Anesthesia, 3*, 11–19.

Brogi, E., Kazan, R., Cyr, S., Giunta, F., & Hemmerling, T. M. (2016). Transversus abdominal plane block for postoperative analgesia: a systematic review and meta-analysis of randomized-controlled trials. *Canadian Journal of Anesthesia/Journal Canadien d'Anesthésie, 63*(10), 1184–1196. https://link.springer.com/content/pdf/10.1007/s12630-016-0679-x.pdf.

Bruel, B. M., Engle, M. P., Rauck, R. L., Weber, T. J., & Kapural, L. (2015). Intrathecal drug delivery for control of pain. In T. Deer, M. Leong, A. Buvanendran, P. Kim & S. Panchal. (Eds.), *Treatment of Chronic Pain by Interventional Approaches*. Springer.

Cheney, F. W., Domino, K. B., Caplan, R. A., & Posner, K. L. (1999). Nerve injury associated with anesthesia: a closed claims analysis. *Journal of the American Society of Anesthesiologists, 90*(4), 1062–1069.

Chin, K. J. (2019). Thoracic wall blocks: from paravertebral to retrolaminar to serratus to erector spinae and back again–A review of evidence. *Best Practice & Research Clinical Anaesthesiology, 33*(1), 67–77.

Chin, K. J., & El-Boghdadly, K. (2021). Mechanisms of action of the erector spinae plane (ESP) block: a narrative review. *Canadian Journal of Anesthesia/Journal Canadien d'Anesthésie*, 1–22.

Chin, K. J., Lirk, P., Hollmann, M. W., & Schwarz, S. K. (2021). Mechanisms of action of fascial plane blocks: a narrative review. *Regional Anesthesia & Pain Medicine, 46*(7), 618–628.

Chin, K. J., McDonnell, J. G., Carvalho, B., Sharkey, A., Pawa, A., & Gadsden, J. (2017). Essentials of our current understanding: abdominal wall blocks. *Regional Anesthesia & Pain Medicine, 42*(2), 133–183.

Chong, M., Berbenetz, N., Kumar, K., & Lin, C. (2019). The serratus plane block for postoperative analgesia in breast and thoracic surgery: a systematic review and meta-analysis. *Regional Anesthesia & Pain Medicine, 44*(12), 1066–1074.

Chou, R., Hashimoto, R., Friedly, J., Fu, R., Bougatsos, C., Dana, T., Sullivan, S. D., & Jarvik, J. (2015). Epidural corticosteroid injections for radiculopathy and spinal stenosis: a systematic review and meta-analysis. *Annals of Internal Medicine, 163*(5), 373–381.

Curatolo, M., Petersen-Felix, S., Arendt-Nielsen, L., & Fisher, D. M. (2000). Sensory assessment of regional analgesia in humans: a review of methods and applications. *The Journal of the American Society of Anesthesiologists, 93*(6), 1517–1530.

De Cassai, A., Bonanno, C., Padrini, R., Geraldini, F., Boscolo, A., Navalesi, P., & Munari, M. (2020). Pharmacokinetics of lidocaine after bilateral ESP block. *Regional Anesthesia & Pain Medicine, 46*(1), 86–89.

Desai, N., Kirkham, K., & Albrecht, E. (2021). Local anaesthetic adjuncts for peripheral regional anaesthesia: a narrative review. *Anaesthesia, 76*, 100–109.

Deshpande, J. P., & Patil, K. N. (2020). Evaluation of magnesium as an adjuvant to ropivacaine-induced axillary brachial plexus block: A prospective, randomised, double-blind study. *Indian Journal of Anaesthesia, 64*(4), 310.

D'Souza, R. S., & Hooten, W. M. (2021). *Neurolytic Blocks*. StatPearls Publishing.

Duckworth, A. D., & McQueen, M. M. (2017). The diagnosis of acute compartment syndrome: a critical analysis review. *JBJS Reviews, 5*(12), e1. https://doi.org/10.2106/jbjs.Rvw.17.00016.

Elbahrawy, K., & El-Deeb, A. (2016). Rectus sheath block for postoperative analgesia in patients with mesenteric vascular occlusion undergoing laparotomy: A randomized single-blinded study. *Anesthesia, Essays and Researches, 10*(3), 516. https://www.aeronline.org/article.asp?issn=0259-1162;year=2016;volume=10;issue=3;spage=516;epage=520;aulast=Elbahrawy.

Eng, H. C., Ghosh, S. M., & Chin, K. J. (2014). Practical use of local anesthetics in regional anesthesia. *Current Opinion in Anesthesiology, 27*(4), 382–387.

Estefan, M. (2021). *Intradiscal Electrothermal Therapy.* StatPearls Publishing.

Gabriel, R. A., & Ilfeld, B. M. (2019). Peripheral nerve blocks for postoperative analgesia: From traditional unencapsulated local anesthetic to liposomes, cryoneurolysis and peripheral nerve stimulation. *Best Practice & Research Clinical Anaesthesiology, 33*(3), 293–302.

Gan, T. J., Belani, K. G., Bergese, S., Chung, F., Diemunsch, P., Habib, A. S., Jin, Z., Kovac, A. L., Meyer, T. A., & Urman, R. D. (2019). Fourth consensus guidelines for the management of postoperative nausea and vomiting. *Anesthesia & Analgesia, 131*(2), 411–448.

Gawęda, B., Borys, M., Belina, B., Bąk, J., Czuczwar, M., Wołoszczuk-Gębicka, B., Kolowca, M., & Widenka, K. (2020). Postoperative pain treatment with erector spinae plane block and pectoralis nerve blocks in patients undergoing mitral/tricuspid valve repair—a randomized controlled trial. *BMC Anesthesiology, 20*(1), 1–9. https://bmcanesthesiol.biomedcentral.com/track/pdf/10.1186/s12871-019-0855-y.pdf.

Gitman, M., Fettiplace, M. R., Weinberg, G. L., Neal, J. M., & Barrington, M. J. (2019). Local anesthetic systemic toxicity: A narrative literature review and clinical update on prevention, diagnosis, and management. *Plastic and Reconstructive Surgery, 144*(3), 783–795.

Goel, V., Patwardhan, A. M., Ibrahim, M., Howe, C. L., Schultz, D. M., & Shankar, H. (2019). Complications associated with stellate ganglion nerve block: a systematic review. *Regional Anesthesia & Pain Medicine, 44*(6), 669–678.

Greengrass, R. A., Narouze, S., Bendtsen, T. F., & Hadzic, A. (2019). Cervical plexus and greater occipital nerve blocks: controversies and technique update. *Regional Anesthesia & Pain Medicine.*

Guay, J., & Kopp, S. (2020). Peripheral nerve blocks for hip fractures in adults. *Cochrane Database of Systematic Reviews, (11).*

Helander, E. M., Kaye, A. J., Eng, M. R., Emelife, P. I., Motejunas, M. W., Bonneval, L. A., Terracciano, J. A., Cornett, E. M., & Kaye, A. D. (2019). Regional nerve blocks—best practice strategies for reduction in complications and comprehensive review. *Current Pain and Headache Reports, 23*(6), 1–9.

Helander, E. M., Webb, M. P., Kendrick, J., Montet, T., Kaye, A. J., Cornett, E. M., & Kaye, A. D. (2019). PECS, serratus plane, erector spinae, and paravertebral blocks: a comprehensive review. *Best Practice & Research Clinical Anaesthesiology, 33*(4), 573–581.

Hermanns, H., Hollmann, M. W., Stevens, M. F., Lirk, P., Brandenburger, T., Piegeler, T., & Werdehausen, R. (2019). Molecular mechanisms of action of systemic lidocaine in acute and chronic pain: a narrative review. *British Journal of Anaesthesia, 123*(3), 335–349. https://bjanaesthesia.org/article/S0007-0912(19)30501-X/pdf.

Hong, S., Kim, H., & Park, J. (2019). Analgesic effectiveness of rectus sheath block during open gastrectomy: a prospective double-blinded randomized controlled clinical trial. *Medicine, 98*(15).

Horlocker, T. T., Vandermeulen, E., Kopp, S. L., Gogarten, W., Leffert, L. R., & Benzon, H. T. (2019). Regional anesthesia in the patient receiving antithrombotic or thrombolytic therapy: American Society of Regional Anesthesia and Pain Medicine Evidence-Based Guidelines. *Obstetric Anesthesia Digest, 39*(1), 28–29.

Hunter, O. O., Kim, T. E., Mariano, E. R., & Harrison, T. K. (2019). Care of the patient with a peripheral nerve block. *Journal of PeriAnesthesia Nursing, 34*(1), 16–26.

Hussain, N., Goldar, G., Ragina, N., Banfield, L., Laffey, J. G., & Abdallah, F. W. (2017). Suprascapular and interscalene nerve block for shoulder surgery: a systematic review and meta-analysis. *Anesthesiology, 127*(6), 998–1013.

Ilfeld, B. M. (2017). Continuous peripheral nerve blocks: an update of the published evidence and comparison with novel, alternative analgesic modalities. *Anesthesia & Analgesia, 124*(1), 308–335.

Ilfeld, B. M., & Gabriel, R. A. (2019). Basal infusion versus intermittent boluses for perineural catheters: should we take the 'continuous' out of 'continuous peripheral nerve blocks'? *Regional Anesthesia & Pain Medicine.*

Ishida, T., Tanaka, S., Sakamoto, A., Hirabayashi, T., & Kawamata, M. (2018). Plasma ropivacaine concentration after TAP block in a patient with cardiac and renal failure. *Local and Regional Anesthesia, 11*, 57.

Ivanusic, J., Konishi, Y., & Barrington, M. J. (2018). A cadaveric study investigating the mechanism of action of erector spinae blockade. *Regional Anesthesia & Pain Medicine, 43*(6), 567–571.

Jack, J., McLellan, E., Versyck, B., Englesakis, M., & Chin, K. (2020). The role of serratus anterior plane and pectoral nerves blocks in cardiac surgery, thoracic surgery and trauma: a qualitative systematic review. *Anaesthesia, 75*(10), 1372–1385.

Jagannathan, R., Niesen, A. D., D'Souza, R. S., & Johnson, R. L. (2019). Intermittent bolus versus continuous infusion techniques for local anesthetic delivery in peripheral and truncal nerve analgesia: the current state of evidence. *Regional Anesthesia & Pain Medicine, 44*(4), 447–451.

Jain, S., Deer, T., Sayed, D., Chopra, P., Wahezi, S., Jassal, N., Weisbein, J., Jameson, J., Malinkowski, M., & Golovac, S. (2020). Minimally invasive lumbar decompression: a review of indications, techniques, efficacy and safety. *Pain Management, 10*(5), 331–348.

Jin, Z., Durrands, T., Li, R., Gan, T. J., & Lin, J. (2020). Pectoral block versus paravertebral block: a systematic review, meta-analysis and trial sequential analysis. *Regional Anesthesia & Pain Medicine, 45*(9), 727–732.

Joubert, F., Gillois, P., Bouaziz, H., Marret, E., Iohom, G., & Albaladejo, P. (2019). Bleeding complications following peripheral regional anaesthesia in patients treated with anticoagulants or antiplatelet agents: A systematic review. *Anaesthesia Critical Care & Pain Medicine, 38*(5), 507–516.

Karaarslan, E., Topal, A., Onur, A., & Uzun, S. T. (2018). Research on the efficacy of the rectus sheath block method.

Kietrys, D. M., Palombaro, K. M., Azzaretto, E., Hubler, R., Schaller, B., Schlussel, J. M., & Tucker, M. (2013). Effectiveness of dry needling for upper-quarter myofascial pain: A systematic review and meta-analysis. *Journal of Orthopaedic & Sports Physical Therapy, 43*(9), 620–634.

Knezevic, N. N., Manchikanti, L., Urits, I., Orhurhu, V., Vangala, B. P., Vanaparthy, R., Sanapati, M. R., Shah, S., Soin, A., & Mahajan, A. (2020). Lack of superiority of epidural injections with lidocaine with steroids compared to without steroids in spinal pain: A systematic review and meta-analysis. *Pain Physician, 23*(4S), 239.

Koniuch, K. L., Buys, M. J., Campbell, B., Gililland, J. M., Pelt, C. E., Pace, N. L., & Johnson, K. B. (2019). Serum ropivacaine levels after local infiltration analgesia during total knee arthroplasty with and without adductor canal block. *Regional Anesthesia & Pain Medicine, 44*(4), 478–482.

Kreutzwiser, D., & Tawfic, Q. A. (2019). Expanding role of NMDA receptor antagonists in the management of pain. *CNS Drugs, 33*(4), 347–374.

Lee, B. H., Kumar, K. K., Wu, E. C., & Wu, C. L. (2019). Role of regional anesthesia and analgesia in the opioid epidemic. *Regional Anesthesia & Pain Medicine.*

Levene, J. L., Weinstein, E. J., Cohen, M. S., Andreae, D. A., Chao, J. Y., Johnson, M., Hall, C. B., & Andreae, M. H. (2019). Local anesthetics and regional anesthesia versus conventional analgesia for preventing persistent postoperative pain in adults and children: a Cochrane systematic review and meta-analysis update. *Journal of Clinical Anesthesia, 55*, 116–127. https://www.ncbi.nlm.nih.gov/pmc/articles/PMC6461051/pdf/nihms-1518484.pdf.

Liu, S. S., Ortolan, S., Sandoval, M. V., Curren, J., Fields, K. G., Memtsoudis, S. G., & YaDeau, J. T. (2016). Cardiac arrest and seizures caused by local anesthetic systemic toxicity after peripheral nerve blocks. *Regional Anesthesia Pain Medicine, 41*, 5–21. https://rapm.bmj.com/content/41/1/5.long.

Lovkov, I., Uvarov, D., Antipin, E., Ushakov, A., Karpunov, A., & Nedashkovskiv, E. (2017). Efficiency and safety of bilateral ultrasound rectus sheath block in urgent laparotomy. *Anesteziologiia i Reanimatologiia, 62*(1), 60–63.

Ma, N., Duncan, J. K., Scarfe, A. J., Schuhmann, S., & Cameron, A. L. (2017). Clinical safety and effectiveness of transversus abdominis plane (TAP) block in post-operative analgesia: a systematic review and meta-analysis. *Journal of Anesthesia, 31*(3), 432–452. https://link.springer.com/article/10.1007%2Fs00540-017-2323-5.

Manchikanti, L., Benyamin, R. M., Falco, F. J., Kaye, A. D., & Hirsch, J. A. (2015). Do epidural injections provide short- and long-term relief for lumbar disc herniation? A systematic review. *Clinical Orthopaedics and Related Research, 473*(6), 1940–1956.

Mayes, J., Davison, E., Panahi, P., Patten, D., Eljelani, F., Womack, J., & Varma, M. (2016). An anatomical evaluation of the serratus anterior plane block. *Anaesthesia, 71*(9), 1064–1069.

Meissner, W., Huygen, F., Neugebauer, E. A., Osterbrink, J., Benhamou, D., Betteridge, N., Coluzzi, F., De Andres, J., Fawcett, W., & Fletcher, D. (2018). Management of acute pain in the postoperative setting: the importance of quality indicators. *Current Medical Research and Opinion, 34*(1), 187–196.

McCormick, Z. L., Marshall, B., Walker, J., McCarthy, R., & Walega, D. R. (2015). Long-term function, pain and medication use outcomes of radiofrequency ablation for lumbar facet syndrome. *International Journal of Anesthetics and Anesthesiology, 2*(2), 028.

Mörwald, E. E., Zubizarreta, N., Cozowicz, C., Poeran, J., & Memtsoudis, S. G. (2017). Incidence of local anesthetic systemic toxicity in orthopedic patients receiving peripheral nerve blocks. *Regional Anesthesia & Pain Medicine, 42*(4), 442–445.

Nagappa, M., Liao, P., Wong, J., Auckley, D., Ramachandran, S. K., Memtsoudis, S., Mokhlesi, B., & Chung, F. (2015). Validation of the STOP-Bang questionnaire as a screening tool for obstructive sleep apnea among different populations: a systematic review and meta-analysis. *PLoS ONE, 10*(12), e0143697.

Nagappa, M., Patra, J., Wong, J., Subramani, Y., Singh, M., Ho, G., Wong, D. T., & Chung, F. (2017). Association of STOP-Bang questionnaire as a screening tool for sleep apnea and postoperative complications: a systematic review and bayesian meta-analysis of prospective and retrospective cohort studies. *Anesthesia & Analgesia, 125*(4), 1301–1308.

Nair, A. S., Poornachand, A., & Kodisharapu, P. K. (2018). Ziconotide: Indications, adverse effects, and limitations in managing refractory chronic pain. *Indian Journal of Palliative Care, 24*(1), 118–119. https://doi.org/10.4103/IJPC.IJPC_113_17.

Neal, J. M., Barrington, M. J., Brull, R., Hadzic, A., Hebl, J. R., Horlocker, T. T., Huntoon, M. A., Kopp, S. L., Rathmell, J. P., & Watson, J. C. (2015). The second ASRA practice advisory on neurologic complications associated with regional anesthesia and pain medicine: Executive summary 2015. *Regional Anesthesia & Pain Medicine, 40*(5), 401–430.

Neal, J. M., Barrington, M. J., Fettiplace, M. R., Gitman, M., Memtsoudis, S. G., Mörwald, E. E., Rubin, D. S., & Weinberg, G. (2018). The third American Society of Regional Anesthesia and Pain Medicine practice advisory on local anesthetic systemic toxicity: Executive summary 2017. *Regional Anesthesia & Pain Medicine, 43*(2), 113–123.

Neal, J. M., Neal, E. J., & Weinberg, G. L. (2021). American Society of Regional Anesthesia and Pain Medicine local anesthetic systemic toxicity checklist: 2020 version. *Regional Anesthesia & Pain Medicine, 46*(1), 81–82.

Odor, P. M., Ster, I. C., Wilkinson, I., & Sage, F. (2017). Effect of admission fascia iliaca compartment blocks on post-operative abbreviated mental test scores in elderly fractured neck of femur patients: a retrospective cohort study. *BMC Anesthesiology, 17*(1), 1–8. https://bmcanesthesiol.biomedcentral.com/track/pdf/10.1186/s12871-016-0295-x.pdf.

Orleans, L., & Urman, R. D. (2019). A contemporary medicolegal analysis of injury related to peripheral nerve blocks. *Pain Physician, 22*, 389–399.

Patel, A., Petrone, B., & Carter, K. R. (2020). *Percutaneous Vertebroplasty and Kyphoplasty.* StatPearls Publishing.

Peek, J., Smeeing, D. P., Hietbrink, F., Houwert, R. M., Marsman, M., & de Jong, M. B. (2019). Comparison of analgesic interventions for traumatic rib fractures: A systematic review and meta-analysis. *European Journal of Trauma and Emergency Surgery, 45*(4), 597–622.

Rahiri, J., Tuhoe, J., Svirskis, D., Lightfoot, N., Lirk, P., & Hill, A. (2017). Systematic review of the systemic concentrations of local anaesthetic after transversus abdominis plane block and rectus sheath block. *BJA: British Journal of Anaesthesia, 118*(4), 517–526.

Riff, C., Guilhaumou, R., Marsot, A., Beaussier, M., Cohen, M., Blin, O., & Francon, D. (2018). Ropivacaine wound infiltration for pain management after breast cancer mastectomy: a population pharmacokinetic analysis. *Clinical Pharmacology in Drug Development, 7*(8), 811–819. https://accp1.onlinelibrary.wiley.com/doi/abs/10.1002/cpdd.452.

Ripollés, J., Mezquita, S. M., Abad, A., & Calvo, J. (2015). Analgesic efficacy of the ultrasound-guided blockade of the transversus abdominis plane-a systematic review. *Revista Brasileira de Anestesiologia, 65*(4), 255–280.

Saad, F. S., El Baradie, S. Y., Aliem, M. A. W. A., Ali, M. M., & Kotb, T. A. M. (2018). Ultrasound-guided serratus anterior plane block versus thoracic paravertebral block for perioperative analgesia in thoracotomy. *Saudi Journal of Anaesthesia, 12*(4), 565.

Salinas, J. D. (2016). Corticosteroid injections of joints and soft tissues. *Medscape.* http://emedicine.medscape.com/article/325370-overview#a1.

Sanderson, B. J., & Doane, M. A. (2018). Transversus abdominis plane catheters for analgesia following abdominal surgery in adults. *Regional Anesthesia & Pain Medicine, 43*(1), 5–13.

Scala, V. A., Lee, L. S., & Atkinson, R. E. (2019). Implementing regional nerve blocks in hip fracture programs: A review of regional nerve blocks, protocols in the literature, and the current protocol at the Queen's Medical Center in Honolulu, HI. *Hawai'i Journal of Health & Social Welfare, 78*(11 Suppl 2), 11.

Scott, N. A., Guo, B., Barton, P. M., & Gerwin, R. D. (2009). Trigger point injections for chronic non-malignant musculoskeletal pain: a systematic review. *Pain Medicine, 10*(1), 54–69.

Shashidhar, Y., Kaushal, R., & Ahirwal, R. (2020). A comparative study on upper limb supraclavicular brachial plexus block: dexmedetomidine with ropivacaine and dexamethasone with ropivacaine and ropivacaine alone. *International Journal of Health and Clinical Research, 3*(12 Suppl), 14–21.

Siddiqui, M. R. S., Sajid, M. S., Uncles, D. R., Cheek, L., & Baig, M. K. (2011). A meta-analysis on the clinical effectiveness of transversus abdominis plane block. *Journal of Clinical Anesthesia, 23*(1), 7–14. https://www.sciencedirect.com/science/article/abs/pii/S0952818010003727?via%3Dihub.

Sondekoppam, R. V., & Tsui, B. C. (2017). Factors associated with risk of neurologic complications after peripheral nerve blocks: a systematic review. *Anesthesia & Analgesia, 124*(2), 645–660.

Su, Y., Zhang, Z., Zhang, Y., Li, H., & Shi, W. (2015). Efficacy of ropivacaine by the concentration of 0.25%, 0.5%, and 0.75% on surgical performance, postoperative analgesia, and patient's satisfaction in inguinal hernioplasty: a randomized controlled trial. *Patient Preference and Adherence, 9,* 1375.

Suzuki, S., Gerner, P., Colvin, A. C., & Binshtok, A. M. (2009). C-fiber-selective peripheral nerve blockade. *The Open Pain Journal, 2*(1).

Suzuki, S., Gerner, P., & Lirk, P. (2019). *Local anesthetics.* In *Pharmacology and Physiology for Anesthesia* (pp. 390–411). Elsevier.

Sviggum, H. P., Jacob, A. K., Mantilla, C. B., Schroeder, D. R., Sperling, J. W., & Hebl, J. R. (2012). Perioperative nerve injury after total shoulder arthroplasty: assessment of risk after regional anesthesia. *Regional Anesthesia & Pain Medicine, 37*(5), 490–494.

Tran, D. Q., Bravo, D., Leurcharusmee, P., & Neal, J. M. (2019). Transversus abdominis plane block: a narrative review. *Anesthesiology, 131*(5), 1166–1190.

Tsai, H.-C., Yoshida, T., Chuang, T.-Y., Yang, S.-F., Chang, C.-C., Yao, H.-Y., Tai, Y.-T., Lin, J.-A., & Chen, K.-Y. (2017). Transversus abdominis plane block: an updated review of anatomy and techniques. *BioMed Research International* 2017.

Turbitt, L. R., McHardy, P. G., Casanova, M., Shapiro, J., Li, L., & Choi, S. (2018). Analysis of inpatient falls after total knee arthroplasty in patients with continuous femoral nerve block. *Anesthesia & Analgesia, 127*(1), 224–227.

Uppal, V., Sancheti, S., & Kalagara, H. (2019). Transversus abdominis plane (TAP) and rectus sheath blocks: a technical description and evidence review. *Current Anesthesiology Reports, 9*(4), 479–487.

Visser, W.A., Lee, R.A., & Gielen, M.J. (2008). Factors affecting the distribution of neural blockade by local anesthetics in epidural anesthesia and a comparison of lumbar versus thoracic epidural anesthesia. *Anesthesia & Analgesia, 107*(2), 708–721.

Waldman, S. D. (2009). *Pain Review* (2nd ed.). Saunders Elsevier.

Wheeler, A. H. (2018). Therapeutic injections for pain management. *Medscape.* https://emedicine.medscape.com/article/1143675-overview#a7.

Willard, F., Vleeming, A., Schuenke, M., Danneels, L., & Schleip, R. (2012). The thoracolumbar fascia: anatomy, function and clinical considerations. *Journal of Anatomy, 221*(6), 507–536. https://www.ncbi.nlm.nih.gov/pmc/articles/PMC3512278/pdf/joa0221-0507.pdf.

Wolfe, R. C., & Spillars, A. (2018). Local anesthetic systemic toxicity: Reviewing updates from the American Society of Regional Anesthesia and Pain Medicine Practice advisory. *Journal of PeriAnesthesia Nursing, 33*(6), 1000–1005. https://www.jopan.org/article/S1089-9472(18)30346-0/fulltext.

Wong, J., Bremer, N., Weyker, P. D., & Webb, C. A. (2016). Ultrasound-guided genicular nerve thermal radiofrequency ablation for chronic knee pain. *Case Reports in Anesthesiology.* https://doi.org/10.1155/2016/8292450.

Xiao, Q., Xu, B., Wang, H., Luo, Z., Yuan, M., Zhou, Z., & Pei, F. (2021). Analgesic effect of single-shot ropivacaine at different layers of the surgical site in primary total hip arthroplasty: a randomised, controlled, observer-blinded study. *Journal of Orthopaedic Surgery and Research, 16*(1), 1–10.

Xie, C., Ran, G., Chen, D., & Lu, Y. (2021). A narrative review of ultrasound-guided serratus anterior plane block. *Annals of Palliative Medicine, 10*(1), 700–706.

Yassen, K., Lotfy, M., Miligi, A., Sallam, A., Hegazi, E. A. R., & Afifi, M. (2019). Patient-controlled analgesia with and without transverse abdominis plane and rectus sheath space block in cirrhotic patients undergoing liver resection. *Journal of Anaesthesiology, Clinical Pharmacology, 35*(1), 58. https://www.joacp.org/article.asp?issn=0970-9185year=2019;volume=35;issue=1;spage=58;epage=64;aulast=Yassen.

Zhang, D., Zhou, C., Wei, D., Ge, L., & Li, Q. (2019). Dexamethasone added to local anesthetics in ultrasound-guided transversus abdominis plain (TAP) block for analgesia after abdominal surgery: A systematic review and meta-analysis of randomized controlled trials. *PLoS ONE, 14*(1), e0209646. https://www.ncbi.nlm.nih.gov/pmc/articles/PMC6324803/pdf/pone.0209646.pdf.

Zhang, F. F., Lv, C., Yang, L. Y., Wang, S. P., Zhang, M., & Guo, X. W. (2019). Pharmacokinetics of ropivacaine in elderly patients receiving fascia iliaca compartment block. *Experimental and Therapeutic Medicine, 18*(4), 2648–2652. https://www.ncbi.nlm.nih.gov/pmc/articles/PMC6755487/pdf/etm-18-04-2648.pdf.

Part 4

Procedural Sedation and Analgesia

Laura Habighorst, BSN, RN, CAPA, CGRN, NPD-BC
Kimberly Wittmayer, MS, APRN, PCNS-BC, PMGT-BC AP-PMN
Maureen F. Cooney, DNP, FNP-BC, ACHPN, AP-PMN*

Introduction

Successful completion of a procedure while maintaining patient comfort is the goal of all procedures and may require procedural sedation and analgesia. This chapter provides evidence-based approaches for safe delivery of procedural care to patients of all ages undergoing procedures.

I. Management of Procedures

A. Efforts should be made to provide optimal comfort for patients of all ages before, during, and after procedures (see pediatric content below for more specific information).
B. Nonpharmacological and pharmacological interventions should be based on type of procedure and patient's age, temperament, coping style, and preference.
C. Procedural sedation should be considered to decrease anxiety and facilitate completion of procedures.

II. Procedural Sedation

A. General Concepts
   1. Definitions
      a. Procedural sedation: administration of pharmacological agents for relief of discomfort, pain, or anxiety which may be experienced during invasive, manipulative, or constraining procedures
      b. Analgesia is often added to the term "procedural sedation" or "moderate sedation" (e.g., procedural sedation and analgesia) to indicate use of medications to decrease pain, as sedation only provides decreased level of consciousness and anxiety.
   2. The American Society of Anesthesiologists' (ASA) goal is for patient to maintain a patent airway with adequate cardiovascular/ventilatory function and to perceive minimal pain or discomfort during designated procedure.
   3. Procedural sedation is a continuum, and patients may experience one or more levels of sedation as identified by ASA (see Section II.B.1 below). Procedural care team should be prepared to rescue patient at the next deeper level of sedation if respiratory or cardiovascular adverse effects arise.
   4. The Joint Commission (TJC) standards for sedation and anesthesia apply to any patient in any setting, for any purpose, by any route, when receiving moderate or deep sedation as well as general, spinal, or any other major regional anesthesia.
      a. Standards do not apply to minimal sedation (anxiolysis).
      b. Standards identify moderate sedation as the second level on a continuum between minimal and deep sedation.
      c. Sedation practices shall be monitored and evaluated by appropriately trained anesthesia providers.
      d. Any hospital providing procedural sedation shall perform an evidence-based assessment in order to decrease risk of complications.
   5. Goals of procedural sedation:
      a. Allow patient to tolerate procedure, while being conscious and cooperative (as appropriate to the procedure).
      b. Decrease patient's fear and anxiety.
      c. Decrease patient's perception of pain.
      d. Maintain consciousness with some degree of amnesia (as appropriate to the procedure).
      e. Minimize variation of vital signs.
      f. Allow for successful completion of procedure.
      g. Provide rapid and safe return to activities of daily living.
B. Levels of Sedation
   1. ASA four levels of sedation
      a. Minimal sedation (anxiolysis)
         1) Patient is awake or arouses easily, yet is under the influence of medication(s).

---

*Section Editor for the chapter.

2) Patient maintains normal respirations, adequate ventilation, intact protective reflexes, and cardiovascular function.
3) Amnesia may or may not be present, and cognitive function or coordination may be impaired.
4) May be administered by any registered healthcare professional (e.g., registered nurse [RN], certified registered nurse anesthetist [CRNA], advanced practice registered nurse [APRN], physician).
b. Moderate sedation (no longer referred to as "conscious sedation")
1) Patient is in pharmacologically controlled state of limited or minimally depressed consciousness and responds appropriately to verbal commands with or without light physical stimulation.
2) Patient independently and continuously maintains a patent airway, spontaneous respirations and ventilation, protective reflexes, and usually, cardiovascular function.
3) Amnesia may or may not be present depending upon medication(s).
4) May be administered by an RN with *demonstrated competency*, physician *credentialed in procedural sedation*, CRNA, or anesthesiologist.
5) Moderate sedation is not synonymous with pain relief; therefore, analgesics and interventions for pain control must also be considered.
c. Deep sedation
1) Deep sedation is a controlled state of depressed consciousness.
2) Patient is not easily aroused but can respond purposefully following repeated painful stimulation.
3) Partial or complete loss of protective reflexes occurs, including ability to independently maintain airway.
4) Loss of spontaneous ventilation may occur; cardiovascular state usually remains stable.
5) Deep sedation may be performed by CRNA, anesthesiologist, emergency department or critical care physician *credentialed in deep sedation*, and, depending on *individual state regulations*, RNs who are deemed competent to administer medications such as propofol for sedation purposes.
d. General anesthesia
1) General anesthesia is controlled state of unconsciousness with a loss of protective reflexes.
2) Airway stabilization is required, and cardiovascular status may or may not be affected.
3) Patient is unable to respond to physical stimuli or verbal commands.

4) General anesthesia is administered *only* by CRNA or anesthesiologist.
C. Procedural Sedation Preparation
1. Patient considerations and assessment
a. Identify populations at greatest risk for respiratory depression or arrest (most common complication associated with procedural sedation).
1) Obstructive sleep apnea
2) Obese
3) Elderly
4) Pediatrics
5) History of substance use or misuse
6) History of chronic obstructive pulmonary disease (COPD)
b. To determine baseline status, suitability for planned procedure and sedation, and potential complications, evaluation should include knowledge of:
1) Medical history
a) History of alcohol, tobacco, and/or illicit substance use
b) History of persistent pain and persistent pain medication use
c) History of cardiovascular/respiratory disease
d) History of bariatric surgery
2) Anesthetic history
a) Difficulty with previous sedation or anesthesia
b) Family history of difficulty with sedation or anesthesia
3) Nothing-by-mouth (NPO) status (Table 20.1)
4) Current medications including prescriptions, over the counter (OTC) medications, vitamins, supplements, and herbal preparations (rationale: may interfere with absorption and clearance of opioids or benzodiazepines used during procedural sedation)
5) Allergies and reactions
6) Mental status including patient expectations and ability to cooperate
c. Physical exam considerations
1) Weight, height, and/or body mass index (BMI)
a) BMI = weight in kilograms divided by height in meters^2
(1) BMI <18.5 = Underweight
(2) BMI 18.5–24.9 = Normal
(3) BMI 25.0–29.9 = Overweight
(4) BMI ≥30.0 = Obese
2) Baseline vital signs including pulse oximetry and end-tidal CO_2
3) ASA classification (Table 20.2)
a) Developed to assist in determining risk of complications during procedures
b) Classes 1 and 2 are considered good candidates for moderate sedation procedures.

Table 20.1

Fasting and Pharmacologic Recommendations

A. Fasting Recommendations*

Ingested Material	Minimum Fasting Period†
• Clear liquids‡	2h
• Breast milk	4h
• Infant formula	6h
• Nonhuman milk§	6h
• Light meal**	6h
• Fried foods, fatty foods, or meat	Additional fasting time (e.g., 8 or more hours) may be needed

B. Pharmacologic Recommendations

Medication Type and Common Examples	Recommendation
Gastrointestinal stimulants:	
• Metoclopramide	May be used/no routine use
Gastric acid secretion blockers:	
• Cimetidine	May be used/no routine use
• Famotidine	May be used/no routine use
• Ranitidine	May be used/no routine use
• Omeprazole	May be used/no routine use
• Lansoprazole	May be used/no routine use
Antacids:	
• Sodium citrate	May be used/no routine use
• Sodium bicarbonate	May be used/no routine use
• Magnesium trisilicate	May be used/no routine use
Antiemetics:	
• Ondansetron	May be used/no routine use
Anticholinergics:	
• Atropine	No use
• Scopolamine	No use
• Glycopyrrolate	No use
Combinations of the medications above:	No routine use

*These recommendations apply to healthy patients who are undergoing elective procedures. They are not intended for women in labor. Following the guidelines does not guarantee complete gastric emptying.

†The fasting periods noted above apply to all ages.

‡Examples of clear liquids include water, fruit juices without pulp, carbonated beverages, clear tea, and black coffee.

§Since nonhuman milk is similar to solids in gastric emptying time, the amount ingested must be considered when determining an appropriate fasting period.

**A light meal typically consists of toast and clear liquids. Meals that include fried or fatty foods or meat may prolong gastric emptying time. Additional fasting time (e.g., 8 or more hours) may be needed in these cases. Both the amount and type of foods ingested must be considered when determining an appropriate fasting period.

From https://pubs.asahq.org/anesthesiology/article/126/3/376/19733/Practice-Guidelines-for-Preoperative-Fasting-and.

From American Society of Anesthesiologists Task Force on Preoperative Fasting and the Use of Pharmacologic Agents to Reduce the Risk of Pulmonary Aspiration. (2017). Practice guidelines for preoperative fasting and the use of pharmacologic agents to reduce the risk of pulmonary aspiration: Application to healthy patients undergoing elective procedures. *Anesthesiology, 126:*376–393. doi: https://doi.org/10.1097/ALN.0000000000001452.

c) Classes 3 and 4 require further assessment of comorbidities which may require special interventions during sedation.

4) Airway assessment to identify risk of respiratory compromise with need for intubation

    a) History of stridor (a harsh, high-pitched wheezing or vibratory sound resulting from a narrowing of central airway or larynx) or other airway concerns

    b) History of obstructive sleep apnea (OSA), reported history of snoring, or positive STOP Bang tool

        (1) STOP Bang tool used to identify high potential for OSA (see Fig. 12.1)

        (2) Based on scoring point system with "yes" or "no" answers

        (3) Score of 3 or more "yes" responses indicates high risk for OSA.

d. Mallampati classes (4) to identify potentially difficult intubation (Fig. 20.1)

    1) Visualization of soft palate, uvula, and pillars

    2) Visualization of soft palate and uvula

    3) Visualization of soft palate and base of uvula

    4) Soft palate not visible at all

e. Other risk factors for difficult intubation

    1) Significant obesity

    2) Facial abnormalities

    3) Head, neck, and jaw deformities

    4) Short neck

    5) Limited neck extension

    6) Neck mass

    7) Cervical spine disease

    8) Tracheal deviation

    9) Mouth deformities

    10) Tonsillar hypertrophy

    11) Small mouth opening

    12) Protruding incisors

    13) Loose or capped teeth

    14) High, arched palate

    15) History of temporalmandibular joint disease (TMJ)

2. Nursing Considerations

  a. RN administering medications used for procedural sedation must have knowledge of type, duration, and intensity of procedure as well as prescribed medications' classification, appropriate dose, onset, peak effectiveness, and duration.

  b. Nurse monitoring patient must:

    1) Have no other responsibilities; however, according to ASA, nurse may assist with minor interruptible tasks after patient has stabilized.

    2) Demonstrate acquired knowledge of anatomy, physiology, pharmacology and cardiac arrhythmia recognition and respiratory physiology including oxygenation and ventilation.

    3) Assess and provide for patient needs before, during, and after administration of sedation and analgesia.

Table 20.2

ASA Physical Status Classification System

ASA PS Classification	Definition	Adult Examples, Including, but not Limited to:	Pediatric Examples, Including but not Limited to:	Obstetric Examples, Including but not Limited to:
ASA I	A normal healthy patient	Healthy, non-smoking, no or minimal alcohol use	Healthy (no acute or chronic disease), normal BMI percentile for age	
ASA II	A patient with mild systemic disease	Mild diseases only without substantive functional limitations. Current smoker, social alcohol drinker, pregnancy, obesity (30<BMI<40), well-controlled DM/HTN, mild lung disease	Asymptomatic congenital cardiac disease, well controlled dysrhythmias, asthma without exacerbation, well controlled epilepsy, non-insulin dependent diabetes mellitus, abnormal BMI percentile for age, mild/moderate OSA, oncologic state in remission, autism with mild limitations	Normal pregnancy*, well controlled gestational HTN, controlled preeclampsia without severe features, diet-controlled gestational DM.
ASA III	A patient with severe systemic disease	Substantive functional limitations; One or more moderate to severe diseases. Poorly controlled DM or HTN, COPD, morbid obesity (BMI ≥40), active hepatitis, alcohol dependence or abuse, implanted pacemaker, moderate reduction of ejection fraction, ESRD undergoing regularly scheduled dialysis, history (>3 months) of MI, CVA, TIA, or CAD/stents.	Uncorrected stable congenital cardiac abnormality, asthma with exacerbation, poorly controlled epilepsy, insulin dependent diabetes mellitus, morbid obesity, malnutrition, severe OSA, oncologic state, renal failure, muscular dystrophy, cystic fibrosis, history of organ transplantation, brain/spinal cord malformation, symptomatic hydrocephalus, premature infant PCA <60 weeks, autism with severe limitations, metabolic disease, difficult airway, long term parenteral nutrition. Full term infants <6 weeks of age.	Preeclampsia with severe features, gestational DM with complications or high insulin requirements, a thrombophilic disease requiring anticoagulation.
ASA IV	A patient with severe systemic disease that is a constant threat to life	Recent (<3 months) MI, CVA, TIA or CAD/stents, ongoing cardiac ischemia or severe valve dysfunction, severe reduction of ejection fraction, shock, sepsis, DIC, ARD or ESRD not undergoing regularly scheduled dialysis	Symptomatic congenital cardiac abnormality, congestive heart failure, active sequelae of prematurity, acute hypoxic-ischemic encephalopathy, shock, sepsis, disseminated intravascular coagulation, automatic implantable cardioverter-defibrillator, ventilator dependence, endocrinopathy, severe trauma, severe respiratory distress, advanced oncologic state.	Preeclampsia with severe features complicated by HELLP or other adverse event, peripartum cardiomyopathy with EF <40, uncorrected/decompensated heart disease, acquired or congenital.
ASA V	A moribund patient who is not expected to survive without the operation	Ruptured abdominal/thoracic aneurysm, massive trauma, intracranial bleed with mass effect, ischemic bowel in the face of significant cardiac pathology or multiple organ/system dysfunction	Massive trauma, intracranial hemorrhage with mass effect, patient requiring ECMO, respiratory failure or arrest, malignant hypertension, decompensated congestive heart failure, hepatic encephalopathy, ischemic bowel or multiple organ/system dysfunction.	Uterine rupture.
ASA VI	A declared brain-dead patient whose organs are being removed for donor purposes			

*Although pregnancy is not a disease, the parturient's physiologic state is significantly altered from when the woman is not pregnant, hence the assignment of ASA 2 for a woman with uncomplicated pregnancy.

**The addition of "E" denotes Emergency surgery: (An emergency is defined as existing when delay in treatment of the patient would lead to a significant increase in the threat to life or body part)

From: https://www.asahq.org/standards-and-practice-parameters/statement-on-asa-physical-status-classification-system.

Excerpted from (Statement on ASA Physical Status Classification System/2020) of the American Society of Anesthesiologists. A copy of the full text can be obtained from ASA, 1061 American Lane Schaumburg, IL 60173-4973 or online at www.asahq.org.

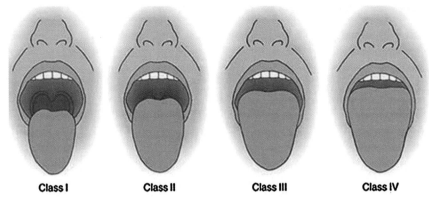

Class I   Class II   Class III   Class IV

Figure 20.1 Mallampati airway classification. (From Fleisher, L.A. [2023]. *Evidence-Based Practice of Anesthesiology,* 4th ed. Philadelphia: Elsevier.)

4) Understand principles and use of a variety of oxygen delivery systems.
5) Recognize potential complications of each type of agent being administered.
6) Possess competency to assess, diagnose, and intervene in event of complications and to provide appropriate interventions in compliance with orders or institutional protocols.

c. Supportive and monitoring equipment must be in room and immediately accessible before administration of any medication:
1) Oxygen and oxygen delivery devices
2) Suction apparatus
3) Noninvasive blood pressure device
4) Electrocardiograph (ECG)
5) Pulse oximeter
   a) Measures blood oxygen saturation
   b) Movement and decreased ventilation may provide false reading.
6) Capnography
   a) Measures ventilation (exchange of carbon dioxide and oxygen during respiration)
   b) Provides early indicator of airway obstruction and hypoventilation
7) Emergency cart with medications and supplies in all appropriate sizes (adult and pediatric) must be immediately available.
   a) Nasal and oral airways
   b) Intubation equipment
   c) Opioid and benzodiazepine reversal agents
      (1) Opioid reversal agent—naloxone
      (2) Benzodiazepine reversal agent—flumazenil
8) Defibrillator

D. Intraprocedural Care
1. RN must only engage in practice of nursing and must only assume those responsibilities within state specific nursing scope of practice; state regulations and laws; and institutional policy, procedures, and protocols in relation to administering

procedural sedation medications. RNs are encouraged to refer to state Board of Nursing (BON) for state in which they are licensed.
2. Monitoring
a. Continuous evaluation of responsiveness to verbal and physical stimulation. If patient is unable to verbally respond to stimulation, "thumbs up" sign may be used for patient to indicate tolerability of procedure.
b. Assess for any signs or symptoms of transition between levels of sedation.
c. Respiratory rate
d. Oxygen saturation using pulse oximetry
e. Ventilation with use of capnography
f. Vital signs: blood pressure, heart rate, and rhythm
g. Continuous electrocardiography
h. Level of sedation
1) Many organizations use sedation scales to assess and document level of sedation and consciousness.
2) Selected sedation scale should be easy to use, monitor changes in level of responsiveness, and be easy to document.
3) Scale should be validated for use in population receiving procedural sedation.
4) Sample scales
   a) University of Michigan Sedation Scale (UMSS) (see Fig. 12.8)
      (1) Simple, efficient tool to assess sedation on continuum
      (2) Uses 0–4 scale with 0 indicating patient awake/alert and 4 indicating unresponsiveness
      (3) Requires patient stimulation to make an assessment
      (4) Validated in pediatrics
   b) Pediatric Sedation State Scale (PSSS) (Fig. 20.2)
      (1) Measures quality and effectiveness of sedation in pediatrics
      (2) Validated for use in pediatric procedural sedation

Pediatric Sedation State Scale (PSSS)	
Behavior	**Score**
Patient is moving (purposefully or nonpurposefully) in a manner that impedes the proceduralist and requires forceful immobilization. This includes crying or shouting during the procedure, but vocalization is not required. Score is based on movement.	5
Moving during the procedure (awake or sedated) that requires gentle immobilization for positioning. May verbalize some discomfort or stress, but there is no crying or shouting that expresses stress or objection.	4
Expression of pain or anxiety on face (may verbalize discomfort), but not moving or impeding completion of the procedure. May require help positioning (as with a lumbar puncture) but does not require restraint to stop movement during the procedure.	3
Quiet (asleep or awake), not moving during procedure, and no frown (or brow furrow) indicating pain or anxiety. No verbalization of any complaint.	2
Deeply asleep with normal vital signs, but requiring airway intervention and/or assistance (e.g., central or obstructive apnea, etc.).	1
Sedation associated with abnormal physiologic parameters that require acute intervention (i.e., oxygen saturation <90%, blood pressure is 30% lower than baseline, bradycardia receiving therapy).	0

Figure 20.2 Pediatric Sedation State Scale (PSSS). (Cravero, J. P., Askins, N., Sriswasdi, P., Tsze, D. S., Zurakowski, D., & Sinnott, S. (2017). Validation of the Pediatric Sedation State Scale. *Pediatrics, 139(5)*, e20162897. https://doi.org/10.1542/peds.2016-2897.)

c) Richmond Agitation Sedation Scale (RASS) (see Fig. 12.10)
   (1) High reliability and validity, and frequently used in sedated patients in ICU setting
   (2) Easy to use
d) Ramsay Sedation Scale (RSS) (see Fig. 12.9)
   (1) Developed and tested for reliability and validity for sedation in ICU patients
   (2) Is widely used during procedural sedation but may lack clarity for procedural sedation
   (3) Uses a 1–6 score to describe sedation level
i. Pain assessment (See Chapter 11 for pain assessment tools.)
j. Skin condition
k. Continuous IV access
3. Changes in condition must be immediately reported to provider.

III. Procedural Sedation Medications

NOTE: Medication administered for procedural sedation should be given in small incremental doses ("titrate to effect"), balancing sedation and pain control with safety. (See pharmacology chapter for additional details.)
A. *Anesthetic* agents
   1. Generally used to provide deep sedation and administered under guidance of anesthesiologists, CRNAs, and credentialed emergency department and critical care physicians. In some situations, where state regulations permit, lower doses of these medications may be used to provide moderate sedation and may be administered by credentialed RN under direct guidance of credentialed physician.
2. Ketamine
   a. Nonbarbiturate anesthetic
   b. Provides analgesia
   c. Monitor patient for emergence reactions (e.g., vivid dreams or visual hallucinations).
   d. Consider premedication (midazolam or diazepam) to reduce potential for side effects.
   e. May increase cerebral spinal fluid (CSF) pressure, respiratory depression, apnea, increased pulmonary secretions, cardiac arrhythmias, brady- or tachycardia, hypo- or hypertension, enhanced skeletal muscle tone
3. Methohexital
   a. Ultra-short-acting barbiturate
   b. Inhibits pain and induces sleep.
   c. May cause drowsiness and a variety of central nervous system (CNS) reactions for up to 12 hours
   d. Concurrent use with antihypertensives and alpha blockers increases risk of *hypo*tension.
   e. Use with caution in older patients and in patients with history of seizures (may induce seizure activity).
   f. Consider administering with lidocaine to reduce incidence of hiccups.
   g. No reversal agent

4. Propofol
   a. Sedative, hypnotic, general anesthetic; induces sedation, does not provide analgesia.
   b. Use with caution in patients with allergies to eggs, egg products, soybeans, or soy products.
   c. Lidocaine prior to IV administration may help to decrease pain on injection.
   d. May cause respiratory depression, bronchospasm, laryngospasm, hypo- or hypertension, arrhythmias, brady- or tachycardia, headache, euphoria, myoclonic/clonic movements, or nausea or vomiting
   e. No reversal agent

B. Benzodiazepines
   1. Benzodiazepines have anticonvulsant, anxiolytics, sedative, muscle relaxant, and amnesic properties and can be administered before, during, and after procedural sedation.
   2. Benzodiazepines do not provide analgesia.
   3. Use with caution in presence of opioids and other sedatives, as effects maybe more profound or longer lasting. May need to decrease dose by 30% to 50% when given with opioids or other CNS depressants.
   4. May cause respiratory depression, bradycardia, hypotension, agitation, confusion, or blurred or diplopia (double vision)
   5. Use with caution in patients with COPD, sleep apnea, or other respiratory diseases.
   6. Contraindicated in patients with narrow angle glaucoma
   7. Paradoxical reactions may occur (e.g., agitation instead of sedation).
   8. Instruct patients effects of benzodiazepines may last 24–48 hours, and driving or operating any machinery should be avoided during this time period.
   9. Reversal agent: flumazenil (see section on reversal agents)
   10. Diazepam
       a. Intramuscular (IM) route of administration not recommended
       b. Potential reactions: phlebitis at site of injection, rash, urticaria
       c. Avoid extravasation.
       d. May be diluted with normal saline to decrease IV irritation
       e. Give slowly (e.g., 1 minute for each 5 mg in adults).
       f. Difficult to titrate and has longer duration of effect
   11. Lorazepam
       a. Dilute with normal saline, sterile water for injection, or D_5W in a 1:1 diluent (1 part lorazepam to 1 part diluent) to decrease IV irritation.
       b. Avoid use in patients with hepatic or renal disease.

12. Midazolam
    a. Short-acting sedative hypnotic; indicated for short procedures
    b. Two to three times more potent than diazepam.
    c. Give slowly to avoid pain at injection site.

C. Opioids
   1. Typically combined with benzodiazepines for procedural sedation. Opioids provide analgesia while benzodiazepines provide anxiolysis and sedation.
   2. Severity of pain is decreased when opioids are administered before procedure.
   3. Considerations with opioids include:
      a. May cause respiratory depression, apnea, bradycardia, or hypotension, and decreases alveolar ventilation.
      b. Use with caution in patients with asthma, COPD, GI obstruction, or ileus.
   4. Reversal agent: naloxone
   5. Fentanyl
      a. Fentanyl is 75–125 times more potent than morphine for analgesia
      b. Rapid onset with shorter duration, indicated for short procedures
      c. Rapid administration of fentanyl may result in chest wall rigidity (flash pulmonary edema, typically seen in young muscular males).
   6. Hydromorphone
      a. Five to six times more potent than morphine
      b. Less histamine release than other opioids (less itching for some patients)
      c. Faster onset of action than morphine
   7. Meperidine
      a. One-tenth as potent as morphine
      b. Use with caution in patients with renal disease or history of seizures due to decreased ability to clear normeperidine (metabolite of meperidine, which may decrease seizure threshold).
      c. Use with caution in patients taking phenothiazines or other CNS depressants, as may increase risk for respiratory depression.
      d. Avoid use in patients on MAOs (isocarboxazid, phenelzine, selegiline, tranylcypromine—FDA approved MAOs), as may cause autonomic instability.
      e. *Because of associated risks, should only be used if other sedating medications cannot be used.*
   8. Morphine
      a. Gold standard for comparison of all opioids
      b. Use with caution in patients with hepatic and renal insufficiency due to clearance issues with metabolites.

D. Alpha-2-adrenergic agonist
   1. Dexmedetomidine
      a. Sedative and anxyoltic properties
      b. Level of sedation is dose dependent and can range from minimal to deep.

c. Has potential analgesic properties owing to reduction in sympathetic tone

d. Less effect on respiratory drive, seldom causes apnea but can impair respiratory responses to hypoxia and hypercapnia; can cause hypo- or hypertension and bradycardia

e. Associated with lower analgesic requirements and higher satisfaction than midazolam in adult patients

f. Has been associated with longer recovery times and fewer side effects and airway concerns in pediatric patients

E. Other Pharmacological Adjuncts Used With Procedural Sedation

1. Other medications may be used to help enhance sedative effects of opioids and benzodiazepines; extreme caution is needed to prevent potential respiratory depression.

2. Diphenhydramine
   a. CNS depressant
   b. Antihistamine
   c. Used as an adjunct in those patients currently receiving opioids or benzodiazepines
   d. Side effects include dry mouth, vertigo, nausea and vomiting, headaches, and urinary retention.

3. Nitrous oxide
   a. Odorless and colorless gas inhaled with oxygen.
   b. Anxiolytic, analgesic, and amnestic properties
   c. Rapid onset and recovery
   d. Side effects may include nausea, vomiting, laryngospasm, or vitamin B12 insufficiency with prolonged nitrous oxide use.

F. Reversal Agents

1. Reversal agents are used to counteract respiratory and sensory effects of opioids and benzodiazepines.

2. Duration of action in reversal agents is less than peak effects of opioids and benzodiazepines.
   a. Extended monitoring of patient after administration of reversal agent is needed, as respiratory depresssion may reoccur.
   b. A repeat dose of reversal(s) may be needed if sedation reoccurs as result of long half-life of opioids (2–4 hours) compared to naloxone (30–60 minutes) and long half-life of benzodizepines (6–8 hours) compared to shorter peak effect of flumazenil (30–60 minutes).

3. Titrate to effect: Low doses will reverse ventilatory effects, whereas higher doses will reverse therapuetic effects of opioids and benzodiazepines.

4. There are no reversal agents for propofol or ketamine.

IV. Procedural Complications

A. *Prevention is key!* Through appropriate assessment, medication management, monitoring, and critical evaluation of assessment parameters, many complications can be prevented.

B. Notify provider immediately of:

1. Rise or fall in systolic blood pressure of 20–30 mm Hg from baseline (for adults)

2. Tachycardia (>150 bpm) or bradycardia (<50 bpm) (for adults)

3. Excessive rise or fall in respiratory rate, <8–10 breaths per minute (for adults)

4. In children, >20% change in vital signs should be reported.

5. Decreased effort or quality of respirations regardless of respiratory rate

6. Oxygen saturation of <90% or significantly (>10% decrease from baseline in children) below presedation level

7. Marked decrease in patient responsiveness to verbal or painful stimulation

8. Signs or symptoms of medication intolerance or allergy

9. Unmet discharge parameters

C. Treatment of respiratory decompensation

1. Administer oxygen.

2. Stimulate patient: verbal or painful stimulus.

3. Instruct patient to take deep breaths.

4. If no spontaneous respiration occurs:
   a. Use a head tilt–jaw lift maneuver.
   b. Use positive-pressure ventilation.
   c. Consider use of oral or nasal airway.

5. Administration of reversal agents as ordered by provider:
   a. Patient should be monitored at least 2 hours after administration of reversal or until peak effect of opioid or benzodiazepine is reached (in some cases as long as 4–6 hours). Sedation may reoccur as soon as 20 minutes to as much as 90 minutes after administration of naloxone or flumazenil.
   b. Reversal agents should be used with caution in patients who have been on opioids or benzodiazepines for longer than one week as rapid reversal may result in withdrawal syndrome.
      1) Naloxone
         a) Opioid antagonist
         b) Onset <2 minutes; duration of action 20–90 minutes
         c) Rapid administration may result in cardiac dysrrhythmias (ventricular fibrillation and tachycardia), pulmonary edema, hypertension, nausea, and vomiting.
      2) Flumazenil
         a) Benzodiazepines antagonist
         b) Onset 1–2 minutes, peak effects within 6–10 minutes

c) Use flumazenil with caution in patients with history of seizures and receiving antiepileptic medications (administration of flumazenil may precipitate seizure activity).

V. Postprocedural Management

A. Recovery and discharge
1. Monitor and document vital signs, respiratory status, pulse oximetry, and mental status in 5- to 15-minute increments until stable at presedation levels or until at least 30 minutes after last sedating medications are given and vital signs are stable.
2. Patient must meet specific discharge criteria as identified by each organization and may include but not be limited to the following:
   a. Stable vital signs
   b. Intact mental status
   c. Tolerable level of pain or discomfort
   d. Denial of nausea or vomiting
3. Return of gag reflex, swallowing, and ability to take fluids
4. Provide verbal and written discharge instructions to patient and responsible adult:
   a. Home medication administration, including any new prescriptions
   b. Dietary instructions
   c. Activity limitations
   d. Procedure findings
   e. Signs and symptoms of complications
   f. Emergency numbers
   g. Follow-up appointment if applicable
5. Patient to be discharged with an adult who will assume care of patient
B. Quality/process improvement
1. Sedation practices should be assessed on a regular basis through a variety of means including procedural audits (concurrent and retrospective) and event/incident/occurrence reports.
2. Policy and procedure should be reviewed on a regular basis and modified as needed based on audit results and recommended guidelines.
3. Considerations when conducting quality review:
   a. Unplanned admissions or prolonged stays
   b. Cardiac or respiratory arrests
   c. Laryngospasm
   d. Use of reversal agents
   e. Assistance with ventilation—airways, positive pressure ventilations
   f. Prolonged periods of desaturations (<85% or <90% in pediatrics)

g. Failure to return to preprocedure vital signs within 20%
h. Progression to general anesthesia
i. Inability to sedate or inability to complete procedure

VI. Considerations for Infants and Children

A. General considerations for pediatric procedural management
1. Painful procedures should be done in a designated treatment or procedure area unless patient/parent requests otherwise. Child's room should be preserved as a *safe zone* when possible.
2. Presence of parents or caregivers should be considered to assist with comforting (not restraining) child.
B. Recommended process for pediatric procedural management (many of these could also apply to adults):
1. Prepare environment:
   a. Ensure privacy.
   b. Adjust lightning.
   c. Decrease noise.
   d. Offer to provide favorite toy or security object.
   e. Ensure supplies for nonpharmacological techniques are readily available.
   f. All appropriate-sized emergency equipment should be immediately available.
2. Prepare child:
   a. Children should not be deceived about painful procedures. They need to be able to trust their parents and healthcare team.
   b. Explanations need to be tailored to child and parent. Some children want little information, while others want extensive information.
   c. A child who is not afraid or in pain will likely be more cooperative and able to remain still for extended period.
   d. Only give choices when choices exist.
3. Prepare parent:
   a. Most children feel more secure with their parent(s) present.
   b. Whenever possible, parent should be present to provide support for their child (not to restrain).
   c. Parents should never be pressured to remain with their child during procedure. If they are not comfortable, they should be allowed to step away to avoid causing more anxiety in the child.
   d. Parents should be prepared appropriately for what they will see and be given simple instructions for what they should do, such as

CHAPTER 20 • Procedural Sedation and Analgesia **327**

hand-holding or talking in soothing voice. Their role in the procedure is to comfort child.
4. During procedure
    a. Use ONE VOICE approach:
        1) **O**ne voice should be heard during procedure.
        2) **N**eed parental involvement (when able and appropriate).
        3) **E**ducate patient before procedure about what is going to happen.
        4) **V**alidate child with words.
        5) **O**ffer most comfortable, nonthreatening position.
        6) **I**ndividualize plan.
        7) **C**hoose appropriate method of distraction.
        8) **E**liminate people not actively involved.
    b. Studies have reported a propensity for children to more quickly advance to deeper levels of sedation than adults. Providers must be prepared to respond swiftly.
5. After procedure
    a. Discuss and evaluate procedure.
    b. Document procedure, including the patient's perspective of the experience.
    c. Develop and implement a comfort plan for after procedure, if needed, and a plan for care at home if indicated.
    d. Parents must be instructed to maintain careful observation of children when discharged after procedures. Two adults are recommended to be in attendance for children having procedures—one to drive and one to observe child. Children may fall asleep in car seats and airway obstruction may occur.
C. Considerations for pediatric procedural sedation
    1. Goal of procedural sedation with children, as with adults, is prevention of pain, relief of anxiety, and possibly behavior modification to prevent patient injury during procedures.
    2. It is imperative procedural pain is individualized and optimally managed every time a procedure is performed. Children are more likely to experience trauma if procedures cause fear and/or pain, making children less likely to cooperate with repeat procedures.
    3. Infants and children are at greater risk.
        a. Pediatric respiratory anatomy differs from adult anatomy resulting in greater risk of respiratory compromise.
            1) Smaller structures and closer proximetry (e.g., "kissing tonsils")
            2) Obligate nose breathers at young ages
            3) Tongue is larger in proportion to oral cavity causing obstruction.
            4) Barrel-chested with smaller lung capacity
            5) Bones more cartilagenous and softer

        6) Shorter oxygenation-hemoglobin dissociation curve in infants and children results in pulse oximetry differences.
    b. Children under 6 years of age are at greater risk for adverse events related to sedating medications:
        1) Medications decrease respiratory drive.
        2) Protective airway reflexes are decreased.
        3) Obstruction may occur.
    c. Studies demonstrate children with developmental delays have a threefold increase in incidence of respiratory depression.
    d. Staff should be competent in pediatric advanced life support.
    4. Choosing appropriate level of sedation
        a. Assess whether procedure is truly needed. Discuss with care team whether results of procedure will offer more benefit than the risk of procedure (and procedural sedation if applicable).
        b. Consultation with appropriate specialists (e.g., anesthesiologists, neonatologists) for more complicated cases is recommended because repeated or lengthy use of general anesthetic and sedating medications for surgery or procedures in children younger than 3 years (or in pregnant women during their third trimester) may affect brain development.
        c. Provider must weigh risks and benefits of diagnostic and therapeutic procedures using sedation/anesthesia, particularly for procedures lasting >3 hours or if multiple procedures are considered.
    5. Medication doses should be weight based and given in small incremental doses ("titrate to effect").
D. Local and topical anesthetics for procedural pain (adult and pediatric patients)
    1. Local anesthetics are used to numb a body surface area and reduce pain sensation. Patients should be told they may feel some sensation of pressure depending on type of procedure being performed.
    2. Local anesthetics may not improve anxiety/fear.
        a. A randomized controlled trial between lidocaine 2.5%/prilocaine 2.5% cream and a needleless lidocaine injection system showed procedural pain scores significantly lower in lidocaine 2.5%/prilocaine 2.5% cream group vs. needless lidocaine injection group. Postprocedure fear scores were significantly lower than pre-procedure fear scores in both treatment groups; however, there was no difference in fear between the two treatment groups.
        b. If present, anxiety requires alternate, appropriate intervention(s).
    3. Eutectic mixture of local anesthetic (lidocaine 2.5%/prilocaine 2.5%):
        a. Many studies confirm efficacy of lidocaine 2.5%/prilocaine 2.5% cream for alleviating pain

from venous cannulation, vaccination, lumbar puncture, and venous port access.

b. Approved for full-term neonates and pediatric patients.

c. Apply a dollop of cream to desired area; cover with occlusive dressing for minimum of 1 hour prior to procedure.

1) May be applied to more than one site at a time, but total area of application should not exceed recommended maximums.

2) Longer application times of 2–4 hours provide deeper local anesthetic penetration.

3) Prolonged application leads to increased absorption which may lead to toxicity in infants.

d. Neonates and infants up to 3 months old should have serum methemoglobin levels monitored.

1) There is risk of methemoglobiniemia in very young children and children who are glucose-6-phosphate dehydrogenase deficient.

2) Methemoglobiniemia can result when hemoglobin oxidizes due to exposure to prilocaine and creates methemglobin, which is not an effective oxygen carrier.

3) In infants younger than 3 months, there is a reduced level of enzyme that converts methemoglobin back to hemoglobin.

4) Lidocaine should not be used in infants younger than 12 months who are receiving methemoglobinemia-inducing agents (e.g., acetaminophen, sulfonamides, nitrates, phenytoin, and class I antiarrhythmics).

4. Liposomal lidocaine cream 4%

a. Available without a prescription

b. Labeled for use in children 2 years and older

c. Lidocaine molecules encapsulated in a lipid layer allow rapid absorption by skin. Dermal analgesia is attained after 20–30 minutes; more invasive procedures require 45 minutes. Further increases in application times may result in decreased local anesthesia because medication dissipates quickly.

d. One-third of intended final dose should be rubbed into skin for approximately 30–60 seconds, and remainder of dose is applied in a thick layer. Occlusive dressing is optional but may deter child from orally ingesting it and help cream stay in place on child. Time to onset of local anesthesia depends on whether occlusive dressing is used.

e. Advantages of liposomal lidocaine cream over lidocaine 2.5%/prilocaine 2.5% cream are faster onset of anesthesia, optional dressing, and no

association with methemoglobiniemia. Studies confirm a 30-minute application is as effective as a 60-minute application of lidocaine 2.5%/prilocaine 2.5% cream for pain relief during venipuncture.

f. Higher success rates for peripheral IV cannulation, shorter procedure times, and less reported pain for children who received liposomal lidocaine 4% compared to those who received placebo have been reported.

g. Liposomal lidocaine 4% provided similar pain reduction compared with buffered lidocaine in randomized trial of children 4–17 years old undergoing peripheral IV insertion.

5. Lidocaine 70 mg and tetracaine 70 mg; topical anesthetic patch

a. Patch is approved for children 3 years and older.

b. Patch contains local anesthetic mixture and an oxygen-activated heating pod to facilitate medication delivery. It should be applied for 20–30 minutes to provide dermal analgesia to intact skin for superficial venous access procedures.

c. Keeping a patch on longer can result in systematic toxicity. Simultaneous or sequential application of more than two patches is not recommended.

d. Significantly decreased pain during venipuncture with a 20-minute application time in 59% of children, compared to 20% of children in placebo patch group, has been reported.

e. Patch must be removed before magnetic resonance imaging (MRI) procedures.

6. Buffered lidocaine

a. Buffered lidocaine (1 part 8.4% sodium bicarbonate to 10 parts 1%–2% lidocaine [i.e., 0.1 mL of sodium bicarbonate to 1 mL of lidocaine]) 0.1 mL or less may be administered as an intradermal injection over intended puncture site using a 30-gauge needle. Suggested maximum dose of lidocaine is 4.5 mg/kg.

b. Greatest advantage is speed of onset.

c. Although method requires two needlesticks, self-reported pain from buffered lidocaine injection has been shown to be lower than that of IV catheter insertion in adults.

d. Alternatively, buffered lidocaine may be administered with a needle-free device that delivers user-loaded buffered lidocaine under skin via a jet of compressed carbon dioxide when placed tightly against skin. Analgesia occurs in 1–3 minutes. To decrease fear and anxiety, prepare child for noise (e.g., like a pop of a soda can being opened) made by device.

7. Lidocaine, epinephrine, tetracaine (LET)

a. LET decreases pain associated with suturing of facial and scalp lacerations. LET solution is placed on wound bed and around its edges for a minimum of 10 minutes and a maximum of 30 minutes. Has also been studied in adults for other laceration locations.

b. LET should not be applied to mucous membranes or end arterioles (i.e., pinna, end of nose, fingers, toes, or penis) because of vasoconstriction and possible ischemia to affected areas.

8. Vapocoolant sprays
   a. Vapocoolants have a short duration of action, less than 1 minute. It may be prudent to have two providers available, one to administer spray and the other to perform procedure. Early studies found use of vapo-coolant spray does not compromise sterility of skin following alcohol prep.
   b. Caution must be exercised to not spray skin for longer than 10 seconds and at a distance of 3–7 inches away from area, as severe local hypothermia with cell death can occur.
   c. In one study, vapocoolant was associated with reduction in pain during IV catheter insertion, and 18% more children reported no or minimal pain with vapo-coolant spray compared to those who received placebo. A cannulation attempt occurred within 60 seconds. A secondary outcome measure showed cannulation on first attempt was more successful with use of vapocoolant spray. Vapo-coolants are useful for immunizations.
   d. *Caution*: Vapocoolant ethyl chloride is flammable.
   e. Pentafluoropropane and tetrafluoroethane work similarly to ethyl chloride; however, they lack flammability concern.
   f. Children have remarked spray is too cold and causes pain itself.
9. Transuretheral 2% lidocaine: mixed literature related to decreasing pain scores with transurethral bladder catheterization in children
10. Atomized nasal-mucosal delivery device
    a. Limited number of medications available via intranasal route
    b. Delivery by this route may be irritating to nasal mucosa, causing burning sensation, or may leave unpleasant aftertaste.
    c. Contraindications
       1) Large volume to be given
       2) Nasal trauma/defect suspected or known
       3) Severe upper respiratory symptoms affecting respiratory status
    d. Procedure
       1) Syringe with desired dose of prescribed medication, plus an additional 0.1 mL (to account

for "dead space" in atomizer) is attached to mucosal atomization device (MAD).
       2) Make sure nasal passage is clear.
       3) Divide dose evenly between both nasal passages, ideally no more than 0.5 mL per side.
E. Nonpharmacological modalities for pediatric procedural pain management
   1. Sucrose
      a. Use of sucrose has been studied in both preterm and term infants; however, bulk of literature is seen in term neonates to 12 months of age.
      b. Sweet taste activates orally mediated endogenous opioid release.
      c. Sucrose 24% can be applied to pacifier to elicit non-nutritive sucking or it can be given orally on tip of tongue 2 minutes prior to procedure. Recent evidence suggests smaller volumes of 0.1–0.2 mL provide similar pain reduction benefits when compared to larger amounts (0.5–1 mL).
      d. Evidence suggests sucrose in combination with adjuvant modalities such as non-nutritive sucking and swaddling have greater effect on pain mangement than sucrose alone. Non-nutrative sucking stimulates nonopioid pathways by way of orotactile and mechanoreceptor mechanisms. Analgesic effect lasts approximately 5 minutes and should be used for short-term procedures.
   2. Behavioral interventions
      a. Low stimulation
      b. Parental presence
      c. Guided imagery
      d. Music therapy
      e. Hypnosis
      f. Distraction
      g. Relaxation techniques
      h. Comfort holds
      i. Kangaroo care
      j. Swaddling
      k. Psychological therapy
      l. Biofeedback
   3. Nonpharmacolgocical measures based on gate control theory
      a. Buzzy®: device is shaped like a bee and provides nonpainful stimulation by way of cold and vibratory sensations, activating large-diameter fibers and closing the gate.
      b. Shot blocker®: Device uses a number of blunt contact points to saturate sensory signals around injection site.

Part 4

VII. Procedural Sedation Considerations for Older Adults

A. Assess for hearing loss and decreased comprehension.
B. Increased caution necessary, as respiratory effort may be compromised due to several factors:
   1. Decreased elasticity of lungs
   2. Decreased alveolar structures, which decrease surface area available for ventilatory exchange
   3. Calcifications of ribs cause stiffer recoil of lungs
   4. Long-term lung disease such as COPD
C. Medications for sedation should be used in small increments with a lower maximum dose.
   1. Start low, go slow.
   2. Renal blood flow decreases by 10% for every decade after age 20, decreasing clearance and increasing accumulation risk.
   3. Liver metabolism may be decreased with increased accumulation of drug metabolites due to decreased blood flow to liver.

VIII. Procedural Sedation Considerations for People With Substance Use Disorder

A. Nearly 10% of all adults over age 12 in United States have a substance use disorder involving alcohol or other substances.
B. Using a nonjudgemental attitude and reassurances of confidentiality, attempt to obtain full disclosure of all substances prior to developing a procedural sedation plan.
C. Addiction specialists may need to be consulted prior to procedures.
D. Patients may require higher doses of opioids and benzodiazepines to induce sedation.
E. Use caution with reversal agents to avoid precipitating wihtdrawal.
F. Ensure clear and explicit instructions for post procedure care.

Bibliography

American Association of Nurse Anesthetists. (2016). Non-anesthesia provider procedural sedation and analgesia: Considerations for policy development. http://www.aana.com/resources2/professionalpractice/Pages/Non-anesthesia-Provider-Procedural-Sedation-and-Analgesia.aspx.

American Association of Nurse Anesthetists. (2018). Discharge after sedation or anesthesia on the day of the procedure: Patient transportation with or without a responsible adult. https://www.aana.com/docs/default-source/practice-aana-com-web-documents-(all)/professional-practice-manual/discharge-after-sedation-or-anesthesia-on-the-day-of-the-procedure.pdf?sfvrsn=ed4a5bb1_4.

American Association of Nurse Anesthetists. (2019). Analgesia and anesthesia for the substance use disorder patient. https://www.aana.com/docs/default-source/practice-aana-com-web-documents-(all)/professional-practice-manual/analgesia-and-anesthesia-for-the-substance-use-disorder-patient.pdf?sfvrsn=3e6b7548_4.

American Society of Anesthesiologists. (2017). Advisory on granting privileges for deep sedation to non-anesthesiologist physicians. Advisory on Granting Privileges for Deep Sedation to Non-Anesthesiologist Physicians | American Society of Anesthesiologists (ASA) (asahq.org). https://www.asahq.org/standards-and-guidelines/advisory-on-granting-privileges-for-deep-sedation-to-non-anesthesiologist-physicians.

American Society of Anesthesiologists. (2018). Distinguishing monitored anesthesia care (MAC) from moderate sedation/analgesia (conscious sedation). https://www.asahq.org/standards-and-guidelines/distinguishing-monitored-anesthesia-care-mac-from-moderate-sedationanalgesia-conscious-sedation.

American Society of Anesthesiologists. (2018). Practice Guidelines for Moderate Procedural Sedation and Analgesia 2018: a report by the American Society of Anesthesiologists Task Force on Moderate Procedural Sedation and Analgesia, the American Association of Oral and Maxillofacial Surgeons, American College of Radiology, American Dental Association, American Society of Dentist Anesthesiologists, and Society of Interventional Radiology. https://pubs.asahq.org/anesthesiology/article/128/3/437/18818/Practice-Guidelines-for-Moderate-Procedural?_ga=2.137164592.1690005981.1630029706-1115868003.1628276874.

American Society of Anesthesiologists. (2019). Continuum of depth of sedation: Definition of general anesthesia and levels of sedation/analgesia. https://www.asahq.org/standards-and-guidelines/continuum-of-depth-of-sedation-definition-of-general-anesthesia-and-levels-of-sedationanalgesia.

American Society of Anesthesiologists. (2020). ASA physical status classification system. https://www.asahq.org/standards-and-guidelines/asa-physical-status-``classification-system.

Aminiahidashti, H., Shafiee, S., Zamani Kiasari, A., & Sazgar, M. (2018). Applications of end-tidal carbon dioxide (ETCO2) monitoring in emergency department: A narrative review. *Emergency (Tehran, Iran)*, 6(1), e5.

Barends, C. R., Absalom, A., van Minnen, B., Vissink, A., & Visser, A. (2017). Dexmedetomidine versus midazolam in procedural sedation. A systematic review of efficacy and safety. *PLoS ONE*, 12(1), e0169525. https://doi.org/10.1371/journal.pone.0169525.

Campbell-Yeo, M., Eriksson, M., & Benoit, B. (2022). Assessment and management of pain in preterm infants: A practice update. *Children (Basel, Switzerland)*, 9(2), 244. https://doi.org/10.3390/children9020244.

Chi, S. I. (2018). Complications caused by nitrous oxide in dental sedation. *Journal of Dental Anesthesia and Pain Medicine*, 18(2), 71–78. https://doi.org/10.17245/jdapm.2018.18.2.71.

Chung, F., Subramanyam, R., Liao, P., Sasaki, E., Shapiro, C., & Sun, Y. (2012). High STOP-Bang score indicates a high probability of obstructive sleep apnea. *British Journal of Anaesthesia*, 108(5), 768–775. doi:10.1093/bja/aes022.

Coté, C. J., & Wilson, S. (2019) American Academy of Pediatrics, American Academy of Pediatric Dentistry. Guidelines for monitoring and management of pediatric patients before, during, and after sedation for diagnostic and therapeutic procedures. *Pediatrics, 143*(6), e20191000. doi:10.1542/peds.2019-1000.

Cravero, J. P., Askins, N., Sriswasdi, P., Tsze, D. S., Zurakowski, D., & Sinnott, S. (2017). Validation of the Pediatric Sedation State Scale. *Pediatrics, 139*(5), e20162897. https://doi.org/10.1542/peds.2016-2897.

Farion, K. J., Splinter, K. L., Newhook, K., Gaboury, I., & Splinter, W. M. (2008). The effect of vapocoolant spray on pain due to intravenous cannulation in children: a randomized controlled trial. *Canadian Medical Association Journal, 179*(1), 31–36. https://doi.org/10.1503/cmaj.070874.

Gallagher, J. J. (2018). Capnography monitoring during procedural sedation and analgesia. *Advance Critical Care Nursing, 29*(4), 405–414. doi:10.4037/aacnacc2018684.

Harjai, M., Alam, S., & Bhaskar, P. (2021). Clinical relevance of Mallampati grading in predicting difficult intubation in the era of various new clinical predictors. *Cureus, 13*(7), e16396. https://doi.org/10.7759/cureus.16396.

Jang, E. K., Lee, H., Jo, K. S., Lee, S. M., Seo, H. J., & Huh, E. J. (2019). Comparison of the pain-relieving effects of human milk, sucrose, and distilled water during examinations for retinopathy of prematurity: A randomized controlled trial. *Child Health Nursing Research, 25*(3), 255–261. https://doi.org/10.4094/chnr.2019.25.3.255.

Jimenez, N., Bradford, H., Seidel, K., Sousa, M., & Lynn, A. (2006). A comparison of a needle-free injection system for local anesthesia versus EMLA for intravenous catheter insertion in the pediatric patient. *Anesthesia & Analgesia, 102*(2), 411–414. doi:10.1213/01.ane.0000194293.10549.62.

Jungquist, C., Quinlan-Cowell, A., Vallerand, A., Carlisle, H., Cooney, M., Dempsey, S., Dunwoody, D., Maly, A., Meloche, K., Meyers, A., Sawyer, J., Singh, N., Sullivan, D., Watson, C., & Polomano, R. (2020). American Society for Pain Management Nursing guidelines on monitoring for opioid-induced advancing sedation and respiratory depression: Revisions. *Pain Management Nursing, 21*, 7–25. doi:10.1016/j.pmn.2019.06.007.

Kahsay, H. (2017). Assessment and treatment of pain in pediatric patients. *Current Pediatric Research, 21*, 148–157.

Kamat, P., McCracken, C., Simon, H., Stormorken, A., Mallory, M., Chumpitazi, C., & Cravero, J. (2020). Trends in outpatient procedural sedation: 2007–2018. *Pediatrics, 145*(5), e20193559. https://doi.org/10.1542/peds.2019-3559.

Mlynek, K., Lyahn, H., Richards, B., Schleicher, W., Bassiri Gharb, B., Procop, G., Tuohy, M., & Zins, J. (2015). Skin sterility after application of a vapocoolant spray part 2. *Aesthetic Plastic Surgery, 39*(4), 597–601. https://doi.org/10.1007/s00266-015-0509-5.

Nagappa, M., Wong, J., Singh, M., Wong, D. T., & Chung, F. (2017). An update on the various practical applications of the STOP-Bang questionnaire in anesthesia, surgery, and perioperative medicine. *Current Opinions in Anaesthesiology, 30*(1), 118–125. doi:10.1097/ACO.0000000000000426. PMID: 27898430; PMCID: PMC5214142.

Schacherer, N. M., Armstrong, T., Perkins, A. M., Poirier, M. P., & Schmidt, J. M. (2019). Propofol versus dexmedetomidine for procedural sedation in a pediatric population. *Southern Medical Journal, 112*(5), 277–282. doi:10.14423/smj.0000000000000973. PMID: 31050796.

Sessler, C., Gosnell, M., Grap, M., Brophy, G., O'Neal, P., Keane, K., Tesoro, E., & Elswick, R. (2002). The Richmond Agitation-Sedation Scale: Validity and reliability in adult intensive care unit patients. *American Journal of Respiratory Critical Care Medicine, 166*(10), 1338–1344. doi:10.1146/rccm.2107138.

Stannard, D., & Krenzischek, D. (2018). *Perianesthesia Nursing Care: A Bedside Guide for Safe Recovery* (2nd ed.). Burlington, MA: Jones & Bartlett Learning.

Stevens, B., Yamada, J., Campbell-Yeo, M., Gibbins, S., Harrison, D., Dionne, K., Taddio, A., McNair, C., Willan, A., Ballantyne, M., Widger, K., Sidani, S., Estabrooks, C., Synnes, A., Squires, J., Victor, C., & Riahi, S. (2018). The minimally effective dose of sucrose for procedural pain relief in neonates: a randomized controlled trial. *BMC Pediatrics, 18*(1), 85. https://doi.org/10.1186/s12887-018-1026-x.

Stoltz, P., & Manworren, R. (2017). Comparison of children's venipuncture fear and pain: Randomized controlled trial of EMLA and J-Tip Needleless Injection System. *Journal of Pediatric Nursing, 37*, 91–96. https://doi.org/10.1016/j.pedn.2017.08.025.

The Joint Commission. (2021). *Comprehensive Accreditation Manual for Hospitals: The Official Handbook*. Oakbrook Terrace, IL: Joint Commission Resources.

United States Department of Health and Human Services, Centers for Disease Control and Prevention. (2016). *Body mass index: Considerations for practitioners*. https://www.cdc.gov/obesity/downloads/BMIforPactitioners.pdf.

United States Food and Drug Administration. (2017). *FDA Drug Safety Communication: FDA approves label changes for use of general anesthetic and sedation drugs in young children*. https://www.fda.gov/drugs/drug-safety-and-availability/fda-drug-safety-communication-fda-approves-label-changes-use-general-anesthetic-and-sedation-drugs.

Williams, M., McKeown, A., Dexter, F., Miner, J., Sessler, D., Vargo, J., Turk, D., & Dworkin, R. (2016). Efficacy outcome measures for procedural sedation clinical trials in adults: An ACTTION systemic review. *Anesthesia & Analgesia, 122*(1), 152–170. doi:10.1213/ANE.0000000000000934.

Part 4

CHAPTER 21

Managing Persistent Pain

Connie Luedtke, MA, RN, BC
Karen V. Macey-Stewart, DNP, AGNP-C, RN-PMGT
Maureen F. Cooney, DNP, FNP-BC, ACHPN, AP-PMN*

Introduction

Persistent pain is complex and can have profound effects on individuals, families, and society. With much still unknown, treatment options for resolving persistent pain require a multidimensional approach. This chapter serves as a guide by providing key components of diagnostic workup (beyond a thorough history and physical) needed in recognizing specific persistent pain syndromes and provides the healthcare community with an armamentarium of pharmacological and nonpharmacological approaches to combat persistent pain.

I. Foundation

A. Persistent pain
1. Pathophysiology of persistent pain process continues to be a subject of intense debate, research, and policy change. Multiple, reproducible pathophysiologic changes have been documented over the past three decades. However, none of these aberrations have been clearly linked to treatments that are more than 30% effective for the average patient.
2. While acute pain decreases overtime as healing occurs, persistent (chronic) pain lasts longer (thought to be longer than 3 months) than typical healing time or recurs intermittently.
3. Postsurgical pain is associated with risk for development of persistent postsurgical pain. To reduce risks of severe postoperative pain and potential for persistent pain processes, Enhanced Recovery after Surgery (ERAS) programs have been adopted. These programs use pre- and intraoperative multimodal pharmacological strategies and regional anesthesia approaches such as epidural injections/infusions and nerve blocks.
4. Emotional distress and functional disability are some psychological components of persistent pain.
5. Persistent pain requires a multidimensional interprofessional approach. Nurses, clinicians,

and researchers (including specialists in metabolic medicine, rehabilitation medicine, psychiatry, and integrative medicine) continue to work to resolve difficulties faced by individuals with complex pain.
6. Persistent pain often co-occurs in individuals with posttraumatic stress disorder (PTSD).
   a. PTSD occurs from traumatic events such as natural disasters, accidents, war/combat, serious injury, threat of death, sexual violence, or terrorist acts.
   b. It has been postulated uncontrolled pain following physical injury is a core trauma in PTSD and PTSD and persistent pain may be mutually maintaining conditions. Therefore, evaluation of PTSD is warranted in many patients with persistent pain.
7. In the areas that follow, a thorough history and physical examination are expected, including pain assessment, psychosocial evaluation, and assessment of substance use. Specific information regarding diagnostic workup is included for each diagnosis.
B. Evidence-Based Guidelines and Clinical Resources for Persistent Pain Diagnoses
1. North American Spine Society (2021; https://www.spine.org/Research-Clinical-Care/Quality)
   a. Provides clinical practice guidelines for management of:
      1) Degenerative spondylolisthesis
      2) Lumbar disc herniation with radiculopathy
      3) Degenerative lumbar spinal stenosis
      4) Cervical radiculopathy from degenerative disorders
      5) Persistent (chronic) low back pain
2. American College of Rheumatology site (rheumatology.org) provides clinical practice guidelines for management of:
   a. Spondyloarthropathies
   b. Osteoarthritis

---

*Section Editor for the chapter.

c. Perioperative management
d. Psoriatic arthritis
e. Rheumatoid arthritis
f. Fibromyalgia
g. Systemic lupus
3. National Institute of Neurological Disorders and Strokes (https://www.ninds.nih.gov) provides educational resources for:
    a. Central pain syndrome
    b. Complex regional pain syndrome (CRPS)
    c. Several other persistent pain conditions
4. National Heart, Lung, and Blood Institute (https://www.nhlbi.nih.gov/health-topics/evidence-based-management-sickle-cell-disease) provides clinical practice guidelines for management of:
    a. Sickle cell disease
    b. Sickle cell crisis
5. International Headache Society (https://ihs-headache.org/en/resources/guidelines/) provides clinical practice guidelines for management of headaches.
6. American Society for Pain Management Nursing (https://aspmn.org/position-statements/) has various position statements, some of which apply to persistent pain. Examples include:
    a. *Pain Assessment in the Patient Unable to Self-Report*
    b. *"As-Needed" Range Orders for Opioid Analgesics in the Management of Pain: A Consensus Statement of the American Society for Pain Management and the American Pain Society*
    c. *Prescribing and Administering Opioid Doses Based Solely on Pain Intensity*
    d. Pain Management at the End of Life
    e. *Deceptive Use of Placebos in the Assessment and Management of Pain*
    f. *Procedural Pain Management: Clinical Practice Recommendations*
    g. *Registered Nurse Management and Monitoring of Analgesia by Cather Technique*
    h. *Position Statement: Pain Management and Substance Use Disorders*

II. Interventions for Persistent Pain

A. Overview
1. Treatment of persistent pain conditions requires consideration for use of multimodal analgesia, which may involve use of a combination of nonpharmacological interventions, pharmacological interventions, interventional pain procedures, and, in some cases, surgical interventions.
2. Interprofessional pain management approach optimizes patient outcomes and reduces risks for harm.

3. Applicable nonpharmacological, pharmacological, and interventional/surgical approaches are listed in subsequent sections for particular persistent pain conditions.
B. Nonpharmacological options
1. General principles
    a. Many, if not all, persistent pain conditions can benefit from nonpharmacological interventions, regardless of underlying diagnosis.
    b. Nonpharmacological interventions are actions used to decrease or manage pain and other associated symptoms in conjunction with or independent of medication use.
    c. Women of childbearing age should work with their healthcare team to plan accordingly when using nonpharmacological interventions as part of their birthing treatment plan.
    d. All interventions listed below should be reviewed with or under supervision of a healthcare provider (HCP) to reduce risk of injury; activities should be introduced gradually. Interventions have various levels of evidence supporting use for various conditions.
2. Patient education
    a. Information about normal body function
    b. Information about disease process
    c. Assistance in recognizing signs and symptoms of disease processes that cause pain
    d. Skills to identify stress triggers and management
    e. Establishment of functional pain goal
    f. Understanding of treatment modality
    g. Review various treatment options.
3. Lifestyle modifications
    a. Dietary modifications when indicated
    b. Smoking cessation/alcohol moderation or cessation
    c. Movement and exercise
    d. Sleep hygiene
4. Physical therapy
    a. Adaptive equipment: braces, canes, kinesiology taping, and other supportive devices
    b. Strengthening and resistance training exercises
    c. Postural training
    d. Exercise pacing
    e. Neuromuscular training
    f. Balance exercise
    g. Manipulation
    h. Myofascial release
    i. Dry needling
    j. Massage
    k. Vibratory stimulus
    l. Transcutaneous electrical nerve stimulation (TENS)
    m. Ultrasound therapy
    n. Mirror therapy

5. Occupational therapy
   a. Paraffin wraps
   b. Fine-motor skills training
   c. Splinting
   d. Use of adaptive equipment
   e. Evaluation of home or workplace modifications
6. Activity/exercise considerations
   a. Moderation training to prevent overexertion or injury is important.
   b. Alternate rest with activity.
   c. Yoga
   d. Tai Chi
   e. Stretching
   f. Water aerobics
   g. Appropriate amounts of sun exposure (while necessary for conversion of vitamin D, excessive exposure can trigger certain pain symptoms, such as systemic lupus erythematosus)
   h. Occlusal appliance therapy
7. Nutrition
   a. Decrease inflammatory foods (trans-fat and sugar).
   b. Nutritionist/dietician
   c. Replacement of essential vitamins and minerals
   d. Decrease or eliminate alcohol and other toxins.
8. Stress management
   a. Self-efficacy
   b. Biofeedback
   c. Relaxation training
   d. Mindfulness
   e. Meditation
   f. Guided imagery
   g. Diaphragmatic breathing
9. Individual or group therapy
   a. Rehabilitation psychologist
   b. Psychological support
   c. Cognitive-behavioral therapy (CBT) or acceptance and commitment therapy (ACT)
   d. Habit reversal
10. Other options
    a. Acupuncture/acupressure
    b. Massage
    c. Heat or ice
    d. TENS
11. Interprofessional pain management approach
C. Pharmacologic options (see Chapter 17)
1. Many persistent pain conditions have nociceptive and neuropathic pain components and are treated with multimodal analgesia (MMA).
2. MMA is rational combination of optimal doses of individual analgesics with differing mechanisms of actions.

3. Many medications used in treatment of persistent pain are used off-label to optimize analgesia while reducing adverse effects associated with higher doses of a single medication.
4. MMA plan must be individualized for each patient to address risks related to age, medical condition, need for follow-up, accessibility, affordability, and other factors.
5. Pharmacological plan often involves a step approach, as additional medications are added depending on response to previous medications.
6. First-line medications used for persistent pain are often nonopioid analgesics and adjuvant medications.
7. Opioids are usually reserved as second-line treatment options for persistent pain and, if necessary, are used as short-term interventions, though may in certain conditions be used long term.
8. The following medication classes are often used in many persistent pain conditions. Choice of medication class should be driven by type of pain, as not all classes are indicated for all types of pain.
   a. Acetaminophen with unclear mechanisms of action but useful in inflammatory processes and in MMA plans
   b. Nonsteroidal anti-inflammatory drugs (NSAIDs) for inflammatory processes
      1) Nonselective cyclooxygenase inhibitors (COX-1 and COX-2 inhibition) (e.g., ibuprofen, naproxen)
      2) Selective cyclooxygenase inhibitors (COX-2 inhibitors) (e.g., celecoxib)
      3) Many available by topical or systemic routes
      4) As with all medications, risks compared to expected benefits must be assessed (e.g., risk of GI bleed may outweigh minimal expected benefit for certain conditions and populations).
   c. Skeletal muscle relaxants for muscle spasm (e.g., cyclobenzaprine, methocarbamol)
   d. Antidepressants for neuropathic pain
      1) Serotonin/norepinephrine inhibitors (SNRIs) (e.g., duloxetine, milnacipran)
      2) Tricyclic antidepressants (e.g., amitriptyline, nortriptyline)
   e. Anticonvulsants for neuropathic pain
      1) Sodium ion channel–blocking agents (e.g., carbamazepine, lamotrigine)
      2) Anticonvulsants with multiple mechanisms of action (e.g., topiramate)
      3) Alpha-2-delta subunit calcium channel binding (e.g., gabapentin, pregabalin)
   f. Corticosteroids for inflammatory processes
   g. Local anesthetics (LAs) for neuropathic pain
   h. Opioids for moderate to severe nociceptive and mixed-type pain in some cases

i. Low-dose naltrexone
   1) Has been used for conditions such as fibromyalgia, Crohn's disease, multiple sclerosis, and chronic repetitive pain syndrome
   2) Tends to be rather inexpensive and well tolerated.
   3) Little evidence to support its efficacy at this time
j. N-Methyl-d-aspartic acid (NMDA) agonist antagonists (e.g., ketamine) for postoperative pain, pain in opioid-tolerant patients, and neuropathic and mixed-type pain
k. Alpha-2 agonists (e.g., clonidine) for neuropathic pain, spasticity, opioid withdrawal, and opioid-induced hyperalgesia

D. Interventional pain procedures (see Chapter 19)
1. Intrathecal and epidural medications
2. Nerve blocks—spinal and peripheral
3. Myofascial trigger point injections
4. Spinal cord and/peripheral nerve stimulation
5. Implanted epidural/intrathecal medication pump delivery devices
6. Tissue engineering: replacements for structures impacted by disease

III. Persistent Joint Pain

A. Persistent joint pain occurs when body repeatedly releases chemicals (e.g., histamines, prostaglandins, and cytokine) to inflamed joint space.
1. Over time, the body's inflammatory response, instead of healing tissues, leads to further deterioration of joint.
2. Persistent joint inflammation can be caused by reinjury to previous joints, infections, severe injury, medications, and surgery.

B. Arachnoiditis
1. Description: persistent inflammation of arachnoid meningeal layer of spinal cord and subarachnoid space
   a. Inflammation may result from variety of factors:
      1) Irritation from chemicals, bacterial or viral infections, spinal injury, spinal surgery, chronic compression of spinal nerves, or other invasive spinal procedures
      2) Accidental intrathecal administration of certain medication solutions such as sulfite-containing preservatives, steroids, blood, and myelographic contrast agents may be neurotoxic.
   b. Adhesions and scar tissue may form due to inflammation, causing spinal nerves to "stick" together.

2. Signs and symptoms
   a. Pain starts as local, continuous, dull, or aching and then progresses to intense, painful, burning sensation.
   b. Neck stiffness and sensory and motor impairments may occur.
   c. Severe pain may occur in upper limb or be diffuse with widespread bilateral symptoms.
   d. When lower back is focal point, pain is distributed to both legs.
   e. Pain is aggravated by movement, coughing, and sneezing and is more intense with bed rest and in morning.
   f. Pain is described as band-like, constricting sensation with increasing pain or as stinging, burning, numbness, aching, or annoying.
   g. Muscle cramps, twitches, or spasms may occur and may become debilitating.
   h. It may affect bladder, bowel, vision, hearing, and sexual function.
3. Diagnostic workup
   a. Labs: Blood and cerebrospinal fluid studies are consistent with infection.
   b. Radiologic evaluation: Magnetic resonance imaging (MRI) or high-resolution computed tomography (CT) scan can demonstrate changes characteristic of arachnoiditis.
4. Treatment options
   a. Acute episodes may require hospitalization for pain control and use of orthopedic brace for immobilization.
   b. Pharmacological options
      1) NSAIDs
      2) Skeletal muscle relaxants
      3) Antidepressants
      4) Anticonvulsants
      5) Corticosteroids
      6) Tetracycline antibiotics
      7) Diuretics
      8) Local anesthetics
      9) Opioids

C. Psoriatic arthritis (PsA)
1. Description: persistent, inflammatory arthritic disease of any joint and wherever ligaments and tendons connect to bone; six subtypes of PsA: peripheral arthritis (oligoarthritis or polyarthritis), enthesitis (inflammation of connection points), dactylitis, or sacroiliitis/spondylitis (inflammation of sacroiliac joint or vertebral joints)
2. Signs and symptoms
   a. Inflammatory arthritis is associated with cutaneous psoriasis.
   b. Tenderness, pain, and swelling over one or more tendons or joints

c. Reduced range of motion

d. Fatigue and morning stiffness

e. Uveitis and redness of eye

f. Skin lesions

3. Classification of psoriatic arthritis (CASPAR) criteria for PsA:

a. Evidence of current arthritis and personal or family history of psoriasis

b. Nail dystrophy: onycholysis (loosening or separation of nail from nail bed close), pitting, or hyperkeratosis

c. Negative rheumatoid factor (RF)

d. Current or history of dactylitis

e. Radiographic evidence of new bone growth near joint margins on plain radiographs of hands or feet

4. Diagnostic workup

a. Labs: human leukocyte antigen (HLA)-B27; RF

b. Radiologic evaluation (radiographs of hands and feet; MRI)

5. Pharmacological options

a. NSAIDs

b. Disease-modifying antirheumatic drugs (DMARDs)

c. Anti–tumor necrosis factor agents

D. Spondyloarthropathies (SpA)

1. Description: Group of inflammatory arthritides, including ankylosing spondylitis (AS), reactive arthritis, arthritis/spondylitis, and arthritis/spondylitis associated with inflammatory bowel diseases.

a. Presence of HLA-B27; inflammatory arthritides of peripheral joints, especially of lower extremities; sacroiliitis, spondylitis, enthesitis, dactylitis, and uveitis; enteric mucosal lesions, and skin lesions are shared expressions of SpA.

b. Most common form of SpA, inflammation of spine, causes stiffening of joint structure in low back and pelvis.

2. Signs and symptoms

a. Chronic inflammatory changes result in gradual onset of low back aching and stiffness.

b. Two to three times more common in males than in females with onset in the 20s and 30s

c. Stiffness and pain occurring in morning and after episodes of inactivity

d. Associated symptoms may include peripheral joint disease, conjunctivitis, and iritis.

e. New York diagnostic criteria for AS are:

1) Limitation of motion of lumbar spine in all three planes (i.e., anterior flexion, lateral flexion, and extension)

2) History of pain at dorsolumbar junction or in lumbar spine

3) Limitation of chest expansion to 2.5 cm (1 inch) or less, measured at level of fourth intercostal space

3. Diagnostic workup

a. Labs: serum HLA-27 (genetic marker)—does not always indicate a positive diagnosis

b. Radiologic evaluation:

1) X-ray may show bilateral symmetrical sacroiliitis (inflammation of sacroiliac joint).

2) Pelvic CT scan used to detect any structural changes. MRI is considered an integral tool in detecting inflammatory changes (e.g., osteitis or bone marrow edema).

4. Pharmacological options

a. NSAIDs

b. Tumor necrosis factor inhibitors (TNFIs) (e.g., adalimumab, infliximab, or etanercept)

c. Corticosteroid injections

IV. Persistent Musculoskeletal and Inflammatory Pain

A. For diagnoses given below, treatment is intended to target symptoms with goals for decreasing swelling and joint tenderness, slow or stop progression of joint deterioration, maintain functioning, and decrease comorbidities.

B. Osteoarthritis (OA)

1. Description: Degenerative joint disease; most common form of noninflammatory arthritis; a slowly progressive disease that affects certain joints of middle-aged to older adults. Joints typically impacted are weight-bearing joints (e.g., knees and hips) and frequently used joints (e.g., hands, feet, spine). Cartilage in between joints breaks down due to mechanical use and biochemical changes in body.

2. Signs and symptoms

a. Deep aching pain results from degenerative process in one or more joints.

b. Severity is related to disease progression.

c. Pain and stiffness can occur at rest when initiating activity and sometimes at night (with disease progression).

d. Morning stiffness occurs due to inactivity.

e. Incidence increases with age (about 25% of world population is affected).

f. Joint line tenderness and crepitus occur on active or passive joint motion.

g. Noninflammatory effusions may be present.

h. Later stages may show gross deformities, bony hypertrophy, and contractures.

3. Diagnostic workup

a. Labs: no specific laboratory tests to diagnose OA

Table 21.1

2010 Diagnostic Criteria

Domain	Description	Number	Score
Joint involvement (swollen/ tender on exam)	• **Median-large joints** (e.g., shoulder, elbow, knee, ankle). • **Small joints** (e.g., metacarpophalangeal, proximal interphalangeal, 2nd through 5th metatarsophalangeal, thumb interphalangeal and wrist joints; excludes distal interphalangeal, 1st carpometacarpal, and 1st tarsometatarsal joints)	1 2–10 1–3 4–10 >10*	0 1 2 3 5
Serology	• No positivity of either RF or anti-CCP • At least one of these tests positive at low titer (above upper limit of normal) • At least one of these tests positive at high titer (>3 times upper limit of normal)		0 2 3
Duration of synovitis	• ≥ 6 weeks		1
Acute phase reactants	• Neither CRP or ESR abnormal • Abnormal CRP or ESR		0 1

*At least one must be a small joint; others may be a combination of large and/or small.

Patients receive highest point value if they fall within domains.

CCP, cyclic citrullinated peptide; *CRP*, C-reactive protein; *ESR*, erythrocyte sedimentation rate; *RF*, rheumatoid factor.

b. Radiologic evaluation:
1) There can be discrepancy between radiological findings and clinical complaints.
2) In later states, radiological evidence shows joint space narrowing, sclerosis, cysts, and reactive osteophytes.
c. Arthrocentesis (joint aspiration) may be diagnostic as well as therapeutic.
d. Differentiate from rapidly advancing OA.
4. Pharmacological options
a. NSAIDs (with or without proton pump inhibitor [PPI] for those at risk for GI bleed)
b. Acetaminophen
c. SNRIs
d. Intraarticular corticosteroid injections
e. Intraarticular hyaluronic acid injection
f. Intraarticular botulinum toxin (conditionally not recommended, but may be appropriate for some individuals)
g. Opioids
C. Rheumatoid arthritis (RA)
1. Description: Common, chronic autoimmune disorder causing pain, swelling, and difficulty moving small joints of feet and hands. It can also affect organs such as skin, lungs, and eyes.
2. Signs and symptoms
a. Pain and stiffness in joints typically worse in morning, sometimes described as burning pain. RA is characterized by symmetrical swelling of movable joints and can lead to progressive destruction of these joints.
b. Pain is accompanied by swelling, tenderness, and decreased range of motion.
c. Frequently associated with chronic fatigue or loss of energy

d. Sometimes associated with hard lumps or rheumatoid nodules growing under skin
e. May be associated with low fevers, dry eyes, and loss of appetite
3. Diagnostic workup (Table 21.1)
a. Physical exam of joints and body organs
b. Labs for:
1) Anemia or decreasing serum albumin
2) Elevated erythrocyte sedimentation rate (ESR) or C-reactive protein (CRP)
3) Positive rheumatoid factor (RF)
4) Anti-citrullinated protein antibodies
5) Thrombocytosis
6) Radiologic evaluation:
a) Radiographs to observe changes in joints, although, in early RA, not many changes will be seen; it is good to get baseline radiographs.
b) MRI, ultrasound, and/or gray-scale Power Doppler can help establish severity of RA.
4. Pharmacological options
a. NSAIDs
b. Acetaminophen
c. Capsaicin
d. DMARDs; If treatment has not been successful within six months, additional biological DMARD should be considered.
e. Opioids
5. Surgical options (e.g., joint replacement, arthrodesis, synovectomy)
D. Systemic lupus erythematosus (SLE)
1. Description: Autoimmune disease with immune dysfunction, inflammation, tissue and organ injury, and variety of additional symptoms, including pain

and fatigue, which may be mild to severe. Skin and joints are frequently impacted, along with other body organs including kidneys, brain, pleura of lungs, and pericardium.

2. Signs and symptoms
   a. Telltale butterfly (malar) rash over checks
   b. Discoid rash—raised oval or round patches
   c. Sores in nose and mouth (for days up to months)
   d. Swollen and tender joints (at least 2) for weeks
   e. Inflammation of lung or heart, causing shortness of breath and chest pain
   f. Protein or blood in urine
   g. May have seizures, a stroke, or psychosis
3. Diagnostic workup
   a. Physical exam: tenderness, effusion, and/or swelling over two or more joints plus morning stiffness for 30 minutes
   b. Labs: complete blood count (CBC), assessing for antinuclear antibodies, anti–double-stranded DNA, and anti-Smith or antiphospholipid antibodies.
   c. Radiologic evaluation: ultrasound, MRI to assess for changes in bone marrow
4. Pharmacological options
   a. Antimalarial medications (e.g., hydroxychloroquine)
   b. Immune suppressants and corticosteroids (e.g., azathioprine, methotrexate, mycophenolate mofetil, cyclophosphamide, rituximab)
   c. NSAIDs
   d. Monoclonal antibody (e.g., belimumab)
E. Temporomandibular joint disorders (TMD)
1. Description: Classified as a musculoskeletal condition associated with structural deformity and/or functional pain processing.
   a. TMD includes anomalies of muscles and joints involved in chewing, causing pain and dysfunction.
   b. TMD is not a diagnosis but rather a broad term that includes various disease processes.
   c. Most common types of TMD focus on pain (myalgia, arthralgia, headaches related to TMD) and disorders related to degeneration or disc displacements, causing difficulties with jaw movements and sounds while opening and closing mouth.
2. Signs and symptoms
   a. Persistent pain in orofacial area
      1) Musculoskeletal, neuropathic or atypical
      2) Pain in face, jaw joint area, neck, shoulders, and in or around ear with speaking or chewing
   b. Decreased ability to open mouth widely
   c. Clicking, popping, or grating sound in jaw with opening or closing mouth or when speaking
   d. Headache
   e. Jaw deviation
   f. Swelling on side of face

   g. Intraoral signs of masticatory dysfunction, including teeth hypermobility and sensitivity, gingival recessions, and teeth impressions on soft tissue and tongue
   h. Depression, decreased quality of life
3. Diagnostic workup
   a. Physical exam: Pay particular attention to cranial nerve exam to exclude tumors.
   b. Labs: no specific labs indicated
   c. Radiologic evaluation: radiography, MRI, and CT
   d. Diagnostic criteria for TMD have been revised with consensus from National Institutes of Health in U.S. and international consensus conferences. Criterion has two domains, a physical Axis I (diagnosis) and a psychosocial Axis II.
      1) Axis 1: Myalgia, joint arthralgia, headache attributed to TMD, joint disorders
      2) Axis 2: Perceived stress, stressful events, catastrophizing, life dissatisfaction
4. Pharmacological options
   a. NSAIDs
   b. Skeletal muscle relaxants
   c. Anticonvulsants
   d. Antidepressants

V. Persistent Degenerative Joint Diseases

A. Persistent joint diseases
1. Description: Disease processes related to injury, inflammation, infection, and degenerative changes can result in pain lasting longer than typical healing time (e.g., lasting up to 3–6 months) or recurs intermittently.
   a. Persistent low back pain occurs in lumbar region (L1–L5) intervertebral disc, ligaments, tendons, muscles, and nerves within spinal column.
   b. As pain progresses, neurochemical, structural, central desensitization, and functional cortical changes of brain occur.
   c. Etiology may be mechanical (e.g., a compression fracture), oncological, infectious, inflammatory, or degenerative. Pain may originate from musculoskeletal sources or viscera (e.g., kidney, renal, or uterus), or pain may be enigmatic.
2. Signs and symptoms are dependent on cause, location, and involved structures (bone, tendons, nerves, ligaments, muscles):
   a. Progressive shock-like pain can lead to motor and/or sensory loss.
   b. Localized tenderness to palpation of spinal process

  c. Psychological: stressors, depression, anxiety, fatigue
  d. Pain precipitated by movement, position change, cough, and sneezing
  e. Muscle spasm
3. Diagnostic workup
  a. Radiologic evaluation: radiography, MRI, CT, or discogram
  b. Labs: no specific labs indicated
  c. Electromyography (EMG) to assess electrical activity of nerves
  d. Nerve conduction studies (NCS) to detect nerve damage
4. Treatment options
  a. Pharmacological options
    1) Acetaminophen
    2) NSAIDs
    3) Antidepressants
    4) Opioids
  b. Interventional pain procedures
    1) Nerve blocks
    2) Epidural injections
    3) Intraarticular injections (e.g., corticosteroid or hyaluronic acid)
  c. Surgical intervention
    1) Implanted nerve stimulators
    2) Joint replacement
B. Facet syndrome
1. Description: Facet joint is an articulation formed by superior articular facet (smooth area of bone) or on adjacent vertebrae's inferior articular facets. Facet syndrome consists of degenerative changes and associated muscle spasm caused by a forced or traumatic twisting sprain of facet joint. Trauma may occur at any intraarticular facet joint level.
2. Signs and symptoms
  a. Lumbar
    1) Pain is described as a dull ache radiating into lower back or hip, buttocks, and posterior or lateral side down to knee; it does *not* occur below knee.
    2) Low back pain, muscle weakness, or stiffness occurs with or without radiation to other areas.
    3) Physical exam should focus on:
      a) Local paralumbar tenderness
      b) Absence of paresthesia
      c) Pain on hyperextension of spine
      d) Depressed deep tendon reflexes; however, there is usually an absence of nerve root tension signs.
  b. Cervical
    1) Neck pain
    2) Headaches
    3) Shoulder pain
    4) Difficulty rotating head

3. Diagnostic workup
  a. Labs: no specific labs indicated
  b. Radiologic evaluation
    1) Plain radiography for correlation with symptoms
    2) CT scan provides better diagnostic results.
    3) MRI may be used to rule out fractures, disc herniation, and degenerative changes.
    4) Single-photon emission computed tomography (SPECT) sometimes used to detect extent of bone involvement
4. Treatment options
  a. Pharmacological options
    1) NSAIDs
    2) Acetaminophen
    3) Skeletal muscle relaxants
    4) Antidepressants
  b. Interventional pain procedure
    1) Facet arthropathy blockade: injection of facet joint with steroids and/or local anesthetic
    2) Facet denervation using radiofrequency lesions or ablation if positive response to blockade
C. Herniated intervertebral disc
1. Description: Mechanical pressure on nerve root resulting in irritation. Intervertebral disc typically comprises annulus fibrosus and nucleus pulposus. A tear in annulus creates bulging of nucleus pulposus, resulting in inflammation or compression of nucleus contents or both. Approximately 95% of herniations occur in lumbar spine, 6% in cervical spine, and 2%–3% in thoracic spine.
2. Signs and symptoms
  a. Lumbar spine
    1) Pain is sudden and severe, sharp and lancinating pain in back.
    2) Pain may radiate in anatomical distribution of affected nerve root.
    3) Compression of nucleus contents at L4–L5 may cause pain radiating to lower portion of legs.
    4) Pain may be associated with neurological symptoms, such as weakness or loss of motor function, diminished or absent deep tendon reflexes, or loss of sensation to affected extremity.
  b. Cervical spine
    1) Neck pain with and without muscle spasms
    2) Deep pain over shoulder blade on affected side
    3) Radiation of pain into shoulder, upper arm, forearm, hands, or fingers depending on nerve affected
    4) Worsening pain with coughing, laughing, or straining
    5) Numbness and muscle weakness

6) Worsening pain with neck bending or turning head to side
7) Decreased range of motion of affected extremity
3. Diagnostic workup
    a. Labs: no specific labs indicated
    b. Physical exam may reveal a decrease or loss of motor function, deep tendon reflexes, or sensation.
    c. Radiologic evaluation: radiography, MRI, CT, myelogram, and/or electromyogram
    d. EMG/NCS may help narrow differential diagnosis.
        1) EMG records electrical activity from muscles and may be helpful in determining which nerve roots are affected.
        2) Needle EMG is required and differentiates between primary muscle disease and abnormalities of anterior horn cell or motor axon.
4. Treatment options:
    a. Pharmacological options
        1) Acetaminophen
        2) NSAIDs
        3) Skeletal muscle relaxants
        4) Corticosteroids
        5) Antidepressants
        6) Anticonvulsants
        7) Opioids
    b. Interventional pain procedures
        1) Epidural injection with local anesthetic and/or corticosteroid
        2) Neuroablation in unresponsive cases
    c. Surgical interventions
        1) Laminotomy
        2) Discectomy
D. Lumbar spondylolysis
    1. Description: Defect of pars interarticularis of vertebrae, not affecting articular processes. Often called a *pars defect*. Exact cause is unclear, but it is hypothesized genetics, overuse, and/or hyperextension of spine is responsible for small stress fractures.
    2. Signs and symptoms
        a. Lumbar spondylolysis occurs more commonly in L5 vertebrae; however, this defect does not always cause pain.
        b. Common in active individuals (males more than females) in their teens
        c. Symptoms are typically bilateral lower back pain and sciatica.
        d. Pain is typically a deep ache, poorly localized in lumbar-sacral region, and gradually recedes with time.
        e. Symptoms usually diminish with decreased activity.
    3. Diagnostic workup
        a. Labs: no specific labs indicated

b. Radiologic evaluation: radiography, MRI, CT
4. Treatment options
    a. Pharmacological options
        1) Skeletal muscle relaxants
        2) Acetaminophen
        3) NSAIDs
        4) Corticosteroids
        5) Antidepressants
        6) Anticonvulsants
        7) Opioids
    b. Interventional pain procedures
        1) Epidural injection with local anesthetic and/or corticosteroid
        2) Facet blockade
    c. Surgical intervention
        1) Surgical stabilization
        2) Surgical replacement of facet joints is in experimental stages.
E. Radiculopathy
    1. Description: Disorder of spinal nerve root. Some causes may be compression of nerve root, diabetes mellitus, herpes zoster, carcinoma, trauma, or an infectious process.
    2. Signs and symptoms
        a. Pain follows a particular nerve or nerve group distribution.
        b. Paresthesia (an abnormal sensation) and dysesthesia (an unpleasant, abnormal sensation) occur such as burning, prickling, tingling, or weakness.
        c. Hyperalgesia (an increased response to normally painful stimuli) and allodynia (extreme sensitivity to nonpainful stimuli) are possible.
        d. Patient may or may not have a loss of sensation or motor function.
    3. Diagnostic workup
        a. Labs: no specific labs indicated
        b. Radiologic evaluation:
            1) MRI to determine if there is direct pressure on a spinal nerve
            2) EMG indicates impairment of a nerve, localizes lesion to one or more nerve roots, and measures severity of condition.
    4. Treatment options
        a. Pharmacological options
            1) Oral corticosteroid steroids for 2–6 weeks
            2) Anticonvulsants
            3) Antidepressants
        b. Interventional pain procedure: epidural steroid injection and other procedures depending on etiology
        c. Surgical intervention
            1) If nerve root impingement, or if symptoms do not resolve or worsen
            2) Procedure depends on etiology.

F. Spinal stenosis
   1. Description: Narrowing of space available for neural elements and most commonly occurs in lower back and neck. Other causes may be disc herniations, ligament thickening, tumors, direct spine injury, congenital spine deformity, and Paget disease.
   2. Signs and symptoms
      a. Persistent back pain and pain in legs and buttocks that gradually increases
      b. Pain is described as deep aching with heavy and numb feeling in leg from buttock to foot.
      c. Pain is worse with activity; in particular, walking causes aching in legs. There is sense of heaviness and clumsiness, which may be associated with frequent falls.
      d. Depending on level of stenosis, associated signs and symptoms may include dermatomal paresthesia, bowel and bladder disturbance, or impotence.
   3. Diagnostic workup
      a. Physical exam shows increased pain with extension of spine, improving with flexion. This may result in a markedly flexed posture of trunk (sometimes referred to as shopping cart sign).
      b. Labs: no specific labs indicated
      c. Radiologic evaluation
         1) Radiography shows diffuse, severe, degenerative disease with facet hypertrophy and decreased anteroposterior diameter of lumbar canal.
         2) MRI, CT, and myelography may indicate a narrowing of spinal canal, osteophytes on intervertebral foramina, or both.
   4. Treatment options
      a. Pharmacological options
         1) Acetaminophen
         2) NSAIDs
         3) Antidepressants
         4) Anticonvulsants
         5) Opioids
      b. Interventional pain procedures
         1) Epidural steroid injections
         2) Minimally invasive lumbar decompression
      c. Surgical decompression

VI. Persistent Myofascial Pain

A. Myofascial pain syndrome (MFS)
   1. Description:
      a. MFS is cue to sensitive or "trigger points" causing pressure-like pain and is associated with dysfunctional CNS pain processing. Pain can occur in individual muscle, groups of muscles, or seemingly unrelated parts of body.
      b. Often occurs after repetitive motions, such as those associated with work or hobbies. Muscle tension related to stress can complicate this pain phenomenon.
      c. May involve localized, ropey band of muscles that act as trigger points, causing flares of pain. This contrasts with fibromyalgia, a similar painful condition, in which pain is widespread.
   2. Mechanisms for trigger point development
      a. Trauma locally tears sarcoplasmic reticulum and releases calcium.
      b. Calcium and available adenosine triphosphate continuously activate local contractile activity. Intense muscle metabolic activity produces substances that sensitize sensory nerve endings.
      c. Restricted range of motion appears with stretching; weakness and atrophy occur without any neurological defect.
      d. Localized vasoconstriction reflex is stimulated to control runaway metabolic activity.
   3. Signs and symptoms
      a. Deep, aching pain and stiffness in muscle
      b. Limited range of motion of affected muscles
      c. Tender knot or taut band in muscle
      d. Demonstration of trigger points within same area of initial pain
      e. Difficulty sleeping or functioning due to pain
   4. Diagnostic workup
      a. Physical exam
         1) Apply gentle finger pressure to area of pain to palpate tense areas or a taut band of painful muscle.
         2) Pressure on primary trigger zone can create a muscle twitch.
         3) Pain may be referred to other areas.
         4) Range of motion is often limited.
      b. Labs: no specific labs indicated
      c. Radiologic evaluation: none specifically indicated
   5. Pharmacological options
      a. Acetaminophen
      b. NSAIDs
      c. Antidepressants
      d. Skeletal muscle relaxants
      e. Sedative hypnotics
      f. Trigger point injections
   6. Nonpharmacological treatments
      a. Stretching and posture training
      b. Massage
      c. Heat
      d. Myofascial release
      e. Dry needling
B. Fibromyalgia
   1. Description: identified by 2010 criteria set by American College of Rheumatology (ACR) and further updated in 2011 and 2016
      a. Centralized pain problem resulting from many factors, including neurochemical imbalances in central nervous system leading

to heightened response to pain and other symptoms

  b. Hyperalgesia, allodynia, and global hypersensitization all seem to be components due to changes in ascending pain pathways, a decrease in inhibition, and other alterations in pain perception.

2. Signs and symptoms
  a. Widespread pain (including hyperalgesia, allodynia, and global hypersensitization)
  b. Severe fatigue
  c. Problems with thinking and memory, often described as "brain fog"
  d. Unrefreshing sleep
  e. Presence of many associated symptoms
  f. Decreased overall functioning and quality of life

3. Diagnostic workup
  a. Self-report measures such as Revised Fibromyalgia Impact Questionnaire
  b. Labs: no specific labs indicated
  c. Radiologic evaluation: no specific radiologic tests indicated
  d. Physical exam
    1) Tender point assessment no longer required
    2) Symptoms must have been present at similar level for at least 3 months.
    3) No other health problems can be cause of above.
    4) Widespread Pain Index (WPI) (Fig. 21.1)
    5) Neurological exam
    6) Joint exam
    7) Assessment of functional status, including physical, emotional, and overall quality of life
  e. 2016 Fibromyalgia diagnosis criteria
    1) WPI > 7 and SSS > 5 OR WPI of 4–6 and SSS > 9
    2) Generalized pain in at least four of five regions must be present. Jaw, chest, and abdominal pain are not included in generalized pain definition.
    3) Symptoms have been generally present for at least 3 months.
    4) A diagnosis of fibromyalgia is valid irrespective of other diagnoses. A diagnosis of fibromyalgia does not exclude presence of other clinically important illnesses.

4. Pharmacological options
  a. Acetaminophen
  b. NSAIDs are not recommended; risks outweigh benefits.
  c. Antidepressants
  d. Anticonvulsants
  e. Tramadol (moderate evidence) but no evidence for full mu opioid agonists (e.g., morphine or oxycodone)
  f. Low-dose naltrexone (LDN)
    1) Orally semisynthetic opiate antagonist shown to mitigate fatigue and stress in fibromyalgia and multiple sclerosis

    2) Reduces inflammatory cytokines, which are elevated in chronic fatigue syndrome

5. Nonpharmacological options
  a. Modified exercise
  b. Physical and occupational therapy
  c. CBT and psychological support

VII. Persistent Neuropathic Pain

A. Syndromes are related to inflammation, ischemia, infarction, or compression injuries of peripheral nerves, resulting in neuropathies.

B. Peripheral neuropathy
1. Description: consists of damage to peripheral nerves
  a. More than 100 types have been identified, each with its own set of symptoms, development, and prognosis. Peripheral neuropathy is related to damage of specific peripheral nerves.
  b. Causes may be inherited (e.g., Charcot-Marie-Tooth disease) or acquired. Acquired causes include physical injury (trauma), tumors, toxins, autoimmune responses, nutritional deficiencies, alcoholism, certain medications, and vascular and metabolic disorders. In many cases, a cause cannot be identified.

2. Signs and symptoms
  a. Vary depending on which nerve(s) are involved
  b. Constant or transient burning, aching, or lancinating limb pain results from disease of peripheral nerves, usually in feet (e.g., sock-like distribution) or hands (e.g., glove-like distribution)
  c. Deep aching pain, especially at night.
  d. Associated with sensory loss, especially to pinprick or dull stimuli and temperature; diminished vibratory sense, occasionally with weakness and muscle atrophy; and loss of reflex, sympathetic tone, or both with development of smooth, fine skin and hair loss
  e. Muscle wasting, paralysis, or organ or gland dysfunction may occur in severe cases.
  f. Impaired digestion, abnormal blood pressure, changes in sweating, sexual dysfunction
  g. Respiratory failure and failure of other organs may develop.

3. Diagnostic workup
  a. Labs: to rule out metabolic and other disease processes
  b. Physical exam with attention to neurological exam
  c. EMG and NCS
  d. Radiologic evaluation—CT, MRI, nerve and skin biopsy
  e. Genetic testing

4. Pharmacological options
  a. Anticonvulsants
  b. Antidepressants

Widespread Pain Index

1. Please indicate the areas you have had pain over the *last week*.				
Left upper region	**Right upper region**	**Left lower region**	**Right lower region**	**Axial region**
☐ Left Jaw*	☐ Right Jaw*	☐ Left Hip/buttock	☐ Right Hip/buttock	☐ Neck
☐ Left Shoulder	☐ Right Shoulder	☐ Upper leg, left	☐ Upper leg, right	☐ Upper back
☐ Left Upper arm	☐ Right Upper arm	☐ Lower leg, left	☐ Lower leg, right	☐ Lower back
☐ Left Lower arm	☐ Right Lower arm			☐ Chest*
				☐ Abdomen*

2. Which of these symptoms have you been bothered by in the *past 6 months*?		
☐ Headache	☐ Pain/cramps in lower abdomen	☐ Depression
☐ TMJ symptoms	☐ Wheezing	☐ Constipation
☐ Muscle weakness	☐ Bladder cramps	☐ Cold intolerance
☐ Numbness/tingling of extremities	☐ Frequent urination	☐ Heat intolerance
☐ Blurred vision	☐ Dry mouth	☐ Multiple sensitivities (lights, smells, foods, medications)
☐ Dry eyes	☐ Oral ulcers	
☐ Hair loss	☐ Loss of/change in taste	☐ Rash
☐ Hearing difficulties	☐ Heartburn	☐ Sun sensitivity
☐ Ringing in the ears	☐ Nausea	☐ Hives
☐ Lightheadedness	☐ Loss of appetitie	☐ Easy bruising
☐ Sense of imbalance	☐ Bowel cramps	☐ Decreased sex drive
☐ Palpitations	☐ Frequent loose stools	☐ Nervousness
☐ Chest discomfort	☐ Increased sweating	☐ Difficulty falling asleep and staying asleep
☐ Shortness of breath		

☐ Depressed mood

SCORING FOR STAFF USE ONLY

Section 1   Widespread pain index (WPI) is total score **from question 1 on front.**   **WPI** _____ **/19**   Number of Pain Regions present (excluding jaw, chest, abdomen)   _____ **/5**

Section 2A
 Symptom severity scale score **from question 2 on front.**
 Score the following three symptoms if they have bothered you over the **past 6 months.**
     0 = Not checked/ not bothersome
     1= Checked/ bothersome
 _____**Headaches** (0-1)
 _____**Pain or cramps in lower abdomen** (0-1)
 _____**Depression** (0-1)
 *Section 2 table was part of 2010 criteria that may still be collected in the patients record but isn't required for scoring according to the 2016 criteria.
 SSS_____**/3**

Section 2B
 Symptom severity scale score.
 Ask the patient **over the past week** the severity of the following symptoms;
     0 = No problem
     1= Slight or mild problems, generally mild or intermittent
     2= Moderate, considerable problems, often present and/or at a moderate level
     3= Severe: pervasive, continuous, life-disturbing problems
       _____**Fatigue** (0-3)
       _____**Waking unrefreshed** (0-3)
       _____**Cognitive Symptoms** (0-3)
 SSS_____**/9**

Symptom Severity Score   Add the total from **Section 2A** (0-3) and the total from **Section 2B** (0-9)   **Section 2A total + Section 2B total**   **SSS score**_____**/12**

Figure 21.1 Widespread Pain Index (WPI)

c. Capsaicin cream

d. Topical local anesthetic

e. Oral local anesthetic agent (e.g., mexiletine)

5. Nonpharmacological options

a. Physical and occupational therapy

b. Mirror therapy

c. CBT and psychological support

d. Acupuncture

e. Progressive muscle relaxation and guided motion therapy

C. Postherpetic neuralgia

1. Description: Pain persisting past stage of healing lesions after acute herpes zoster infection. Pain usually diminishes with time (3 months). Risk factors include being 50 years or older (immune senescence) or with defective cellular immunity (e.g., HIV infection, malignant lymphoma).

2. Signs and symptoms

a. Persistent pain and skin changes in a dermatomal distribution after acute herpes zoster infection

b. Pain is mild to severe with burning, sharp sensations. May have brief, intense shooting pains. Other words used to describe pain are twisting, boring, jabbing, and buzzing.

c. Dysesthesia, allodynia, and hyperesthesia occur.

3. Diagnostic workup

a. Thermograms may show heat emission in affected dermatomes.

b. Labs:

1) Viral cultures during active phase may indicate herpetic infection.

2) Serological antibody test

c. Radiologic evaluation: no radiologic tests indicated

4. Pharmacological options

a. Antiviral agents, if started within 72 hours after onset of rash, may reduce pain severity and duration and hasten rash resolution.

b. Antidepressants

c. Anticonvulsants

d. Oral local anesthetic agents

e. Capsaicin cream after lesions resolve

f. Topical local anesthetic (e.g., lidocaine) after lesions resolve

g. Opioids

D. Mononeuropathies or plexopathies

1. Description: include brachial plexus neuropathies, brachial mononeuropathies, lumbosacral plexopathies, crural mononeuropathies, and entrapment neuropathies

2. Signs and symptoms

a. Constant or transient burning, aching, stabbing, shooting, electrical, heat or cold sensations, or lancinating pain involving area supplied by nerve. At night, pain can be profound and aching

b. Associated with sensory loss, especially to pinprick or dull touch and temperature; diminished vibratory sense, sometimes with weakness, and muscle atrophy

c. Occasionally, loss or diminished deep tendon reflex, sympathetic tone, or both with development of smooth, fine skin and hair loss in affected area

d. Muscle atrophy occurs in late stages.

3. Diagnostic workup

a. Physical exam with attention to neurological exam

b. Labs: no specific labs indicated

c. Radiologic evaluation: none specially indicated

d. EMG and nerve conduction studies to assess for muscle denervation

4. Pharmacological options

a. Anticonvulsants

b. Antidepressants

c. Oral local anesthetic agents

d. Topical capsaicin cream

e. Topical local anesthetic

E. Trigeminal neuralgia (tic douloureux)

1. Description: Consists of pain along second or third division of trigeminal nerve. It may be caused by pressure from a blood vessel on trigeminal nerve as it exits brainstem. It may also be caused by other disorders that damage nerve sheath.

2. Signs and symptoms

a. Pain:

1) Sudden onset, brief, stabbing, recurrent pain in distribution of fifth cranial nerve most often causing pain to cheekbone, nose, upper lip, and upper teeth (can include chin)

2) Unilateral and more frequent on right side

3) Described as sharp, agonizing, electric shock-like stabs of pain felt superficially in skin or buccal mucosa

4) Characteristically occurs in brief, repetitive bursts for several seconds to two minutes followed by refractory period of 30 seconds to a few minutes

5) Associated with mild flush during episodes

b. Episodes occur intermittently, often several times daily, and are rarely continuous. Duration occurs from a few weeks to 2 months, followed by pain-free period and then recurrence.

c. Psychosocial: Isolation, depression, and sleep disturbance often occur.

3. Diagnostic workup

a. Neurological exam

b. Hypoesthesia on face or absence of corneal reflex

c. If sensory deficit is present, diagnostic workup for causation needs to be completed.

d. Labs: no specific labs indicated

e. Radiologic evaluation: none specifically indicated
4. Treatment options
   a. Pharmacological options
      1) Anticonvulsants (gabapentin, pregabalin)
      2) Antidepressants
      3) NSAIDs
      4) Skeletal muscle relaxants
      5) Topical local anesthetics
   b. Nonpharmacological options
      1) Pressure around areas may be helpful during a flare.
      2) Protection from cold wind
   c. Interventional pain procedures
      1) Local anesthetic infiltration into trigeminal ganglion
      2) Glycerol injection
      3) Radiofrequency thermal lesioning
      4) Microvascular decompression
      5) Gamma knife radiosurgery
F. Painful cranial neuropathies
1. Description: Include persistent facial pains and headaches. Pain in head and neck is mediated by afferent fibers in trigeminal, glossopharyngeal, nervus intermedius, and vagus nerves and upper cervical roots via occipital nerves. Stimulation of nerves can cause pain in innervated areas, which include:
   a. Bell's palsy
   b. Glossopharyngeal neuralgia
   c. Nervus intermedius neuralgia
   d. Occipital neuralgia
   e. Optic neuritis
   f. Ischemic ocular motor nerve palsy
   g. Tolosa-Hunt syndrome
   h. Paratrigeminal oculosympathetic (Raeder) syndrome
   i. Recurrent painful ophthalmoplegic neuropathy
   j. Burning mouth syndrome (BMS)
   k. Persistent idiopathic facial pain (PIFP)
   l. Central neuropathic pain
   m. Persistent idiopathic facial pain
2. Signs and symptoms
   a. Vary based on affected nerve
   b. Numbness and tingling sensation
   c. Hypoesthesia (decrease in sensation to temperature and touch)
   d. Muscle weakness or paralysis
   e. Visual changes
3. Diagnostic workup
   a. Physical exam focused on neurological assessment
   b. EMG to assess electrical impulse of muscles
   c. Labs: no labs specifically indicated
   d. Radiologic evaluation: CT or MRI of brain
   e. Skin and nerve biopsy

f. Auditory testing
4. Pharmacological options vary and will be dependent on identified cause.
   a. NSAIDs
   b. Skeletal muscle relaxants
   c. Anticonvulsants
   d. Antidepressants
5. Interventional pain procedures
   a. Nerve block with local anesthetic depending on location of specific nerve involvement
   b. Radiofrequency nerve ablation
G. Human immunodeficiency virus (HIV) and acquired immunodeficiency syndrome (AIDS) related neuropathic pain
1. Description: may involve average of two or more types of pain at any given time
2. Types of pain
   a. Oral pain secondary to:
      1) Candidiasis
      2) Dental caries
      3) Herpes simplex virus (HSV)
      4) Cytomegalovirus (CMV)
      5) Epstein-Barr virus
      6) Mycobacterium infection
      7) Cryptococcal infection
      8) Histoplasmosis
      9) Kaposi sarcoma
   b. Esophageal pain secondary to:
      1) Candidiasis
      2) Other fungal infections
      3) CMV
      4) HSV
   c. Abdominal pain secondary to:
      1) Cryptosporidial diarrhea
      2) *Shigella* infection
      3) *Salmonella* infection
      4) *Campylobacter enteritis*
      5) CMV ileitis and colitis
      6) Lymphoma
      7) Kaposi sarcoma
   d. Biliary and pancreatic pain secondary to:
      1) Coincidental cholelithiasis
      2) Acalculous cholecystitis related to *Cryptosporidium*
      3) CMV
      4) Mycobacterial infection
      5) Kaposi sarcoma
      6) Sclerosing cholangitis related to CMV and *Cryptosporidium*
      7) Pancreatitis associated with medication therapy, in particular, pentamidine and antiretroviral agents
      8) Acute pancreatitis associated with CMV
   e. Anorectal pain secondary to:
      1) Perirectal abscesses
      2) Kaposi sarcoma

3) CMV proctitis
4) Fissures
5) HSV
6) Cancer
7) Genital warts
f. Neurological pain secondary to:
1) Headaches related to primary HIV syndromes
2) HIV encephalitis
3) Atypical septic meningitis
4) Viral and nonviral nervous system infections
5) AIDS-related neoplasms
6) Common migraines
g. Peripheral neuropathy
1) Symmetrical sensory neuropathies can constitute 16% to 50% of pain diagnoses.
2) Distal peripheral neuropathy is most common neuropathy in HIV infection and occurs in about 50% of patients.
   a) HIV neuropathies are characterized by tingling, numbness, or pins and needles.
   b) Cramping, stabbing, aching, and burning may be present.
   c) Decreased or absent ankle jerks and decreased pinprick and vibration sensations in lower extremities are common.
   d) Upper extremity involvement may be present in advanced cases.
   e) Several antiretroviral agents can cause painful peripheral neuropathy (e.g., nucleoside reverse transcriptase inhibitors [NRTIs] such as didanosine and zalcitabine; dapsone, isoniazid, vincristine, and stavudine).
3) Kaposi sarcoma results in lower extremity pain in 45% of patients.
4) Demyelinating polyneuropathies are caused by:
   a) Guillain-Barre syndrome
   b) Chronic mononeuritis
   c) Multiples, progressive inflammatory polyradiculopathy of lower limbs
h. Rheumatological pain secondary to:
1) Reactive arthritis
2) Arthropathies
3) PsA
4) Septic arthritis
5) Myopathy and myositis, possibly related to medication therapy
6) Unknown etiology
i. Pain related to HIV therapy can occur from:
1) Medications
2) Chemotherapy
3) Radiation therapy
4) Procedures
5) Surgery
j. Pain related to concomitant problems (e.g., persistent low back pain, diabetic neuropathy)
3. Diagnostic workup (as appropriate to patient)
a. Labs: based on site of pain and symptomatology
b. Skin biopsy
c. Radiologic evaluation: based on symptomatology
d. EMG and NCS
4. Treatment options
a. Treat cause of pain when known.
1) Same interventions are appropriate in patients with and without HIV infection, although few studies have been conducted specifically in patients with HIV. Choice of pain therapy depends on type of pain.
2) Caution is needed when choosing medications because antiretroviral medications are associated with drug–drug interactions.
b. Pharmacological options
1) Acetaminophen
2) NSAIDs and salicylates
3) Antidepressants
4) Anticonvulsants
5) Corticosteroids
6) Methadone (drug–drug interaction risk), buprenorphine, ketamine, and lidocaine IV infusion with use guided by a specialist who has expertise in this area

VIII. Persistent Postsurgical Pain

A. Generally defined as pain persisting for longer than 3 months after surgical procedure that was not present before surgical intervention or was present before surgery with difference in characteristic or intensity seen in postoperative phase of recovery
1. Pain is often localized to surgical site, but referred pain can be present.
2. Mechanism triggering persistent postsurgical pain is unclear, but literature supports it can develop secondary to muscle injury, scarring, pain sensitization, and/or deconditioning.
3. Risk factors include type of surgery, surgical technique, intraoperative nerve damage, psychosocial factors, genetics, preexisting health conditions, history of persistent pain, and gender. Several types of persistent postsurgical pain are presented below.
B. Postamputation pain
1. Description: Formerly known as "stump pain," is due to sensory abnormalities that cause hyperalgesia and allodynia. At end of stump, nerve fibers

become a mass or neuroma that sends signals to brain and elicits pain. This type of persistent pain can be caused by infection, underlying chronic disease (e.g., diabetes), surgical trauma, neuroma, nerve entrapment, and poor blood circulation.

2. Signs and symptoms
   a. Dependent on cause of pain
   b. Skin may be sensitive.
3. Diagnostic workup
   a. History
   b. Physical examination of residual limb
   c. Labs: vary but may be used to help determine cause
   d. Radiologic evaluation: MRI, CT, and radiography to rule out other potential causes
4. Treatment options
   a. Pharmacological options
      1) Acetaminophen
      2) Antidepressants
      3) Anticonvulsants
      4) Skeletal muscle relaxants
      5) Local anesthetics
      6) Alpha-2-adrenergic agonist (e.g., clonidine)
      7) Beta-blockers
      8) Opioids
      9) NMDA agonist (e.g., ketamine)
   b. Interventional pain procedure
      1) Peripheral nerve block
      2) Neuromodulation (spinal or peripheral nerve stimulation)
   c. Surgical options
      1) Removal of a neuroma is often ineffective because it grows back.
      2) Revision of prosthesis
C. Phantom limb pain
   1. Description: May be associated with residual limb pain, but cause of phantom pain is unclear and seems to originate in brain.
      a. Mixed signals in brain are thought by many experts to explain phantom pain at least partially. Damaged nerve endings, scar tissue at amputation site, and memory of preamputation pain may also contribute to phantom pain.
      b. Risk factors include pain before amputation, stump pain, and poorly fitting prosthesis.
   2. Signs and symptoms
      a. Follows amputation and may start at time of amputation or occur months to years later
      b. Pain:
         1) Occurs in missing body part
         2) Severity varies among individuals.
         3) Persists indefinitely and often with gradual reduction over years

4) May be intermittent or continuous
5) Described as cramping, aching, squeezing, throbbing, or burning with transient shock-like pain
6) May feel like phantom part is forced into an uncomfortable position
7) May be felt at other body sites
8) May be associated with a distorted image of lost part
9) May be triggered by weather changes, pressure on remaining part of limb, or emotional stress
   3. Diagnostic workup
      a. History
      b. Physical examination of residual limb
      c. Labs: vary but used to help determine cause
      d. Radiologic evaluation: MRI, CT, and radiography to rule out other potential causes
   4. Pharmacological options
      a. Anticonvulsants
      b. Antidepressants
      c. NMDA receptor antagonist (e.g., ketamine)
      d. Oral local anesthetic agents
   5. Interventional pain procedures
      a. Neuromodulation
      b. Sympathetic nerve block
D. Postmastectomy pain syndrome
   1. Description: Pain lasting longer than 3 months after acute phase and caused by surgical trauma to intercostobrachial and other upper thoracic nerves. It may occur at brachial plexus during an axillary node dissection.
   2. Risk factors
      a. Age <40 years old
      b. Female
      c. Elevated BMI
      d. Smoking
      e. Late-stage disease process
      f. Tumor in upper lateral quadrant of breast
      g. Type of surgery and postoperative complication
      h. Adjuvant therapy: radiation, chemotherapy
      i. Pain: perioperative pain, persistent pain before surgery, acute postoperative pain
      j. Pain regimen used during surgery may impact risk of postmastectomy pain syndrome development.
      k. Psychosocial factors: depression, anxiety, poor sleep hygiene, catastrophizing
      l. Axillary lymph node dissection
   3. Signs and symptoms
      a. Pain may begin immediately or start many months after surgery and may last for years.
      b. Pain may involve ipsilateral arm, axilla, and anterior chest, and it may be in area of surgical scar.

Part 4

c. Pain is described as burning, constant, tingling, stabbing, numbness, pins and needles, and pulling and may be unresponsive to analgesics.

d. Aggravated by prosthesis, clothing, straining, sudden movement, tiredness, cold weather, coughing, or touch

e. May be associated with emotional lability and avoidance of sexual encounters.

f. Hyperesthesia to pinprick, patchy anesthesia, and allodynia

g. Trigger point tenderness over area

4. Diagnostic workup
   a. Labs: no specific labs indicated
   b. Radiologic evaluation: MRI, CT, or bone scan to rule out presence of recurrent tumor or metastases

5. Pharmacological options
   a. Antidepressants
   b. Anticonvulsants
   c. Capsaicin cream
   d. Topical anesthetics (e.g., lidocaine patch)
   e. Botulinum toxin
   f. Lidocaine injection or infusion
   g. Opioids

6. Interventional pain procedures
   a. Paravertebral block
   b. Serratus block

E. Post-thoracotomy pain syndrome
1. Description: Results from operative trauma to intercostal nerves or ribs and is defined as pain that recurs or persists along thoracotomy incision more than two months after surgical procedure. It can affect about 25% to 57% of postsurgical patients.

2. Risk factors
   a. Advanced age
   b. Female sex
   c. Non-White ethnicity
   d. Low socioeconomic status
   e. Comorbidities
   f. Genetics
   g. Preexisting psychiatric disease

3. Signs and symptoms
   a. Pain:
      1) Recurs or persists along a thoracotomy scar for at least 2 months after surgery. Pain beyond this time may have burning, electrical shock component, with itching or tightening of skin.
      2) Described as aching sensation in distribution of incision
      3) Increased by movement of ipsilateral shoulder
   b. Sensory loss and absence of sweating occur along surgical scar lines.

4. Diagnostic workup
   a. History
   b. Physical exam
   c. Labs: no specific labs indicated
   d. Radiologic evaluation: none specifically indicated

5. Pharmacological options
   a. Acetaminophen
   b. NSAIDs
   c. Ketamine
   d. Antidepressants
   e. Anticonvulsants
   f. Topical local anesthetics
   g. Capsaicin
   h. Opioids

6. Interventional pain procedures
   a. Epidural steroid injections
   b. Paravertebral nerve block
   c. Intercostal nerve blocks
   d. Erector spinae blocks
   e. Neuroablative procedures

F. Post-radical neck dissection pain syndrome
1. Description: Caused by operative trauma to superficial cervical plexus. May always also involve regional myofascial pain. Some patients experience both types of pain.

2. Signs and symptoms
   a. Persistent moderate or severe pain starts after radical neck dissection.
   b. Pain may be reported within distribution of superficial cervical plexus, trigeminal nerve distribution, C2–C8 distribution, mandibular angle and inferior border of jaw, and lateral side of neck.
   c. Duration can be years, and pain may decrease with time.
   d. Pain is aggravated by clothing or touch.
   e. Patchy anesthesia may be present.
   f. Trigger point tenderness in sternocleidomastoid, trapezius, splenius capitis, splenius cervicis, and semispinalis cervicis muscles may be present.
   g. Pain is described as burning or shooting; it may be constant or variable.
   h. Pain nonresponsive to opioid analgesics

3. Diagnostic workup
   a. Labs: no specific labs indicated
   b. Radiologic evaluation: none specifically indicated

4. Pharmacological options
   a. NSAIDs
   b. Antidepressants
   c. Anticonvulsant agents
   d. Oral local anesthetic agents
   e. Skeletal muscle relaxants

f. Capsaicin
g. Topical local anesthetics (e.g., lidocaine patch)
5. Interventional pain procedures
  a. Channel neurolysis of superior cervical plexus nerve
  b. Trigger point injections

IX. Persistent Central Pain

A. Disease processes in persistent central pain typically occur after stroke; demyelinating disease; or trauma to brain, brainstem, or spinal cord. It can also occur after a syrinx formation on brainstem, or spinal cord.
1. Can be difficult to determine central pain from peripheral or musculoskeletal pain in people who have neurologic impairment
2. Patients with brain or spinal cord injury can have both central pain and pain as result of other pain generators.
3. Central pain is different than central sensitization; central pain occurs only as direct result of injury to CNS. Central sensitization is process of irreversible changes in pain pathways.
4. Not a fatal disorder, but pain and suffering can be quite debilitating. Pain is typically constant but can range from mild to severe.

B. Central pain syndrome (CPS)
1. Description: neurological disorder involving pain associated with ischemia or lesions in CNS including spinal cord, brainstem, or brain, resulting in impaired communication between sensory thalamus and sensory cortex could be caused by a stroke, traumatic brain injury (TBI), multiple sclerosis (MS), tumors, brain or spinal cord trauma, epilepsy, Parkinson disease, or CNS surgery
2. Signs and symptoms
  a. Due to multiple etiologies, central pain varies greatly, with degree of pain and symptoms directly related to area of injury or CNS damage. Pain and numbness are usually worse on hands and feet.
  b. Pain:
    1) Typically occurs within a few weeks to 2 years after initial injury but may start months or years later, especially after a stroke
    2) May be localized to specific body area or widespread; constant or intermittent and mild to excruciating
    3) Described as pins and needles, lancinating, burning, uncomfortably cold, aching, pressing, itching, painful numbness or sharp, searing extreme burst of pain similar to pain of dental probe on nerve

    4) Evoked by light touch, cold or heat, movements, increased anxiety, or emotional arousal; can also be activated by visceral activity like micturition
    5) May be associated with typical hemiparesis, most often with motor impairments and sensory deficits in affected areas. Sensation associated with light touch is impaired.
  c. Patients often have heightened response to other painful stimuli.
  d. Vasomotor and sudomotor atrophic changes are often present.
  e. Anxiety and depression often occur.
3. Diagnostic workup
  a. History and examination to differentiate central pain from other pain types.
  b. Assess for pinprick and/or temperature sensation of impacted limb. For pain to be classified as CPS, there must be pain within region of body affected by CNS insult. If pinprick and temperature sensations are within normal limits, then CPS can be ruled out.
  c. For patients with multiple sclerosis, ascertain main symptoms at time of diagnosis. Patients have higher likelihood of developing CPS if pain was part of their original complex of symptoms.
  d. Labs: no specific labs indicated
  e. Radiologic evaluation: none specifically indicated
4. Pharmacological options
  a. CPSs have wide array of pathophysiology, and there have been few successful studies, leaving a gap in evidence-based guidelines for medication.
  b. An individualized approach is necessary (Table 21.2).
5. Interventional pain procedures: Investigational studies are promising, including extradural cortical stimulation, transcranial magnetic stimulation (TMS), and transcranial direct current stimulation (tDCS) of affected area.

C. Spinal cord injury (SCI)
1. Pain depends on level of spinal cord impact and may be associated with varied types of pain (Table 21.3).
2. Signs and symptoms
  a. Localized, radicular or diffuse; constant or intermittent; at, above, or below injury level. Level of SCI may be associated with sites of pain.
  b. Injuries at higher spinal levels are more likely to result in upper extremity pain consistent with dermatomal distribution of pain at level of injury.
  c. Lower body pain tends to be described as more intense.

Table 21.2

Practical Dosing Recommendations for Medications With Randomized Controlled Trial Data Supporting Their Use in Central Pain Syndromes

Agent	Usual Starting Dosage	Dosing	Effective Dosage In Central Pain Rcts	Maximum Dosage	Precautions	Common And Notable Adverse Effects
Gabapentin	300 mg at bedtime (100-mg increments available for slower titration)	Increase by 300-mg increments every 4–7 d initially to 3 times daily, then to goal of 1800 mg/d	At least 1800 mg/d	Increase as necessary to 3600 mg/d (split risk 3 times daily)	Renal insufficiency (dosage adjust); risk of seizure if abruptly stopped	Sedation, dizziness, confusion, edema, tremor
Pregabalin	75 mg twice daily (25-mg and 50-mg dosing available for slower titration)	Increase by 75 mg after 4–7 d to goal of 300 mg/d	Mean dosage of 410–460 mg/d	Increase as necessary to 600 mg/d	Renal insufficiency (dosage adjust); risk of seizure if abruptly stopped; psychiatric disease or addiction history (euphoria risk)	Sedation, dizziness, confusion, edema, tremor, euphoria
Lamotrigine	25 mg/d for 2 wk	Increase to 25 mg twice daily for 2 wk, then increase weekly by 25 mg twice daily to goal of at least 100 mg twice daily	Mean dosage of 200–400 mg/d	400 mg/d	Dose adjust with liver disease or renal impairment; patients taking medications such as valproic acid that inhibit hepatic P450 system require slower titration regimen; risk of seizure if abruptly stopped	Rash (Stevens-Johnson syndrome); abdominal pain; diarrhea; headache; dizziness Slow titration to minimize the risk of toxicities
Carbamazepine	200 mg once daily	Increase by 200 mg every 4–7 d to twice daily, then thrice daily, and as necessary 4 times daily (extended-release formulations allow twice-daily dosing of same total daily dosage)	500–760 mg/d	1200 mg/d	Test for inherited allelic variant *HLA-B* 1502* in patients of Asian descent and if present do not use carbamazepine; risk of seizure if abruptly stopped	Stevens-Johnson syndrome; hematologic suppression (monitor CBC); hepatic dysfunction (monitor LFTs); hyponatremia; nausea; dizziness; drowsiness

Continued

Table 21.2

Practical Dosing Recommendations for Medications With Randomized Controlled Trial Data Supporting Their use in Central Pain Syndromes—cont'd

Agent	Usual Starting Dosage	Dosing	Effective Dosage In Central Pain Rcts	Maximum Dosage	Precautions	Common And Notable Adverse Effects
Amitriptyline	10–25 mg at bedtime	Increase every 4–7 d to goal of 100 mg at bedtime	At least 75 mg/d	150 mg/d	Risk of emerging suicidality (children/young adults—see boxed warning); risk of serotonin syndrome; use with caution if patent has cardiac disease or dysrhythmia history	Sedation, dry mouth, orthostatism, confusion, weight gain, urinary retention, constipation, blurred vision
Duloxetine	20–30 mg once daily	Increase weekly by same dosage to goal of 60 mg/d	60 mg/d	120 mg/d (split BID)	Risk of emerging suicidality (children/young adults—see boxed warning); risk of serotonin syndrome; increased bleeding risk (use cautiously with anticoagulants); withdrawal syndromes with abrupt discontinuation; use with caution in patients with hepatic failure	Sedation, fatigue, nausea, hyperhidrosis, dizziness
Cannabinoids	Dosing and relative proportion of tetrahydrocannabinol and cannabidiol (the two most common medical cannabinoids) were highly variable in RCTs. Form of administration varied in RCTs. No recommendations possible.				Federally illegal for medicinal usage (Schedule I drug), but increasing number of states have legalized medical cannabinoids	Palpitations hypotension, dry mouth, dizziness, depression, inattention, hallucinations, paranoia, addiction

Note: All doses are for reference only and based on adult dosing (not pediatric).

BID, twice a day; *CBC,* complete blood cell count; *LFT,* liver function test; *RCT,* randomized controlled trial.

From Watson, J. C., & Sandroni, P. (2016). Central neuropathic pain syndromes. *Mayo Clinic Proceedings, 91*(3), 372–385. https://doi.org/10.1016/j.mayocp.2016.01.01.

Table 21.3

Pain Related to Spinal Cord Injury

Term	Location	Features
Neuropathic		
Below level	Diffusely below level of injury	Sharp, shooting, burning, electrical, abnormal responsiveness (hyperesthesia, hyperalgesia); may respond to anticonvulsants
At level	In segment pattern at level of injury	
Above level	In region of sensory preservation	
Nociceptive		
Musculoskeletal	In bones, joints, muscles	Dull, aching, movement related, eased by rest; responds to opioids and NSAIDs
Visceral	In abdominal region with preserved innervation	Dull, cramping; may or may not respond to NSAIDs

NSAID, nonsteroidal anti-inflammatory drug.

d. High-intensity pain may occur over multiple body locations and may have multiple pain generators.

e. SCI pain due to trauma (e.g. diving or motor vehicle accidents) often occurs below level of injury: torso, hips, and groin and may extend to legs, feet, and toes. May have sensation of cramping in feet, feeling feet are deformed, or sensations of sitting on a hot fire or having a mass in rectum.

f. Other causes of SCI pain are vascular or skeletal pathology, inflammatory lesions, neoplasms, demyelinating diseases, iatrogenic perisurgical causes, abscesses, and congenital lesions.

g. SCI may result in painful pressure sores and spasticity.

3. Diagnostic workup
    a. Assess for allodynia, hypoesthesia, *hypo*analgesia, *hyper*pathia, dysesthesia, and neurological signs of damage to affected region.
    b. Labs: cultures as indicated
    c. Radiologic evaluation: as indicated
    d. Biopsies as indicated

4. Pharmacological options
    a. Anticonvulsants
    b. Antidepressants
    c. Skeletal muscle relaxants
    d. Opioids

5. Interventional pain procedures
    a. Neurolytic therapies are controversial.
    b. Neuromodulation with motor cortex stimulation (MCS) and deep brain stimulation (DBS), but long-term stimulation therapies are still controversial.

D. Syringomyelia disorder (syrinx)
    1. Description: Fluid-filled cavitation or cyst is formed within spinal cord. Cyst expands and elongates over time, resulting in destruction of spinal cord from center outward.
    2. A number of medical conditions can create obstruction in normal CSF flow, redirecting it into central canal and ultimately into spinal cord itself. Redirected CSF fills expanding central canal and results in syrinx formation. Pressure differences along spine cause fluid to move within cyst. It is thought this continual movement of fluid builds pressure around and inside spinal cord and results in cyst growth and further damage to spinal cord tissue. Chiari I malformation is most common cause of syrinx. This congenital anatomical abnormality causes lower part of cerebellum to protrude from its normal location in back of head into cervical or neck portion of spinal canal.
    3. Signs and symptoms
        a. May begin in childhood or early adulthood, especially if due to Chiari malformation
        b. Symptoms may develop slowly or suddenly with cough or sneeze.
        c. Symptoms vary depending on location and size of syrinx and involved spinal nerves.
        d. Syrinx pain is neuropathic and dysesthetic pain similar to CRPS or radicular pain. When syrinx is in cervical area, pain may be in "cape-like" distribution.
        e. Pain may be experienced as interscapular pain and may spread upward from syrinx site.
        f. May be described as sensation of "skin stretching"
        g. Pain and stiffness (back, shoulders, arms, legs)
        h. Weakness
        i. Headaches
        j. Loss of ability to feel hot or cold on one or both sides of body
        k. Similar to CRPS, sweating, skin coldness, and/or pallor may be experienced.
        l. Progressive loss of sensation
        m. Sexual dysfunction and subsequent bowel and bladder impairment
    4. Diagnostic workup
        a. EMG
        b. Labs: lumbar puncture to measure CSF pressure and analyze CSF
        c. Radiologic evaluation: MRI is usually diagnostic; CT may be indicated
    5. Treatment options
        a. No treatment is necessary if asymptomatic.
        b. If symptomatic, surgical intervention. If symptomatic syrinx is not treated surgically, syringomyelia often leads to SCI with incumbent symptoms and severe, persistent pain.

c. Avoid activities associated with straining.

6. Pharmacological options: conventional analgesics and neuropathic medications provide little or no relief.

7. Interventional pain procedures: sympathetic nerve blocks (e.g., stellate ganglion or lumbar sympathetic)

X. Headaches

A. Categories of headache:
   1. Primary headaches (with four subcategories)
   2. Secondary headaches
   3. Painful cranial neuropathies, other facial pains, and other headaches

B. Primary headaches
   1. Migraines:
      a. Migraines affect approximately 12% of population: 18% of females and 6% of males.
      b. Includes chronic daily headaches (>15 days per month), episodic (<15 days per month), and migraine with and without aura
      c. Pain is associated with changes in cranial vasculature and impacts neurological, gastrointestinal, and autonomic nervous systems.
      d. Migraine *without* aura (previously identified by hemicranias simplex or common migraine)
         1) Characterized by specific headache features and associated symptoms
         2) Signs and symptoms
            a) Headache pain, predominantly unilateral, but not always
            b) Pulsating quality
            c) Moderate to severe pain intensity
            d) Nausea and/or vomiting
            e) Sensitivity to light and/or sound
         3) Diagnostic criteria
            a) Five or more attacks
            b) Headache duration between 4 and 72 hours if untreated
            c) Headache with at least two of the following, but *not* weakness:
               (1) Unilateral location
               (2) Pulsating
               (3) Moderate to severe Intensity
               (4) Aggravated by routine physical activity
            d) Has at least one of the following:
               (1) Phonophobia
               (2) Photophobia
               (3) Nausea
               (4) Emesis
            e) Does not fit better under other criteria
      e. Migraine *with* aura
         1) Previously identified as classic or classical migraine, hemiparanesthetic, hemiplegic, ophthalmic, aphasic migraine, migraine accompagnée, or complicated migraine
         2) Primarily transitory focal neurological symptoms that may occur before or during headache
         3) May have premonitory phase hours or days before headache, followed by resolution phase
         4) Premonitory phase and resolution symptoms may include hyper- or hypoactivity, depression, yawning, food cravings, fatigue, neck stiffness, and pain.
         5) Signs and symptoms
            a) Focal neurological sensations may occur prior to or along with headache.
            b) Recurrent attacks
            c) Visual aura (most common) may be bright spots, dark spots, zigzag shapes, sharp edges, double or distorted vision, blind spots, and tunnel vision.
            d) Sensory distortion (next most common)—numbness, tingling, and paresthesia in one arm or on one side of body; vertigo or weakness
            e) Less frequent are speech disturbances such as aphasia, but these are often hard to categorize; aversion to odors
         6) Diagnostic criteria
            a) At least two headaches that also fulfill characteristics of migraine without aura
            b) Headaches usually follow aura but may begin with it and last 4–72 hours if left untreated.
            c) At least one of several reversible symptoms lasting between 4 and 60 minutes but with no weakness
            d) Positive (adding to field) or negative (removing from field) visual symptoms such as flashing lights, diminished visual field, blind spots, or blurred vision
            e) Positive or negative sensory symptoms such as numbness or tingling
      f. Basilar migraine
         1) Migraine whose aura seems to involve both right and left hemispheres of brain or originates from brainstem
         2) Signs and symptoms
            a) Two or more headaches with an aura whose symptoms are reversible and localized to brainstem or impact both brain hemispheres, but without weakness
            b) Dysarthria—speech impairment caused by muscle weakness

c) Vertigo or dizziness

d) Bilateral visual symptoms may include temporary blindness, double vision, or nystagmus.

e) Poor coordination and difficulty walking

f) Altered consciousness

g) Bilateral numbness and tingling

h) Tinnitus with or without decreased hearing

g. Diagnostic workup for all types of migraine

1) Suggestive clinic history

a) Headache diary—assess frequency, episode intensity, and duration (i.e., headache days/month)

b) Self-reported disability measure (Migraine Disability Assessment [MIDAS]), which assesses impact of migraine across all areas to determine impact on functioning and quality of life

c) Six-item Headache Impact Test (HIT-6): rating frequency of HA severity over past 4 weeks, numeric rating scale with points per item, and summary score of all six items

2) Physical exam—focus on neurological exam including motor function examination, sensory testing, and coordination

3) Diagnostic evaluation: possible CT scan, MRI, MRA, EEG

4) Labs: lumbar puncture, ESR if temporal arteritis is part of differential diagnosis

5) Any diagnostic testing to exclude a secondary cause

h. Treatment options for all migraines

1) Avoid triggers—foods high in tyramine (e.g., chocolate, aged cheeses, yogurt, sour cream, soy sauce, avocados, nuts, and yeast products), foods high in nitrates (hot dogs; salami; bacon; sausage; corned beef; canned, smoked, or aged meats), certain food additives (e.g., monosodium glutamate [MSG], aspartame), alcoholic beverages

2) Increase lifestyle choices that help decrease frequency or severity of migraines.

3) Avoid opioids and barbiturates.

4) Pharmacological options

a) Abortive (treatment) medications: ergotamines; triptans, NSAIDs; combination therapy of caffeine, aspirin, and acetaminophen; intranasal lidocaine

b) Preventive (prophylactic) medications: calcium channel blockers, amine modulators, beta-blockers, TCAs, anticonvulsants (many are off-label use); neurotoxic protein to inhibit spasms (e.g., botulinum toxin)

c) Controversial: CGRP receptor antagonist and monoclonal antibodies: results vary; CGRP monoclonal antibodies studies under way

2. Tension-type headache (TTH)

a. Most common form of headache with estimated lifetime prevalence between 30% and 78% worldwide. TTH results from combination of many factors, including peripheral excitability, muscle pain and hyperalgesia, changes in neurotransmitters, and genetic and psychological factors.

b. Subtypes of TTH: *chronic* and *episodic*; episodic form is further subdivided by time criteria into *infrequent* (less than one episode per month) and *frequent*

c. TTH previously called tension headache, muscle contraction headache, psychomyogenic headache, stress headache, ordinary headache, essential headache, idiopathic headache, and psychogenic headache

d. Diagnostic criteria

1) Headache lasts 30 minutes to 7 days

2) At least two of the following characteristics:

a) Tightening or pressing (nonpulsating) quality

b) Mild to moderate intensity

c) Occurs bilaterally

d) Not aggravated by regular physical activities

e) Both of the following:

(1) Absence of nausea and vomiting

(2) Absence of light or sound sensitivity

f) Headache is not due to another disorder

3) Specific diagnostic criteria for an *infrequent episodic* TTH:

a) Less than 12 episodes per year

b) Typically separated by several weeks (less than 1 day per month)

4) Specific diagnostic criteria for *frequent episodic* TTH: At least 10 episodes occur on more than 1 day but less than 15 days per month, for at least 3 months (e.g., more than 12 days and less than 180 days per year).

5) Specific diagnostic criteria for *chronic* TTH: Headache occurs on more than 15 days per month on average for more than 3 months (e.g.. more than 180 days per year).

6) Specific diagnostic criteria for *probable* TTH: Episodes fulfill all but one of criteria for TTH and do not fulfill criteria for migraine without aura.

e. Diagnostic workup

1) History—frequency of headaches may change over time; therefore, classification may change.

2) Physical exam including motor function, cranial nerves, sensory response, and coordination.

3) If symptoms are not consistent with above-mentioned criteria, diagnostic tests such as CT, MRI, MRA, lumbar puncture, EEG, and ESR may be indicated to rule out temporal arteritis.

f. Pharmacologic options:

1) *Abortive* (treatment) medications: skeletal muscle relaxants, antidepressants

2) *Preventive* (prophylactic) medications: NSAIDs, acetaminophen, aspirin, caffeine-containing products, TCAs, NMDA, skeletal muscle relaxants

3) Botulinum toxin

3. Trigeminal autonomic cephalgia (TAC)

a. Cluster headaches, paroxysmal hemicranias, and hemicranias continua—a group of uncommon headaches described as most disabling and painful headache

b. Often present with unilateral trigeminal distribution pathway that occurs with ipsilateral cranial autonomic features

c. Cluster headache has two forms: episodic and persistent.

1) Episodic attacks occur in periods lasting 7 days to 1 year separated by pain-free periods lasting 1 month or longer.

2) Persistent attacks occur for more than 1 year without remission or with remissions lasting less than 1 month.

d. Signs and symptoms

1) Unilateral headache

2) Excruciating pain occurring around orbital and temporal regions

3) Headache lasts from 15 minutes to 3 hours.

4) Pain is accompanied by autonomic symptoms (e.g., tearing, nasal congestion, pinpoint pupils, eyelid drooping, and facial flushing).

e. Diagnostic criteria

1) Severe unilateral orbital or supraorbital pain, or a combination of both, lasting 15–180 minutes if untreated

2) Frequency of attack is from once every other day up to eight times per day.

3) Pain is accompanied by at least one of these autonomic symptoms present on painful side:

a) Redness in eye

b) Tearing

c) Runny nose

d) Sweating of forehead or entire face

e) Sensation of fullness in ear

f) Pinpoint pupil or drooping eyelid

g) Edema of eyelid

h) Restlessness or agitation

f. Diagnostic workup

1) Motor function assessment, sensory and coordination testing

2) Labs: Lumbar puncture and serum chemistry may be indicated.

3) Radiologic evaluation: CT, MRI, MRA

4) EEG and baseline ECG may be indicated.

g. Treatment options

1) Acute measures

a) 100% oxygen for 15–20 minutes

b) Pharmacologic options

(1) Abortive (treatment) medications (e.g., triptans)

(2) Intranasal lidocaine

(3) Dihydroergotamine

2) Preventive pharmacologic options

a) Avoiding triggers (e.g., alcohol, medication overuse)

b) Calcium channel blockers

c) NSAIDs (can be both abortive and preventative)

d) Ergotamine, dihydroergotamine (can be both abortive and preventative)

e) Corticosteroids

f) Melatonin

g) Anticonvulsants

h) Capsaicin

3) Interventional pain procedures

a) Occipital nerve block and stimulator

b) Trigeminal sensory root rhizotomy

c) Deep brain stimulation (DBS)

d) Radiofrequency thermocoagulation of trigeminal ganglion

4. Other primary headaches

a. Includes various headaches not associated with structural lesion

b. May mimic secondary headaches, so must be thoroughly assessed

c. Subcategories include:

1) Primary stabbing headache

2) Primary cough headache

3) Primary exercise headache

4) Primary headache associated with sexual activity

5) Hypnic headache (dull headache awakes person from sleep, known as alarm clock headache)

6) Primary thunderclap headache (acute-onset, high-intensity headache resembles a ruptured cerebral aneurysm for which immediate emergent neurology referral may be indicated)

7) Cold-stimulus headache
8) External pressure headache
9) Nummular headache (also referred to as coin-shaped headache): pain of highly variable duration, but often persistent in a small circumscribed area of scalp in absence of underlying structural lesion
10) New daily persistent headache
d. Diagnostic workup: This is diagnosis of exclusion, based on symptomatology.
e. Treatment: dependent on specific subcategory
f. Pharmacological options
1) Calcium channel blockers
2) NSAIDs
3) Acetaminophen
4) Beta-blockers
5) Skeletal muscle relaxants
6) Opioids
C. Secondary headaches
1. Usually occur as result of other health conditions
2. May also be reclassified later or treated as primary headache; for instance, if a trauma makes migraine worse, headache should be treated as migraine. Usually disappear or are greatly reduced spontaneously within 3 months, with treatment or after remission of causative disorder.
3. Potential causes:
a. Head and neck trauma: posttraumatic headache (PTH)–often these headaches are most disabling component of traumatic brain injuries (TBIs) and common with military veterans
b. Cranial or cervical vascular disorders
c. Nonvascular intracranial disorders
d. Substance use or its withdrawal
e. Infection
f. Disorder of homeostasis
g. Disorders of cranium, neck, eyes, ears, nose, sinuses, teeth, mouth, or other facial structures
h. Psychiatric disorders
D. Painful cranial neuropathies, other facial pains, and other headaches
1. Pain in head and neck is mediated by afferent fibers in trigeminal, glossopharyngeal, nervous intermedius, and vagus nerves and upper cervical roots via occipital nerves. Stimulation of these nerves can cause pain in innervated areas.
2. Painful conditions include:
a. Trigeminal neuralgia
b. Glossopharyngeal neuralgia
c. Nervus intermedius neuralgia
d. Occipital neuralgia
e. Optic neuritis
f. Headache attributed to ischemic ocular motor nerve palsy
g. Tolosa-Hung syndrome

h. Paratrigeminal oculosympathetic (Raeder) syndrome
i. Recurrent painful ophthalmoplegic neuropathy
j. Burning mouth syndrome (BMS)
k. Persistent idiopathic facial pain (PIFP)
l. Central neuropathic pain
E. When is a headache an emergency?
1. Concerning symptoms include:
a. Sudden, intense, "thunderclap" headache
b. Severe or sharp pain occurring for first time
c. Pain associated with temperature of 102°F or above, fainting, stiffness in neck
d. Pain that wakes person from sleep
e. Pain associated with confusion or difficulty speaking, hearing, or walking
f. Pain associated with droopiness on one side of face or weakness on one side of body
2. Emergent headaches may be associated with:
a. High blood pressure, TIAs, or stroke
b. Meningococcal disease
c. Head injury
d. Heat stroke
e. Preeclampsia
f. Brain tumor, aneurysm, or hemorrhage
g. Infection from cat or dog bite

XI. Complex Regional Pain Syndrome (CRPS)

A. Overview
1. Previously known as reflex sympathetic dystrophy (RSD or CRPS I) and causalgia (CRPS II)
2. Poorly understood condition accompanied by multifactorial persistent pain likely involving excessive firing of peripheral C-fiber nerves transmitting messages to brain. Excessive or prolonged firing can decrease immune response in affected extremity.
3. Can be either acute (lasting less than 6 months) or persistent (lasting more than 6 months)
4. Generally involves sensory, motor, and autonomic system but can also have neuropsychological component that affects extremities
5. Duration varies from weeks in mild cases to indefinitely in others. Some patients may have remissions for weeks, months, or years followed by exacerbations.
B. Causes
1. Approximately 90% of patients experience a specific trauma, such as fracture, sprain, soft tissue injury, limb immobilization, or surgery.
2. Abnormalities of unmyelinated and thinly myelinated nerve fibers are found with CRPS.
a. These small nerve fibers communicate with blood vessels and may trigger symptoms of

inflammation and other blood vessel abnormalities of CRPS.
- b. Abnormal neurological function in spinal cord and brain triggered by abnormal peripheral nerves may lead to complex disorders of higher cortical function.

3. Blood vessel changes:
   - a. May dilate resulting in fluid leaking into tissue, causing flushing
   - b. May constrict, causing cold, white, or blueish skin
   - c. Tissue can be deprived of oxygen and other nutrients, causing muscle and joint damage and pain.

4. Immune system changes:
   - a. Tissues with high levels of inflammatory chemicals (cytokines)
   - b. Increased cytokine levels may also lead to redness, swelling, and warmth reported by many patients.
   - c. CRPS is more common in those with other inflammatory and autoimmune conditions.

5. Genetics and environment may play a role, as clusters of CRPS have been noted in some families.

6. Chronic diseases lead to either nerve damage or inflammation (e.g., diabetes, asthma).

C. Signs and symptoms
1. Pain
   - a. Initial pain in one or more extremities and described as severe, continuous burning; deep ache; or both without involvement of major nerve
   - b. All tactile sensations may be painful (allodynia).
   - c. Repetitive tactile stimulation may cause increasing pain with each tap, and pain may continue after simulation is stopped (hyperpathia).
   - d. Muscles of affected area may have diffuse tenderness or point tender spots due to small muscle spasms called muscle trigger points (MTPs).
   - e. Spontaneous, sharp jabs of pain that seem to come from nowhere may occur in affected region (paroxysmal dysesthesias and lancinating pain).
   - f. Pain is aggravated by use of affected part and relieved by immobilization.

2. Edema
   - a. Diffuse edema is pitting or hard and localized to painful region.
   - b. Edema sharply demarcated on surface of skin along line is highly suggestive of CRPS.

3. Skin changes
   - a. Atrophy of skin on appendages and cool, red, clammy skin may be variably present.
   - b. Skin may appear shiny, dry, or scaly.
   - c. Nails may grow faster initially and then grow slower. Faster growing nails are highly suggestive of CRPS.
   - d. Hair may grow coarse and then thin.
   - e. Skin may be pale, mottled, red, purple, or blue.
   - f. CRPS is associated with skin disorders, such as rashes, ulcers, and pustules.

4. Movement disorder
   - a. Movement causes pain.
   - b. Direct inhibitory effect on muscle contractions is possible.
   - c. Patients have difficulty initiating movement and describe "stiffness "in joints.
   - d. Tremors or involuntary jerk may be present.
   - e. Debilitating, severe muscle cramps with sudden onset may occur.
   - f. Increased muscle tone in extremity, described by some patients as a slow "drawing up of muscles" may result in hand and fingers or foot and toes, drawing into fixed position (dystonia).
   - g. Psychological distress may exacerbate symptoms.
   - h. Patients can exhibit seemingly bizarre movements and might be inaccurately diagnosed with a psychogenic movement disorder.
   - i. Progression of disease
     1) There is possibility of spreading to other extremities with disease progression.
     2) With progression, demineralization of bone may occur.
     3) Progressive symptoms may include persistent coldness, pallor, cyanosis, Raynaud's phenomenon, atrophy of skin and nails, loss of hair in affected area, atrophy of tissues, and stiffness of joints.
     4) All symptoms may not be present at same time.

D. Diagnostic workup
1. Labs: none indicated
2. Radiologic evaluation: MRI, radiography, or bone scan may identify bone demineralization.
3. Rule out other causes of underlying diseases, such as deep vein thrombosis, cellulitis, or diabetes.
4. Nerve conduction studies can identify some CRPS but not all.
5. Sympathetic block may be used diagnostically.

E. Pharmacological options
1. Acetaminophen
2. NSAIDs
3. Anticonvulsants
4. Antidepressants
5. Bisphosphonates (e.g., alendronate or pamidronate)
6. Local anesthetics (lidocaine patch)
7. Capsaicin

8. High doses of corticosteroids often used in early phase of disease
9. Nasal calcitonin, for deep bone pain
10. NMDA agonist (e.g., ketamine, dextromethorphan)
11. Opioids
12. Intravenous immunoglobulin (IVIG)
13. Botulinum toxin injections

F. Interventional pain procedures
1. Sympathetic nerve block
2. Regional block
3. Spinal cord stimulation
4. Implanted intrathecal pumps with single drug or mixture (e.g., baclofen, opioids, local anesthetic agents, and clonidine)
5. Other types of neural stimulation (e.g., repetitive transcranial magnetic stimulation; deep brain stimulators; motor cortex stimulation with electrodes; peripheral nerve stimulators)
6. Plasma exchange treatment

XII. Persistent Gastrointestinal and Genitourinary Pain

A. There are innumerable differential diagnoses for persistent abdominal and pelvic floor conditions. Collaboration with interprofessional colleagues is essential.

B. Persistent abdominal pain
1. Description: defined as intermittent or continuous abdominal pain lasting 6 months or longer
   a. Can develop as result of gastrointestinal disorders or from adjoining organs, such as pancreas, biliary tract, genitourinary, or gynecological origins
   b. Often associated with functional syndrome and may result from central sensitization
2. Persistent (chronic) or functional abdominal pain (FAP)
   a. Functional dyspepsia
   b. Irritable bowel syndrome (IBS) diarrhea predominant, constipation predominant, or mixed
3. Differential diagnosis: organic etiologies
   a. Pancreatitis
   b. Cholecystitis, cholelithiasis
   c. Hepatomegaly
   d. Splenomegaly
   e. Peptic ulcer disease
   f. Esophagitis/gastritis
   g. Intestinal colic
   h. Crohn's disease
   i. Neoplasms
   j. Pelvic inflammatory disease
   k. Endometriosis

l. Uterine obstruction
m. Ovarian cyst torsion
n. Ovulatory pain
o. Ruptured ovarian cyst
p. Dysfunction of pelvic floor muscles
q. Chronic gastrointestinal conditions: functional etiologies

4. Signs and symptoms
   a. Pain, burning, or discomfort in upper or lower abdomen
   b. Gas, distention, and bloating
   c. Indigestion, uncomfortable fullness, early satiety, food intolerances
   d. Diarrhea, constipation, or both
   e. May have associated symptoms that commonly occur with central sensitization (e.g., headache, bladder dysfunction, sleep disturbance, fatigue, pain in other area, anxiety, depression)

5. Diagnostic workup
   a. Manual abdominal and pelvic exam
   b. Labs: CBC, liver function tests, hepatitis screen, carcinoembryonic antigen (CEA)
   c. Radiologic evaluation: abdominal ultrasound, radiography, CT and MRI, endoscopy, colonoscopy, and MR cholangiopancreatography (MRCP)
   d. Laparoscopy and laparotomy as indicated

6. Treatment options
   a. Treat organic cause if/when identified
   b. Pharmacological options:
      1) Acetaminophen
      2) NSAIDs (consider cause before prescribing)
      3) Antidepressants
      4) Anticonvulsants
      5) Skeletal muscle relaxants
      6) Opioids
      7) Serotonergic agents are effective for treating IBS, chronic constipation, and diarrhea.
      8) There is promising research on agents that may impact gut microbiome and decrease GI symptoms.
   c. Interventional pain procedures: celiac or sympathetic nerve block for diagnosis and pain relief

C. Persistent pancreatitis pain
1. Description: Progressive and persistent inflammatory disease of pancreas creating scarring, irreversible damage of pancreas leading to loss of exocrine and endocrine function and chronic abdominal pain. Previously thought to be due to anatomical or structural changes in pancreas, but now considered problem related to central sensitization.
2. Causes of *chronic* pancreatitis
   a. Heavy alcohol use/abuse

b. Recurrent episodes of acute pancreatitis

c. Genetic abnormalities/family history of chronic pancreatitis

d. Blockage or strictures of pancreatic duct

e. Cystic fibrosis

f. Very high triglyceride levels

g. Hypercalcemia

h. Hyperlipidemia

i. Tumors

j. Medications (e.g., anticonvulsants)

3. Signs and symptoms

   a. Chronic or intermittent abdominal pain

     1) Individual variation; may be intermittent, frequent, or persistent and can range from mild to moderate to severe

     2) Located in upper abdomen

     3) Often described as sharp and intense or slowly progressing and gnawing, frequently radiates to back

     4) Aggravated by trigger foods or alcohol

   b. Symptoms may include fever, nausea and vomiting, and rapid heart rate.

   c. Weight loss often occurs due to inability to maintain adequate intake during flares.

   d. Associated with diabetes

   e. Associated with alcohol use

   f. Patient may have digestive problems, including malabsorption and/or fatty-food intolerance.

   g. Patient may have steatorrhea (foul-smelling, greasy stools).

4. Diagnostic workup

   a. STEP-wise algorithm approach outlined in American Pancreatic Association Practice Guideline, evidenced-based report on diagnostic criteria:

     1) **Step 1**: CT scan; if inconclusive or nondiagnostic, continue to step 2.

     2) **Step 2**: MRI with secretin enhancement; if inconclusive or nondiagnostic, continue to step 3.

     3) **Step 3**: Endoscopic ultrasound with quantification of parenchymal and ductal criteria; if inconclusive or nondiagnostic, continue to step 4.

     4) **Step 4**: Pancreas function test (with secretin gastroduodenal or endoscopic collection method); if inconclusive or nondiagnostic, continue to step 5.

     5) **Step 5**: Endoscopic retrograde cholangiopancreatography (ERCP): if inconclusive or nondiagnostic, monitor symptoms and repeat process in 6 months to a year.

   b. Labs: carbohydrate antigen 19-9, glucose tolerance test, and amylase (which may or may not be elevated)

5. Pharmacological options:

   a. Acetaminophen

   b. Antidepressants

   c. Antioxidant therapy (e.g., selenium, beta carotene, vitamin C, methionine, and vitamin E)

   d. Opioids

6. Interventional pain procedures

   a. Celiac plexus block

   b. Endoscopic treatment to place stents may be helpful.

7. Nutritional options include:

   a. Low-fat diet, diabetic diet

   b. Instruct on small, frequent meals

   c. Address malabsorption issues

   d. Address pancreatic dysfunction

D. Complex pelvic pain (CPP)

1. Description: non–menstrual-related pain lasting 6 months or longer, contributing to functional disability or requiring medical or surgical intervention

   a. Can involve pelvis, anterior abdominal wall, and buttocks and can be intermittent or continuous

   b. Does not exclusively occur with menstruation, during intercourse, or with pregnancy

   c. Pain is often serious enough to cause disability. Exact pain mechanisms in CPP are unknown but thought to be associated with central sensitization.

   d. Associated pain syndromes include painful bladder syndrome, irritable bowel syndrome, endometriosis, fibroids, and adhesions.

   e. Associated comorbidities include obesity, asthma, cardiovascular disease, other painful areas (back, neck), and psychiatric conditions.

2. Differential diagnosis

   a. Irritable bowel syndrome

   b. Neoplasm

   c. Pelvic inflammatory disease

   d. Endometriosis

   e. Uterine obstruction

   f. Ovarian cyst torsion or ruptured ovarian cysts

   g. Ovulatory pain

   h. Dysfunction of pelvic floor muscles

3. Signs and symptoms

   a. Pain

   b. Urinary and fecal incontinence

   c. Pelvic organ collapse

   d. Constipation

   e. Incomplete relief with most treatments

   f. Significant impairment of daily functioning at home and/or work

4. Diagnostic workup

   a. History

   b. Physical exam

   c. Psychosocial assessment (include smoking history)

d. Physical and sexual abuse history
e. Manual abdominal and pelvic exam
f. Radiologic evaluation: pelvic, transvaginal transperineal or transrectal ultrasound; CT or MRI
g. Endoscopic evaluation if lesion is suspected
h. Laparoscopy and laparotomy
i. Labs: CEA, cancer antigen (CA-125), liver function tests, renal function tests, and CBC
j. Diagnostic nerve blocks
5. Treatment options
a. Treat underlying cause when identifiable.
b. Pharmacological options
1) Acetaminophen
2) NSAIDs
3) Antidepressants
4) Anticonvulsants
5) Opioids
c. Interventional pain procedures
1) Trigger point injections
2) Pudendal nerve block
3) Hypogastric nerve block
d. Nonpharmacological
1) Pelvic floor physical therapy with intravaginal myofascial release
2) Combined with cognitive-behavioral interventions for incontinence and organ prolapse
E. Interstitial cystitis/bladder pain syndrome (IC/BPS)
1. Description: unpleasant sensation perceived to be related to bladder; associated with lower urinary tract symptoms of more than 6 weeks' duration in absence of infection or other identifiable causes
2. Signs and symptoms
a. Mild burning to excruciating pain in bladder, lower abdomen, perineum, vagina, low back, and thighs
b. Pain becomes worse as bladder fills.
c. Associated with incontinence
d. Associated with gastrointestinal symptoms
e. Microscopic to gross hematuria/white blood cells in urine without bacteria
f. Gynecological signs and symptoms
3. Diagnostic workup
a. History
b. Pelvic and rectal exam
c. Labs: CBC, CMP, erythrocyte sedimentation rate (ESR), C-reactive protein (CRP), blood culture, urine cytology
d. Radiologic evaluation: urodynamic studies
e. Cystoscopy
f. Laparoscopy
g. Specialist referral (urologic or other as indicated)
4. Treatment options
a. First-line treatment

1) Diet and behavioral changes
a) Reduce intake of alcohol, coffee, tea, chocolate, and spicy foods.
b) Dietary management of constipation
c) Adequate fluid intake
2) Pelvic floor relaxation exercises
3) Bladder training
4) Stress management and general relaxation training
b. Second-line treatment
1) Physical therapy to release myofascial trigger points
2) TENS
c. Pharmacologic options
1) Pentosan polysulfate: FDA approved for IC/BPS to decrease pain, frequency, and urgency of urination
2) TCAs
3) Histamine and leukotriene receptor inhibitors (e.g., cimetidine, hydroxyzine, montelukast)
4) Rosiptor (AQX-1125): oral medication being studied but has identified many side effects
d. Third-line treatments
1) Cystoscopy under anesthesia with hydrodistension (therapeutic instillation via a urinary catheter)
2) Intravesical medications: Dimethyl sulfoxide is commonly used, but no clear guidelines for use have been outlined. Studies include use of heparin, pentosan polysulfate, chondroitin sulfate, and hyaluronic acid for intravesicular use.
3) Ablation of Hunner lesions if found
e. Fourth-line treatments
1) Intradetrusor injection of botulinum toxin A (FDA approved for treatment of incontinence): studies show limited efficacy with considerable risk of side effects, including urinary retention
2) Neuromodulation: proximal treatment by sacral nerve stimulation; limitations: expensive, limited efficacy, and may be painful
f. Fifth-line treatments
1) Cyclosporine A: only if IC/BPS is refractory to all other treatments, as may be nephrotoxic and lead to reduced renal function and possible hypertension
g. Sixth-line treatment—surgery
1) Partial supratrigonal cystectomy with augmentation cystoplasty: reports to improve pain, decrease urinary symptoms, and improve quality of life
2) Urinary diversion with or without cystectomy: improves symptoms, but some patients still have pain
3) Substitution cystoplasty

XIII. Persistent Sickle Cell Pain (Table. 21.4)

A. Description: Sickle cell disease (SCD) is an inherited disorder that refers to a group of complex, chronic genetic hemolytic disorders resulting in varying degrees of anemia and intermittent and persistent pain syndrome. This disease can have life-threatening illnesses due to multisystem complications if persistent pain is not treated.

1. Persistent pain can begin in children as early as 5 months old. Risk for persistent pain increases over time due to frequent acute pain episodes, nociceptive pain from vaso-occlusive crisis, inflammatory pain, and opioid-induced hyperalgesia.

2. Medical advancements have contributed to estimated increased survival rate of more than 90% of children entering adulthood today and living into their 60s and 70s.

3. Signs and symptoms
   a. Pain may be severe and is usually present in bones, joints, chest, and abdomen.
   b. Children may experience sickle cell dactylitis, causing swelling in hands and feet dorsal surfaces.
   c. There may be ischemic manifestations, such as hemolytic crisis, priapism, renal failure, jaundice, hepatomegaly, ischemic leg ulcers, cerebral vasculopathy, or stroke.
   d. Acute chest pain syndrome, with or without fever, can occur in association with a pulmonary infiltrate caused by lung or rib infarction.
   e. Abdominal pain due to splenic sequestration
   f. Neuropathic pain may present with reports of numbness, tingling, electric, pins, and needle sensation.

4. Diagnostic workup
   a. History including:
      1) Psychiatric disorders (mood disorders, anxiety, pain catastrophizing, PTSD, and substance use disorder)
      2) Autoimmune diseases such as rheumatoid arthritis, Crohn's disease, juvenile idiopathic arthritis
      3) Medication use at home, including nonopioids, opioids, antidepressants, anticonvulsants, skeletal muscle relaxants, herbal, alternative substances, other OTC medications, and illicit substances
      4) History of nonpharmacological interventions for managing pain, including meditation, music, religion, and family
   b. Physical assessment for ischemic manifestations and other complications
   c. A ventilation-perfusion (VQ) scan to rule out pulmonary embolism
   d. Radiologic evaluation:
      1) CT scan to rule out osteonecrosis, sclerosis, collapse of femoral head, or bone and soft tissue abscesses.
      2) MRI to identify infarct-related changes in bone and soft tissue of lower extremities
      3) Chest radiography to rule out pneumonia and bone fractures
   e. Labs:
      1) Coagulation studies
      2) Hemoglobin and hematocrit individualized to patient
      3) Autoimmune markers—antinuclear antibody titers (ANA), CRP, ESR

5. Pharmacological options:
   a. Oral therapy to reduce number of vaso-occlusive crises such as hemoglobin oxygen-affinity modulators (voxelotor), nutritionals (glutamine), miscellaneous antineoplastic agent (hydroxyurea), and P-selectin inhibitors (crizanlizumab)
   b. Acetaminophen
   c. Opioids
   d. NSAIDs
   e. Ketamine infusion
   f. Lidocaine infusion

6. Nonpharmacological options for children and adults
   a. In community
      1) Monthly visits with hematologist
      2) Community resources, social support, and care coordinator

Table 21.4		
Three Types of Pain Experienced with Sickle Cell Disease		
Type of Pain	**Characteristics**	**Considerations**
Vaso-occlusive crisis pain	Recurrent; inflammation and tissue damage; repetitive nociceptive injury	Hypoxic ischemic reperfusion injury of bones and tissues due to vaso-occlusion
Central sensitization	Hyperalgesia; allodynia; opioid induced hyperalgesia; neuropathic pain	Increased nociceptor response to stimuli (pain and non-painful)
Recurrent opioid withdrawal	Cycles of increased pain followed by opioid withdrawal due to too rapid tapering or discontinuation	Often not recognized by patient or providers

3) Pain management specialist for medication management

4) Psychiatry for management of depression, anxiety, PTSD, and attention deficit hyperactivity disorder (ADHD)

5) Recommended guidelines: dental visits, immunizations, annual physical exams, pulmonary screening, cardiology visit, eye exam and psychology for social support, coping with a chronic illness, and possible Cognitive Behavioral Therapy (See chapters 3 and 16 for more information).

b. In emergency department during crisis

1) Assess pain based on patient's self-report; include patient's functional pain level before vaso-occlusive crisis started.

2) Assess current analgesic use at home (opioids and nonopioid medications).

3) Rapidly administer analgesics within 30 minutes of triage and within 60 minutes of registration.

a) Choose analgesia based on patients' knowledge of effective analgesic doses, outpatient analgesic use, and pain assessment.

b) Use parenteral analgesics first; if unable to obtain access, administer subcutaneously until intravenous access is obtained.

c) Individualize analgesic regimen with care team's collaboration including emergency department, hematologist, and pain management specialist.

d) Calculate parenteral dose based on total daily dose of short-acting analgesic. If this dose is not adequate, recommend increasing by increments of 25% for optimal pain relief.

e) Reassess pain every 15 minutes, and administer analgesics every 30 minutes until pain is relieved, as reported by patient.

4) Start patient-controlled analgesia (PCA)

a) Be aware of patient's status with regard to opioid tolerance; higher doses may be indicated.

b) Use patient's home medications as basal rate (e.g., long-acting morphine, sustained release, or scheduled morphine q4h) for around-the-clock continuous pain management. If unable to tolerate oral medications or does not use oral opioids at home, consider adding low-dose continuous infusion to PCA.

5) Administer NSAIDs and other adjuvant analgesics.

6) Oral antihistamines to be offered as needed every 4–6 hours for pruritus

7) Hypotonic or hypertonic fluids for rehydration due to fever, dehydration, and consideration of other comorbidities

c. At discharge from hospital

1) Resume home opioids at previous home dose.

2) Preventative treatment: Restart hydroxyurea, glutamine, and other medications to decrease number of vaso-occlusive crises if prescribed prior to or during admission.

3) Hydration as an outpatient

4) Follow-up appointment with hematologist within 2 weeks of discharge home

5) Behavioral treatment

a) Exercise

b) Relaxation therapies, deep breathing, biofeedback, and behavior modification

d. Psychological treatment

1) Social support

2) Cognitive therapies, hypnotherapy, visual imagery, and distraction

e. Physical treatment

1) Hydration

2) Oxygen

3) Heat, massage, hydrotherapy, ultrasound, acupuncture, TENS, and physical therapy

f. Education

1) Teach patient about disease, signs and symptoms of acute episodes, treatment options, precipitating factors, exercise options, stress management, and psychological support systems.

2) Give instructions on home pain management, including:

a) Importance of rest, hydration, diet, and avoidance of precipitating factors

b) Medication regimen and National Institutes of Health guidelines

c) Opioid taper at discharge

XIV. COIVD-19–Related Persistent Pain

A. Description: According to CDC, long term post-COVID-19 conditions, or "long COVID" is used to describe spectrum of physical and mental health consequences that persist for at least 4 weeks after initial onset of COVID-19. Likely, there is more than one subtype of long COVID syndrome.

B. Signs and symptoms

1. Pain

a. Headaches

b. General myalgias and joint pain

c. Abdominal pain

d. Chest pain

e. Various other types of pain

2. Fatigue
3. Tinnitus
4. Brain fog
5. Dizziness and orthostatic intolerance
6. Muscle weakness
7. Shortness of breath
8. Sleep disturbances
9. Anxiety and depression
10. Additional symptoms from studies include the following, in no particular order: cognitive dysfunction (brain fog), palpitations, numbness/tingling, generalized weakness, temperature changes, restless legs/sleep, sensitivities to lights/sounds/smells/foods, bladder symptoms, appetite changes, nausea, diarrhea/constipation swelling in legs, tinnitus, and blurred vision.

C. Diagnostic workup (to rule out active infection and other unidentified medical conditions)
1. Labs to check for low blood levels, signs of infection, or hypoglycemia
2. Radiologic evaluation: chest radiography or chest CT
3. Pulmonary function tests
4. Echocardiogram
5. Tilt-table tests and other tests for autonomic dysfunction

D. Pharmacological options include:
1. Treat acute COVID infection.
2. Treat according to symptomatology.

E. Nonpharmacological options include:
1. Medical management to treat/stabilize any acute issue
2. Physical therapy and rehabilitation to improve physical stamina and reverse deconditioning
3. Stress management and relaxation
4. Cognitive-behavioral therapies
5. Integrative therapies—yoga, massage, mindfulness, acupuncture, biofeedback
6. Occupational therapies and work hardening if needed to improve patients overall

XV. Interprofessional Approach to Persistent Pain Conditions

A. Persistent pain is multifactorial, impacting almost every area of patients' lives; interprofessional collaboration is thought to be best approach to address multitude of interconnected issues.

B. International Association for the Study of Pain (IASP) has identified different types of programs for pain and established set characteristics and guidelines to help consumers gain the most benefit.
1. An interprofessional pain center is largest and most complex of facilities for treatment of pain.
2. Generally, includes research, teaching, and care for people with acute or persistent pain; often located

within teaching hospital or associated with medical school
3. An interprofessional team of individuals collaborate together to meet patient needs. May include physicians, scientists, psychologists, nurses, physical and occupational therapists, vocational counselors, social workers, and chaplains. Healthcare providers communicate regularly regarding patient assessment and ongoing care.
4. Goals are typically to reduce pain and/or improve pain coping skills; improve functioning and overall quality of life, which, when possible, includes return to work; reduce healthcare utilization; and resolve medication issues.
5. There is moderate evidence of pain reduction and improved functioning as result of participation in interprofessional care program compared to other treatment modalities. However, these programs demonstrated greater impact on functioning such as in return to work, decreased utilization of healthcare resources, and closing disability claims. Physical therapy is one critical component identified as necessary for successful outcomes.

Bibliography

Addis, D. R., DeBerry, J. J., & Aggarwal, S. (2020). Pain in HIV. *Molecular Pain*(16), 1–11.

Adler-Neal, A., & Zeidan, F. (2017). Mindfulness meditation for fibromyalgia: mechanistic and clinical considerations. *Current Rheumatological Reports*, 4–9.

Amaniti, A., Sardeli, C., Fyntanidou, V., Papakonstantinou, P., Dalakakis, I., Mylonas, A., Sapalidis, K., Kosmidis, C., Katsaounis, A., Giannakidis, D., Koulouris, C., Aidoni, Z., Michalopoulos, N., Zarogoulidis, P., Kesisoglou, I., Ioannidis, A., Vagionas, A., Romanidis, K., Oikonomou, P., & Grosomanidis, V. (2019). Pharmacologic and non-pharmacologic interventions for HIV-neuropathy pain: A systematic review and a meta-analysis. *Medicina, 55*(12), 762. https://doi.org/10.3390/medicina55120762.

Ambrose, K. R., & Golightly, Y. M. (2015). Physical exercise as non-pharmacological treatment of chronic pain: Why and when. *Best Practice & Research Clinical Rheumatology, 29*, 120–130.

Atsawarungruangkit, A., & Pongprasobchai, S. (2015). Current understanding of the neuropathophysiology of pain in chronic pancreatitis. *World Journal of Gastrointenstinal Pathophysiology, 6*(4), 193–202. doi:10.4291/wjgp.v6.i4.193.

Anderson, T. L., Morris, J. M., Wald, J. T., & Kotsenas, A. L. (2017). Imaging appearance of advanced chronic adhesive arachnoiditis: A retrospective review. *American Journal of Roentgenology, 209*(3), 648–655. doi:10.2214/AJR.16.16704.

Anastasi, J. K., & Pakhomova, A. M. (2020). Assessment and management of HIV distal sensory peripheral neuropathy: Understanding the symptoms. *Journal for Nurse Practitioners, 16*(4), 276–280. https://doi.org/10.1016/j.nurpra.2019.12.019.

Arnold, L. M., Choy, E., Clauw, D. J., Goldenberg, D. L., Harris, R. E., Helfenstein, M., Jr., Jensen, T. S., Noguchi, K., Silverman, S.

L., Ushida, T., & Wang, G. (2016). Fibromyalgia and chronic pain syndromes: A white paper detailing current challenges in the field. *Clinical Journal of Pain, 32*(9), 737–746. https://doi.org/10.1097/AJP.0000000000000354.

Ballas, S. K. (2014). Pathophysiology and principles of management of the many faces of the acute vaso-occlusive crisis in patients with sickle cell disease. *European Journal of Hematology, 95,* 113–123. doi:10.1111/ejh.12460.

Bruta, K., Vanshika, Bhasin, K., & Bhawana (2021). The role of serotonin and diet in the prevalence of irritable bowel syndrome: a systematic review. *Translational Medicine Communications, 6*(1), 1–9. https://doi.org/10.1186/s41231-020-00081-y.

Burmester, G. R., & Pope, J. E. (2017). Novel treatment strategies in rheumatoid arthritis. *Lancet, 389*(10086), 2338–2348. https://doi.org/10.1016/S0140-6736(17)31491-5.

Buch, N. S., Qerama, E., Brix Finnerup, N., & Nikolajsen, L. (2020). Neuromas and postamputation pain. *Pain, 161*(1), 147–155. doi:10.1097/j.pain.0000000000001705.

Capuco, A., Urits, I., Orhurhu, V., Chun, R., Shukla, B., Kaye, R. J., Garcia, A. J., Kaye, A. D., & Viswanath, O. (2020). Comprehensive review of the diagnosis, treatment, and management of postmastectomy pain syndrome. *Current Pain Headache Report, 24,* 41. https://doi.org/10.1007/s11916-020-00876-6.

Casiano, V. E., Dydyk, A. M., & Varacallo, M. (2020). Back Pain. In: StatPearls StatPearls Publishing. https://www.ncbi.nlm.nih.gov/books/NBK538173/.

Canavero, S., & Bonicalzi, V. (2015). Pain myths and genesis of central pain. *Pain Medicine, 16*(2), 240–248.

Center for Disease Control and Prevention. (2019). Data and statistics on sickle cell disease. https://www.cdc.gov/ncbddd/sicklecell/data.html.

Center for Disease Control and Prevention (2021). Background: Evaluating and caring for patients with Post-COVID Conditions: Interim Guidance. https://www.cdc.gov/coronavirus/2019-ncov/hcp/clinical-care/post-covid-background.html.

Centner, C. M., Little, F., Van Der Watt, J. J., Vermaak, J. R., Dave, J. A., Levitt, N. S., & Heckmann, J. M. (2018). Evolution of sensory neuropathy after initiation of antiretroviral therapy. *Muscle & Nerve, 57*(3), 371–379. https://doi.org/10.1002/mus.25710.

Chappell, A. G., Bai, J., Yuksel, S., & Ellis, M. F. (2020). Postmastectomy pain syndrome: defining perioperative etiologies to guide new methods of prevention for plastic surgeons. *World Journal of Plastic Surgery, 9*(3), 247–253. https://doi.org/10.29252/wjps.9.3.247.

Conwell, D. L., Lee, L. S., Yadav, D., Longnecker, D. S., Miller, F. H., Mortele, K. J., et al. (2014). American Pancreatic Association practice guidelines in chronic pancreatitis: evidenced-based report on diagnostic guidelines. *Pancreas, 42*(8), 1143–1162.

Costelloe, C., Burns, S., Yong, R. J., Kaye, A. D., & Urman, R. D. (2020). An analysis of predictors of persistent postoperative pain in spine surgery. *Current Pain Headache Reports, 24*(11). https://doi.org/10.1007/s11916-020-0842-5.

Colvin, L. A. (2019). Chemotherapy-induced peripheral neuropathy (CIPN): where are we now? *Pain, 160*(Suppl 1), S1–S10. doi:10.1097/j.pain.0000000000001540. http://europepmc.org/backend/ptpmcrender.fcgi?accid=PMC6499732&blobtype=pdf.

Dydyk, A. M., Ngnitewe Massa, R., & Mesfin, F. B. (Updated January 2023). Disc Herniation. In *StatPearls.* StatPearls Publishing. Available from: https://www.ncbi.nlm.nih.gov/books/NBK441822/.

Dydyk, A. M., Khan, M. Z., & M Das, J. (Updated October 2022). *Radicular Back Pain.* In *StatPearls.* StatPearls Publishing.

Eldeufani, J., Elahmer, N., & Blaise, G. (2020). A medical mystery of complex regional pain syndrome. *Heliyon, 6*(2), E003329.

Esses, S. I., & Morley, T. P. (2021). Spinal arachnoiditis. *Canadian Journal of Neurological Sciences.* https://www.cambridge.org/core/services/aop-cambridge-core/content/view/6E08668235D-735CFEE360CD6D392EA17/S0317167100044486a.pdf/div-class-title-spinal-arachnoiditis-div.pdf.

Fleming, K., & Volcheck, M. (2015). Central sensitization syndrome and the initial evaluation of a patient with fibromyalgia: A review. *Rambam Maimonides Medical Journal, 6*(2).

Forde, G. (2018). Migraine. In C. E. Argoff, A. Dubin, & J. G. Pilitsis (Eds.), *Pain management secrets* (4th ed., pp. 46–56). Elsevier. ISBN: 978-0-323-27791-4, E-ISBN: 978-0-323-41386-2.

Fornari, M., Robertson, S. C., Pereira, P., Zileli, M., Anania, C. D., Ferreira, A., Ferrari, S., Gatti, R., & Costa, F. (2020). Conservative treatment and percutaneous pain relief techniques in patients with lumbar spinal stenosis: WFNS Spine Committee recommendations. *World Neurosurgery: X, 7,* 100079. https://doi.org/10.1016/j.wnsx.2020.100079.

Gardner, T. B., Douglas, A. G., Forsmark, C. E., Bryan, S. G., Taylor, J. R., & Whitcomb, D. C. (2020). International consensus guidelines on the role of diagnostic endoscopic ultrasound in the management of chronic pancreatitis. Recommendations from the working group for the international consensus guidelines for chronic pancreatitis in collaboration with the International association of Pancreatology, the American Pancreatic Association, the Japan Pancreas Society and European Pancreatic Club. *The American Journal of Gastroenterology, 115*(3), 322–339. doi:10.14309/ajg.000000000000053.

Garzon, S., Lagana, A. S., Casarin, J., Raffaelli, R., Cromi, A., Sturla, D., Ranchi, M., & Ghezzi, F. (2020). An update on treatment options for interstitial cystitis. *Menopause Review, 19*(1), 35–43.

Gong, Y., Tan, Q., Qin, Q., & Wei, C. (2020). Prevalence of postmastectomy pain syndrome and associated risk factors: A large single-institution cohort study. *Medicine, 99*(20), e19834. https://doi.org/10.1097/MD.0000000000019834.

Gross, G. E., Eisert, L., Doerr, H. W., Fickenscher, H., Knur, M., Maier, P., Maschke, M., Muller, R., Uwe, P., Schafer, M., Sunderkotter, C., Werner, R. N., Wutzler, P., & Nast, A. (2020). S2k guidelines for diagnosis and treatment of herpes zoster and postherpetic neuralgia. *Journal of German Society of Dermatology, 18*(1), 55–78. https://doi.org/10.1111/ddg.14013.

Gupta, P., Gaines, N., Sirls, L. T., & Peters, K. M. (2015). A multidisciplinary approach to the evaluation and management of interstitial cystitis/bladder pain syndrome: an ideal model of care. *Translational Andrology and Urology, 4*(6), 611–619.

Gupta, R., Van de Ven, T., & Pyati, S. (2020). Post-thoracotomy pain: Current strategies for prevention and treatment. *Drugs, 80,* 1677–1684. https://doi.org/10.1007/s40265-020-01390-0.

Halicka, M., Vittersø, A. D., Proulx, M. J., & Bultitude, J. H. (2020). Neuropsychological changes in complex regional pain syndrome (CRPS). *Behavioral Neurology.* Article 4561831. https://doi.org/10.1155/2020/4561831.

Hooten, W. M. (2016). Chronic pain and mental health disorders: shared neural mechanisms, epidemiology, and treatment. *Mayo Clinic Proceedings, 91*(7), 955–970. doi:10.1016/j.mayocp.2016.04.029.

Kälin, S., Rausch-Osthoff, A. K., & Bauer, C. M. (2016). What is the effect of sensory discrimination training on chronic low back pain? A systematic review. *BMC Musculoskeletal Disorders, 17*, 143. https://doi.org/10.1186/s12891-016-0997-8.

Khanna, S. (2020). *Mayo Clinic on disgestive health* (4th Edition). Mayo Clinic Press.

Kolasinski, S. L., Neogi, T., Hochberg, M. C., Oatis, C., Guyatt, G., Block, J., Callahan, L., Copenhaver, C., Dodge, C., Felson, D., Gellar, K., Harvey, W. F., Hawker, G., Herzig, E., Kwoh, C. K., Nelson, A. E., Samuesl, J., Scanzello, C., White, D., Wise, B., Altman, R. D., DiRenzo, D., Fontanarosa, J., Giradi, G., Ishimori, M., Misra, D., Shah, A. A., Shmagel, A. K., Thoma, L. M., Turgunbaev., M., Turner, A. S., & Reston, J. (2020). 2019 American College of Rheumatology/Arthritis Foundation guideline for management of osetoarthritis of the hand, hip, and knee. *Arthritis Care & Research, 72*(2), 149–162. doi:10.1002/acr.24131.

List, J., & Jensen, H. (2017). Temporomandibular disorders: Old ideas and new concepts. *Cephalagia, 37*(7), 692–704.

McGeary, D (2021). Headache. In S. Pangakrkar, Q. Pham, & B. Eapen (Eds.), *Pain care essentials and innovations* (pp. 15–31). Elsevier Inc. ISBN: 978-0-323-72216-2\.

Modest, J. M., Raducha, J. E., Testa, E. J., & Eberson, C. P. (2020). Management of post-amputation pain. *Rhode Island Medical Journal*. http://rimed.org/rimedicaljournal/2020/05/2020-05-19-pain-modest.pdf.

Moini, J., & Piran, P. (2020). Spinal cord lesions and disorders. In J. Moini & P. Piran (Eds.), *Functional and clinical neuroanatomy* (pp. 617–646). Academic Press. doi:10.1016/B978-0-12-817424-1.00020-3. Retrieved from https://www.sciencedirect.com/science/article/pii/B9780128174241000203.

Murphy, M. K., MacBarb, R. F., Wong, M. E., & Athanasiou, K. A. (2015). Temporomandibular joint disorders: A review of etiology, clinical management, and tissue engineering strategies. *Internal Journal Oral Maxillofacial Implants, 37*(7), 692–704.

National Heart, Lung, and Blood Institute. (2014). Evidence-Based Management of Sickle Cell Disease. Retrieved from https://www.nhlbi.nih.gov/health-topics/evidence-based-management-sickle-cell-disease.

National Institute on Drug Abuse. (2020). What is the impact of medication for opioid use disorder treatment on HIV/HCV outcomes? Retrieved from https://www.drugabuse.gov/publications/research-reports/medications-to-treat-opioid-addiction/what-impact-medication-opioid-use-disorder-treatment-hivhcv-outcomes.

Ohtake, P. J., & Borello-France, D. (2017). Rehabilitation for women and men with pelvic-floor dysfunction. *Physical Therapy, 97*(4), 390–392.

Parker, L. (2020). Symptoms and diagnosis of facet joint disorders. *Spine-health*. https://www.spine-health.com/conditions/arthritis/symptoms-and-diagnosis-facet-joint-disorders.

Parkitny, L., & Younger, J. (2017). Reduced pro-inflammatory cytokines after eight weeks of low-dose naltrexone for fibromyalgia. *Biomedicines, 5*(2), 16.

Peng, H., & Conermann, T. (2021). Arachnoiditis. In *StatPearls [Internet]*. Treasure Island (F.L.): StatPearls Publishing. 2021

Jan-. Available from: https://www.ncbi.nlm.nih.gov/books/NBK555973/.

Perolat, R., Kastler, A., Nicot, B., Pellat, J. M., Tahon, F., Attye, A., Heck, O., Boubagra, K., Grand, S., & Krainik, A. (2018). Facet joint syndrome: from diagnosis to interventional management. *Insights Into Imaging, 9*(5), 773–789. doi:10.1007/s13244-018-0638-x.

Pisetshy, D. S., Eudy, A. M., Clowse, M. E. B., & Rogers, J. L. (2021). The categorization of pain in systemic lupus erythematosus. *Rheumatic Disease Clinics of North America, 47*, 215–228. https://doi.org/10.1016/j.rdc.2020.12.004.

Poddubnyy, D. (2020). Classification vs diagnostic criteria: the challenge of diagnosing axial spondyloarthritis. *Rheumatology, 59*(Suppl4), iv6–iv17. https://doi.org/10.1093/rheumatology/keaa250.

Ritchlin, C. T., Colbert, R. A., & Gladman, D. D. (2017). Psoriatic arthritis. *New England Journal of Medicine, 376*(10), 957–970.

Rozental, J. M. (2018). Migraine headache and the trigeminal autonomic cephalalgias. In H. T. Benzon, S. N. Raga, S. S. Liu, S. M. Fishman, & S. P. Cohen (Eds.), *Essentials of pain medicine* (4th ed, pp. 157–164). Elsevier. ISBN: 978-0-323-40196-8.

Sahni, S., & Khan, J. (2021). Persistent breast cancer pain. In M. F. Valarmathi (Ed.), *Breast cancer*. IntechOpen Publishing https://www.intechopen.com/online-first/persistent-breast-cancer-pain.

Schug, S. A, Lavand'homme, P., Barke, A., Korwisi, B., Rief, W., & Treede, R. (2019). The IASP taskforce for the classification of chronic pain the IASP classification of chronic pain for ICD-11: chronic postsurgical or posttraumatic pain. *Pain, 160*(1), 45–52. doi:10.1097/j.pain.0000000000001413.

Shamrock., A. G., Donnally, C. J., III, & Varacallo, M. (2020). Lumbar spondylolysis and spondylolisthesis. In *StatPearls*. StatPearls Publishing. https://www.ncbi.nlm.nih.gov/books/NBK448122/.

Sluka, K. A. (2016). Introduction: definitions, concepts, and models of pain. In K. Sluka (Ed.), *Mechanisms and management of pain for the physical therapist* (2nd edition). New York, N.Y: IASP Press.

Szok, D., Tajti, J., Nyári, A., & Vécsei, L. (2019). Therapeutic approaches for peripheral and central neuropathic pain. *Behavioral Neurology*. https://doi.org/10.1155/2019/8685954.

Taurog, J. D., Chhabra, A., & Colbert, R. A. (2016). Ankylosing spondylitis and axial spondyloarthritis. *New England Journal of Medicine, 375*(13), 1303. https://doi.org/10.1056/NEJMc1609622.

Tennant, F. (2016). Arachnoiditis: Diagnosis and treatment. *Practical Pain Management, 16*(5). https://www.practicalpainmanagement.com/pain/spine/arachnoiditis-diagnosis-treatment.

Thapa, P., & Euasobhon, P. (2018). Chronic postsurgical pain: Current evidence for prevention and management. *Korean Journal of Pain, 31*(3), 155–173. https://doi.org/10.3344/kjp.2018.31.3.155.

Travell, J. G., & Simons, D. G. (1983). *Myofacial pain and dysfunction: The trigger point manual*. Baltimore: Williams & Wilkins.

U.S. Department of Health and Human Services. Genetic and Rare Diseases Information Center. (2021). Arachnoiditis. https://rarediseases.info.nih.gov/diseases/5839/arachnoiditis.

Van Deun, L., de Witte, M., Goessens, T., Halewyck, S., Ketelaer, M., Matic, M., Moens, M., Vaes, P., Van Lint, M., & Versijpt, J.

Part 4

(2020). Facial pain: A comprehensive review and proposal for a pragmatic diagnostic approach. *European Neurology, 83,* 5–16. doi:10.1159/000505727.

Watson, J. C., & Sandroni, P. (2016). Central neuropathic pain syndromes. *Mayo Clinic Proceedings, 91*(3), 372–385.

Wenker, K. J., & Quint, J. M. (2020). Ankylosing spondylitis. In *StatPearls*. StatPearls Publishing. https://www.ncbi.nlm.nih.gov/books/NBK470173/.

Wilcox, C. M., Gress, T., Boermeester, M., Masamune, A., Levy, P., Syham, T., Varadarajulu, S., Irisawa, A., Levy, M., Kitano, M., Garg, P., Shimosegawa, T., Sheel, A., Whitcomb, D. C., & Neoptolemus, J. P. (2020). Consensus guidelines for chronic pancreatitis. *Pancreatotomy, 20*(5), 822–827.

Yawn, B. P., Buchanan, G. R., Afenyi-Annan, A. N., Ballas, S. K., Hassell, K. L., James, A. H., & John-Sowah, J. (2014). Management of sickle cell disease: Summary of the 2014 evidence-based report by expert panel members. *Journal of the American Medical Association, 312,* 1033–1048. doi:10.1001/jama.2014.1051.

Yosef, A., Ahmed, A. G., Al-Hussaini, T., Abdellah, M. S., Cua, G., & Bedaiwy, M. A. (2016). Chronic pelvic pain: pathogenesis and validated assessment. *Middle East Fertility Society Journal, 21,* 205–221.

Younger, J., Parkitny, L., & McLain, D. (2014). The use of low-dose naltrexone (LDN) as a novel anti-inflammatory treatment for chronic pain. *Clinical Rheumatology, 33,* 451–459.

Zhu, W., He, X., Cheng, K., Zhang, L., Chen, D., Wang, X., Qiu, G., Cao, X., & Weng, X. (2019). Ankylosing spondylitis: etiology, pathogenesis, and treatments. *Bone Research, 7,* 22. https://doi.org/10.1038/s41413-019-0057-8.

CHAPTER 22
Managing Pain in the Context of Substance Use Disorder

Timothy Joseph Sowicz, Ph.D., RN
Marian Wilson, PhD, MPH, RN, PMGT-RN
Maureen F. Cooney, DNP, FNP-BC, ACHPN, AP-PMN*

Introduction

This chapter will provide important information necessary to treat pain within the context of substance use disorders (SUDs) and risks for substance misuse. The scope of the problem, definitions, clinical recommendations, and barriers to appropriate pain management will be covered. Principles of assessment, screening, and treatment for SUD and comorbid pain are outlined along with recommendations for pain management based on ethical principles, guidelines from expert authorities, and available research evidence.

I. Definitions and Context

A. The United States declared a public health emergency in 2017 in response to a crisis of opioid misuse, addiction, and overdose deaths.
   1. The crisis followed a rise in opioid prescriptions that occurred in the 1990s as pharmaceutical companies assured healthcare providers (HCPs) opioids were not addictive when prescribed for pain.
   2. As it became clear both prescribed and illegal opioids have high addictive potential, changes occurred in policy, law, and clinical practice that altered patient access to opioid-based pain management.
B. HCPs who are knowledgeable about pain management and SUD can provide safe and effective pain care.
C. Barriers to pain management in persons with SUD include:
   1. Patients' characteristics, beliefs, and access to appropriate treatments
   2. HCPs' lack of knowledge: professionals have acknowledged they need more knowledge about SUDs and access to other supports/collaborators.
   3. HCPs' personal biases and adoption of societal stigma

a. Historically, HCPs have reported negative attitudes about people with SUDs.
b. Negative attitudes may stem from perceptions about people with SUDs as not safe, responsible, or motivated and that fear they may be aggressive or violent.
c. Even among nurses who believe they have an ethical duty to provide care and be sympathetic to people living with SUDs, negative thoughts and feelings have been reported.
d. How nurses perceive pain management may be influenced by their experiences with people with SUDs, including difficulty reconciling nurses' assessments of pain and patients' requests for pain medication.
   4. Stigma
a. Earnshaw (2020) defines stigma as "a social process that exists when labeling, stereotyping, separation, status loss, and discrimination occur within a power context."
b. Structural- and individual-level factors create and reinforce stigma for people living with SUDs.
      1) Criminalization of people experiencing SUDs is an example of how stigma is manifested at the structural level.
      2) An example of how stigma is manifested at the individual level might include stereotypes such as "all people living with SUDs are dangerous."
      3) Access to resources (e.g., housing), psychological resources to assist with responses to stigma (e.g., coping), and reducing social isolation have been identified as potentially improving outcomes in people with SUDs.
         a) Contextual factors (e.g., a person's cultural identity), personal factors (e.g., age), and access to resources that promote resilience (e.g., social support) influence how stigma is manifested and impacts patient outcomes.

---

*Section Editor for the chapter.

Table 22.1
Challenges Associated With Substance Use Disorders

Challenges

- Ongoing use despite negative impacts on physical or psychological health (e.g., using despite it being physically dangerous settings)
- Ongoing use resulting in social and interpersonal consequences (e.g., limited social or recreational activities)
- Difficulty meeting professional obligations at school or work
- Exaggerate amounts of time to obtain opioids or recover from them
- Taking more than intended
- Cravings
- Inability to decrease amount used
- Tolerance
- Substance-specific withdrawal

---

b) Several recommendations for confronting stigma regarding people living with SUDs have been proposed for mental health professionals; many can be adapted and adopted by nurses in administrative, clinical, educational, and research positions.

    (1) Nurses can confront stigma by carefully selecting the language they use when discussing people with SUDs.

    (2) Words and phrases such as "addict" and "dirty urine" perpetuate stigma; these can be replaced with "people with a substance use disorder" and "cocaine was detected in urinalysis."

D. Defining pain management and SUD terms is important to reduce stigmatizing language and provide clear communication with colleagues, patients, and the public. Preferred terminology can be accessed at https://nida.nih.gov/research-topics/addiction-science/words-matter-preferred-language-talking-about-addiction.

  1. The following terms should be continually examined for both clarity and stigmatization within patient care settings, as changes in meaning can occur over time:

    a. Physical dependence refers to the body's adaptation to regular use of a drug, resulting in withdrawal symptoms when the drug is stopped. It can occur with use of many substances (e.g., opioids, benzodiazepines, nicotine), even when taken as prescribed, and in and of itself does not signify SUD.

    b. Tolerance refers to a normal, expected physiologic process causing reduced response to a drug with repeated use, requiring a higher dose to achieve the same effect, and in and of itself does not signify SUD.

    c. Withdrawal symptoms are unpleasant physiological and cognitive reactions unique to the substance one has developed dependency for, often accompanied by cravings for the drug to relieve uncomfortable symptoms. Duration, intensity, and type of withdrawal symptoms will differ based on the drug used, method of use, level of dependency, and if any co-occurring disorders are present. Presence of withdrawal symptoms is expected with abrupt cessation after regular use and in and of itself does not signify SUD.

    d. Substance use disorder

     1) The American Psychiatric Association updated the *Diagnostic and Statistical Manual of Mental Disorders, Fifth Edition (DSM-5)* in 2013 to introduce substance use disorder (SUD) to replace previous terms "substance dependence" and "substance abuse."

     2) Older stigmatizing terms and labels (e.g., "drug abuser," "drug addict," or "alcoholic") should be avoided.

      a) Addiction has been defined in the not-too-distant past as a disease of the brain that is chronic, relapsing, and treatable and that is characterized by cravings, dysfunctional behaviors, and an inability to control impulses despite harmful consequences.

      b) The term "addiction" is not used in *DSM-5*, but it is used by other organizations, including National Institute on Drug Abuse, which uses it interchangeably with more severe levels of SUD.

     3) Diagnostic criteria for SUD in *DSM-5* include three criteria-based subclassifications for all SUDs:

      a) Mild (presence of 2 or 3 symptoms)

      b) Moderate (presence of 4 or 5 symptoms)

      c) Severe (presence of 6 or more symptoms)

      d) Refer to *DSM-5* for specific criteria; also see Table 22.1.

4) SUDs are often progressive and can result in disability or premature death.

5) Treatment will depend on severity of SUD and an individual's preferences.

e. Unhealthy drug use refers to use of substances (other than alcohol or tobacco products) illegally obtained and includes nonmedical use of prescription psychoactive medications.

f. Use disorder refers to when use becomes problematic and meets *DSM-5* criteria for mild, moderate, or severe disorder and is defined by impaired control, social impairment, risky use, and pharmacological criteria.

1) Use disorder may be applied to specific substances (e.g., alcohol use disorder [AUD], opioid use disorder [OUD], cannabis use disorder [CUD]).

2) Use disorders have similar diagnostic criteria outlined in *DSM-5* (see Table 22.1).

3) OUD is preferred term for problematic pattern of opioid use that causes significant impairment or distress and can develop with inappropriate use of both legally prescribed opioid medicines or illegally obtained opioids (i.e., heroin, fentanyl, or prescription opioids purchased illegally).

4) Dependence, tolerance, and withdrawal are *not* criteria for OUD when individuals are taking prescribed opioids under medical supervision as part of prescribed agonist maintenance therapy (e.g., methadone, buprenorphine) or when in a controlled environment where access to opioids is restricted.

g. "Substance misuse" is a general term applied to overindulgence or inappropriate use of legal substances (such as alcohol and prescribed opioids) and use of illegal drugs (such as heroin).

1) The term misuse can be applied to taking medications for reasons other than those for which they were intended, indicated, or prescribed (e.g., taking opioids for sleep or anxiety; crushing or snorting prescribed long-acting medications to receive bolus effect).

2) Misuse occurs when more medication than prescribed is taken or when sharing doses. Misuse alone does not meet diagnostic criteria for SUD.

3) Pain relief is the most common reason for misuse of opioids and in 2015 was reported by 12.5% of people with an opioid prescription in a national survey of 51,200 U.S. adults.

4) Substance Abuse and Mental Health Services Administration (SAMHSA)

estimated 10.1 million people aged 12 years or older misused opioids in 2019.

E. Laws and policies

1. National legislation and policy

a. Nurses should be familiar with laws added over time to address opioid overdose crisis: https://www.hhs.gov/opioids/treatment/resources-opioid-treatment-providers/index.html.

b. Comprehensive Addiction and Recovery Act (CARA)

1) Allowed nurse practitioners and physician assistants (PAs) to prescribe buprenorphine for treatment of OUD.

2) Those who prescribed buprenorphine for treatment of OUD had to obtain an X-waiver from the U.S. Drug Enforcement Administration (DEA).

a) Continuing education requirements and limitations on the number of patients a prescriber can treat have been modified since initial CARA publication to increase patient access to treatment.

b) State laws regulating the practice of these providers may have had other stipulations related to prescribing buprenorphine.

c) States not permitting full practice authority may have required nurse practitioners to have a collaborative agreement with a physician who also has an X-waiver.

c. Substance Use Disorder Prevention that Promotes Opioid Recovery and Treatment (SUPPORT) Act of 2018

1) Expanded provisions of CARA and definition of HCPs qualified to prescribe buprenorphine to include Certified Nurse Midwives, Certified Registered Nurse Anesthetists, and Clinical Nurse Specialists until October 1, 2023. At the time of this writing, extension of this act could not be confirmed.

2) Loosened some restrictions on the number of patients practitioners may treat

3) Allowed all X-waivered advanced practice registered nurses (APRNs) to prescribe buprenorphine for no more than 100 patients in the first year. After the first year, APRNs could apply to treat up to 275 patients.

4) Consolidated Appropriations Act, 2023 removed federal requirement that APRNs and PAs complete 24 hours of specialized training to receive a waiver from SAMHSA to prescribe buprenorphine for treatment of OUD (i.e., the X-wavier) and added a training requirement for anyone who has a DEA

registration to prescribe Schedule II through IV medications.

2. State legislation and policy
   a. State laws and regulations direct RN and APRN practices. RNs' practices are regulated by the nurse practice act in their state; in some states, APRNs' practices are regulated by other state regulatory bodies, such as medical boards, in addition to boards of nursing.
   b. States may have full, reduced, or restricted regulatory structures guiding APRN practice.
   c. APRNs should also adhere to terms of their professional service employment agreements, regardless of whether their state has full, reduced, or restricted practice structures.
   d. State-specific APRN practice information is regularly updated by state boards of nursing (or other regulatory bodies) with information about scopes of practice regarding people with SUDs and specifically about medical management of SUDs.
   e. Nurses should be aware of state-specific guidelines, law, and policy surrounding opioid prescribing. In some cases, pain management specialists are required for high-dose opioid prescriptions, and dosing limits are detailed.

F. Nursing organizations
   1. American Society for Pain Management Nursing (ASPMN)
      a. A professional nursing organization with a mission to foster best nursing practices for people living with pain
      b. Membership requires payment.
      c. Publications:
         1) *ASPMN Core Curriculum for Pain Management Nursing*
         2) *Pain Management Nursing* is a peer-reviewed journal published every 2 months.
         3) Several education and professional development resources and position papers on topics relevant to pain management are available at aspmn.org.
      d. This present chapter is an updated version of the position paper *Pain Management and Risks Associated with Substance Use: Practice Recommendations,* (2022), jointly written and endorsed by ASPMN and International Nurses Society on Addictions (IntNSA).
         1) Central message of this position paper is that every person has the right to be treated with dignity and respect and to receive high-quality pain assessment and management; in addition, pain and SUDs should be treated concurrently.
         2) Position statement includes recommendations for all patients with persistent pain

and those who are at low, moderate, or high risk for developing an SUD; it includes a table that describes attributes of patients that may increase their risk for developing an SUD (e.g., past or current SUD, family history of SUD, presence of a mental health disorder, and social support).
   e. Certification opportunities
      1) Pain Management Nursing (PMGT-BC) certification through American Nursing Credentialing Center (ANCC)
      2) Advanced Practice Recognition in Pain Management Nursing (AP-PMN) recognition through ASPMN

   2. International Nurses Society on Addictions (IntNSA)
      a. A professional nursing organization whose goal is to aid nurses in providing care for those living with addictions
      b. Membership requires payment.
      c. Publications:
         1) *Journal of Addictions Nursing* is a peer-reviewed journal published quarterly.
         2) Several position papers on topics relevant to addictions nursing are available (e.g., *The Prescribing of Buprenorphine by Advanced Practice Addictions Nurses*).
      d. Education and professional development resources are available through IntNSA's virtual classroom at intnsa.org.
      e. Certification opportunities available through Addictions Nursing Certification Board
         1) Certified Addiction Registered Nurse (CARN)
         2) Certified Addiction Registered Nurse–Advanced Practice (CARN-AP)

II. Prevalence of Co-Occurring Pain and Substance Use Disorders

A. Alcohol use disorder
   1. AUD affects approximately 14.8 million American adults.
   2. About 28% of people with persistent pain report using alcohol to alleviate suffering.
B. Cannabis use disorder
   1. Common SUD affecting approximately 4.8 million people 12 years or older in the United States
   2. Adults with pain have been found to be at increased risk for CUD.
C. Opioid use disorder
   1. National Survey on Drug Use and Health (NSDUH) provides data about substance use and

SUDs (including OUD) from youths and adults. For this survey, respondents who met diagnostic criteria for heroin use disorder or prescription pain reliever use disorder (or both) were categorized as having OUD. Data from 2020 showed:

   a. More than 2.7 million Americans 12 years and older reported an OUD.

   b. Approximately 691,000 Americans 12 years and older reported a heroin use disorder.

   c. More than 1.3 million Americans 12 years and older reported a prescription pain reliever use disorder.

2. Estimates regarding comorbid OUD and persistent pain are challenging due to heterogeneity in defining addiction in research studies.

   a. Persistent pain is highly prevalent in adults with OUD at rates up to 60%.

   b. Rates of OUD in patients taking opioids for persistent pain have been reported at 8% to 12%, yet some studies find as many as 26% of people with persistent pain exhibit misuse patterns that can be a precursor to SUD.

D. Other SUDs in patients with pain can co-occur with substances such as amphetamines, benzodiazepines, stimulants, and polysubstance use (i.e., use of more than one substance).

1. In a study of 951,000 U.S. adults:

   a. Most patients with a SUD had a comorbid persistent pain condition. Specifically, patients with persistent pain reported SUD involving:

      1) Opioids: 74.7%

      2) Sedatives: 72.3%

      3) Cannabis: 64.3%

      4) Alcohol: 58.7%

      5) Tobacco: 59.5%

   b. Prevalence of persistent pain was greater in females than males for most SUD diagnoses.

   c. Presence of persistent pain was associated with more mental health disorders and chronic medical conditions among each SUD group.

2. The 2019 NSDUH includes data about prescription sedatives and tranquilizers classified as benzodiazepines.

   a. Sedative use disorder was reported by 162,000 Americans 12 years and older.

   b. Tranquilizer use disorder was reported by 586,000 Americans 12 years and older.

E. Select populations

1. Children and adolescents

   a. Understanding differences in physiology, development, and social factors is important in context of children and adolescents with pain and/or substance use.

   b. Acute and persistent pain episodes add stress for young people and exposure to opioids and other addictive medications, both of which can increase future risks of substance use and misuse.

   c. World Health Organization (WHO) recognized persistent pain in children as a significant public health problem affecting one-quarter to one-third of all children, with 1 in 20 experiencing high pain-related disability.

      1) WHO published guidelines in 2020 noting most pain recommendations are for adults and may not be appropriate for children.

      2) Guidelines emphasized concept of opioid stewardship such that:

         a) Opioids are used appropriately and prescribed by trained providers with careful ongoing assessment of benefits and risks.

         b) Child and family are included in clear plan for continuation, tapering, or discontinuation of opioids according to child's condition.

         c) Attention is given to procurement, storage, and disposal of unused opioids.

   d. Concerns about youth exposure to opioids are heightened by evidence that legitimate use of opioids among adolescents before high school graduation has been found to be correlated with 33% increase in risk of future nonmedical opioid use when reaching young adulthood.

   e. More recently, data from National Longitudinal Study of Adolescent to Adult Health (N = 14,784) examined longitudinal relationship between history of adolescent persistent pain and odds of misusing prescription opioids in adulthood.

      1) Persistent pain during adolescence was found to be an independent risk factor for opioid misuse in adulthood, over and above other known risk factors.

      2) Among those with adolescent persistent pain, substance use, exposure to trauma, and race were associated with opioid misuse.

      3) Prescription opioid misuse in the United States is most prevalent among young adults 18 to 26 years of age.

2. Pregnancy

   a. Pain during pregnancy is common, and pain management is complex due to potential for adverse fetal and pregnancy outcomes with certain analgesics.

      1) Evidence-based guidelines to assist clinicians in pain management are lacking in this population.

      2) Medications should be given at lowest therapeutic dose for shortest duration with discussion of risks and benefits.

Part 4

b. Screening for substance use is recommended as routine part of comprehensive obstetric care at first prenatal visit.

1) Exposure to substances during prenatal period can cross placenta and expose developing fetus to harms, including stillbirth, miscarriage, birth defects, and lifelong behavioral and learning problems.

2) Specific resources to address substance use and pain in pregnancy are available at Centers for Disease Control and Prevention (CDC) website.

c. Rise in pregnant women using opioids for pain and with OUD has accompanied rising trends in the general population. Women have reported using pain medicines during pregnancy, including opioids, at rates above 50%.

1) For persistent pain in pregnancy, recommended strategies are to avoid or minimize use of opioids for pain and highlight non-pharmacological (e.g., exercise, physical therapy, behavioral approaches) and non-opioid pharmacological treatments.

2) For acute pain care in pregnancy, labor, and delivery, planning should include discussion of addictive substances, including risks to mother and baby.

3) For pregnant women with OUD, opioid agonist pharmacotherapy is recommended and preferred over medically supervised withdrawal. Withdrawal is associated with high relapse rates, which can lead to worse outcomes for mother and infant, according to American College of Obstetricians and Gynecologists (ACOG).

4) OUD during pregnancy is linked with negative health outcomes for pregnant women and babies, including preterm birth, stillbirth, maternal mortality, and neonatal abstinence syndrome (NAS). NAS is a group of withdrawal symptoms most commonly occurring in newborns after exposure to opioids or other substances during pregnancy. Neonatal opioid withdrawal syndrome is group of withdrawal symptoms specifically related to opioid exposure alone.

d. Cannabis use among pregnant women is estimated at 1 in 10; many use cannabis daily and meet criteria for CUD.

1) Due to insufficient research to understand health effects for mother and baby, both CDC and ACOG recommend against cannabis use in pregnancy.

2) Pain is one of most common reasons given by women for using cannabis in pregnancy.

Belief in cannabis safety has increased among pregnant women, along with ease of its access due to expanding legalization.

3. Racial and ethnic minorities

a. Racial and ethnic differences occur in the experience of pain, and racial and ethnic disparities occur in assessment and treatment of pain and SUD.

b. Black and Hispanic patients in the United States have been found to be less likely than Whites to receive analgesia for acute pain in emergency settings.

c. Racial disparities exist in treatment services and outcomes for SUDs, with more severe consequences of SUDs and less initiation of treatment services among non-Whites.

1) African Americans began to exceed Whites in opioid-related overdose deaths from 2013 to 2021. Disparities in opioid prescribing for African Americans were thought to explain prior lags in overdose deaths.

2) A proliferation of illegal use of manufactured fentanyl increased among non-Hispanic Blacks and Hispanics along with increases in overdose deaths.

4. Veterans

a. Given significant problems of SUDs and pain among U.S. veterans, routine screening to detect and treat SUDs is recommended.

b. U.S. military veterans (particularly veterans who served during recent conflicts) have higher prevalence of severe pain occurring "most days" or "every day" than do members of the general population.

c. U.S. military veterans also suffer disproportionately from SUDs, with percentages of AUDs and drug use disorders reported to be higher than those among civilian counterparts.

III. Neuromechanisms of Brain With Substance Use Disorders and Pain

A. Brain disease model of addiction

1. Research over the past three decades has supported brain disease model of addiction (BDMA) identifying SUD primarily as disease caused by and impacting structure and neurocircuitry of the brain.

a. Model serves to encourage individuals to seek and accept treatment by decreasing self-recrimination and attitudes that addiction was result of moral failing or weak character.

b. BDMA explains relationships between brain circuits disrupted by addictive substances and changes in brain circuitry involved in multiple behaviors, including self-control, reward, motivation, decision-making, inhibition, executive control, and memory.

c. BDMA established understanding of addiction as disease beyond an individual's control or willpower. Biological mechanisms include alteration in the brain's reward circuit, causing euphoria with use of the addictive substance and flooding the brain with chemical messenger dopamine.

d. Viewing SUD as brain disease aligns well with medication approaches that address biological changes occurring within brain synapses.

   1) Substances trigger dopamine release that is reinforcing and at the same time decreases activity occurring in area of the brain associated with decision-making and judgment.

   2) With repeated exposure to rewards, environmental cues paired with drug use are reinforced.

   3) Persons with SUDs also become less motivated by everyday stimuli that once was rewarding (e.g., relationships and activities).

2. Challenges to BDMA have raised concern that a disease model may simplify SUD to a problem focused on brain chemistry alone and favors biomedical treatments.

3. Proponents note BDMA provided advances in health policy so patients can receive treatment for SUD and have insurances cover it. Additionally, BDMA does not negate role of psychological, social, and socioeconomic processes involved in SUD development and consequences.

B. Shared neurophysiological patterns with SUD and pain

1. Overlap exists between brain regions engaged by ongoing pain, addictive drugs, and analgesics. Both pain and addiction share neural systems associated with dopamine surges, reward, motivation, and learning centers.

2. Persistent pain and SUD both involve abnormal neural processing.

a. These common neuronal pathways can complicate distinctions between pain relief behaviors and addictive behaviors.

b. Both pain relief and addictive drugs are reinforcing in brain's circuitry and can lead to preoccupation or craving for consumption of analgesic drugs.

c. Discerning pain behaviors from SUD behaviors is an important distinction yet can be quite difficult.

C. Treating persistent pain and SUD as separate entities may miss the complexity of the whole individual. As coexisting problems, they interact with each other in complex ways and thus necessitate an integrated, multidimensional therapeutic approach. Both pain and SUD deserve and require attention.

IV. Screening for and Assessment of Substance Use Disorder

A. Nursing assessment considerations

1. Because SUDs can occur at higher frequency among populations with pain than general populations, SUD screening should be integrated routinely into pain management care plans. Unfortunately, few tools have been well-validated for use in populations with concurrent pain and OUD; care should be given in interpreting findings. Very brief screening tools for opioid misuse are available for use in paper or electronic forms.

2. SUD screening should occur before potentially addictive substances are prescribed, and patients should be fully informed of risks and benefits.

3. Research findings suggest certain demographic, physical, and psychosocial factors can predict opioid misuse among patients with persistent pain.

a. Pain

   1) Causing or contributing to an inability to function

   2) Pain for which cause is unclear or unknown

b. History of substance use

   1) Family or personal history

   2) History of treatment for SUD

   3) Tobacco use

c. Emotional or mental state

   1) Psychological disease, stress, and/or trauma

   2) Mood swings

   3) Use of psychotropic substances

   4) Prescription drug craving

   5) Focusing on opioids

d. Childhood experiences

   1) Adversity

   2) Sexual abuse

e. Other

   1) Inadequate social support

   2) Legal concerns

   3) Young age

4. *Pain Management Nursing: Scope and Standards of Practice* described here comes from the American Nurses Association (ANA) and ASPMN.

a. See chapter 11 for general information regarding comprehensive pain assessment.

b. Within context of SUD or potential SUD:

1) Assessment of SUD may be challenging if patients are reluctant to engage because of fear of losing access to their opioid prescriptions.

2) Compassionate, nonjudgmental care respecting patient's pain experience is essential.

3) Nurses must take time to establish trusting relationships and work in conjunction with patient preferences for pain treatment, whether or not it occurs in conjunction with SUD.

4) When assessing patients, clinicians must be careful to avoid assuming pain relief–seeking behaviors are attributable to SUDs.

5. U.S. Preventive Services Task Force (USPSTF) published a final recommendation for screening for unhealthy drug use in adolescents and adults in June 2020.

   a. Screening is recommended for adults 18 years and older and applies to adolescents and those who are pregnant and postpartum regardless of presence of risk factors for unhealthy drug use.

   b. USPSTF recommends asking questions about unhealthy drug use; nurses can use existing screening tools (see sections below).

   c. Currently, evidence is insufficient about when to initiate screening for unhealthy drug use or frequency of screening.

6. Addictions nursing:

   a. IntNSA and ANA, in *Pain Management Nursing: Scope and Standards of Practice,* define assessment as the process by which addictions nurse collects comprehensive data pertinent to healthcare consumer's health and/or situation.

   b. Select assessment competencies related to SUDs include:

     1) Collect data about substance use, including type, amount, frequency, and pattern of use.

     2) Use appropriate screening and assessment tools and document-assessment findings.

B. Substance abuse disorder screening and assessment tools

1. Numerous screening tools are available to assess for use of alcohol, opioids, tobacco, cannabis, and other substances.

2. National Institute on Drug Abuse provides a Screening and Assessment Tools chart with evidence-based free screening tools available at https://www.drugabuse.gov/nidamed-medical-health-professionals/screening-tools-resources/chart-screening-tools.

3. Specific tools are based on patients' age (i.e., adults, adolescents), substance type (i.e., drugs, alcohol), and tool administration type (i.e., self- or clinician-administered).

4. The Tobacco, Alcohol, Prescription medication, and other Substance use (TAPS) Tool is validated for use with adults to generate a risk level for each substance class. It can be self-administered or conducted via clinician interview.

5. Screening, Brief Intervention, and Referral to Treatment (SBIRT)

   a. Evidence-based approach to delivery of early intervention and treatment services for people with SUDs and those at risk of developing these disorders

   b. Online training is available through SAMHSA website https://www.samhasa.gov/sbirt. Steps involve:

     1) Brief screening to assess severity of substances

     2) Identification of appropriate level of treatment

     3) Brief intervention focused on increasing insight and awareness of substance use

     4) Nurses can begin conversations by assessing patients' interest in changing substance use with tools such as "readiness ruler" (https://iprc.iu.edu/sbirtapp/mi/ruler.php).

     5) Referral to treatment appropriate for situation, with specialty care as needed

     6) Reimbursement for SBIRT is available through commercial insurance, Medicare, and Medicaid.

C. Screening for opioid withdrawal

1. Clinical Opiate Withdrawal Scale

   a. Scale with 11 items to rate withdrawal symptoms in both inpatient and outpatient settings and to monitor symptoms over time

   b. Summed total score uses combination of self-reported symptoms (e.g., anxiety, bone or joint aches, gastrointestinal upset) along with those observed by trained clinician (e.g., pupil size, pulse, sweating).

2. Adjective Rating Scale for Withdrawal is a 16-item self-report scale used to assess severity of opiate withdrawal symptoms.

3. See chapter 12 "Risk Assessments Related to Pain Management" for additional tools.

D. Screening for associated symptoms

1. People living with SUD may experience co-occurring mental health disorders (also known as dual diagnosis or dual disorders), such as generalized anxiety disorder and major depressive disorder; these may increase risk for suicide.

2. Nurses should routinely assess for signs and symptoms of co-occurring mental health disorders.

   a. Several reliable and valid tools are available. For each co-occurring disorder below, one screening tool is presented, but more exist.

b. Nurses should adopt tools appropriate for their practice settings and types of patients served within them.

c. Tools below serve as screening instruments only, and a positive screen is not synonymous with a medical diagnosis.

d. Patients who have a positive screen should be further evaluated by a qualified HCP.

3. Screening for anxiety: Generalized Anxiety Disorder Screener-7 (GAD-7) is used to screen for GAD.

a. Patients are asked to rate how bothered they have been by certain problems (e.g., trouble relaxing) in last 2 weeks on 4-point scale (0 = not at all; 3 = nearly every day).

b. Scoring of 7 items ranges from 0 to 21. Score of 0 to 4 indicates minimal level of anxiety severity; 5 to 9, mild severity; 10 to 14, moderate severity; and 15 to 21, severe severity.

c. If any problems are selected, patients are asked to rate how difficult the problems affect their ability to do their work, take care of things at home, or get along with other people.

4. Screening for depression: Patient Health Questionnaire (PHQ)-9 is self-administered tool to measure depressive symptoms.

a. Patients are asked how often they have been bothered by 9 symptoms/problems in previous 2 weeks.

b. Ranges from 0 (not at all) to 3 (nearly every day) for each symptom/problem.

c. Total score is calculated, and if any symptoms/problems are endorsed, patients are asked to rate how difficult they made it "to do your work, take care of things at home, or get along with other people" by selecting not difficult at all, somewhat difficult, very difficult, or extremely difficult.

d. Total score ranges from 0 to 27; if patient selects "more than half the days" or "nearly every day" for at least 5 symptoms/problems (and one of the symptoms/problems is depressed mood), then major depression can be diagnosed.

5. Screening for Posttraumatic Stress Disorder (PTSD): Trauma Screening Questionnaire (TSQ).

a. Consists of 10 items that assess re-experiencing and arousal symptoms and are answered as either yes or no

b. Items include reactions to traumatic events, for example "upsetting thoughts or memories about the event that have come into your mind against your will."

c. Answering yes to 6 or more items is considered a positive screen.

d. It is recommended TSQ be administered approximately 3 weeks after traumatic event.

6. Screening for sleep disturbance

a. Sleep disturbance is common among people with pain and with SUD. Inadequate sleep can worsen pain and increase risk for substance use relapse.

b. Pittsburgh Sleep Quality Index (PSQI) is 10-item self-report screening tool on which respondents indicate most accurate response for most days and nights in past month to series of questions pertaining to their sleep. PSQI items are used to calculate 7 component scores and a single global score of sleep quality.

c. Epworth Sleepiness Scale (ESS) is a simple, 8-item measure of daytime sleepiness in which respondents rate their likelihood of dozing or falling asleep in 8 different situations.

1) Responses are provided on scale of 0 to 3 (never, slight, moderate, and high).

2) Summation of scores provides composite score and describes extent of daytime sleepiness.

3) ESS is commonly given in clinical setting to patients who are suspected of having a sleep disorder.

7. Screening for suicide

a. Increased suicide risk has been linked to opioid and benzodiazepine use, persistent pain, SUD, and other mental health disorders.

b. Risk Stratification Table developed by Rocky Mountain Mental Illness, Research, Education, and Clinical Center aids nurses in stratifying suicide risk.

1) Risk is categorized as either acute or chronic, then as high, intermediate, or low based on essential features and common warning signs and risk factors.

2) Tool provides actions nurses should take based on risk stratification. For example, a person with no current suicidal intent, no specific or current suicidal plan, and no preparatory behaviors along with collective high confidence that the person can independently maintain safety would be classified as low acute risk. This person could be managed by their primary care provider or be referred to a mental health provider for evaluation and treatment.

V. Nursing Diagnosis

A. Select NANDA International (NANDA-I) nursing diagnoses related to SUD and pain

1. Nursing diagnoses include a diagnosis label, definition, defining characteristics, risk factors, and related factors.
2. Diagnosis is second standard of practice for addictions nursing.
3. Nursing diagnoses are categorized into 13 broad domains and within narrower classes for each domain. For example, Domain 12 is "comfort," which includes three classes: physical comfort (class 1), environmental comfort (class 2), and social comfort (class 3).
4. Select NANDA-I diagnoses for pain. Diagnoses below are part of Domain 12, comfort, and are included in Class 1, physical comfort:
   a. Acute pain
   b. Chronic (persistent) pain
   c. Labor pain
   d. Chronic (persistent) pain syndrome
5. There are no NANDA-I diagnoses specific to SUD.
   a. "Substance abuse," "history of substance abuse," "insufficient knowledge about substance abuse," "genetic predisposition to substance abuse," and "family substance abuse" are included as related factors, risk factors, or defining characteristics for several nursing diagnoses across 12 domains.
   b. For example, "substance abuse" is a risk factor for the nursing diagnosis, "risk for impaired liver function," which is a diagnosis under Domain 2, nutrition.
   c. Additionally, "substance abuse" is included as example of "mental health issue" (a related factor) for some nursing diagnoses.

VI. Interventions

A. Considerations when planning or implementing pain interventions for people with SUD
   1. An integrative approach with concurrent, coordinated management of addiction/dependence, comorbidities, and persistent pain is needed.
   2. Treating pain and SUD as two separate problems is often unsuccessful because multiple psychological, psychiatric, and medical problems coincide and overlap.
   3. Programs specifically developed for use in comorbid pain and SUD populations are uncommon although they show promise and are supported by theory.
   4. A multidimensional approach using a combination of pharmacotherapy, behavioral therapies, and pain self-management strategies needs further development and research.

B. Tapering opioids
   1. Several reasons for discontinuing long-term opioid therapy exist, including adverse effects unable to be mitigated, simultaneous use of other central nervous system depressants with associated increased overdose risk, and lack of functional improvement.
   2. Before a tapering protocol (either to lower dose or discontinue opioid therapy) is implemented, several factors should be considered, including:
      a. Patient's willingness to taper
      b. Speed of taper
      c. Management of withdrawal symptoms
      d. Availability of team-based care to assist with taper (e.g., primary care, pain care, pharmacy, and addiction care)
   3. Length of tapering protocols may vary from days to years.
      a. Clinicians should refer to most current evidence-based guidelines when creating tapering protocols.
      b. U.S. Department of Veterans Affairs provides guidance for reducing doses based on length of taper and intervals for follow-up throughout taper.
      c. CDC has also developed tapering guidelines stressing the need to taper slowly, adjust rate of taper depending on person's response, and avoid abrupt or sudden discontinuation of opioids. Visit www.cdc.gov for most current guidelines: https://www.cdc.gov/drugoverdose/pdf/clinical_pocket_guide_tapering-a.pdf.

C. Medication-assisted treatment (MAT)
   1. MAT is approach to SUD treatment involving use of medications and behavioral therapies. All MATs should be accompanied by psychological support, although specific certification in counseling is not required, with exception of methadone treatment for OUD.
   2. Purposes:
      a. Returning balance to normal reward pathways in brain
      b. Restoring emotional and decision-making capacities
      c. Controlling symptoms of withdrawal
      d. Suppressing drug cravings
   3. Benefits:
      a. MAT can reduce substance use relapse and block positive-reinforcing effects of ongoing drug use. Because of these benefits, MAT can facilitate successful engagement in recovery oriented activities and assist in successful employment and meeting social and family obligations.
      b. MAT has been shown to reduce morbidity, mortality, and criminal activity.

c. MAT can also reduce risk of contracting human immunodeficiency virus (HIV) or hepatitis C virus (HCV).

d. Some MATs also have pain-relieving benefits. Therefore, nurses can advocate for and prescribe MAT to patients with comorbid SUD and pain when licensed to do so.

4. MAT for alcohol use disorder

   a. Three commonly used U.S. Food and Drug Administration (FDA)-approved medications are available to treat AUD and work via different mechanisms.

     1) Disulfiram discourages drinking using an aversive effect. It makes a person physically ill when they drink alcohol.

     2) Acamprosate reduces post-acute withdrawal symptoms. The person may avoid a negative or aversive event (withdrawal symptoms) by using this medication.

     3) Naltrexone discourages drinking by blocking opioid receptors, which reduces euphoria when alcohol is consumed. This reduces positive reinforcement.

   b. Best option will depend on individual's unique situation and preferences.

5. MAT for opioid use disorder

   a. FDA-approved medications for OUD include:

     1) Buprenorphine

       a) Available in multiple formulations

       b) Buprenorphine/naloxone

         (1) Combination products that can deter misuse

         (2) Formulations include sublingual tablets or film, injections, implants.

       c) Long-term studies of newer medications are lacking.

       d) Caution is needed when initiating treatment with buprenorphine products or when transferring from other opioids because precipitated withdrawal can occur if opioids are in the person's system.

     2) Methadone

       a) Has specific eligibility criteria when used for SUD:

         (1) Unlike buprenorphine, methadone used for SUD must be dispensed as part of an opioid treatment program and not from a pharmacy.

         (2) Initial induction is generally done under daily observation, in person, and treatment requires mandatory counseling.

       b) Can prolong QT intervals; electrocardiograms should be done prior to starting it and periodically throughout treatment

       c) Multiple drug interactions are possible; therefore, close monitoring is needed.

       d) More than 40 years of data support safety and efficacy, yet stigma persists, including that methadone is "substituting one drug for another."

     3) Naltrexone

       a) Approved for AUD and OUD, so may be a good choice for a person with both conditions

       b) As an opioid antagonist, naltrexone blocks opioid receptors and reverses or prevents opioid euphoric effects.

       c) Precipitates withdrawal if opioids are in the system

       d) Various formulations are available, including oral and injectable. A once-monthly intramuscular depot formulation is also available.

6. MAT for cannabis use disorder

   a. No FDA-approved medications exist to treat CUD.

   b. Only scant evidence supports use of any specific medications. Research is needed to explore interventions for CUD in the context of pain conditions.

D. Nonpharmacological interventions

1. A variety of psychological options can be offered, including:

   a. Cognitive behavioral therapy

   b. Peer-based 12-step programs that include social support (i.e., Alcoholics Anonymous and Narcotics Anonymous)

   c. Mind-body interventions, including relaxation and mindfulness interventions and guided imagery

2. Treatments helpful for pain are likely also useful in context of all types of SUD and pain, including physical therapy, acupuncture, and massage (see other chapters for more on nonpharmacological options).

3. Patient and family education

   a. One standard of practice for addictions nursing is implementation, which includes two substandards: coordination of care and health teaching and health promotion.

   b. Sources for educational materials related to drug disposal, drug storage, and naloxone are provided below.

     1)

       a) Drug disposal: FDA website includes several webpages used for health teaching.

Part 4

b) Webpage, "Disposal of Unused Medicines: What You Should Know," includes:
   (1) Video and infographic about drug disposal options
   (2) Links to other webpages for information about drug take back locations (including link to search for disposal locations provided by DEA)
   (3) FDA's flush list (drugs that can be safely flushed down toilet)
   (4) Ways to dispose of drugs not included on flush list (e.g., mixing the drugs with cat litter or used coffee grounds).

2) Drug storage
   a) CDC's "Up and Away and Out of Sight" (www.UpAndAway.org) initiative is an educational program about storing medications safely. Website includes resources used for health teaching such as:
      (1) Videos
      (2) Tip sheets (e.g., for storing medications safely when traveling)
      (3) Coloring book
      (4) Poison Help telephone number (800-222-1222)

3) Naloxone
   a) Naloxone is an opioid antagonist used to rapidly reverse an opioid overdose. Intravenous, intramuscular, intranasal, and subcutaneous routes of administration are available.
   b) Recommended or required in some states when high-dose opioids are prescribed, following an overdose, or following a period of abstinence (e.g., after incarceration).
   c) FDA recommends the following people be prescribed naloxone:
      (1) Those prescribed opioids
      (2) Those prescribed medications to treat OUD
      (3) Those at risk for opioid overdose, even if they are no longer prescribed an opioid or using medication to treat OUD
      (4) Those taking central nervous system depressants, with history of OUD, or having experienced past opioid overdose
      (5) Those on opioid therapy living with others at risk for accidental poisoning from opioids, such as children

   d) Naloxone may be administered by healthcare providers, first responders, law enforcement personnel, friends, relatives, and bystanders.
   e) "How to Use Naloxone" is a brief video created by the American Medical Association and provides instructions for administering formulations of the drug such as the nasal spray (Narcan®), and intramuscular needle syringe.
   f) Nurses and others responding to an opioid overdose should call 9-1-1 immediately after administering a dose of naloxone. If there is no rapid response, follow product instructions to repeat the dose.

4) Harm reduction strategies
   a) Syringe service programs (SSPs) or syringe exchange programs provide several services for people who inject drugs including:
      (1) Sterile syringes and injection equipment
      (2) Testing for HCV and HIV
      (3) Linking people to treatment for HCV, HIV, and SUD treatment
      (4) Recently, it has been reported the number of SSPs in the United States increased from 141 in 2015 to 292 in 2018. During the same time, the number of sterile syringes purchased by SSPs increased from 42.2 million in 2015 to 87.5 million in 2018.
      (5) Dave Purchase Project is a harm-reduction organization.
         (a) One of the Project's initiatives, North American Syringe Exchange Network (NASEN), assists in providing harm-reduction materials to SSPs nationally.
         (b) NASEN website includes directory of SSP locations. Nurses can use directory to locate SSPs and refer people who inject drugs to these SSPs.

5) National Harm Reduction Coalition is another organization with a website nurses can use to assist patients with learning about and accessing harm-reduction measures, such as naloxone.
   a) Harm-reduction models also recognize substance use reduction (versus abstinence) may be appropriate goal for some people.
      (1) Nurses can share information specific to substance use to improve patient knowledge regarding harms.

(2) For example, patients can be taught mixing alcohol with acetaminophen can cause acute liver failure; alcohol and aspirin increase risk for gastric bleeding; and alcohol increases effects of opioids, increasing risk for overdose.

E. Clinical practice guidelines

1. Diagnosis of SUD for a person experiencing pain requires thorough evaluation, which can include both objective (i.e., physical examination, urine drug testing, medical record audits) and self-reported patient information.

2. CDC provides guidelines for treating persistent pain in adults that include considerations for SUD risks when prescribing opioids. Guidelines can be accessed in full at https://www.cdc.gov/drugoverdose/prescribing/guideline.html and key points are summarized below:

   a. Because of its punitive tone and implications of a legal document, the term "pain contract" is no longer recommended. "Pain agreements" may be initiated by clinicians to establish boundaries with patients and reduce risks of drug diversion.

      1) They often include formally written agreements between prescribers and patients defining key aspects of opioid therapy, including potential risks and benefits of treatment.

      2) Providers may outline expected behaviors, such as to use only one provider and only one pharmacy for all opioid prescriptions, and may outline consequences of violating agreement.

      3) Intention should be to promote patient safety and reduce clinicians' liability.

      4) Little research has been done to determine whether these agreements improve pain outcomes or reduce risks. They may have negative effects on patient-clinician relationships.

   b. Prescription drug monitoring programs (PDMPs) are statewide electronic databases used to monitor controlled prescription medications filled by patients.

      1) They can be used to monitor patient adherence with pain agreements and identify suspected medication misuse or diversion.

      2) States vary regarding who can access information in PDMPs, and they are limited in ability to share or report information in real time across states.

   c. Urine drug screens should occur prior to prescribing opioids and at regular intervals thereafter to confirm presence of prescribed drug and detect other drugs that might work synergistically to reduce respirations and increase overdose risk.

      1) Identification of such risks will require greater caution, closer follow-up, and patient education (potentially including opioid antagonist training).

      2) Urine drug screens are just one of many tools to assess patient status. Clinicians should be aware errors can occur in interpreting urine drug screening.

3. Standardized guidelines

   a. Due to highly addictive nature of prescription opioids, many U.S. clinics establish standardized guidelines, such as those listed above, for prescribing opioids intended to reduce drug diversion, misuse, illegal drug use, and addiction.

   b. Such planned oversight can reduce individualized care and may result in unintended feelings of mistrust and/or humiliation from people seeking pain relief.

      1) Building trust with active listening, a non-judgmental approach, and accepting the pain experience as credible shows patients the relationship between caregiver and patient is based on caring and empathy.

      2) Feeling stigmatized can inhibit open communication and limit the supportive relationship needed between patients with pain or SUDs and their HCPs.

      3) HCPs must consider anger and defensiveness from patients may stem from past negative clinical encounters.

      4) Nurses should be compassionate and empathic to facilitate these relationships.

F. Considerations in context of SUD

1. Tolerance

   a. Tolerance is normal physiologic response and should be considered by providers who prescribe medications (such as opioids) to decrease or alleviate pain and improve and maximize function.

   b. Patients should be educated about this phenomenon when beginning opioid therapy and regularly throughout treatment.

   c. Patients requiring higher or more frequent doses of opioids should not be labeled as "drug seeking" or described using other pejorative language.

   d. Tolerance should be considered when:

      1) Pain intensity is no longer acceptable for patients

      2) Functionality plateaus or decreases

      3) Self-reported quality of life decreases

   4) Participation in activities of daily living is impaired
2. Opioid-induced hyperalgesia (OIH)
   a. OIH may occur in people using long-term opioid therapy.
   b. Symptoms of OIH may include:
      1) An increase in pain (as opposed to a decrease in pain) with higher opioid doses.
      2) Myalgias
      3) Abdominal pain
      4) Cramping
   c. Symptoms associated with OIH may be like those of tolerance or withdrawal, but OIH is a distinct condition.
   d. Treatment options for OIH may include:
      1) Tapering opioids to a lower dose, or to off completely.
      2) Changing opioid (opioid rotation)
      3) Adding non-opioid adjuvant drugs
      4) Adding N-methyl-D-aspartate receptor antagonists (e.g., ketamine, methadone, dextromethorphan) or other medications (e.g., buprenorphine, naloxone)
      5) Further evaluation by pain management and/or addiction medicine providers
3. Co-occurring disorders
   a. Term co-occurring disorder (or dual disorders, dual diagnosis, or comorbid condition) refers to experience of living with both SUD and a mental health disorder (e.g., generalized anxiety disorder or major depressive disorder).
   b. Many combinations of co-occurring disorders exist and are common in people with persistent pain.
      1) As part of comprehensive assessment, patients seeking treatment for SUD should be evaluated for mental health disorders; similarly, people being treated for mental health disorders should be assessed for SUD.
      2) Both disorders should be treated simultaneously using evidence-based therapies.
      3) Treating co-occurring disorders may require coordination among several providers, including those with expertise in primary care, mental health and psychiatry, addiction medicine, clinical psychology, and social work.
      4) SAMHSA provides guidance for integrating treatment for co-occurring disorders.

Bibliography

American Association of Nurse Practitioners. (n.d.). *Comprehensive Addiction and Recovery Act (CARA)*. https:// www.aanp.org/advocacy/recent-legislative-changes/comprehensive-addiction-and-recovery-act-cara.

American Association of Nurse Practitioners. (2021, January 1). *State practice environment*. https://www.aanp.org/advocacy/state/state-practice-environment.

American College of Obstetricians and Gynecologists. (2017). Opioid use and opioid use disorder in pregnancy: Committee opinion, No. 711. *Obstetrics & Gynecology, 130*(2), e81–e94. https://doi.org/10.1097/AOG.0000000000002235.

American Nurses Association and International Nurses Society on Addictions. (2013). *Addictions nursing: Scope and Standards of Practice*. Nursesbooks.org.

American Psychiatric Association. (2013). *Diagnostic and Statistical Manual of Mental Disorders* (Ed. 5). American Psychiatric Association. https://doi.org/10.1176/appi.books.9780890425596.

American Public Health Association. (2021). *Substance Misuse*. https://www.apha.org/topics-and-issues/substance-misuse.

American Society of Addiction Medicine. (2015, June 1). *The ASAM national practice guideline for the treatment for the use of medications in the treatment of addiction involving opioids*. https://www.asam.org/docs/default-source/practice-support/guidelines-and-consensus-docs/asam-national-practice-guideline-supplement.pdf?sfvrsn=24#search= "in disability or premature death".

Black, E., Khor, K. E., Kennedy, D., Chutatape, A., Sharma, S., Vancaillie, T., et al. (2019). Medication use and pain management in pregnancy: a critical review. *Pain Practice: The Official Journal of World Institute of Pain, 19*(8), 875–899. https://doi.org/10.1111/papr.12814.

Brewin, C. R., Rose, S., Andrews, B., Green, J., Tata, P., Turner, S., & Foa, E. B. (2002). Brief screening instrument for post-traumatic stress disorder. *The British Journal of Psychiatry, 181*(2), 158–162. https://doi.org/10.1192/bjp.181.2.158.

Broyles, L. M., Binswanger, I. A., Jenkins, J. A., Finnell, D. S., Faseru, B., Cavaiola, A., Pugatch, M., & Gordon, A. J. (2014). Confronting inadvertent stigma and pejorative language in addiction scholarship: A recognition and response. *Substance Abuse, 35*(3), 217–221. https://doi.org/10.1080/08897077.2014.930372.

Buysse, D. J., Reynolds, C. F., Monk, T. H., Berman, S. R., & Kupfer, D. J. (1989). The Pittsburgh sleep quality index: A new instrument for psychiatric practice and research. *Psychiatry Research, 28*(2), 193–213. https://doi.org/10.1016/0165-1781(89)90047-4.

Centers for Disease Control and Prevention. (n.d.). Module 5: Assessing and addressing opioid use disorder (OUD). https://www.cdc.gov/drugoverdose/training/oud/accessible/index.html.

Centers for Disease Control and Prevention. (2020a, April 30). *Up and Away Campaign*. https://www.cdc.gov/medicationsafety/protect/campaign.html.

Centers for Disease Control and Prevention. (2020b, July 15). *Substance use during pregnancy*. https://www.cdc.gov/reproductivehealth/maternalinfanthealth/substance-abuse/substance-abuse-during-pregnancy.htm.

Centers for Disease Control and Prevention. (2021, January 26). *Commonly used terms*. Retrieved February 3, 2021 from www.cdc.gov/drugoverdose/opioids/terms.html.

Coughlin, L. N., Ilgen, M. A., Jannausch, M., Walton, M. A., & Bohnert, K. M. (2021). Progression of cannabis withdrawal symptoms in people using medical cannabis for chronic pain. *Addiction.* Advance online publication. https://doi.org/10.1111/add.15370.

Dave Purchase Project. (2021). *About us. Pioneering harm-reduction strategies since 1988.* https://www.davepurchaseproject.org/about-us.

Des Jarlais, D. C., Feelemyer, J., LaKosky, P., Szymanowski, K., & Arasteh, K. (2020). Expansion of syringe service programs in the United States, 2015-2018. *American Journal of Public Health, 110*(4), 517–519. https://doi.org/10.2105/AJPH.2019.305515.

Earnshaw, V. A. (2020). Stigma and substance use disorders: A clinical, research, and advocacy agenda. *The American Psychologist, 75*(9), 1300–1311. https://doi.org/10.1037/amp0000744.

Elman, I., & Borsook, D. (2016). Common brain mechanisms of chronic pain and addiction. *Neuron, 89*(1), 11–36. https://doi.org/10.1016/j.neuron.2015.11.027.

Furr-Holden, D., Milam, A. J., Wang, L., & Sadler, R. (2021). African Americans now outpace whites in opioid-involved overdose deaths: A comparison of temporal trends from 1999–2018. *Addiction, 116*(3), 677–683. https://doi.org/10.1111/add.15233.

Groenewald, C. B., Law, E. F., Fisher, E., Beals-Erickson, S. E., & Palermo, T. M. (2019). Associations between adolescent chronic pain and prescription opioid misuse in adulthood. *The Journal of Pain, 20*(1), 28–37. https://doi.org/10.1016/j.jpain.2018.07.007.

Han, B., Compton, W. M., Blanco, C., Crane, E., Lee, J., & Jones, C. M. (2017). Prescription opioid use, misuse, and use disorders in U.S. adults: 2015 National Survey on Drug Use and Health. *Annals of Intern Medicine, 167*(5), 293–301. https://doi.org/10.7326/M17-0865.

Hasin, D. S., Sarvet, A. L., Cerd, M., Keyes, K. M., Stohl, M., Galea, S., et al. (2017). U.S. adult illicit cannabis use, cannabis use disorder, and medical marijuana laws: 1991-1992 to 2012–2013. *JAMA Psychiatry, 74*(6), 579–588. https://doi.org/10.1001/jamapsychiatry.2017.0724.

Hasin, D. S., Shmulewitz, D., Cerdá, M., Keyes, K. M., Olfson, M., Sarvet, A. L., et al. (2020). U.S. adults with pain, a group increasingly vulnerable to non-medical cannabis use and cannabis use disorder: 2001-2002 and 2012-2013. *The American Journal of Psychiatry, 177*(7), 611–618. https://doi.org/10.1176/appi.ajp.2019.19030284.

Herdman, T. H., Kamitsuru, S., & North American Nursing Diagnosis Association. (2014). *Nursing diagnoses: Definitions and classification 2015-2017* (10th ed.). Wiley-Blackwell.

Hser, Y. I., Mooney, L. J., Saxon, A. J., Miotto, K., Bell, D. S., & Huang, D. (2017). Chronic pain among patients with opioid use disorder: Results from electronic health records data. *Journal of Substance Abuse Treatment, 77*, 26–30. https://doi.org/10.1016/j.jsat.2017.03.006.

John, W. S., & Wu, L. T. (2020). Chronic non-cancer pain among adults with substance use disorders: Prevalence, characteristics, and association with opioid overdose and healthcare utilization. *Drug and Alcohol Dependence, 209*, 1–9. https://doi.org/10.1016/j.drugalcdep.2020.107902.

Johns, M. W. (1991). A new method for measuring daytime sleepiness: The Epworth sleepiness scale. *Sleep, 14*(6), 540–545. https://doi.org/10.1093/sleep/14.6.540.

Kaye, A. D., Kandregula, S., Kosty, J., Sin, A., Guthikonda, B., Ghali, G. E., et al. (2020). Chronic pain and substance abuse disorders: Preoperative assessment and optimization strategies. *Best Practice & Research Clinical Anaesthesiology, 34*(2), 255–267. https://doi.org/10.1016/j.bpa.2020.04.014.

Kondo, K., Morasco, B. J., Nugent, S., Ayers, C., O'Neil, M. E., Freeman, M., Paynte, R., & Kansagara, D. (2020). Pharmacotherapy for the treatment of cannabis use disorder: A systematic review. *Annals of Internal Medicine, 172*(6), 398–412. https://doi.org/10.7326/M19-1105.

Kroenke, K., Spitzer, R. L., & Williams, J. B. W. (2001). The PHQ-9: Validity of a brief depression severity measure. *Journal of General Internal Medicine, 16*(9), 606–613. https://doi.org/10.1046/j.1525-1497.2001.016009606.x.

Lan, C. W., Fiellin, D. A., Barry, D. T., Bryant, K. J., Gordon, A. J., Edelman, E. J., Gaither, J. R., Maisto, S. A., & Marshall, B. D. (2016). The epidemiology of substance use disorders in U.S. Veterans: A systematic review and analysis of assessment methods. *The American Journal on Addictions, 25*(1), 7–24. https://doi.org/10.1111/ajad.12319.

Lee, P., Le Saux, M., Siegel, R., Goyal, M., Chen, C., Ma, Y., et al. (2019). Racial and ethnic disparities in the management of acute pain in U.S. emergency departments: Meta-analysis and systematic review. *The American Journal of Emergency Medicine, 37*(9), 1770–1777. https://doi.org/10.1016/j.ajem.2019.06.014.

Lippold, K. M., Jones, C. M., Olsen, E. O., & Giroir, B. P. (2019). Racial/ethnic and age group differences in opioid and synthetic opioid-involved overdose deaths among adults aged ≥18 years in metropolitan areas - United States, 2015–2017. *Morbidity and Mortality Weekly Report, 68*(43), 967–973. https://doi.org/10.15585/mmwr.mm6843a3.

Manhapra, A., & Becker, W. C. (2018). Pain and addiction: An integrative therapeutic approach. *Medical Clinics of North America, 102*(4), 745–763. https://doi.org/10.1016/j.mcna.2018.02.013.

Metz, T. D., & Borgelt, L. M. (2018). Marijuana use in pregnancy and while breastfeeding. *Obstetrics and Gynecology, 132*(5), 1198–1210. https://doi.org/10.1097/AOG.0000000000002878.

Miech, R., Johnston, L., O'Malley, P. M., Keyes, K. M., & Heard, K. (2015). Prescription opioids in adolescence and future opioid misuse. *Pediatrics, 136*(5), e1169–e1177. https://doi.org/10.1542/peds.2015-1364.

Nahin, R. L. (2017). Severe pain in Veterans: The effect of age and sex, and comparisons with the general population. *The Journal of Pain, 18*(3), 247–254. https://doi.org/10.1016/j.jpain.2016.10.021.

National Harm Reduction Coalition. (2021). https://harmreduction.org.

National Institute on Alcohol Abuse and Alcoholism. (n.d.). *Alcohol use disorder.* https://www.niaaa.nih.gov/alcohols-effects-health/alcohol-use-disorder.

National Institute on Drug Abuse. (2016, February 25). *Adjective rating scale for withdrawal.* https://datashare.nida.nih.gov/instrument/adjective-rating-scale-for-withdrawal.

National Institute on Drug Abuse. (2018a, July). *The science of drug use and addiction: The basics.* https://www.drugabuse.gov/publications/media-guide/science-drug-use-addiction-basics.

National Institute on Drug Abuse. (2018b, November 26). *Screening for substance use in the pain management setting.* https://www.drugabuse.gov/nidamed-medical-health-professionals/science-to-medicine/screening-substance-use/in-pain-management-setting.

National Institute on Drug Abuse. (2020, July). *Marijuana research report: Is marijuana addictive?* https://www.drugabuse.gov/publications/research-reports/marijuana/marijuana-addictive.

National Institute on Drug Abuse. (2021, January 28). *Words matter–Terms to use and avoid when talking about addiction.* https://www.drugabuse.gov/nidamed-medical-health-professionals/health-professions-education/words-matter-terms-to-use-avoid-when-talking-about-addiction.

North America Syringe Exchange Network. (2021). *Map.* https://www.nasen.rog/map/.

Patel, J., & Marwaha, R. (2020). *Cannabis use disorder.* StatPearls. https://www.statpearls.com/ArticleLibrary/viewarticle/18815.

Sowicz, T., Compton, P., Matteliano, D., Oliver, J., Strobbe, S., St. Marie, B., et al. (2021). Position Statement: Pain Management and Substance Use Disorders. https://aspmn.org/aspmn-joint-statements/.

Spitzer, R. L., Kroenke, K., Williams, J. B. W., & Bernd, Löwe (2006). A brief measure for assessing generalized anxiety disorder: The GAD-7. *Archives of Internal Medicine, 166*(10), 1092–1097. https://doi.ORG/10.1001/archinte.166.10.1092.

Substance Abuse and Mental Health Services Administration. (n.d.). *Integrated treatment for co-occurring disorders: Evidence-based practices (EBP) KIT.* https://store.samhsa.gov/product/Integrated-Treatment-for-Co-Occurring-Disorders-Evidence-Based-Practices-EBP-KIT/SMA08-4366?referer=from_search_result.

Substance Abuse and Mental Health Services Administration (n.d.-b). *Risk and protective factors.* https://www.samhsa.gov/sites/default/files/20190718-samhsa-risk-protective-factors.pdf.

Substance Abuse and Mental Health Services Administration. (2020a, April 16). *About screening, brief intervention, and referral to treatment (SBIRT).* https://www.samhsa.gov/sbirt/about.

Substance Abuse and Mental Health Services Administration. (2021, October). Key Substance Use and Mental Health Indicators in the United States: Results from the 2020 National Survey on Drug Use and Health. https://www.samhsa.gov/data/sites/default/files/reports/rpt35325/NSDUHFFRPDFWHTMLFiles2020/2020NSDUHFFR1PDFW102121.pdf.

Substance Abuse and Mental Health Services Administration. (2020c, September 11). *2019 NSDUH detailed tables.* https://www.samhsa.gov/data/report/2019-nsduh-detailed-tables.

Substance Abuse and Mental Health Services Administration. (2020d, October 7). *Statutes, regulations, and guidelines.* https://www.samhsa.gov/medication-assisted-treatment/statutes-regulations-guidelines#support.

Substance Abuse and Mental Health Services Administration. (2021, January 4). *Medication-assisted treatment (MAT).* https://www.samhsa.gov/medication-assisted-treatment.

Teeters, J. B., Lancaster, C. L., Brown, D. G., & Back, S. E. (2017). Substance use disorders in military veterans: Prevalence and treatment challenges. *Substance Abuse and Rehabilitation, 8,* 69–77. https://doi.org/10.2147/SAR.S116720.

U.S. Department of Health and Human Services. (2021, February 19). *What is the U.S. opioid epidemic?* https://www.hhs.gov/opioids/about-the-epidemic/index.html.

U.S. Department of Veterans Affairs. (2017). *VA/DoD clinical practice guidelines. Management of opioid therapy (OT) for chronic pain. Patient-provider tools: Tapering and discontinuing opioids.* https://www.qmo.amedd.army.mil/OT/OpioidTaperingBooklet_FINAL_508.pdf.

U.S. Department of Veterans Affairs. (2019a). *Pain management opioid taper decision tool: A VA clinician's guide.* https://bit.ly/3imYaHe.

U.S. Department of Veterans Affairs. (2019b). *Rocky Mountain MIRECC for suicide prevention. Therapeutic risk management–risk stratification table.* https://bit.ly/3bOYduq.

U.S. Food & Drug Administration. (2020, October 01). *Disposal of unused medicines: What you should know.* https://www.fda.gov/drugs/safe-disposal-medicines/disposal-unused-medicines-what-you-should-know.

U.S. Preventive Services Task Force. (2020). Screening for unhealthy drug use: U.S. Preventive Services Task Force recommendation statement. *Jama, 323*(22), 2301–2309. https://doi.org/10.1001/jama.2020.8020.

Valentino, R. J., & Volkow, N. D. (2020). Drugs, sleep, and the addicted brain. *Neuropsychopharmacology: Official Publication of the American College of Neuropsychopharmacology, 45*(1), 3–5. https://doi.org/10.1038/s41386-019-0465-x.

Volkow, N., Benveniste, H., & McLellan, A. T. (2018). Use and misuse of opioids in chronic pain. *Annual Review of Medicine, 69,* 451–465. https://doi.org/10.1146/annurev-med-011817-044739.

Volkow, N. D., Koob, G. F., & McLellan, A. T. (2016). Neurobiologic advances from the brain disease model of addiction. *The New England Journal of Medicine, 374*(4), 363–371. https://ntserver1.wsulibs.wsu.edu:2137/10.1056/NEJMra1511480.

Webster, L. R. (2017). Risk factors for opioid-use disorder and overdose. *Anesthesia and Analgesia, 125*(5), 1741–1748. https://doi.org/10.1213/ANE.0000000000002496.

Wesson, D. R., & Ling, W. (2003). The clinical opiate withdrawal scale (COWS). *Journal of Psychoactive Drugs, 35*(2), 253–259.

Wilson, M. (2019). Revisiting pain assessments amid the opioid crisis. *Pain Management Nursing, 20*(5), 399–401. https://doi.org/10.1016/j.pmn.2019.10.002.

Wilson, M., Shaw, M. R., & Roberts, M. (2018). Opioid initiation to substance use treatment: "They just want to feel normal.". *Nursing Research, 67*(5), 369–378. https://doi.org/10.1097/NNR.0000000000000298.

World Health Organization (2020, December 22). *Guidelines on the management of chronic pain in children.* https://www.who.int/publications/i/item/9789240017870.

Yi, P., & Pryzbylkowski, P. (2015). Opioid induced hyperalgesia. *Pain Medicine, 16*(S1), S32–S36. https://doi.org/10.1111/pme.12914.

INDEX

Note: Page numbers followed by *f* indicate figures, *t* indicates tables, and *b* indicate boxes.